The Practice of Veterinary Anesthesia:
Small Animals, Birds, Fish and Reptiles

The Practice of Veterinary Anesthesia:
Small Animals, Birds, Fish and Reptiles

Donald C. Sawyer, DVM, PhD, DACVA

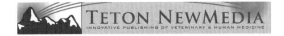

Executive Editor: Carroll C. Cann
Development Editor: Susan L. Hunsberger
Creative Director: Sue Haun www.fiftysixforty.com
Production Manager: Mike Albiniak www.fiftysixforty.com

Teton NewMedia
P.O. Box 4833
Jackson, WY 83001

1-888-770-3165
tetonnm.com

Printed in the United States of America

Print Number 5 4 3 2 1

Library of Congress Cataloging-in-Publication Data on file.

Contributing Authors

David B Brunson, DVM, MS, DACVA
Pfizer Animal Health, Veterinary Specialty Team
Adjunct Professor, Department of Surgical Sciences
School of Veterinary Medicine
University of Wisconsin
Madison, WI 53711
Subject: Birds

Paul A. Flecknell, MA, VetMB, PhD, DLAS, DECLAM, DECVA
Professor (of Laboratory Animal Science)
University of Newcastle
Medical School, Framlington Place
Newcastle, Tyne and Wear, UK, NE2 4HH
England
Subject: Guinea Pigs, Hamsters, Rats, Mice, Gerbils and Rabbits

Edward G. Foster, DVM
For 38 years, owned and operated the Town and Country Animal Hospital, Inc.,
Charlotte, Michigan
Home address: 316 Beech Street,
Charlotte, Michigan 48813-1006
Subject: Brachycephalic breeds and dogs with problem airways

Elizabeth A. Leece BVSc, MRCVS, CVA, DECVA
Animal Health Trust
Lanwades Park
Newmarket
Suffolk
CB8 7UU, UK
England
Subject: Neuromuscular blockade, Local Anesthesia and Regional Anesthesia.

Juergen P. Schumacher, DMV, DACZM
Associate Professor in Avian and Zoological Medicine
Department of Small Animal Clinical Sciences
College of Veterinary Medicine
The University of Tennessee
Knoxville, Tennessee 37901
Subject: Reptiles: Lizards, Snakes, Turtles, Tortoises and Crocodilians

Charles E. Short, DVM, PhD, DACVA, DECVA
Professor Emeritus, Cornell University
Adjunct Professor of Anesthesiology
Center for Management of Animal Pain
College of Veterinary Medicine, University of Tennessee
Home address: 1800 Shady Hollow Lane
Knoxville, Tennessee 37922
Subject: Alpha$_2$ Receptor Agonists and Antagonists, Risk Assessment and Pain Score

James G. Sikarskie, DVM, MS, DACZM
Associate Professor, Zoo and Wildlife Medicine
Department of Small Animal Clinical Sciences
College of Veterinary Medicine
Michigan State University
East Lansing, Michigan 48824
Subject: Small Non-Domestic Carnivores

Polly Taylor, MA VetMB PhD DVA DECVA MRCA MRCVS
Taylor Monroe
Gravel Head Farm
Downham Common
Little Downham, Nr Ely
Cambs CB6 2TY
England
Subject: Non Steroidal Anti-inflammatory Drugs

Alistair I. Webb, BVSc, PhD, FRCVS, DVA, DACVA
Professor of Clinical Pharmacology & Anesthesiology
Department of Physiological Sciences
University of Florida
P.O. Box 100144
Gainesville, FL 32610-0144
Subject: Blood Gases and Acid - Base Relationships

Walter E. Weirich, DVM, PhD, DACVS
Professor Emeritus, Purdue University
Home address: 7957 W. Juniper Shadows Way
Tucson, AZ 85743
Subject: Electrocardiography; Pain from a surgeon's perspective

Thomas D. Williams, DVM
Monterey Bay Aquarium
886 Cannery Row,
Monterey, CA 93940
Practice: Aquajito Veterinary Hospital
1221 10th St.
Monterey, CA 93940
Subject: Freshwater and Saltwater Fishes

Preface

This book is designed to provide insights into procedures and problems associated with anesthesia of small animals and other pets. This includes preemptive methodology and ways of dealing with specific situations associated with anesthesia. It has been prepared for small animal veterinarians, technicians and students not only to provide practical information about anesthesia and pain management but problem solving issues about breeds, surgical procedures, geriatrics and disease conditions that place certain patients at higher risk for anesthesia. Modern methods of monitoring the anesthetized patient are described to help in this process as well. Although the book is primarily focused on dogs and cats, it includes information on restraint, preanesthetics, anesthetic procedures, monitoring and use of analgesics for birds, exotic cats, skunks, ferrets, raccoons, guinea pigs, hamsters, rats, mice, gerbils, rabbits, fish, and reptiles. The text is presented by chapters in sequence as one would do anesthesia: Preanesthesia; Induction; Maintenance; Predictable Problems; Other Small Animals including birds, fish and reptiles; Emergency Procedures; and Recovery. Methods of pain management are placed in the first chapter because effective treatment of pain begins before anesthesia and surgery start. The book includes suggested anesthetic protocols in tabular form that clinicians will find useful. In addition, anesthetics, analgesics, sedatives, tranquilizers and non-steroidal anti-inflammatory drugs are not only those available in North America but Europe, United Kingdom and other countries as well. For this purpose, it makes it easier to refer to drugs by generic name rather than only by brand name. The content is well referenced but this is not intended to be a reference text. However, it is presented in a manner that makes information easy to find and easy to read to make anesthesia safe as possible for those who deal with one of the most fascinating and challenging deciplines in veterinary practice.

Acknowledgements

I am very grateful for the expertise of each and every one of the contributing authors in the development of this book. They all accepted the challenge and the information provided is outstanding. Without their help, this book would not have been completed in its present format. In particular, my friend and colleague Charlie Short has been a big supporter and provided a great deal of encouragement to get the job done. Special thanks are extended to Cheryl Blaze who provided the most complete review that could be expected. Her special contribution is greatly appreciated. Over the time that I have worked on this text, many people have helped in a variety of ways. I would like to extend my sincere gratitude to the following individuals and colleagues: Gail Whiting; Marlee Langham, LVT; Elaine Striler, LVT; Audra Guikema, BS, LVT; Rob Durham, BS, MS, PhD; Shannon Briggs, BS, PhD; William Spielman, PhD; and the Clinical Faculty, College of Veterinary Medicine, Michigan State University.

Dedication

To my wife Judy.

Contents

Chapter 1
The Pre-anesthetic Period

General Considerations

The need for general anesthesia, defined as loss of sensation to pain with unconsciousness, is based on two essential requirements: first is to provide analgesia, the other is to induce partial or complete immobility. The requirement for analgesia with or without loss of consciousness may apply to elective or non-elective surgery or for patient examination that may produce discomfort and perhaps pain. The need for immobility may be the only requirement, but concurrent loss of consciousness is produced by most anesthetics and some analgesics. In this respect, requirements for anesthetic drugs are broader in veterinary medicine than in human medicine because for most human subjects, restraint is often accomplished by self control and communication. Perhaps the closest comparison can be made between veterinary anesthesia and anesthesia for pediatric and senile human patients.

The use of general anesthetics can be confusing in the control of animal pain. To many, anesthesia is synonymous with analgesia. Unfortunately, for many anesthetic procedures, even though the animal is not moving during the surgical procedure and may be assumed to be pain free, significant changes in cardiopulmonary and neurologic variables may be evoked by inadequate depth or lack of concurrent use of analgesics. As a rule, all volatile liquid anesthetics and most injectable anesthetics provide little or no analgesia. An understanding of pain perception is a key to better anesthetic management. One of the outstanding current considerations is the use of regional and systemic analgesics in combination with general anesthesia for more profound pain control and less CNS depression.

Physical Status

Estimation of the patient's anesthetic risk is based on a number of factors. A minimum database should be established for patients in various categories. A modification of the classification by the American Society of Anesthesiologists (ASA) is recommended to select patients on the basis of risk (Table 1-1).

Table 1-1

Classification of Pre-anesthesia Risk Status

P1 Excellent	An animal with no organic disease or systemic disturbance or an animal submitted for elective surgery in excellent health would be considered an excellent risk for anesthesia.
P2 Good	An animal with slight to moderate systemic disturbance would be a member of this group. Patients with minor fractures, slight dehydration, and obesity, and some older patients tend to fit this category.
P3 Fair	Animals with moderate to major systemic disturbance, such as chronic heart disease, anemia, open or severe fracture subsequent to trauma, and mild pneumonia would be included in this group.
P4 Poor	Patients with extreme systemic disturbance fit this group. Such a disturbance is severe enough to result in death for which surgical or medical intervention requiring anesthesia may be necessary to change the course. Ruptures of an abdominal viscus, or strangulated and diaphragmatic hernias are examples. In some cases, severe airway problems may be part of the clinical picture.
P5 Critical	Animals in a moribund state are in the worst category because they are close to death or in the process of dying without intervention. Patients with gastric dilatation/volvulus of over one hour's duration, severe hypotension due to hemorrhage, or comatose conditions due to any cause may be categorized as critical. Animals with acute trauma and in severe shock should be placed in this group.

Patient Evaluation
Criteria Used to Determine Risk Status

Determination of health status can be made from a variety of criteria. A complete history and physical examination will provide valuable information.

History

A preanesthetic history should be provided by the client. Table 1-2 contains a Preanesthetic History Checklist that will help begin the patient evaluation process. This information should be reviewed before the patient is admitted for physical examination. Weakness, fatigue, lethargy, and reduced exercise tolerance are common to many diseases. Cardiovascular disease with a resultant decrease in cardiac output and peripheral perfusion is but one cause. Reduced exercise tolerance is the common denominator in nearly every form of heart disease but it is not pathognomonic for same. Respiratory signs occur frequently in animals with cardiovascular disease. However, respiratory signs are in general more frequent in animals with diseases of the airway and lungs than they are in animals with heart disease. Cough is produced by inflammatory, mechanical, chemical, and thermal stimulation of cough receptors. The history and physical examination can generally determine whether the cough is upper or lower airway in origin, and combined with the history can frequently occur together, and one causes exacerbations of the other. Dyspnea, difficult breathing which is frequently labored breathing, is a cardinal sign of diseases affecting the cardiorespiratory system. Cardiac dyspnea usually begins as difficulty in breathing with strenuous exertion, and over a course of months or years progresses until the patient is dyspneic at rest.

Physical Examination

A defined physical should follow a specific format that includes a description of the examination for each body system. Gaining information using guidelines contained on the form presented in Table 1-3 is an excellent way of developing consistency. Essential information includes breed, age, sex, body weight, vaccination status, body temperature, assessment of nutritional status, heart rate, respiratory rate, respiratory pattern, general health (well or sick or sustained trauma), attitude, activity level, external appearance, appearance of mucous membranes, capillary refill time, and auscultation of thorax for respiratory and heart sounds, chest radiographs, non-invasive blood pressure (NIBP) measurements, and electrocardiogram. Evidence of pain should be noted as well. Observation of the animal's general body condition, temperament, attitude, and ability to ambulate should be made noting any abnormalities. Observations that may suggest the presence of heart disease include weakness, loss of muscle mass, poor condition of skin and hair coat, abdominal distension, abducted elbows, dyspnea, hyperpnea, or other abnormalities in respiratory rate, effort or regularity. Mucous membranes of the eyes and oral cavities should be compared to those in the posterior aspects of the body.

Patients with cardiac or cardiocirculatory disease may be asymptomatic. It is more and more common to detect cardiac disease as a result of some abnormal physical finding such as heart murmur, enlarged cardiac silhouette on the chest radiograph, or abnormal ECG findings detected during the "wellness" examination or when examining an animal for some other complaint. It is also recognized that dyspnea, one of the cardinal manifestations of diminished cardiac reserve, is not just limited to heart disease, but is characteristic of conditions such as pulmonary disease, marked obesity, and anxiety/excitement. Examination of the jugular veins gives an indication of central venous pressure (CVP) as well as valuable information about right-side cardiac events (Ross 2005). Jugular veins can be examined with the animal standing, sitting, or in sternal recumbency. Elevating the animal's chin and turning the head slightly to the left facilitates inspection of the right jugular vein. While a thick hair coat can sometimes obscure jugular venous distension, the hairs often move with jugular pulsations and facilitate the identification of the various pulse waves. CVP is estimated by determining the height the jugular vein is distended about right atrial level. By occluding the vein at the thoracic inlet, it easily can be identified as it becomes distended through filling from above. If veins are collapsed in a recumbent animal, CVP is subnormal and

Table 1-2

Pre-Anesthetic History Checklist

Owner's Name: _____   Pet's Name: _____   Date: _____

☐ Dog   ☐ Cat   Age: _____

	No	Mild	Moderate	Severe	When did problem begin?
1) Weight gain____ Weightloss____					
2) Appetite: Increase____ Decrease____					
3) Vomiting____ Diarrhea____					
4) Constipation / difficult defecation					
5) Increased drinking____ Increased urination___					
6) Lumps / tumors____ Skin problems____ Describe:					
7) Bad breath / Sore gums / Difficulty chewing					
8) Decreased awareness – gets confused/lost					
9) House soiling____ Spraying____ Describe:					
10) Decreased recognition of people, animals or previously learned commands Describe:					
11) Decreased affection / interaction with owners					
12) Chewing, licking, eating non-food items Describe:					
13) Increased irritability / aggression					
14) Increased fear / anxiety					
15) Decreased tolerance of handling					
16) Decreased hearing or "selective hearing"					
17) Repetitive behaviors, e.g. pacing, over-grooming Describe:					
18) Decreased grooming or self care					
19) Muscle tremors/shaking					
20) Weakness / incoordination					
21) Difficulty climbing stairs / increased stiffness					
22) Decreased activity – sleeps more					
23) Excessive vocalization: Day____ Night____					
24) Waking owners at night					
25) Evidence of pain or discomfort					

Other problems / concerns; _____

Medications: _____

Existing medical problems: _____

Information contributed by Dr. Ilona Rodan of the Cat Care Clinic

Pre-Anesthetic Examination Form

Table 1-3

Client: _____ Patient: _____ Date: _____

Examined by: _____ Technician / Assistant: _____

1. ATTITUDE
- ○ Normal / Alert   ○ Other_____

2. HYDRATION
- ○ Normal   ○ Other_____

3. COAT & SKIN
- ○ Normal   ○ Flea comb negative
- ○ Other_____

4. EYES
- ○ Normal   ○ Other_____

5. EARS
- ○ Normal   ○ Other_____

6. NOSE & THROAT
- ○ Normal   ○ Other_____

7. MOUTH, TEETH & GUMS
- ○ Normal
- ○ Tartar   ○ Mild ○ Mod   ○ Severe
- ○ Gingivitis ○ MIld ○ Mod   ○ Severe
- ○ Mucus membrane color   ○ Pink
- ○ Pigmented
- ○ Other_____

8. LEGS & PAWS
- ○ Normal   ○ Other_____

9. WEIGHT
- ○ Normal   ○ Other_____
- ○ Overweight by_____
- ○ Underweight by_____

10. HEART
- ○ Normal   ○ Slow   ○ Fast (HR=)
- ○ Murmur Grade (/VI)
- ○ Other_____

11. LUNGS
- ○ Normal   ○ Other_____

12. ABDOMEN
- ○ Normal   ○ Other_____

13. GASTROINTESTINAL SYSTEM
- ○ Normal   ○ Other_____

14. UROGENITAL SYSTEM
- ○ Normal   ○ Other_____

15. LYMPH NODES, TONSILS, & THYROID GLANDS
- ○ Normal   ○ Other_____

16. CENTRAL NERVOUS SYSTEM
- ○ Normal   ○ Other_____

17. PAIN SCORE 0-10:_____

DESCRIPTION (Use same numbers as above for corresponding descriptions below)
_____
_____
_____
_____
_____
_____

Weight_____ Temp_____
Age_____ F FS M MN
Diet_____

Feline

Canine

Assessment
_____
_____
_____
_____

Recommendations
_____
_____
_____
_____

Next visit
_____

blood volume is frequently inadequate (Ross 2005). If height of venous distension is above right atrial level, this is a relatively accurate reflection of CVP. CVP is estimated by measuring the vertical distance between the top of the oscillating venous column and the thoracic inlet, adding the necessary figure for distance from the thoracic inlet to the middle of the right atrium. Normal range would be 3 to 5cm depending on size of animal.

It is ultimately important that an accurate assessment of the cardiovascular system be part of the physical examination. Using one's hands, eyes, and ears to maximal advantage in diagnosis, need for noninvasive procedures such as ECG, thoracic radiographs, echocardiography, non-invasive blood pressure and occasionally invasive procedures such as cardiac catheterization can be utilized. The question needs to be answered whether the patient is healthy enough for the anesthetic procedure. If surgery is essential for survival, information can be obtained rather quickly to provide the best assessment of anesthetic risk and establishment of the most appropriate anesthetic protocol to achieve a successful outcome.

Age

Age is an important factor in patient assessment because the margin of safety with patient responses to anesthetic drugs is wider in young patients compared with that for old animals. Young adult and middle age patients will be expected to react in a more predictable manner than will neonatal, pediatric, senior, or geriatric patients. Meyer (1987) suggests that the newly born and nearly dead represent the widest extremes of the life experience. Very young and very old patients are in a changing physiological status, maturation for the young and degeneration for the old. Therefore it would be expected that the margin of safety would be narrow for these patients and the degree of uncertainty the greatest. Perhaps as a general rule, patients less than 12 weeks of age can be categorized as pediatric and should be evaluated very carefully because not only are body functions at risk but most of the time, size is a factor.

Increasing physiological age may not parallel increasing chronological age for all species and breeds. Definitions of the neonatal and geriatric periods are required. The neonatal period is defined for canine and feline species as the first 2 weeks of life and the pediatric period as the first 12 weeks of postnatal life (Robinson 1983). Transition from young adult to middle age to old age cannot be arbitrarily defined but life expectancy of the species or breed in question must be taken into consideration. The last quarter of anticipated natural life span has been suggested as the geriatric phase of life for dogs (Dodman 1984) and that is a reasonable estimate for cats as well. For example, a sporting dog such as Labrador Retriever might have an average life expectancy of 10 to 12 years, thus their geriatric period might begin at 9 years of age. However, a large working dog, e.g., Great Dane, would start that period at about 6 years of age and be considered aged at 9 years. Cats are a little more difficult to classify, as there appears to be few if any feline breeds that have short life spans. Domestic cats might have fewer stresses on their life but cats over 14 years of age should be considered starting their geriatric period.

When considering age as part of the criteria for assessing preanesthetic risk status for dogs and cats, it is helpful to compare age of animals to that of human years. In this regard, both age and size (body weight) are necessary to classify pets as adult, senior, or geriatric. The comparative information developed by Dr. Fred Metzger is presented in Table 1-4.

To summarize, the neonatal period is the first 2 weeks of life. Companion animals are considered kittens and puppies (pediatric) until they are 3 months old. From 3 to 18 months of age, they would be referred to as young adults. Thereafter, they would be called adults until they become senior citizens at age 6 for dogs over 50 pounds or 9 years for smaller dogs and cats. The geriatric period begins when animals reach 10 to 14 years, depending on body weight.

Is your pet a senior citizen?

Table 1-4

Patient: _____ Weight: _____ Date: _____

☐ Dog   ☐ Cat   Breed: _____

Age	0-20	21-50	51-90	>90
5	36	38	40	42
6	40	42	45	49
7	44	47	50	56
8	48	51	55	64
9	52	56	61	71
10	56	60	66	78
11	60	65	72	86
12	64	69	77	93
13	68	74	82	101
14	72	78	88	108
15	76	83	93	115
16	80	87	99	123
17	84	92	104	
18	88	96	109	☐ Adult
19	92	101	115	▨ Senior
20	96	105	120	▧ Geriatric

Relative age of your pet in "human years"

In order to maintain your companion's health, it is important to understand where he or she is in the "life stage" cycle.

Both age and size (weight) are necessary information to classify your pet as young, adult, senior or geriatric. Depending on your pet's life stage classification, he or she may have different health and diet needs.

This table was developed to help you determine your pet's life stage.

Following the table, you can locate your pet's age in years. Now, match the age in years with your pet's weight and the corresponding color code will identify your pet's life stage. For example, a 9-year old dog weighing 70 pounds is 61 in "human years" and is classified as a senior citizen.

Information for life

09-62386-00

Chart courtesy of Fred L. Metzger. DVM, Dipl. ABVP

Hematology and Blood Chemistry

Laboratory tests provide useful information not only in helping evaluate patient status but also during and following the anesthetic procedure. In-hospital analytical blood testing capability now produces on-site results in a matter of minutes. Table 1-5 lists criteria for laboratory analyses pre-anesthesia. These are guidelines that should be used based on history and clinical examination and may be expanded as individual circumstances dictate.

Reference standards are available from all clinical laboratories for in-hospital testing equipment and should be used as general guidelines for normal ranges. Whenever possible, test results should be interpreted by comparing the patient's values to a normal range for the species tested. If tests are done at laboratories that infrequently test animal blood, they will not have species-specific reference standards. In this case, veterinarians must use published data as a guide for interpreting results.

Table 1-5

Guidelines for Pre-anesthetic Diagnostic Data

| | | Patient Age | |
Physical Status	3 Mo to < 6 Years	Senior	Geriatric
P1. Excellent	PAP	PAP, CBC, EL	GHP, CBC, EL
P2. Good	PAP, CBC, EL	GHP, CBC, EL	GHP, CBC, EL
P3. Fair	GHP, CBC, EL, UA	GHP, CBC, EL, UA	GHP, CBC, EL, UA
P4. Poor	GHP, CBC, EL, UA	GHP, CBC, EL, UA	GHP, CBC, EL, UA
P5. Critical	GHP, CBC, EL, UA	GHP, CBC, EL, UA	GHP, CBC, EL, UA

PAP (Pre-anesthetic Profile) = TP, Glu, BUN, Creatinine, ALT, Alk Phos, PCV + CBC

GHP (General Health Profile)= BUN, ALT, Albumin, Amylase, Creatinine, Glucose, Total Bilirubin, Cholesterol, ALKP, TP, Phosphorus, Calcium

CBC (Complete Blood Count) Total white and red blood cell count, differential, platelet appearance.

UA (Urine Analysis); includes color, turbidity, specific gravity, pH, protein, glucose, ketones, bilirubin, occult blood, urobilinogen, blood cells, casts, bacteria, sperm, and crystals)

EL (Blood Electrolytes) = Sodium, Potassium, Chloride

PCV = Packed Cell Volume

TP = Total Protein

Senior and Geriatric (Defined by age and body weight, Table 1-4)

Pre-anesthesia Electrocardiogram

A resting awake electrocardiogram can provide absolutely vital information to the clinician when making a decision on the anesthetic protocol for a patient. This is most important in the patient over 5 years of age and has diminishing returns in the young healthy patient unless there are indications from the history and physical examination. Breeds of both dogs and cats that are prone to cardiomyopathy should have an ECG recorded prior to any anesthetic event. Breeds at greatest risk are the Doberman, Great Dane, Saint Bernard, Newfoundland and Boxer dogs; Persian and Siamese cats. Other recognized breeds as well as mixed breeds can develop cardiomy-opathy but do so with a lesser frequency.

An ECG that is completely within normal ranges for the species can provide a great deal of information. This can be most useful when considering the ECG data in light of the procedure for which the anesthesia is required. As an example, if the patient is to have surgery on tissues that have a high degree of vagal influence such as the respiratory or GI systems and the awake, resting ECG shows prominent vagal influence such as slow heart rate or sinus arrhythmia, anticholinergics to block or reduce vagal influence should be employed. Nor should the anesthetic protocol be one that tends to cause bradycardia. If the patient has fast heart rates on the resting, non-sedated ECG, it might be wise not to try to further block the vagal influence or use anesthetics that tend to induce faster heart rates. If abnormal resting ECG tracings are encountered, those problems must be addressed before the anesthetic is administered.

In an emergency situation, a pre-anesthetic ECG can be very helpful in planning for possible problems that may arise during the anesthetic period. It should be noted that 40 to 50% of dogs that have hit by car history have heart and lung trauma that can lead to potentially fatal cardiac arrhythmias and ventilation/perfusion problems that may have to be dealt with during anesthesia in the early post traumatic period. Another high risk emergency patient is the post gastric dilation volvulus (GDV) patient. They may develop ventricular cardiac arrhythmias during the post surgical period up to 72 hours after corrective surgery. The clinician should be particularly alert for these arrhythmias in these large breed dogs as they also have a propensity to develop cardiomyopathy as well as GDV.

Pre-anesthesia Radiographs
When there is any indication from the history or physical examination that there may be potential pulmonary or cardiac problems, thoracic radiographs would be indicated. This would be especially true for impact trauma patients in which pneumothorax is an expected sequel. If lung sounds are not normal or cardiac enlargement is detected, radiographs will be very useful in helping to make decisions on anesthetic risk and appropriate anesthesic and analgesic protocols.

Pre-anesthesia Blood Pressure
Non invasive blood pressure (NIBP) and pulse rate (PR) measurements can be invaluable in assessment of patient status especially based on history and physical examination. This is particularly important in aged animals, those with systemic disease, or patients with any history of cardiac problems. Detection of hypertension that may be due to pain, dehydration, or renal disease especially in geriatric patients should lead to further diagnostics and corrective therapy. Assessment of hypotension is equally important as it would not be in the best interest of achieving a successful anesthetic outcome with the patient in a compromised status at the outset. Most anesthetic protocols include drugs that have the potential of producing myocardial depression and changing peripheral resistance that will further aggravate the situation. Knowledge of the pre-anesthesia pulse rate will help determine the appropriate use of anticholinergics and other drugs that may induce changes in rate and rhythym. Some animals, especially cats, will have elevated heart rate and blood pressure just from the stress and anxiety of being in the unfamiliar environment of the veterinary hospital.

Risk Assessment of the Injured Patient
Anesthetic and pain management for the injured patient can be divided into three general areas: animal-to-animal physical contact (bite wounds); human-to-animal blunt trauma (vehicle impact); and human-to-animal penetrating injuries (gunshot or arrow wounds). Depending on the extent and type of injury, patients may be classified in any of the five anesthetic risk categories (Table 1-1). This can range from a fall from a couch to blunt trauma from a moving vehicle to penetrating wounds. Minor to extensive tissue damage may have occurred. Injury initiates the release of neuropeptides including prostaglandin and substance P that intensify pain response and release of endogenous opiates such as β-endorphins and enkephalins that modulate natural body responses to reduce pain. Physiology of the body is usually very unstable and most often there is an elevation in body temperature.

With tissue damage, there is associated inflammation and tissue swelling. Reduced tissue perfusion may result especially if the injury has caused sufficient damage to blood vessels to initiate both inflammation and hematoma formation. The extent of damage may include both soft tissue and bone. Control of hemorrhage is often needed at the site of injury but attention must also be given to the possibility of bleeding elsewhere such as a ruptured spleen, liver, kidney, urinary bladder, or other internal organ. Traumatic myocarditis often results from moving vehicle injuries not necessarily from the first impact but rather from the ground or other object following body propulsion. The most obvious injury may not be the problem of greatest risk to the patient. One should be aware that risk may not diminish until at least 3 days post injury.

Animal-to-animal injuries involving cats are mostly puncture wounds and may not have significant influence on risk status when they are presented in the acute phase. For cat fight wounds of longer duration, both pain and infection may be factors that will increase risk to anesthesia. Untreated cat bite wounds often become infected and abscessed due to the penetrating nature of wounds. Dog fight wounds may be associated with severe tissue damage. Extent of injury may include major hemorrhage such as puncture of an artery, penetration of the thoracic wall which might occur from a large dog attack on a small dog, or trauma to the trachea. Usually wounds to the head and ears result in considerable blood loss.

Most penetrating injuries in dogs and cats are gunshot wounds. Some shotgun blasts result in multiple pellet penetration of skin and muscle. In contrast rifle, pistol, or shotgun slugs usually inflict major damage that results in considerable discomfort. The primary problem may be pain, life-threatening wounds, hemorrhage, or combination of these. Pain management must be part of the initial therapy along with life saving measures until the patient is stabilized. Focus should be to carefully evaluate each patient and if surgery is determined to be necessary for survival, the risk status will likely be high.

Risk assessment must be made and proper drugs selected to manage patients in order to achieve a successful outcome. Anesthetic protocols for P1 and P2 patients will often not be appropriate for patients in P3, P4, or P5. Therefore, it is of utmost importance to properly evaluate each patient in the preanesthetic period.

Hospitalization
Inpatient Surgery
Whenever possible, animals should be hospitalized the day before surgery. The extra day allows more time for evaluation and laboratory analysis of health status as well as acclimatization to the hospital environment. Usually, animals so treated are better able to accept their situation than those admitted the day of surgery. An exception to this might be senior or geriatric patients who might be better off at home the night before surgery. If an animal is hospitalized the day before anesthesia, food should be provided at the regular feeding time, which may occur either at home or at the hospital. It is recommended that water be provided *ad libitum* to allow inpatients to drink as needed to provide proper hydration before anesthesia.

For seriously ill patients or those who have sustained trauma, food intake may have been restricted or limited because of diagnostic procedures or inappetence. At major referral centers, it is not uncommon for animals to be without food for 2 or 3 days unless attention is given to feeding them separately. For example, an animal hit by car may be referred for treatment to another hospital the day after admission to the primary hospital. It may not have been fed the day of the accident. Depending upon the travel distance to and diagnostic work-up at the referral hospital, the animal might miss the normal feeding time and go the second day without food. On the day of surgery, the procedure may not be performed until afternoon. Thus, the animal would have gone without food for 3 days. Therefore, it is well to give attention to the history of food and water intake so that proper nutrition and hydration can be maintained during and following anesthesia.

Outpatient Surgery

Most small animal practices admit patients the morning of surgery and are released a few hours following recovery (Wagner 2000). If animals are treated strictly as outpatients and scheduled for admission to the hospital the same day as surgery, the excitement at home, trip to the hospital, and an unfamiliar environment all serve to produce fear and anxiety. Young animals may tolerate the hospitalization process better than older pets but attitude of the patient pre-anesthesia is a major determinant of patient behavior and attitude during recovery as well. Some companion animals vocalize and show other hypersensitive activities in recovery even without pain, especially if they are unfamiliar with the recovery area or feel threatened by personnel or other patients. Early attempts to comfort these patients by holding, stroking, or other caring techniques may help reduce anxiety. The use of tranquilizers in these cases may reduce fear and stress but do not relieve pain.

It is important that animals undergo a peaceful induction of anesthesia in order for a smooth recovery to follow. Observation and assessment of the patient 30 to 60 minutes before induction will provide the clinician and technician with valuable knowledge as to how the animal will behave during induction and recovery. It is important to consider that the first thing an animal will recall will likely be the last event that occurred before becoming unconscious. Pain induced from surgery will be superimposed on this undesirable behavior that is not conducive to an uneventful smooth recovery.

Another important consideration is the protocol of withholding food and water pre-anesthesia. For outpatient surgeries, e.g., animals not hospitalized overnight, food should be withheld overnight by the owner but water can be provided *ad libitum*. However, once admitted to the hospital, providing water to the animal *ad libitum* is not advised. Nervous drinking of a high volume of water could promote emesis during induction or recovery. For older patients with potential for or compensated renal disease, controlled amounts of water can be provided.

What should be done if an animal is fed the morning of surgery? Gastric emptying time depends on the quantity of food ingested, whether it is liquid or semi-solid, time interval before surgery, excitement of the animal, and concurrent drugs administered. Gastric emptying of liquids and solids resides in different areas of the stomach. The oral portion is thought to control emptying of liquids while solid foods need to be reduced in size by the distal stomach before passing through the pylorus (Miyabayasi and Morgan 1984). Onset of gastric emptying of liquids usually begins within 15 minutes of ingestion but movement of the solid phase may not start for as long as 60 minutes. A small meal will tend to take longer to initiate gastric emptying compared to a larger amount of food. Mean gastric emptying time of the dog was reported to be slightly more than 50 minutes with a maximum a little less than 90 minutes (Leib 1985). Normal emptying time in dogs with a full meal can be as long as five to ten hours (Miyabayashi 1984). It appears that the sympathetic nervous system does not greatly influence normal gastric emptying time but does decrease gastric motor activity and emptying during stressful situations. Lieb et al (1985) demonstrated that acepromazine when given preanesthesia did not influence gastric emptying time in dogs. In contrast, when acepromazine (0.1mg/kg) was combined with butorphanol (0.05mg/kg) gastrointestinal motility was decreased and gastric emptying time prolonged for as much as 5 hours (Scrivani et al 1998).

Drugs that induce vomiting may not completely empty the stomach. Therefore, use of emetics will give one a false sense of security. However, in circumstances in which there would be an increased risk to the patient by delaying surgery, keeping the animal in a quiet environment and perhaps sedated, waiting 2 hours or more will allow the stomach to empty liquids and at least a portion of solid food. The subject should then be treated as a full stomach patient, as would be done for emergency surgery. Postponing surgery 24 hours is a good alternative. Use of pre-anesthetic medication to induce emesis is based not on a pharmacologic need but rather on the fact that vomiting is a side effect of drugs such as morphine sulfate, xylazine, and medotomidine. However, sedatives and analgesics that both induce emesis and provide preemptive analgesia may have benefits in selected cases. Although apomorphine has a primary action of inducing vomiting, it has some analgesic and CNS depressant properties as well.

Pain Management: *It starts before anesthesia!*

Veterinarians are a compassionate group of professionals who care about the welfare of animals. It is recognized that animals experience pain essentially to the same extent as humans and that there are numerous ways to alleviate any imposed discomfort (Dohoo & Dohoo 1996a&b, Capner et al 1999, Lascelles et al. 1999). Many new pain management modalities have been developed for humans and a similar development process has taken place for veterinary patients, especially small animals. Treatment of animals in pain from surgical intervention, from injury or in association with acute or chronic disease processes should be paramount as part of any therapeutic protocol. There is no question that in order to manage animal pain effectively, veterinarians must have a basic knowledge concerning underlying physiological processes, pharmacology of analgesics and effective methods that can be applied under various circumstances. There has been a concerted effort to provide information to practitioners published in professional journals and presented at local, state, national and international veterinary meetings (Davis 1968, Heavner 1970, Sawyer 1985, Short 1987b, Thurmon et al. 1996, Flecknell 2000, others too numerous to mention). In addition, articles have been written in lay journals (Sawyer 1992) and information on pain management has been included in national magazines and via radio and television. As a result, animal owners are more informed than ever that animals experience pain and that effective analgesic drugs and methods are available.

Yoxall published a key paper in 1978 regarding recognition and control of animal pain that received little attention at the time. He introduced many concepts that were rediscovered over the next 10 to 20 years. In 1983, Kitchell and Davis, editors of the book *Animal Pain*, provided information on control of pain in dogs and cats as well as species differences in drug disposition as factors in alleviation of pain. Significant advances were made at the 1990 symposium, *Animal Pain and Its Control*, chaired by Charles E. Short. This meeting brought together participants from human medicine, government, industry, and veterinary medicine to develop a mutual understanding regarding knowledge of pain in animals. The subsequent text edited by CE Short and A Van Poznak (1992) provided a review of pain in animals and served as a resource for clinical management.

Most recently, *Pain Management in Animals*, edited by Paul Flecknell and Avril Waterman-Pearson (2000), is an excellent text authored by a faculty of international experts that provide the reader with essential, understandable and clinically applicable information. Other excellent sources of information are *Pain Management for the Small Animal Practioner* by Tranquilli et al. (2004), *Physiology of Pain* (Lamont et al. 2000) and *Veterinary Anesthesia and Pain Management Secrets* by Greene (2002).

With increased availability of resources regarding proper use of analgesics in small animals and studies to describe their effectiveness, use of appropriate drugs to alleviate pain has greatly improved over the past 10 years. However, it may not be a common protocol in many veterinary practices, especially for elective procedures. The consequences of pain are many and none of these responses can be considered beneficial for optimizing successful outcome (Figure 1). Only 9.6% of Australian veterinarians responded to a survey conducted in 1996. Results indicated that 80% of respondents generally used analgesic drugs for potentially painful surgical procedures with doses usually given after surgery but before recovery. Use of analgesic drugs varied and was 94% for patients with acute severe trauma, 60% following cruciate ligament repair, 29% for perineal herniorrhaphy, and only 5% for OHE and canine castration (Watson et al. 1996).

13

Consequences of Pain

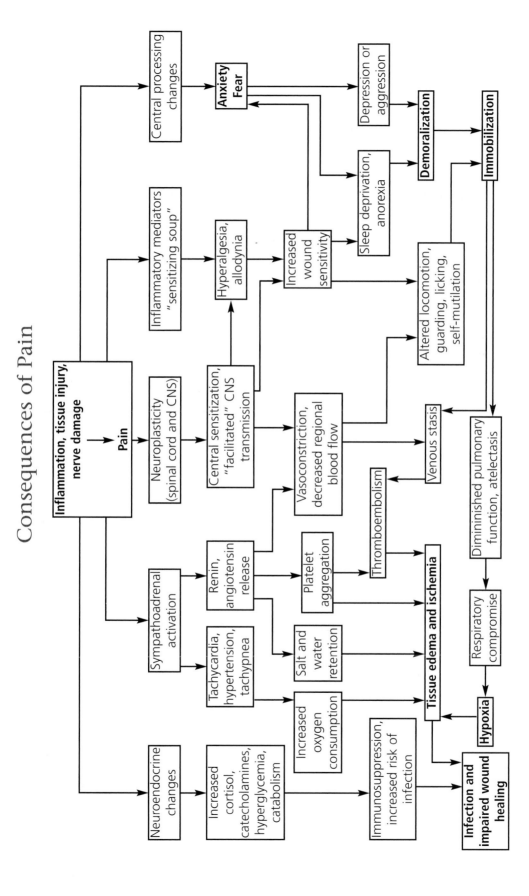

Figure 1-1 Consequences of Pain. (Reprinted by permission from Handbook of Veterinary Pain Management, J. Gaynor and W. Muir III, 2002, Mosby).

From a survey of veterinarians in the United Kingdom, it was reported that only 50% of dogs and 26% cats received analgesic drugs after elective ovariohysterectomy (OHE) and relatively few used combinations of different classes of analgesics either before or after surgery (Capner et al. 1999, Lascelles et al.1999). A survey of 1,083 Colorado State University veterinary alumni resulted in a response rate of 32% (Wagner & Hellyer 2000). Most were practitioners located mainly in cities with populations greater than 100,000 or in suburban areas. A key finding in this study was that 75% of veterinarians or their staff promoted the importance of postoperative pain management to their clients. However, clinical implementation was less common. They reported that only 21 to 45% routinely administered analgesics following elective procedures such as castration or OHE in dogs and cats. From a survey of South African veterinarians in 1999 with a 27% response rate, analgesic agents were only administered to 14% of cats and 19% of dogs (Joubert 2001). Ketamine or xylazine were frequently used for preanesthetic medication but no specific drugs were administered for post-operative pain.

For his PhD thesis research, Dr. Steve Fox conducted an extensive study of dogs undergoing OHE using various anesthetic protocols (Fox 1995). Over 160 behaviors were identified as possible indices of post-operative pain-induced distress in the bitch. Of these behaviors, 90 were used to clearly demonstrate that analgesic therapy is warranted for this most common elective procedure (Fox et al. 2000).

Feline onychectomy is a common procedure performed by veterinarians in the U.S. In the Wagner/Hellyer survey, 70% of practitioners included local and systemic analgesics as part of their protocol. Dentistry is commonly performed in private practice but use of analgesic techniques such as local blocks and analgesic drugs is relatively uncommon.

For human patients, the Joint Commission on Accreditation of Healthcare Organizations (JCAHO) mandated in 2000 that human hospitals in the US measure pain in patients and take steps to manage pain appropriately (Phillips 2000). Nurses and assistants in human hospitals are often more aware of pain but can only provide treatment per "doctor's" orders. Thus JCAHO has mandated that pain be considered the fifth vital sign, in addition to temperature, pulse, respiration, and blood pressure. So instead of just taking vitals of TPR, it is better to do PA + TPR, pain assessment plus TPR.

Including pain assessment on the preanesthetic history checklist and physical examination form will be very helpful in determining dosage levels and treatment intervals for analgesics (see Tables 1-2 and 1-3). All animals do not require the same dosage nor do they have the same pharmacokinetic uptake, distribution and elimination phases of medications. As a result, re-evaluation at appropriate intervals for acute or chronic pain is desirable. Therefore, it is very helpful to include pain as a vital sign and establish a score not only preanesthesia and but following use of pain management protocols as well. As a guide, a numerical range of 1 to 10 can be used where 10 indicates the worst severe pain and 1 no detectable pain (Figure 1-2).

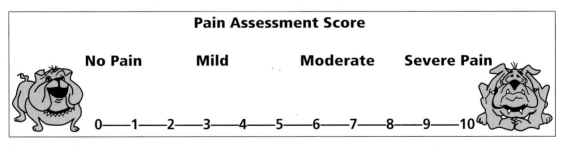

Figure 1-2 Pain score schematic used to rank pain; no pain = 0, most pain = 10.

Why is it that analgesics are not part of treatment protocols in some veterinary practices? Perhaps it is because of the mistaken concept that pain in animals is good or that signs of pain are not recognized when they develop (Hill 1995, Hansen 1997). Some have supported the philosophy that pain is not an important issue in animals and if patients are painful, there is not much that can or should be done about it. One might argue that veterinarians may not always be able to provide complete analgesia post-operatively because they do not have personnel, equipment, or financial support to provide monitoring services needed to properly use analgesic drugs and techniques for pain management. It would appear, however, that if veterinarians have the expertise, instrumentation, and facilities to perform major or minor surgical procedures, they must also be in a position to use advanced drugs and methods. Because animals respond to noxious stimuli and to conditions that cause tissue damage, the use of pain control measures is one of the most noble goals and keys to the practice of veterinary surgery and medicine.

Use of analgesics to relieve painful situations in research animals is mandated under the jurisdiction of diplomates of the American College of Laboratory Animal Medicine (Hubbel and Muir 1996). In fact, it is almost impossible to receive review committee approval for a research study in which painful procedures would be performed without the appropriate use of analgesic drugs. There is no single drug ("magic bullet") available to treat all types of pain in all patients under all conditions. However, there are many types and classes of analgesics that can be used alone or in combination to prevent and manage pain. It is acknowledged that pain is complex but treatment modalities are not too complex and time-consuming to obviate their application. Peter Hellyer (2002) suggested that practitioners must be willing to do two things. First, if an analgesic protocol does not work in a specific circumstance, veterinarians must be willing to take time to analyse the situation and problem-solve. Second, practitioners must periodically re-examine analgesic protocols as new information is provided and more effective techniques are developed. Both are consistent with being a professional and are just good medical practices.

As is discussed in more detail in this chapter, waiting to treat pain after the fact is far more difficult and less effective than administering analgesic drugs before surgery, i.e., preemptive analgesia. It is for this very reason that pain management is discussed in the first chapter of this book. Veterinary anesthesiologists are responsible for providing and teaching proper anesthetic and analgesic management of patients, so students who have graduated since the early to mid-1990 have been exposed to this advanced knowledge. Veterinary technicians and assistants are the practice caregivers who administer drugs and provide comfort for such animals under the supervision of veterinarians. Technicians and assistants well know signs of pain when it is present. A happy hospital staff is one where there are aggressive pain management protocols being practiced.

Clients expect that pain management is a service provided for their pets as part of good medical practice and are willing to support the expense. As is the case in many practices, analgesia or pain treatment is a separate listing on the client billing form. There is no question that pain management should be an identified profit center in any veterinary practice.

Pain Mechanisms

Significant advances have been made in the science and art of pain management. Analgesics, tranquilizers, and anesthetics that are commonly used to sedate, immobilize, or anesthetize different animal species often induce different drug effects and cardiovascular responses (Stanley 1987, Dubner 1987). Reasons for these different requirements and effects are influenced by a whole range of factors including heightened or depressed ability to perceive pain, stress, excitement, age, weight, health status, and whether the animal has any experience of confinement.

Subjective responses to pain experienced by humans are compared to those found in animals using analogies based on anatomical, physiological, and pathological studies. Pain is based on personal experience. It is a perception, not a physical entity and perception of pain depends on a functioning cerebral cortex. No single area of the brain is specifically responsible for the perception of pain. Complex neural mechanisms are responsible for processing of information from nociceptors that lead to the sensation of pain. These mechanisms include neural circuits within the dorsal horn of the spinal cord and of the medulla oblongata, ascending tracts, nuclei of the thalamus, and cerebral cortex (Willis and Chung 1987). Pain is identified as a feeling that is opposite to that of pleasure–hurt. The term noxious describes stimuli that, if perceived, give rise to pain.

Pain is mediated by functionally distinctive components. It may involve acute high threshold stimuli (thermal, mechanical, or chemically damaged tissue); protracted afferent input (long-lasting hyperalgesia); or low threshold input (allodynia related to pain from light touch). Behavioral patterns will be associated with the effects of noxious stimuli on excitatory transmitters. Studies using mechanical, thermal (cold pressor test), audio-evoked potentials, or other noxious stimuli during anesthesia and analgesia provided clues to perception of pain in animals that helped in the establishment of guidelines for the clinical relief of animal pain (Wall 1992). There is a better understanding of cutaneous somatosensory responses than of deep sensation (e.g., subcutaneous tissue, muscle, bone, viscera). The prevention or treatment of pain can best be accomplished when there is anticipation of pain and a diagnosis based on evidence of sensory dysfunction involving a peripheral nerve, plexus, nerve root, or central pathway. This evidence can be found by using different modalities for quantitative sensory testing. Anatomical studies have demonstrated that unmyelinated primary afferent fibers contain a variety of neuroactive substances that may be released by high intensity peripheral stimulation. Injury or disease processes in deeper tissue or in visceral areas with extensive innervation may result in pain thresholds not completely controlled by current available analgesics or at their recommended dosage levels. These issues are complex and diagnosis is even more difficult due to species and breed differences in outward expression to painful insult. Medications now and in the future will be targeted for specific receptors.

Sensory nerves carry impulses to the level of the dorsal horn of the grey matter of the spinal cord. This is the first major site where chemical neurotransmitters are involved in the process. The spinal cord also houses synapses that make up the reflex arc for simple motor withdrawal from a painful stimulus. To better understand how impulses are sent to the brain via the spinal cord, the gate theory was proposed by Melzack and Wall (1965) (Fig 1-3). Further modified in 1992, signals transmitted to the brain are a summation of excitatory and inhibitory inputs from different levels in the spinal cord (Wall 1992). It is not clear where noxious stimuli are perceived as pain within the brain but it is most likely to be at the level of the thalamus (Livingston and Chambers 2000).

Neurotransmitters are located in the brain and spinal cord to facilitate transfer of nerve impulses at various sites (Figure 1-3). These include glutamate, noradrenaline, 5-hydroxytryptamine (5-HT, serotonin), (GABA), substance P, and endogenous opioid peptides, e.g., β-endorphins and enkephalins. It is not surprising that analgesic drugs have been developed or found in a natural state that either inhance or inhibit transmitters involved in pain processing.

Specific sites responsive to noxious stimuli are termed nociceptors. A stimulus must reach a certain level before a nociceptor will generate nerve impulses. The level of this stimulation is called the nociceptive threshold. Once the noxious stimulation is perceived, it is referred to as the pain detection threshold. Pragmatically, if a dog grasps your hand in its mouth, you probably would not be in any hurry to remove it if you had never been bitten or observed such an act. Once the animal exerts enough pressure to crush or penetrate tissue, the pain detection threshold is reached and most of the time, a verbal expression of pain occurs!

The stimulus needed to exceed the pain detection threshold is quite variable and is probably higher in individuals who have experienced pain previously. Some animals (and humans) are very tolerant to noxious stimuli while others are very sensitive (hyperalgesic). It is interesting to note that some animals recovering from anesthesia and surgery exhibit very little or no response to

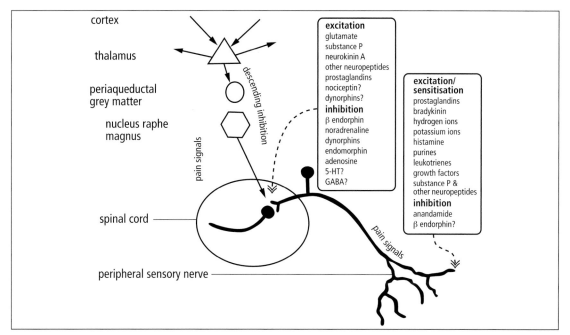

Figure 1-3 Pain pathways. A wide variety of substances can increase or decrease the frequency of firing in neurons carrying pain signals. This is particularly important at the level of the spinal cord, where the signal is "gated"; however, "gating" probably occurs at several different levels, especially at the thalamus. The higher up the CNS the signal goes, the more complex the processing becomes and the less certain is our knowledge of what is happening.
Reprinted by permission from Pain Management in Animals, W.B. Saunders. Edited by Paul Flecknell and Avril Waterman-Pearson.

what would be considered a noxious stimulus and thus may have a high pain tolerance threshold. Other animals have a very low threshold meaning that they just have a lower tolerance to pain. It is important to be sensitive to both extremes and to recognize individual animals that are in pain but demonstrate discomfort by being quiet and withdrawn instead of crying or being overactive.

Expressions of pain by animals can either be seen or heard and must be learned by humans. Any lack or uncertainty of pain perception that leads to denial that pain exists in animals is logically and empirically unfounded. Animals feel pain to the same extent as humans and have a wide variation in tolerance to pain stimuli. Animals may express pain or discomfort in two extremes. Excessive activity and relative lethargy are both reflections of a painful state. Moaning, groaning, crying, whimpering, looking at the painful area, licking or biting, or simply decreases in activity are all expressions of pain. The issue is not if a painful state develops in animals but whether the symptoms of pain will be recognized and appropriate therapy provided. Veterinarians have an ethical obligation to alleviate pain and suffering in animals. Lloyd Davis (1983) expressed that pain and suffering constitute the only situation in which, if in doubt, one should go ahead and treat.

In animals, pain from high threshold afferent stimuli with sustained input is often of concern since it is more easily diagnosed and more likely to respond to currently available therapy. Fortunately, along with receptors that are affected by noxious stimuli there are other receptors that are acted upon by several medications that modify pain behavior. Among these are the opioid, adrenergic, dopamine, serotonin, adenosine, GABA, cholinergic, neuropeptide Y, neurotensin, and glutamate receptors with respective active agents (Guyton 1991).

Pain stimulation from tissue damage in a number of organ systems may produce similar levels of discomfort. Is there a real difference between severe colic pain from intestinal blockage and ischemia versus acute renal blockage? Can one distinguish between the severity of dental pain and a luxated intravertebral cervical disc? It is certainly easier to diagnose the difference in chronic and acute pain. Signs of pain that may be observed by veterinarians, technicians or owners are listed in Table 1-6. Some of these would be obvious by casual observation while others may be evident with other testing methods.

Table 1-6

Visible Symptoms of Pain in the Dog and Cat

	Physiologic	Neurologic	Metabolic
Frightened when usually friendly	Change in heart rate, usually tachycardia	Increase in brain wave activity	Fluid and electrolyte imbalance due to alteration in fluid intake and discharge
Aggressive behavior	Change in blood pressure, usually hypertension	Increase in cerebral metabolism and cerebral blood flow	Weight loss due to lack of nutrient intake
Hyperexcitable	Change in capillary refill time	Hypersensive to touch, sound, or temperature change	Diabetic symptoms due to imbalance between food intake and insulin administration
Lack of physical activity	Change in mucous membrane color	Not sleeping	Increase in epinephrine
Unusual response to owner or other animals	Change in cardiac output, peripheral resistance, and blood flow	Attempts to find a comfortable place to ly down in cage	Increase in norepinephrine
Self-mutilation	Change in respiratory frequency, usually increase in rate	May lick at incision site or front paws.	Increased cortisol
Vocalization	Tidal volume may be decrease due to pain	Harsh barking or growling: cats hiss	Increased ACTH due to pain related stress
Hiding	Back of cage, usually head down position	Shivering / trembling	Potential shock-like syndrome
Anxious facial expression	Apprehensive	Lack of contentment	Anorexia

Non-Pharmacological Methods of Pain Management

Most often, small animals undergoing surgical procedures are in the foreign environment of a veterinary hospital or clinic. They are exposed to strange smells and the presence of other animals may provoke unusual behavior. Animals are cared for by professional staff that is also strange to them so they may naturally be apprehensive, excited and sometimes aggressive. Seniors and geriatrics may be the most sensitive and being attentive to this circumstance can be helpful. Keeping animals comfortable and within view of people in the pre-op/post-op area may be advantageous. Placing animals on the floor with comfortable padding in view of people rather than being put in cages during the initial stages of anesthesia recovery will reduce imposed stresses. Having background music or radio going in the area may be helpful along with being in a warm place, covered by towels warmed in a microwave oven and any number of comfort items can help with the post-operative process of managing acute pain.

Acupuncture has been used as a non-pharmacologic means of acute pain relief with varying success. This is done by placing needles in specific points of the body to cause a type of stress-induced analgesia (Shoen 1994). For detailed information on the use of acupuncture for treatment of acute pain, please refer to other resources such as that provided by the International Veterinary Acupuncture Society and Acupuncture References (Klein and Trachtenberg 1998).

Analgesia

Pain is understood to be a protective mechanism to avoid catastrophic consequences that occur just in the process of living. As described briefly before, there are intrinsic mechanisms within the body to allow escape and then provide some degree of pain relief. Literally translated, analgesia means without pain. From a clinical perspective, it is possible to make patients pain free following surgery. However, it is usually not necessary to achieve such a level. The primary goal is to create a situation in which the patient can tolerate discomfort and to either eliminate or keep to a minimum undesirable physiological responses such as tachycardia, arterial hypertension, vasoconstriction, and ventricular dysrhythmias.

Analgesics are considered to be drugs that alleviate pain. This may be accomplished by raising the pain detection threshold or by reversing the cascade of a lowered threshold response such as might accompany an inflammatory process (Nolan 2000). Most analgesic drugs used in association with anesthesia and surgery in small animals are hypoalgesic. Although this is a dose dependent process, they reduce pain rather than abolish it completely. The five main classes of analgesics are: opioids, alpha$_2$ adrenoceptor agonists, non-steroidal anti-inflammatory drugs (NSAIDs), local anesthetics, and miscellaneous (NMDA receptor agonists, e.g., ketamine).

Preemptive Analgesia

If sensation to pain did not exist in the body, damage to tissue would not be detected which could lead to severe injury and infection. This is a lifesaving process designed to impede or prevent major injury, multiple organ failure, and death. Once pain gets a head start, it is tough to catch and treat effectively. Aggressive therapy is often needed in animals that have sustained traumatic injury, disease, and developing infection. However, when surgery is performed for elective procedures or as a means of providing therapeutic measures, pain is an unavoidable consequence. Until modern time, the protocol for giving an analgesic for treatment of pain was to wait until the patient demonstrated overt discomfort. Most commonly with a complaining patient, doses are high and more frequent and everyone becomes stressed including the patient. Faster acting inhalation anesthetics such as isoflurane and sevoflurane allow patients to recover quicker but in doing so, the onset and realization of a painful state by patients during recovery is also more rapid. General anesthetics do not prevent transmission of nociceptive impulses from the operative site to the spinal cord and release of the excitatory neurotransmitter glutamate. Thus light levels of general anesthesia, as is commonly practiced, cannot prevent the creation of hyperexcitability in the CNS.

The use of incisional infiltration of local anesthetics following elective cholecystectomy in human patients was shown to improve pulmonary function and produce less atelectasis in the recovery period. In 1988, a clinical study in humans demonstrated that there was a better outcome if patients received opioid premedication and were given a local block before surgery compared to postsurgical therapy (McQuay 1988). The addition of local anesthesia to general anesthesia for patients undergoing inguinal herniorrhaphy resulted in an increase in the postoperative time to the first request for analgesic from 1 hour to 9 hours (Tverskoy et al., 1990). This effect could not be explained by the prolonged presence of a local anesthetic in the body because pain relief was still evident 48 hours later and with pressure-induced incisional pain even 10 days after surgery. Human patients given fentanyl before inguinal herniorrhaphy compared to postsurgical administration but before recovery, required lower doses of an alternative opioid and less frequent patient controlled analgesia (PCA) injections during the immediate surgical recovery period. Preincisional infiltration of tonsils with a local anesthetic resulted in a better outcome in managing pain following tonsillectomy (Jebeles 1991). Katz et al (1992) evaluated the efficacy of preemptive opioid analgesia and specific contribution of sugical incision and rib retraction in 30 human patients scheduled for elective thoracic surgery through a posterolateral thoracotomy incision.

They found that epidural administration of fentanyl given before surgical incision resulted in lower postoperative pain scores and reduced postoperative rescue morphine requirements when compared with the same dose and route of administration given just 15 minutes after incision. Thus preemptive analgesia was found to attenuate or prevent development of central sensitization induced by surgical incision and later maintained by inputs from rib retraction at the wound site. From animal studies and numerous clinical trials, clinicians found that patients did better if they received analgesics before surgery.

Without preemptive analgesia, signals travel through peripheral sensory nerves from the site of injury to the spinal cord and brain. Because of the resulting increased activity from the site of injury, receptors become bombarded by impulses during the surgical procedure to become hyperactive along with expansion of receptive fields of CNS neurons. The inflammatory process continues following surgery to aggravate the situation such that the resultant condition produces more discomfort, more distress and more pain to the patient. Perception of pain by the brain does not just involve a moment-to-moment analysis of afferent noxious input, but rather involves a dynamic process that is influenced by the effects of past experiences. Sensory stimuli act on neural systems that have been modified by past inputs and the behavioral output is significantly influenced by the memory of these prior events (Melzack et al. 2001).

Peripheral tissue injury from any source provokes changes in responsiveness of the nervous system. One type of change is peripheral sensitization, a process of lowering the nociceptive threshold in afferent peripheral nerve terminals. A second change is the process of increased excitability and modulation of spinal neurons called central sensitization (Woolf and Chong 1993). These two modifications contribute to the postoperative pain hypersensitivity condition that increases body responses to noxious stimuli and a lowering of the pain detection threshold. This occurs both at the site of injury (primary hyperalgesia) and in surrounding uninjured tissue (secondary hyperalgesia). Sensory pain signals that evolve during surgery are not obtunded by modern injectable or inhalation anesthetics and trigger a prolonged state of increased excitability in the CNS. Windup is a term used to describe this increased excitability in the spinal cord and brain.

A key component in this process are N-methyl-D-aspartate receptors (NMDAR) located in brain and spinal cord. These were first identified in the late 1980's and now recognized for development of dorsal horn neuron hyperexcitability or wind-up and induction of central sensitization (Pozzi et al. 2006). By giving regional local anesthesia before surgery or by using opioid premedication, postoperative pain is reduced by preventing the establishment of central sensitization (Woolf and Chong 1993). This was a good beginning but it was later found that for surgical procedures that result in severe pain, it was even better to give analgesics preoperatively, intraoperatively as well as postoperatively to block the surgery-induced afferent barrage and establishment of the pain hypersensitivity process. This would include analgesics given locally, systemically and by spinal or epidural injection. The intent of these protocols is to provide therapeutic intervention in advance of the pain rather than as a reaction to it (Shafford et al. 2001).

Demerol (pethidine) was shown to prevent development of surgically induced hyperalgesia when it was given pre-emptively in rats undergoing ovariohysterectomy (Lascelles et al 1995). Lascelles et al. (1998) also determined that preoperative administration of carprofen had a greater analgesic effect than postoperative administration in dogs undergoing OHE. Dogs undergoing OHE induced to anesthesia with thiopental and maintained with halothane benefited from medetomidine analgesia administered preanesthesia (Ko et al. 2000). Others have demonstrated preemptive effects of opioids in dogs and cats including buprenorphine, butorphanol, fentanyl, oxymorphone and morphine (Roughan et al., 1999; Broadbelt et al., 1997; Stanway et al., 2002; Halder 2001). More recently, prevention or reduction of central sensitization can be achieved by blocking NMDARs before or soon after pain is established (Pozzi et al. 2006). Ketamine and tiletamine are NMDAR antagonists and both are commonly used for anesthesia induction along with minor tranquilizers.

When used in combination with opioids and NSAIDs, better approaches to pain management can be assured. For severe pain, it would be advisable to continue analgesic therapy during the initial healing process to prevent the reestablishment of central sensitization. Thus, *preemptive analgesia* means treating postoperative pain by preventing establishment of central sensitization.

Preanesthetic Medication
Anticholinergics

The question pertaining to the benefits of anticholinergics given preanesthesia has received attention in recent years. Perhaps the widespread use of atropine with thiobarbiturates and modern inhalation anesthetics is a carryover from its use to prevent bradycardia mediated by opioids such as morphine and meperidine and inhalation anesthesia with diethyl ether. In the 1960's and 1970's, morphine premedication was a common adjunct prior to induction and maintenance with sodium pentobarbital. The use of atropine with diethyl ether was to prevent excessive salivation.

Anticholinergics are lytic to the parasympathetic nervous system thus their action is to block acetylcholine at the postganglionic terminations of cholinergic fibers. Their muscarinic action is to depress salivary and bronchial secretions, cause pupillary dilation, and possibly increase heart rate due to partial blockade of vagal tone (Beleslin 1984). Large doses inhibit parasympathetic responses to the urinary bladder and decreased peristalsis of the gastrointestinal tract. Normal doses will decrease motility somewhat and will reduce gastric secretions.

The primary goal in using anticholinergics prior to anesthesia induction is to prevent severe bradycardia that may result from vagal stimulation (Takabashi 1983). This may occur subsequent to tracheal intubation or as a side effect of certain drugs such as opioids and alpha$_2$ agonists, e.g., oxymorphone, xylazine, and medetomidine (Hsu 1985). With careful attention to proper dosages, this can be done without inducing profound tachycardia (Kantilip 1985; Rigel 1984). Another reason for giving anticholinergics would be to decrease or prevent salivary and bronchial secretions that may be induced by a drug such as ketamine or occur as animals recover from anesthesia. Bronchodilation occurs along with increased physiological and anatomical dead space. Blocking cholinergic fibers of ciliary nerves except in birds produces papillary dilatation.

Anticholinergics should either be used with great caution or avoided in patients with existing sinus tachycardia (Muir 1978). They should also be used at appropriate doses so as not to induce tachycardia. In patients with pre-existing tachycardia or premature ventricular contractions, care must be taken not to place patients in a compromised situation of significantly reducing the percentage of time the heart spends in diastole thus reducing coronary sinus refill (Conrad 1981). For situations in which tachycardia is present, e.g., rates in excess of 150 beats per minute (bpm), and the use of an anticholinergic is required for such procedures as thoracic or abdominal laparotomy, the anticholinergic of choice should be administered after the patient is anesthetized. The tachycardic response of anticholinergics is known to be suppressed by inhalation anesthetics such as halothane or isoflurane. Anticholinergics should not be administered indiscriminately. Anticholinergics should be given preanesthesia only after patient evaluation and assessment of the anticipated response to anesthetic and analgesic drugs and the surgical procedure, the tendency of specific species and breeds to develop bradycardia and the possibility of excessive salivation during recovery. A selective guide is not to give anticholinergics preanesthesia to dogs with heart rates above 140 bpm and more than 160 bpm in cats. This will, in general, avoid potentially dangerous tachycardia. Monitoring heart rate must still be done but prevention of severe bradycardia, which may be initiated by tracheal intubation, visceral manipulation, or drug action is an important criterion for use of this class of drugs in dogs and cats. In addition, the antisialagogue effect is useful during intubation and recovery and chances of vomiting and regurgitation are minimized.

Atropine sulfate and glycopyrrolate are the two anticholinergic agents that have been evaluated for clinical use in small animal patients (Short 1983a, 1983b). Atropine sulfate is extracted from plants such as *Atrpa belladonna* and *Jimsonweed*. Glycopyrrolate is a synthetic quaternary ammonium compound that can be used as a substitute for the belladonna alkaloid. The latter has increased in popularity since its introduction but both are commonly used in clinical small animal practice.

Atropine Sulfate
Atropine can be given subcutaneously (SQ), intramuscularly (IM), or intravenously (IV). The recommended dose for the dog and cat is 0.04mg/kg SQ, 0.02mg/kg IM, and 0.01mg/kg IV. It should be given SQ 15 to 30 minutes before induction; effects are present within 10 minutes following IM injection. This drug should be given as premedication in which opioids or ketamine are included. The half-life of atropine is 2 hours. As a guide, a repeat dose should be given at one-half of the preanesthetic dose. Pupillary dilatation will still be present during recovery so intense lighting in the area should be avoided.

Glycopyrrolate
Glycopyrrolate may be given to dogs and cats SQ, IM, or IV at doses of 0.02, 0.01, and 0.005mg/kg, respectively (Short 1987a). There appears to be a greater tendency to produce sinus tachycardia and ventricular arrhythmias with atropine than with glycopyrrolate (Short 1978). As a result, the use of this drug has increased over the past 20 years. There are other advantages in specific situations such as a longer duration of decreased gastrointestinal motility, and gyclopyrolate is less likely to cross the placental barrier or cause an excessive increase in heart rate (Proakis 1978). Thus, it is preferred over atropine for cesarean section (McIntyre 1982). The increase in gastric pH induced by gyclopyrrolate versus atropine is advantageous in the event aspiration of vomited gastric contents should occur which is problematic in certain breeds such as brachycephalics. The anticipated half-life of glycopyrrolate is about 4 hours and the repeat dose should be reduced by 50%.

Tranquilizers
Major
Fear and apprehension are present in most veterinary patients admitted to a hospital or clinic and are easily recognized by those experienced in animal behavior. Adversive behavior will be manifested by cowering in a cage or run, hiding under bedding, snarling, snapping, shaking, and casting a doubtful or distrustful looks.

Use of tranquilizers and sedatives in veterinary practice has contributed greatly to decreased morbidity and mortality in patients undergoing anesthesia and surgery. Fear and apprehension cause increased levels of catecholamines that induce potentially dangerous drug interactions with some anesthetics and subsequent ventricular dysrhythmias (Price 1980). Calming of fractious animals not only stabilizes physiological responses prior to anesthesia but it also creates a less stressful and safer environment for veterinarians, technicians, and assistants. Two major classes of psychoactive drugs are used in humans and these are for antianxiety (benzodiazepines) and antipsychosis (phenothiazines and butyrophenones). These terms provide an appreciation of how these two classes of drugs act in different ways in animals, specifically dogs and cats.

Phenothiazines
Phenothiazines constitute the major group of tranquilizing drugs for domestic animals. They are widely used to make animals more tractable when given preanesthesia while at the same time serving as antiemetics. This group includes chlorpromazine, promazine, acetylpromazine, perphenazine, trimeprazine, propriopromazine, triflupromazine, and piperacetazine. Chlorpromazine is the oldest of this group and the most frequently studied representative of phenothiazines. However, acetylpromazine is the most widely applied representative in this group for dogs and cats. The phenothiazines can be effective in suppressing types of aggressive behavior that do not reflect fear reactions.

Phenothiazines act on the CNS by depressing the brain stem and connections to the cerebral cortex (Booth 1982). This results in a general calming with reduction in motor activity. The structure of phenothiazines is similar to that of dopamine. At least some of the activity for this group of drugs is associated with antagonism of dopamine excitatory receptors. The emetic action of opioids in dogs may be due to stimulation of dopamine excitatory receptors and antagonism of this emetic action is one reason why phenothiazines have been used with opioids in neurolep-tanalgesic combinations.

High doses of phenothiazines should be avoided as they may cause extrapyramidal signs, such as rigidity, tremor and catalepsy. Aggressive behavior has been reported following the labeled dose of acetylpromazine, which is 1.1mg/kg (0.5mg/lb.). It was reported that 15 minutes after an IM injection of 13mg acepromazine in an 11kg dog (1.18mg/kg), the dog suddenly became vicious. While carrying the dog to the surgical area, the patient proceeded to attack the veterinarian inflicting 64 puncture wounds and lacerations to both hands plus one lost fingernail (Waechter 1982). The veterinarian also reported aggressive behavior in a 1.5 year old 3.5kg Chihuahua given 4mg acepromazine IM (1.14mg/kg). Although the clinician had been using this dose for more than 20 years, no undesirable reactions had been observed in this practice. However, it would be considered to be a very high dose today in the way this drug should be used as a pre-anesthetic alone, in combination with opioids, or with other adjunctive drugs. Dose related arterial hypotension is due to CNS depression and peripheral alpha adrenergic receptor blockade. At doses of acepromazine equal to or less than 0.1mg/kg in young healthy patients, vasodilation and mild hypotension are possible. However, in animals dehydrated as a result of disease or because of unavailability of water, hypotension may be severe and can lead to circulatory shock, especially in the presence of anesthetic drugs. Balanced electrolytes add volume to the dilated vascular bed and increase venous return to allow maintenance of cardiac output.

Hypothermia may be accelerated by phenothiazines during anesthesia due to depression of thermoregulation that may be due to depletion of catecholamines in the region of the hypothalamic thermoregulatory center (Booth 1982). However, the beneficial effects of phenothiazines outweigh this side effect and slowing of the temperature decrease can be off-set by placing anesthetized animals on heated circulating water pads or using other forms of external heating.

Use of epinephrine is contraindicated because of peripheral alpha blockade induced by phenothiazine tranquilizers. The pressor receptors are blocked by acetylpromazine but not the depressor receptors; thus there is stimulation of the depressor receptors resulting in a further fall in blood pressure (Lumb 1973). Treatment is best provided by IV fluids and a beta stimulant such as norepinepherine, or a α_1 vasoconstrictor such as methoaxamine or phenylephrine.

Some dogs are fear biters, domain protectors, or simply mean and aggressive. The attitude of mean and aggressive animals is not influenced by tranquilization even at high doses, as all that may be affected is the aim and quickness of the bite. Therefore, a tranquilizer-opioid combination to achieve neuroleptanalgesia will usually effect the desired degree of chemical restraint. It is imperative when using such a combination that the dog not be confronted or aroused for at least 20 minutes following injection because drug effects may be over-ridden before the full response is achieved.

Acetylpromazine has been shown to have a protective effect on epinephrine-induced ventricular dysrhythmias (Muir et al. 1975) (Booth 1982). This antidysrhythmic action of phenothiazines has been attributed to sympathetic blockade, local anesthetic-like action, and quinidine-like action (Muir 1981). The use of phenothiazines given preanesthesia is advisable when drugs known to sensitize the myocardium are used, e.g., halothane or catecholamines. This may also be the case when catecholamines are endogenously released due to stress and anxiety. In dogs given epidural or spinal anesthesia that would induce both a sensory and motor block, phenothiazine tranquilization should be avoided (Booth 1982). The normal physiological response to segmental anesthesia is compensatory vasoconstriction in unanesthetized segments and increased cardiac output. This response is obtunded by phenothiazines and their use may lead to severe hypotension.

Phenothiazines have been shown to cause thrombocytopenia and platelet dysfunction but until the significance of this in clinical veterinary anesthesia is clarified, these drugs should not be used in animals known to have a platelet disorder (Davenport 1982). Certain phenothiazines are potent antihistaminics. Thus, these drugs must be avoided in animals undergoing intradermal skin testing for allergies because the response to the allergen may be masked during the test. Their antihistaminic properties may be useful in patients undergoing mast cell tumor removal, where manipulation of the tumor may cause degranulation of mast cells and consequent histamine release.

In studies using malignant hyperthermic (MH) susceptible pigs, acetylpromazine was shown to have a protective effect at doses exceeding 1.1mg/kg. This drug is not known to trigger MH but it will not necessarily prevent it other than by indirectly depressing the stress response.

A characteristic physical sign of phenothiazine induced sedation is protrusion of the nictitating membrane. In addition, phenothiazines must be used with caution in patients with severe hepatic disease because their action may be prolonged subsequent to the depressed function of liver enzymes. Practitioners have long been cautious about using acepromazine in Boxer dogs. There is no published evidence that there is breed sensitivity to this drug but it may be that clinicians have had profound responses subsequent to doses higher than 0.1mg/kg. In healthy P1 animals, adverse effects should not occur as long as the dose is kept at or below 0.1mg/kg. Phenothiazines have been shown to lower the threshold to seizure activity from a variety of etiologies (Holliday 1980). Although this paper did not specifically consider acetlypromazine, it has been a long-time practice to avoid the use of any phenothiazine tranquilizer in patients with a history of seizures. It may also be prudent not to use drugs in patients undergoing cervical myelography as injection of a radiographic contrast agent is known to induce seizures (Hall 1983). This is especially important in dogs with cervical abnormalities preventing redistribution of contrast media.

Finally, acetylpromazine has been shown not to have analgesic effects in the dog and cat (Sawyer 1992). However, phenothiazines are known to augment, e.g., be additive or synergistic to the analgesic effects of opioids (Briggs et al. 1998). It has long been known that the neuroleptic component of this class of tranquilizers plays an important role in combination with opioids for a state of well-being and sedation. Augmentation of opioid induced analgesia by representatives of this group makes it even more important to use them in combination.

Acetylpromazine
For sedation and relief of anxiety, tranquilization is recommended using light doses of acetylpromazine (Acepromazine, Ft Dodge), 0.02 to 0.1mg/kg IM or SC 20 to 60 minutes pre-anesthesia induction. Doses in the lower range are advised when used in combination with opioids such as butorphanol, hydromorphone or oxymorphone. At doses below 0.1mg/kg, a remarkable change in attitude will result with much easier management for the anesthetist and patient. With rare exception, the top dose should not exceed 3mg in any patient when used as a pre-anesthetic.

Butyrophenones
Representatives of this group include droperidol, azaperone, fluanisone and lenperone. Although they have higher therapeutic ratios, they have never reached the same popularity as phenothiazines in dogs and cats. Drugs in either class have sympatholytic characteristics and produce tranquilization in the form of indifference to their surroundings and decreased motor activity.

Droperidol
Droperidol is a butyrophenone tranquilizer with properties similar to those of acetylpromazine. Droperidol is not marketed for sole use in animals but was available in a fixed ratio with fentanyl

in the proprietary neuroleptanalgesic combination Innovar-Vet®. The dose of droperidol for dogs is 0.7-1.7mg/kg IV and 2.2-2.9mg/kg IM (Gleed 1987). Lenperone has been reported for use in dogs (Muir 1985). The dosage is 0.22-0.88mg/kg IV; 0.44-1.8mg/kg IM; 0.55-2.2mg/kg PO. Fluanisone has been used in combination with fentanyl (10 mg/ml and 0.34mg/ml, respectively) in the propri-etary neuroleptanalgesic Hypnorm®. Azaperone (Stresnil®) is marketed in the UK for use in swine but is no longer available in the USA.

Because of the popularity of acetylpromazine and lack of significant differences between the two classes of major tranquilizers, representatives of the butyrophenones are not used very much as anesthetic adjuncts in dogs and cats. In addition, the neuroleptic containing droperidol, Innovar-Vet®, is no longer available.

Minor
Benzodiazepine Derivatives

The history of the benzodiazepines as anxiolytics can be divided into two phases. The first was characterized by a very rapid increase in their clinical use in the late 60's and early 70's but with very little understanding of their mechanism of action. The second phase began in 1977 with the identification of specific receptors in the brain. It is now known that virtually all of the major pharmacological actions of benzodiazepines are mediated through gamma-aminobutyric acid (GABA) receptors (Hobbs et al 1996). These receptors have been demonstrated in a wide variety of species and no major differences in the biochemical or pharmacological characteristics of these receptors have been demonstrated. The major GABA receptor, $GABA_A$, is an integral membrane chloride channel that mediates inhibitory neurotransmission in the CNS (Pritchett et al., 1989).

Benzodiazepine tranquilizers have five distinct pharmacologic properties: antianxiety, anticonvul-sant, sedation, centrally mediated muscle relaxation and amnesia. This class of drugs has been widely studied and their use in human medicine is primarily as anxiolytics. Midazolam is commonly used for preanesthetic and intraoperative medication. The use and abuse of diazepam in people has received considerable attention. The anticonvulsant properties are useful in companion animals when treating drug induced seizures associated with myelographic procedures. It must be assumed that there is retrograde amnesia associated with benzodiazepine drugs in animals based on responses in humans but it is very difficult to demonstrate the scientific basis for this effect in dogs and cats. This leaves the other characteristics of antianxiety, centrally mediated muscle relaxation and sedation as the primary effects of this class of drugs in veterinary patients.

Benzodiazepines undergo hepatic metabolism by several different microsomal enzyme systems with both the parent drug and their active metabolites having a high affinity for protein binding. Active metabolites, such as would be associated with diazepam, are biotransformed more slowly resulting in a longer duration of action. In contrast, when drugs such as midazolam, that are inactivated by the initial reaction of α-hydroxylation, there a much shorter duration of action due to lack of metabolites and extensive protein binding in dogs (Court and Greenblatt 1992). It was also demonstrated that midazolam was completely absorbed when given by IM injection.

The cardiovascular effects of benzodiazepines are minor in healthy small animal patients. At preanesthetic doses, a slight decrease in blood pressure and increase in heart rate may be noticed. With midazolam, the effects appear to be secondary to a decrease in peripheral resistance (Nugent et al. 1982).

Effects of benzodiadepines can be reduced or prevented by prior treatment with antagonists at the $GABA_A$ receptor. Flumazenil is one such antagonist available for clinical application to selectively block both high-affinity binding and biological effects by benzodiazepines. It has been shown to reduce analgesic effects of diazepam as equated by changes in isoflurane minimum alveolar concentrations (MAC) in dogs (Hellyer et al. 2001) and to reverse experimental midazolam-induced cortical activity during isoflurane anesthesia in dogs (Keegan et al., 1993). Tranquilli et al. (1990) demonstrated that clinical signs of CNS depression induced by midazolam and xylazine could be completely reversed by simultaneous injections of flumazenil and yohimbine. In another study, flumazenil combined with naloxone or butorphanol was used to reverse the depressant effects of oxymorphone-diazepam in dogs (Lemke et al., 1996). These studies support the use of flumazenil to reverse effects of benzodiazepines when used with other CNS depressants (Gross et al., 1992). However, it is not a common procedure to reverse effects of either diazepam or midazolam premedication when used in association with surgical anesthesia. The recommended dose of flumazenil is .001mg/kg IV or 1/3rd to 1/2 of the tranquilizer dosage.

Diazepam

This benzodiazepine derivative received approval in the US for use in dogs in 1993 and is a valuable adjunct when used with ketamine and opioids. This drug is classified by the US Drug Enforcement Administration (DEA) as a C-IV controlled drug. Because the base drug is not water soluble, the parenteral preparation has propylene glycol as the solubilizing agent and is marketed in several formulations. The recommended dose range is 0.2-0.5mg/kg in the dog and cat. It has great value as an induction agent when combined with 100mg/ml ketamine in a 50:50 by volume ratio, or when given simultaneously, but in separate syringes, with an opioid such as oxymorphone. (See chapter 2, Injectable anesthetic procedures, for further details.)

Midazolam

Under the brand name in the US of Versed (Roche Pharmaceuticals) and Hypnovel in the UK, midazolam is marketed as a human drug at a concentrations 1, 2 and 5mg/ml. Midazolam is a water-soluble benzodiazeipine that can be given alone or in combination with other sedatives and hypnotics. A pre-anesthetic dose of 0.1mg/kg in dogs reduced thiamylal requirement for anesthesia induction by 16% (Greene et al., 1993). In a similar manner, midazolam decreased isoflurane anesthesia requirement (MAC) in dogs (Takeuchi et al., 1991). Following premedication with 0.1mg/kg midazolam in dogs, mask induction with sevoflurane or isoflurane produced a smooth rapid onset without episodes of induction-related complications such as struggling or breath-holding (Mutoh et al. 2001). At higher doses, e.g., 0.5mg/kg, marked changes in behavioral responses were observed in dogs such as profound weakness, ataxia, and transient agitation followed by a period of quiesence (Court and Greenblatt 1992). Ilkiw et al. (1996a) studied the onset of action and behavioral effects following IV and IM administration of doses ranging from 0.05 to 5.0mg/kg in cats. Onset of action was rapid following both routes of administration with some cats becoming ataxic while others were recumbent. Even at the highest dose, anesthesia was not induced with swallowing and response to tail clamp still present. In addition, adverse behavior can be expected at doses above 0.5mg/kg that include restlessness, vocalization, and difficulties with restraint. As a result, if used alone midazolam should be used at doses below 0.5mg/kg. It would be advisable to use this drug as a premedicant in combination with opioids or alpha$_2$ agonists.

Midazolam is a generic drug distributed by a number of different companies in a number of different formulations. It does not have a veterinary label but experience from using this drug in both cats and dogs have been extremely positive. Because of its numerous advantages over diazepam as a preanesthetic, it is one of the most useful adjunctive anesthetic drugs to have in small animal hospital. In situations when the use of acepromazine may be contraindicated for pre-anesthetic sedation such as in patients at risk, with a seizure history, or for senior and geriatric patients, midazolam has great application. In these situations, it is often combined with butorphanol and atropine and given IM. 20 to 30 minutes pre-anesthesia. In dogs recovering from surgery and anesthesia, there are occasions when patients are seemingly dysphoric or their behavior is not conducive to a smooth recovery. This is usually manifested by moaning or crying and persists even after the animal has been comforted or after additional analgesic therapy has been given. A low dose of midazolam (0.1mg/kg) given IV is an effective method of relieving this form of anxiety that has worked numerous times very well. It has also great application when combined with ketamine (Ilkiw et al. 1996b). Recommended dosage of midazolam in the dog and cat are 0.1 to 0.3mg/ kg IV or IM.

Opioids

The term opioid refers to all natural and synthetic drugs that have morphine-like actions or actions that are mediated through opioid receptors. In contrast, opiate is more specific referring to naturally occurring alkaloids obtained from opium poppy sap which contains morphine, codeine among other alkaloids. Opioid receptors are normal sites of action of several endogenous substances. Enkephalins are found in areas of the brain that are related to the perception of pain. Endorphins are found in the pituitary gland and hypothalamus. These compounds function as neurotransmitters, modulators of neurotransmission, or neurohormones. It is assumed that exogenous opioids, such as butorphanol, morphine, fentanyl, buprenorphine, hydromorphone and oxymorphone, produce their effects by mimicking actions of the endogenous enkephalins and endorphins. In some species, certain doses of exogenous opioids may have actions on receptors that are not strongly activated by their own endogenous opioid like compounds. This may explain why excitation and seizure-like activity may be induced by opioids in some animals, i.e., cat and horse. The existence of these endogenous substances may also explain why there are such diverse tolerances to pain. However, this does not mean that opioids cannot be used in cats. Mu opioid agonists are generally considered to be the best analgesics so with refinements in dosing, many different opioids can be used successfully for pain management in cats (Robertson & Taylor 2004).

Two major types of opioid receptors are designated as mu and kappa. Delta receptors have also been identified and are similar to mu receptors. Epsilon receptors respond specifically to endoge-nous peptides, endorphins. There are a number of mu receptors, e.g., mu-1, mu-2, etc., that are involved with supraspinal analgesia, respiratory depression, mydriasis, euphoria, sedation and physical dependence. Kappa receptors are responsible for spinal analgesia, miosis, a modest degree of sedation and some respiratory depression. Sigma receptor activation produces euphoria and hallucinations as well as respiratory and vasomotor stimulatory effects. Most opioids and opioid antagonists have different affinities for different receptors.

Drugs such as morphine, meperidine, fentanyl, hydromorphone and oxymorphone are mu opioid receptor agonists and are all classified as DEA C-II drugs in the U.S. Naloxone is a pure opioid antagonist that, in a competitive manner, attaches to all receptors to reverse effects of opioids by displacing them from the receptors. Drugs that bind specifically to these receptors compete with other substances for these sites and may either exert no action or have only limited effects. Certain opioids have both agonist and antagonist affects. Most commonly, opioids with diverse actions exert agonist actions at receptors to provide analgesia and varying degrees of sedation. They also have antagonist effects at receptors; thus terms agonist antagonist analgesics or mixed opioid agonists are used to describe this complex pattern of action. Nalorphine, nalbuphine, butorphanol and pentazocine are agonist to kappa and mu receptors at low doses but exert antagonist actions at mu receptors with higher doses. Buprenorphine is a mu agonist but has minor antagonist affects on kappa receptors. Some drugs with mixed effects are better agonists while others are better antagonists. The pure antagonist, naloxone, can be used to reverse all of the effects exerted by both opioid receptor agonists and agonist-antagonist analgesics by competing for attachment at the same receptor sites.

Opioids produce their major effects on the CNS and gut. These include analgesia, sedation, respiratory depression, depressed gastrointestinal motility, nausea, vomiting, and alterations of the endocrine and autonomic nervous systems. These drugs act as agonists, interacting with binding sites or receptors in the brain and other tissues. The affinity of many opioids for binding sites correlates well with their potency as analgesics.

Analgesia produced by exogenous opioids is rather selective as other modalities such as vision, hearing and other senses are not obtunded. Animals may respond to noise and initiate muscular movement while still having reduced nociceptive responses. The goal in pain management is to make patients feel comfortable: that is, to allow them to accept discomfort. Animals cannot anticipate their destiny. Therefore, it is not possible to convince an animal that pain or discomfort, which occurs subsequent to surgery, is to be expected and that it will only be temporary. Animals recovering from surgery are often surprised and confused because they hurt. Therefore sedation along with analgesia is often desirable and necessary. It must also be realized that continuous dull pain is more easily treated than sharp intermittent pain. The former is most often associated with visceral pain while the latter is more typical of somatic pain (muscle and skin).

Opioid Receptor Agonists (Table 1-7)
Fentanyl
This mu receptor agonist is 75-100 times more potent than morphine and 500 times more potent than meperidine (Jaffe and Martin 1990). It is a C-II DEA controlled drug in the U.S. It is the most prevalent opioid used in conjunction with anesthesia in humans and does have application in dogs. Fentanyl may be used alone for analgesia in the dog at a dose of 0.001-0.005mg/kg IM. If given IV repeat doses may be needed every 20 minutes or by continuous infusion of 0.003-0.10mg/kg/hr. (Dobromylskyj et al. 2000). Fentanyl does not have a veterinary label in parenteral or transdermal preparations.

Transdermal fentanyl is available in preparations that release the opioid at different rates of 25, 50, 75 and 100µg/hr. This can be an effective method used preanesthesia, intraoperatively and post-anesthesia for sustained pain management in dogs and cats as long as adequate time is provided for drug uptake from transdermal administration (Kyles 1996, Kyles 1998). However, certain precautions are advised. Patches should be applied to areas where hair is clipped close to skin and deoiled with alcohol. The skin must be dry before applying the patch. It should be covered with an occlusive non-porous dressing as a barrier to the pet and children (Robinson 1999). Positioning is most common over the shoulder, dorsal cervical region, chest wall, hips, or flank area to avoid removal by the animal. Uptake of transdermal fentanyl is slow and adequate blood levels may take up to 20 hours to occur in dogs. Lag time for decay of blood levels after removal is about 12 hours. Care should be taken to not use in animals with fever which will result in increased absorption. In anesthetized animals with a patch, the area should not be placed on a heated surface such as water blanket as this may cause localized vasodilation and increased uptake of the drug.

Lee et al. (2000) studied the pharmacokinetics of fentanyl after 25µg IV and 25µg/h transdermal administration in cats. They found that fentanyl was rapidly distributed and eliminated following IV administration. Mean distribution was about 30 minutes and elimination-half life 2.3 hours which was considerably shorter than values reported for dogs, e.g., 45 min and 6 hours, respectively (Kyles 1996). Following application of the fentanyl patch, plasma concentrations increased gradually to a maximum at 44 hours. Overall guidelines in cats is as follows: onset of detectable plasma concentrations 0 to 6 hours; interval to steady-state values 12 to 18 hours; duration of steady-state conditions 18 to 100 hours; median rate of delivery was 36 % of theoretical rate for the 25µg/h patch. As a result, if transdermal fentanyl is used for preemptive analgesia, it must be applied 12 to 18 hours prior to surgery. Postoperative respiratory depression in animals does not appear to be a significant problem with the fentanyl patch (Welch et al. 2002).

Transdermal patches should not be left in position for more than 100 hours. After removal in dogs, fentanyl concentrations decrease rapidly with a half-life of 1.4 hours (Kyles 1996). Plasma concentrations in cats decrease much slower than in dogs. Patches were removed in the Lee study at 100 hours and appreciable levels of the drug were still present 8 hours later. There have not been studies to document alteration of the surface area of absorption to decrease rate of

Common Opioid Dosages and Indications

Table 1-7

Opioid	Dose/Route	Duration (IM)*	Indications	Comments
Buprenorphine	Dog: 0.01-0.02mg/kg; IM, IV Cat: 0.005-0.015mg/kg; IM, IV	3-8 hrs 3-8 hrs	Mild to moderate pain	Provides more sedation than other opioids. May be difficult to antagonize.
Butorphanol	Dog: 0.1-0.2mg/kg;IM, IV, SC Cat: 0.1-0.2mg/kg; IM, IV, SC	45-90 min 2-5 hrs	Mild to moderate pain	Mild sedation in dogs. Little or no sedation in cats. Mu antagonist at 0.4mg/kg or more.
Fentanyl	Dog: 0.002-0.01mg/kg; IV, IM Cat: 0.001-0.005mg/kg; IV, IM 5 - 20µg/kg/hr IV CRI**	Up to 0.5 hr Up to 0.5 hr Up to 0.5 hr after termination of infusion	Mild to moderate pain **CRI needed for long term analgesia	Sedation,respiratory depression, slow heart rate, nausea; inadequate duration of analgesia following single IV bolus or IM injection
Transdermal Fentanyl	Dog: 0.005mg/kg/hr; transdermal Cat: 0.005mg/kg/hr; transdermal	3 days 3-5 days	Mild to moderate chronic pain	Onset of effect is quite variable: 6-12 in dogs, may be longer in cats.
Hydromorphone	Dog: 0.1-0.2mg/kg IM; 0.03-0.1mg/kg IV Cat: 0.05-0.1mg/kg IM; 0.02-0.1mg/kg IV	2-4 hrs 30-45 min 2-4 hrs 30-45 min	Moderate to severe pain	Similar effects as those with oxymorphone
Morphine	Dog: 0.2-2.0mg/kg; IM, SC 0.05-0.4mg/kg IV*** Cat: 0.05-0.1mg/kg IM, SC	1-2 hrs 1-2 hrs	Moderate to severe pain	Sedation, respiratory depression, slow heart rate, nausea, vomiting, dysphoria or excitement in larger dosages
Oxymorphone	Dog: 0.03-0.2mg/kg; IM, IV, SC Cat: 0.03-0.1mg/kg; IM, IV, SC	2-4 hrs 2-4 hrs	Moderate to severe pain	Only FDA CVM approved opioid for dogs and cats; sedation, mild respiratory depression
Tramadol	Dog: 0.1-0.2mg/kg IM, IV 1-3mg/kg PO Cat: 0.05-0.1mg/kg IM, IV 1-2mg/kg PO	2-4 hrs 2-4 hrs	Mild to moderate pain	Has not been associated with abuse potential and does not have usual side-effects of other mu opioids.

* Duration varies with dosage and route of administration. If given IV, onset is more rapid and shorter duration, while SQ usually results in slower onset and longer duration than if given IM. Sedation lasts longer than analgesia. Opioid agonists and agonist/antagonist effects may be reversed with naloxone at 1-10 g/kg IV or IM.   ** CRI = Constant Rate Infusion   *** IV use may cause histamine release

delivery of fentanyl. The drug must pass through the system-skin interface to the stratum corneum, epidermis, and dermis where it absorbed into the circulation. Because of so many variables involved in this process, one can expect great differences in outcome from patient to patient. Other problems include changes in drug delivery affected by skin temperature, skin blood flow, failure of patches to remain attached to skin, dermatitis under the patch, and human abuse. Because of the risk of patches being eaten by animals or children, discretionary use in a non-hospital setting must be taken with great caution. Having a good understanding with the owner of potential problems is of paramount importance.

Hydromorphone

This potent mu opioid receptor agonist has been available for use in pain management of human patients since the late 60's and early 70's (Halpern et al. 1996; Rapp-Suzanne et al. 1996; Chan-Wei Hung et al. 1999). It is a C-II DEA controlled drug under the brand name of Dilaudid®, is approximately 5 times as potent as morphine on a milligram basis in humans (Coda B et al. 1997) and appears to have the same potency as oxymorphone in dogs and cats. When oxymorphone became more difficult to obtain in North America, clinical evaluations in dogs identified hydromorphone as a reasonable substitute. Smith et al. (2001) reported that hydromorphone was comparable to oxymorphone as a preanesthetic in dogs and that sedation was enhanced by acepromazine without complication. Neither opioid increased plasma histamine concentrations. Machado and Dyson (2002) compared effects of 0.05mg/kg IV oxymorphone followed by 0.2mg diazepam / kg to 0.1mg/kg IV hydromorphone with the same dose of diazepam. They found these two opioid/diazepam combinations to be comparable in hypovolemic dogs. Postoperative respiratory depression of butorphanol (0.4mg/kg) or hydromorphone (0.2mg/kg) combined with acepromazine (0.02mg/kg) and glycopyrrolate (0.01mg/kg) given IM preoperatively was evaluated in healthy dogs (Campbell et al 2002). Although hypoventilation was more evident with hydromorphone, these changes were not clinically significant. Hydromorphone was found to have antinociceptive effects in cats without dysphoria or changes in behavior (Lascelles & Robertson 2004).

Clinical experiences with hydromorphone suggest a dose range of 0.05 to 0.2mg/kg for preanesthetic medication in dogs and 0.05 to 0.1mg/kg for cats. It can be used with acepromazine or midazolam to provide greater sedation when needed. When hydromorphone is used during anesthesia for supplemental analgesia, 0.1 to 0.2mg/kg can be given IV in small incremental doses. There appears to be a low incidence of hyperthermia in cats given hydromorphone that can reach 105-106°F during recovery and it may not be easily recognized. If the skin is hot to touch, measure with a rectal probe and treat accordingly.

Meperidine

The effects of meperidine on the cardiovascular, respiratory, and gastrointestinal systems are similar to those of morphine but as a general rule, meperidine does not stimulate chemoreceptors in the brain to induce nausea, vomiting, or defecation. Because analgesia in both the cat and dog is provided for less than 60 minutes, this drug is better suited for analgesia and sedation pre-anesthesia rather than for treatment of post operative pain. For this purpose, a dose range of 3-10mg/kg may be given IM along with an anticholinergic and repeated every 2-3 hours (Dobromyskyj 2000). Intravenous administration of meperidine is not advised in order to avoid severe hypotension and other responses caused by histamine release.

Morphine Sulfate

This was the first opioid to be purified and as a result, all other drugs with similar properties are compared to it. It is also the most widely used mu opioid throughout the world. Morphine produces analgesia and CNS depression in the dog but at high doses; excitement, tonic spasms, histamine release, and change in behavior may be observed. Following SC injection in dogs, there is a brief period of excitement, restlessness, and salivation followed by nausea, vomiting, and defecation. Thereafter, sedation and analgesia are induced. The effect of morphine on the gastrointestinal (GI) system occurs in two phases. Nausea, vomiting, and defecation occur as a result of direct stimulation. Thereafter, there is a slowing of GI motility. Most of these side effects are moderated by using low doses and when combined with tranquilizers and sedatives.

Mild respiratory depression occurs and is dose related. Reductions in respiratory rate and tidal volume at high doses both contribute to elevation of arterial carbon dioxide ($PaCO_2$). There are minimal effects on the cardiovascular system induced by morphine. Bradycardia may occur if an anticholinergic is not given. Analgesia and sedation will be produced using 0.2-0.5mg/kg given IM or SC in the dog. A dose of 0.2mg/kg should provide 45 to 60 min of analgesia in dogs. In the cat, 0.1mg/kg has been advocated for postoperative pain (Heavner 1970). To reduce the undesirable gastrointestinal and cardiovascular effects of morphine, an anticholinergic such as atropine or glycopyrrolate should be used.

Oxymorphone HCl

This semisynthetic opioid was approved for use in the dog and cat in 1961 and continues as the only FDA approved mu opioid agonist in companion animals in the U.S. It is a DEA C-II controlled drug and availability is limited to the U.S. It has 70 to 130 times the potency of morphine and produces more sedation in the dog than morphine or meperidine (Sawyer et al. 1992). Respiratory depression is mild and there is little depression of the cough reflex (Copland and Haskins 1987). This is an advantage when this drug is used for postoperative pain management and also as a component of neuroleptanalgesia for bronchoscopy. Oxymorphone can be used effectively as premedication with midazolam in canine geriatric or canine patients at risk (P-3, 4, 5). If used in cats, the oxymorphone dose must be at or below 0.1mg/kg. With diazepam or midazolam given concurrently for induction, oxymorphone may be injected slowly IV over 60-90 seconds at a dose of 0.1mg/kg to the desired effect. The dose is determined by the patient's physical status and whether it will be used as a component for anesthesia. In cases where a major tranquilizer is indicated, 0.02 to 0.05mg/kg acepromazine may be given prior to induction along with oxymorphone at doses ranging from 0.05 to 0.2mg/kg. For treatment of postsurgical pain, pre-anesthetic medicaton with oxymorphone (0.01 to 0.1mg/kg IM or IV) can provide analgesia for 2-4 hours. Unlike morphine and meperidine, Robinson et al. (1988) found that histamine values did not increase at any time after IV oxymorphone administration in dogs. As pre-anesthetic medication, it is best to give the analgesic at doses of 0.05 to 0.1mg/kg IM or SQ 15 to 30 minutes before induction. For post-surgical analgesia, additional doses may be given as needed at 2-4 hour intervals.

Opioid Receptor Agonists with Antagonist Properties
Buprenorphine

This opioid is classified as an agonist-antagonist analgesic that is a partial agonist to the mu receptor with antagonist properties to the kappa receptor. However, in the late 70's, buprenorphine was known more for its low abuse potential and utility in treating narcotic addiction in humans (Jasinski et al. 1978). Methadone was not available in the U.S. for treating addicts so buprenorphine was a welcome alternative (Bickel et al. 1988). It was reported to be longer acting and 25 to 50 times more potent than morphine. Buprenorphine is unlike most other opioids in that its association and dissociation with receptors is much slower. Even when given IV, onset of action may take 30 minutes or longer.

Results of a study comparing sublingual buprenorphine with morphine given IM indicated slower onset of analgesic effects but much longer duration without serious side effects (Edge et al. 1979; Bullingham et al. 1981). Subsequently, this mixed opioid was evaluated and marketed as a perioperative analgesic given systemically and by intrathecal injection in adults and children (Abrahamsson et al 1983; Capogna et al. 1988; Maunuksela et al. 1988). In a study conducted in the U.K. comparing pentazocine, buprenorphine, and morphine in dogs, Taylor (1984) found that all three analgesics were effective without adverse effects. Two years later, combinations of meperidine (3.3mg/kg) or buprenorphine (.009mg/kg) with acepromazine (.07mg/kg) were evaluated in dogs undergoing radiography (Taylor 1986). Both combinations provided effective and safe sedation.

Pre-operative buprenorphine (0.01mg/kg IM) and 0.1mg/kg morphine IM combined with 0.05mg/kg acepromazine were evaluated in cats (Stanway et al. 2002). They found that both analgesics were useful but that the buprenorphine/ace combination was superior to morphine/ace. One caution with pre-anesthetic administration of buprenorphine is the long period for uptake that may take as long as 60 min. Based on the availability of a sublingual buprenorphine tablet that is widely used in human patients, Robertson et al. (2001) found that the buccal route can be used in cats and is similar to IV and IM dosing. Buprenorphine solution was administered into the side of the cat's mouth at a dose of 0.01mg/kg. They found that the solution was well accepted without salivation or resentment. Comparative plasma half-life for buccal, IV and IM routes of administration was 347 ± 83 min, 470 ± 133 min, and 380 ± 131 min, respectively. Some sources have suggested duration of analgesia is up to 12 hours in dogs and cats but those data are not supported by published reports. Clinically useful duration is recognized to be 4 to 6 hours. Repeat doses at 6 to 8 hour intervals for 24 to 48 hours have not been associated with undesirable effects (Dobromylskyj et al. 2000). Its longer duration of effect is due to the slow dissociation from receptors and the tight binding to receptors makes it more difficult to antagonize with naloxone. Recommended dose for cat and dog is 0.01-0.02mg/kg IM or SC.

Buprenorphine is a Schedule 3 controlled drug in the UK (Misuse of Drugs Act, 1991). It is a C-V controlled drug by the US-DEA marketed under the brand name of Buprenex for humans and in the UK; it is marketed for dogs under the veterinary label of Vetergesic. It has become the most commonly used analgesic in small animals in the UK but is not approved for animals in the US. It has been used to some extent in small animal practices and is becoming more popular as a useful analgesic for pain management in a variety of animals.

Butorphanol

Butorphanol (Torbugesic™, Ft Dodge) is a synthetic opioid analgesic with kappa and mu receptor agonist properties and 3 to 5 times the potency of morphine. If used as a mu opioid antagonist, butorphanol is 50 times less potent than naloxone and those effects are best found at doses at or above 0.44mg/kg (Lemke et al 1996). Butorphanol has an interesting history. It was first approved for its antitussive properties in dogs and because of its potential as an opioid analgesic, investigation was started in the early 1980's to develop a visceral pain model in cats to evaluate the benefits of butorphanol (Sawyer & Rech 1987; Sawyer et al. 1990). Based on negative hot plate tests in small rodents, it was felt that determining antinociceptive thresholds with butorphanol using thermal stimulation would be ineffective; a colorectal distension model was subsequently developed. At low doses, the respiratory depressant properties are less than those seen with morphine but as is typical with this class of drugs, a "ceiling effect" is reached where higher doses do not produce further depression or analgesia. The ceiling for cats is between 0.2-0.4mg/kg and in dogs, increased doses above 0.4mg/kg does not necessarily provide added antinociception (Houghton et al 1991; Sawyer et al 1991).

When evaluating comparative reports about the use of butorphanol either with other opioids or drugs of other classes, one should carefully evaluate clinical relevance when the dose of butorphanol is 0.4mg/kg or higher (Carroll et al. 2005; Al-Gizawly and Rude 2004). For example, antinociceptive effects of oxymorphone-butorphanol combination was found to be additive or even synergistic in cats with the dose up to 0.2mg/kg (Briggs et al 1998) whereas when butorphanol (0.4mg/kg) and hydromorphone were used together in cats, decreased intensity of antinociception from butorphanol was felt to decrease level of analgesia provided by hydromorphone (Lascelles & Robertson 2004b). Butorphanol (0.1 to 0.3mg/kg IV) reduced enflurane MAC in dogs but higher doses did not reduce MAC any further. Doses of butorphanol (0.2, 0.4 and 0.8mg/kg) did not have a halothane-sparing effect in dogs (Quandt et al. 1994) but both 0.08

and 0.8mg/kg infused IV decreased isoflurane MAC in cats (Ilkiw et al. 2002). Route of administration does not appear to make any difference as the pharmacokinetics was the same with either IM or SQ administration in dogs (Pfeffer et al 1980). Therefore, when using this drug for postsurgical pain, 0.05 to 0.2mg/kg is best administered pre-anesthesia in the dog or cat (Campbell et al. 2003; Caulkett et al. 2003; Cornick & Hartsfield 1992; Dyson 1992; Fox 1995; Itamoto et al. 2000; Muir et al. 1999; Sawyer 1991, Sawyer 1993, Sawyer 1998). The lower doses should be used if acepromazine is given in combination. Analgesia should last 45 min to 1.5 hours in the dog and more than twice that duration in cats (Sawyer et al. 1993). If additional visceral analgesia is needed during recovery, the initial dose can be given IV, IM, or SQ. However, preference is for a mu opioid agonist such as fentanyl, morphine, oxymorphone, hydromorphone, or buprenorphine for moderate to severe somatic or visceral pain.

High doses of butorphanol infusion (0.1 and 0.2mg/kg/min) produce significant depression in heart rate, blood pressure, and cardiac output (Sederberg et al. 1981). Occasionally, dysphoria may occur when given alone, expressed as increased irritability and disorientation (Lascelles et al. 2004a). This is the major reason why butorphanol has not gained much popularity in the recovery room for human patients.

Butorphanol, acepromazine, and glycopyrrolate may be compounded in a multiple dose bottle as follows: 4ml (40mg) Torbugesic [butorphanol], 0.5ml of acepromazine (5mg), 5ml of Robinul [glycopyrrolate] (1mg), and the balance sterile water or saline to provide a 20ml mixture of "BAG". Atropine may be substituted for glycopyrrolate. In this case, the same amount of butorphanol and acepromazine is used, but 8ml of atropine (0.5mg/ml) is added in place of glycopyrrolate and the balance sterile water or saline to yield a 20ml mixture of BAA. The mixture with atropine is still called "BAG" because it just sounds like a better word associated with anesthesia than "BAA". Stability studies have not been reported for this mixture. It is best given as pre-anesthetic medication in the cat or dog at a dose of 0.1ml/kg IM or SQ 20 to 30 minutes prior to induction. For older dogs and those over 40kg, only 0.25ml of acepromazine is used in the mixture. In senior or geriatric patients, acepromazine is not advised because of their higher susceptibility to induced hypotension. Instead, midazolam is a good substitute.

A unique method of dispensing butorphanol for clinical use in dogs and cats was provided by Dr. Charles Baldwin from Lebanon Animal Hospital in Lebanon, CT (2002). Scientific study of this method has not been documented and this is likely to be buccal absorption, not oral. One ml of butorphanol (2mg/ml) is mixed with 30ml of Pet-Tinic, an oral vitamin preparation (Pfizer). In small dogs and cats, 1ml is given in the mouth BID or TID with a small bulb syringe. For geriatric cats and small dogs, 0.5ml is given BID. In 50lb dogs and larger, 2 to 3ml of the mixture is given BID and can be dosed TID as needed. Just based on his experience and client feedback, Dr. Baldwin found this to be an effective means of providing pain relief for mild to moderate pain. It would seem reasonable to use this method of giving butorphanol at home for mild to moderate pain relief and preemptive analgesia prior to scheduled surgery.

Nalbuphine

Nalbuphine (Nubain™)* is a mixed agonist/antagonist structurally related to the opioid agonist oxymorphone and opioid antagonist naloxone. In human patients, nalbuphine's relative analgesic potency appears to be somewhat less than that of morphine but it has a slightly longer duration of action. It produces minimal sedation and respiratory depression, and as an opioid antagonist, it is about one-fourth as potent as nalorphine. Studies indicate that nalbuphine may be given at doses between 0.75 to 3mg/kg IM or IV (Sawyer 1987). It can be given pre-anesthesia with sedation provided by acetylpromazine as part of a balanced anesthesia regimen. Experience with this drug has shown that it does not provide as effective analgesia as butorphanol because of its weaker action as an opioid receptor agonist. However, it has stronger opioid antagonist properties than butorphanol. It is not controlled by the DEA in the U.S. and is often used as an opioid antagonist instead of naloxone, administered IV in equal mg's of the drug per mg of opioid.

Pentazocine Lactate

Pentazocine (Talwin™) has been reported to be an effective analgesic for many animals including dogs and cats but its duration of pain relief is very short (Sawyer 1987). Plasma half life for pentazocine in the dog is only 22 minutes (Davis 1983). The drug has minimal effects on the cardiovascular system and is a mild respiratory depressant. The dose for the dog is 2mg/kg IM or SQ. This drug is a weak analgesic in the cat at doses from 0.75 to 1.5mg/kg (Sawyer 1987). Although it produces analgesia at 3.0mg/kg IV, the excitatory effects preclude its use in the cat.

Atypical Opioid Agonist

Tramadol HCl

Tramadol is one of the most prescribed centrally acting analgesics in the world (Lai et al. 1996). The brand name in European countries is *Tramal*. It is manufactured by Grunenthal, Aachen, Germany, has approval for use in humans in more than 100 countries but does not have a veterinary label in any country. Prior to 1990, tramadol was thought to produce its effects exclusively through an opioid mechanism. However, subsequent studies suggested an additional contribution from a non-opioid mechanism that is now understood to be due to inhibition of serotonin and noradrenalin reuptake (Giusti et al. 1997). Comprised of two enantiomers, the positive molecule shows affinity for the μ opioid receptor with its agonist effects being blocked or reversed by naloxone. The negative enantiomer is less effective on opioid receptors and the serotonin system but inhibits noradrenalin reuptake. The analgesic and antinociceptive potency is 5 to 10 times lower than that of morphine (Lehmann et al. 1990). Its acute therapeutic use in man is not associated with side effects such as respiratory depression, sedation, nausea, gastrointestinal motor function, or dysphoria. Further, long-term clinical trials in human patients have not been associated with significant side-effects. Chronic studies have shown an absence of abuse potential that supports it not being listed as a controlled drug by the US-DEA. It is possible for it to not be listed as a controlled substance by any country.

Tramadol is available in both oral and parenteral formulations. The oral form is provided in 50 and 100mg tablets but only 50mg tablets are available in the U.S (*Ultram*, Johnson & Johnson). Owing to its good water solublity, tramadol is absorbed rapidly being limited only by transit time through the stomach. Onset time is 15-20 minutes. For injection, 50mg tramadol/ml is prepared in a water/Na acetate buffered solution, without perservatives, with a pH of 6.8. Toxicity studies in dogs show that this drug is very safe. Lethal dose given orally is 450mg/kg and 50-100mg/kg IM or IV (unpublished company data).

In a clinical study conducted in Modena, Italy, 0.1mg/kg tramadol was combined with 0.01mg/kg acepromazine and 0.05mg/kg atropine for preanesthetic medication in dogs (Ronchetti et al. 2002). Over the subsequent 3 days, 1mg/kg was given orally bid. In young dogs, the dose was increased to 2-4mg/kg. Comparative results of analgesia provided by tramadol, butorphanol and carprofen are presented in Figures 1-4, 1-5, 1-6, and 1-7. This protocol was found to be an effective means of managing surgical pain in dogs. In another study, tramadol (0.2mg/kg IV) or morphine (0.2mg/kg IV) was used to modulate neuroendocrine response in 30 dogs treated surgically for pyometritis (Mastrocinque and Fantoni 2001). Cortisol levels increased in both groups but glucose and catecholamine levels did not change. Based on reports regarding epidural use of tramadol in humans, Halder and Bose (2000) administered xylazine (0.75mg/kg) alone and in combination with tramadol (2mg/kg) epidurally in 18 healthy dogs. They found that coadministration of xylazine and tramadol was an effective means of controlling postoperative pain.

Tramadol can be given orally at a dose of 1-3mg/kg bid to dogs and cats one to two days presurgery with the presumption that preemptive analgesia will be accomplished (Ronchetti 2003, personal communication). However, there have not been any studies to support this contention. Just based on clinical experience, tramadol can be used effectively to control postsurgical acute pain when given orally two or three times daily at doses up to 5mg/kg. It has also been used by small animal practitioners for chronic pain management including terminal cancer patients.

Observation	Score	Observation about Patient
Vocalization	0	No vocalization
	1	Vocalization, respond to comforting
	2	Vocalization, no interaction
Movement	0	None
	1	Frequent change in position
	2	Trashing
Distress	0	Calm or sleeping
	1	Light agitation
	2	Moderate agitation
	3	Strong agitation
Total Score	0 - 2	Excellent analgesia
	3 - 5	Good analgesia
	6 - 8	Poor analgesia
	9	Unacceptable

Figure 1-4 Scoring system to evaluate effects of tramadol, carprofen and butorphanol for postsurgical pain in dogs.

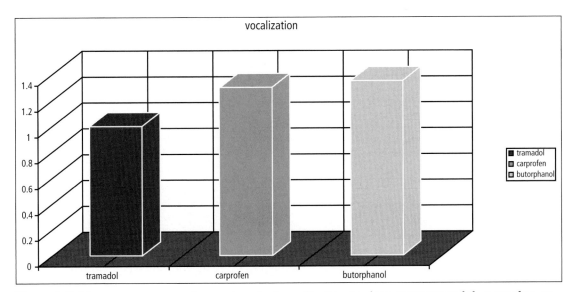

Figure 1-5 Mean scores comparing postsurgical vocalization in dogs given tramadol, carprofen, or butorphanol.

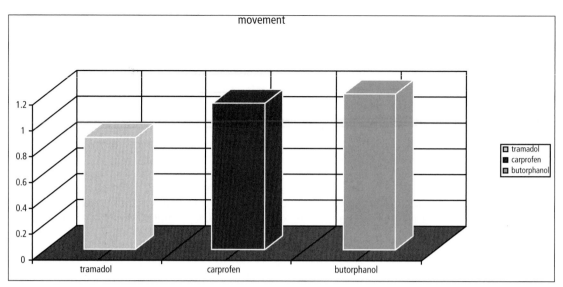

Figure 1-6 Mean scores comparing postsurgical movement in dogs given tramadol, carprofen, or butorphanol.

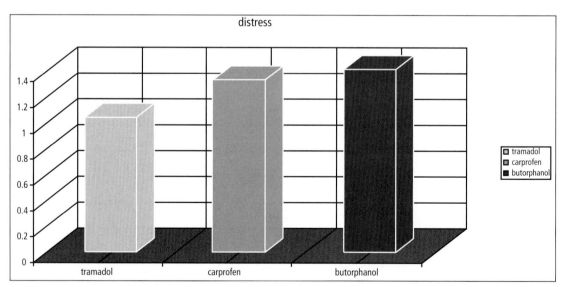

Figure 1-7 Mean scores comparing postsurgical distress in dogs given tramadol, carprofen, or butorphanol.

Alpha₂ Adrenergic Receptor Agonists

Drugs included in this class serve an important role in the management of veterinary patients because they improve handling of patients by reducing fear, anxiety, and stress. This ultimately contributes to improved comfort of animals. Alpha₂ adrenoceptors are located in brain, spinal cord, and other tissues throughout the body. Activation of these receptors induces inhibitory effects including analgesia, sedation, bradycardia, hypotension, mydriasis, and relief of anxiety (Weinger et al. 1989). Emesis is frequently observed and is more prevalent in cats than dogs. Alpha₂ agonists inhibit release of acetylcholine in intestinal smooth muscle and this results in decreased gut motility. Alpha₂ agonists are commonly used for diagnostic and minor procedures or as pre-anesthetic agents before injectable or inhalation anesthesia. They produce mild to deep sedation in a dose dependent manner. The dosage of anesthetic is reduced proportionately because of CNS depression caused by alpha₂ agonists. Worldwide, the two alpha₂ adrenergic agonists most used in small animal practice are xylazine and medetomidine. They are followed by romifidine and most recently dexmedetomidine was approved in Europe.

Four alpha₂ agonists are used to modify animal pain. Clonidine is the classical substance of the group but not used in animals. Xylazine has been the drug used in veterinary practice for more than 30 years. Two relatively new compounds have been developed: detomidine (Dormosedan) for horses and cattle and medetomidine (Domitor) for cats, dogs and various small animals (Table 1-8). These drugs share some common structural features. By the nature of the heterocyclic ring, molecules can be separated into three categories: detomidine and medetomidine are closely related imidazole derivatives, whereas, clonidine is an imidazoline and zylazine is classified as a thiazole.

Alpha₂ agonists may be safely and effectively used as pre-anesthetics providing the influence of these medications on the dosage, expected responses to anesthetics and drug interactions are understood. The most important consideration is dose reduction of the anesthetic. First, the pre-anesthetic dosage of the alpha₂ agonist is normally only 10-30% of the dosage used as a sole medication for sedation and analgesia or for diagnostic or minor surgery. As dosage of the alpha₂ agonist is increased, there will be a direct proportional 10-90% decrease in anesthetic requirements. For example, 5µ/kg medetomidine will reduce dosage of propofol in the dog by 30-35% while 10µ/kg will reduce propofol requirements by 60-67%.

The combinations of these medications with anesthetics can provide additional sedation and analgesic quality, prolonging sleep time and contributing to post anesthetic patient comfort especially following short anesthetic/ surgical procedures. It is recognized that the use of multiple combined medications contribute to balanced anesthesia and reducing unwanted side effects, but there is no substitute for attentive patient monitoring to assure desired results with these or any other anesthetic combination.

Xylazine

Xylazine is an alpha₂ adrenoreceptor agonist with sedative, analgesic, and muscle relaxant properties. Its analgesic characteristics are mild to moderate lasting less than 30 minutes in both dog and cat. The sedative effects will outlast analgesia. From cardiopulmonary studies in dogs, heart rate and aortic blood flow are reduced following an initial increase in blood pressure and peripheral vascular resistance (Klide 1975). Xylazine induces hyperglycemia in cats and dogs as a result of inhibition of insulin secretion.

Xylazine-induced atrioventricular block can be prevented by prior administration of an anticholinergic. Emesis occurs occasionally in dogs but is more common side-effect in cats. Acute abdominal distension may occur in large breed dogs as a consequence of aerophagia or parasympatholytic activity resulting in gastrointestinal atony and gas accumulation. As a result, xylazine should especially be avoided in deep chested dogs, i.e., Great Danes, Irish setters and others.

Table 1-8

Alpha$_2$ Agonist Dosages and Indications

Alpha$_2$ agonists	Dosage / Route*	Duration (IM)**	Indications	Comments
Xylazine	Dog and Cat: 0.1-0.5mg/kg IM, IV, SC	0.5 hr	Mild pain	Sedation, slow heart rate, minimal respiratory depression, emesis
Medetomidine	Dog: 5-15µg/kg IM, IV, SC Cat: 10-20µg/kg IM, IV, SC	0.5-1.5 hr 0.5-1.5 hr	Mild pain	Sedation, slow heart rate, minimal respiratory depression, occasional emesis
Medetomidine	Dog: 15-60µg/kg IM, IV, SC Cat: 20-80µg/kg IM, IV, SC	1-3 hr 1-3 hr	Moderate to severe pain	Sedation, slow heart rate, minimal respiratory depression, occasional emesis
Dexmedetomidine	Same as medetomidine at 50% of the medetomidine dosage guidelines.	See above	Mild pain	Dexmedetomidine has twice the potency in µg/kg as medetomidine.
Romifidine	Dog: 10-30 µg/kg IV Cat: 20-40 µg/kg IM	0.5-1.0 hr	Mild pain	Same as others
Romifidine	Dog: 30-120 µg/kg IV Cat: 40-160 µg/kg IM	0.5-1.5 hr	Moderate pain	Same as others

* The highest dosages suggested are based on approved levels when used as a sole medication. When used in combination with opioids, anesthetics or other CNS depressants, careful consideration to the reduction of dosages of medications used in combination must be practiced.

** Duration of analgesia varies with dosage and route of administration. IV administration generally results in a more rapid onset and shorter duration, while SQ administration usually results in a slower onset and longer duration than listed above for IM administration. The dose range for medetomidine is 20-60µg/kg for most dogs with smaller dogs requiring higher dosages. The medetomidine dosage of 5 and 10µg/kg IM was evaluated as a preanesthetic to propofol anesthesia. Effects of alpha$_2$ agonists may be reversed with atipamezole 25-300µg/kg IM (5x the administered dose of medetomidine).

Xylazine has been shown to sensitize the myocardium which lowers the threshold to epinephrine induced ventricular dysrrhythmias (Muir 1975). From its effects on the cardiovascular system, xylazine should be avoided in mean, excited, or aggressive dogs and cats. If used as a pre-anesthetic, doses of an induction agent such as thiopental must be reduced 50 to 90%. It should not be used in high-risk patients. Dose for the cat and dog is 0.5 to 1mg/kg IV and 1 to 2mg/kg IM.

Medetomidine

Following the widespread acceptance of xylazine, additional efforts were made to develop other alpha$_2$ adrenoreceptor agents for sedation and analgesia. This resulted in development of new products as well as a better knowledge and understanding of alpha$_2$ adrenergic agents. The new products are more receptor specific having a higher pharmacologic affinity for alpha$_2$ receptors. Medetomidine, a very potent alpha$_2$ drug, was developed for use in dogs and cats. Atipamezole, a corresponding alpha$_2$ antagonist, was developed to reverse the effects of medetomidine by competing with medetomidine at alpha$_2$ receptors. The anxiolytic action of medetomidine was first reported in 1986 (Lammintausta 1986). Chemistry and neurochemistry of medetomidine were determined and reported (Laine 1986, Turpeinen 1988, MacDonald 1988). In 1989, the pharmacokinetics of uptake, distribution, metabolism and elimination of medetomidine and atipamezole were determined and reported (Virtanen 1989). Medetomidine and atipamezole are widely used in many countries.

Medetomidine is a highly selective and potent alpha$_2$ adrenergic agonist. Receptor binding assays show that it has a $\alpha 2$: $\alpha 1$ adrenoreceptor selectivity ratio of 1,620 compared with 260 for detomidine (Virtanen 1989). Medetomidine is 10 times more potent than detomidine in inhibiting spontaneous locomotor activity in rats. Central nervous system neurotransmission characterized by norepinephrine turnover is inhibited at low doses, whereas brain dopamine and serotonin turnover are inhibited at higher doses in medetomidine-treated rats. In 1989, it was reported that medetomidine is a full agonist at both presynaptic and postsynaptic alpha$_2$ adrenoceptors (Virtanen 1989). Alpha$_2$ agonists potentiate injectable and inhalation anesthetics. Because arousal is coupled with elimination of drug from brain, it is possible to make judgements on neurologic evaluation using clinical parameters.

Medetomidine is a clinically effective sedative/analgesic in dogs and cats (Clark 1989a, Clark 1989b, Hamlin 1989, Vaha-Vahe 1989a, Vaha-Vahe 1989b). Studies of the neurologic responses to medetomidine as a sole agent for sedation and analgesia or in conjunction with other medications for anesthesia have been completed in dogs. Reports of its use in several wildlife species and birds have been favorable and support use of alpha$_2$ medications for sedation, analgesia and immobilization in wildlife populations (Jalanka 1989). Medetomidine produces sedation in dogs and cats 5 to 10 min after IM injection and very rapid sedation (1 to 3 min) when given IV. There is significant depression of brain activity as demonstrated by reduction in total amplitude and shifts in frequency distribution of the EEG. Changes in EEG records following medetomidine administration in dogs correspond to clinical signs of depression, sedation and analgesia (Short 1992b). In addition to sedation, higher dosages of medetomidine allow completion of more involved diagnostic and minor surgical procedures, e.g., cleaning and repair of wounds and lacerations, radiographs, examination of the ears and bandage changes (Raiha 1989a, b, c). Since medetomidine is not an anesthetic, combining it with a local anesthetic increases medetomidine's utility for minor surgery (e.g., more extensive wound repair).

As with other alpha$_2$ adrenergic agonists, medetomidine initially causes arterial hypertension followed by bradycardia with or without atrioventricular heart block. This change usually self-corrects without medication. Hemodynamic effects are initiated by the activation of alpha$_2$ adrenoceptors. As blood pressure increases, a slower heart rate and decreased blood flow results. The decrease in heart rate is due, in part, to baroreceptor response to increased blood pressure (Scheinin 1988). Ketamine with its associated increase in heart rate often will prevent much of the trend to bradycardia. In addition, administration of a thiobarbiturate following medetomidine premedication often will reduce duration of hypertension and bradycardia induced by medetomidine. Atipamezole reversal of medetomidine sedation will also reverse changes in heart rate and blood pressure. High medetomidine doses can result in prolonged sedation. Caution is advised in animals with cardiopulmonary, CNS, or endocrine dysfunction. Numerous combinations of alpha$_2$ agonists and opioids have been reported. Such combinations can result in profound sedation and analgesia to achieve an anesthetic-like condition.

Use of Medetomidine as a Pre-anesthetic
Medetomidine, given IM or IV at 5 to 10µg/kg pre-anesthesia, results in sedation and a reduction of the anesthetic induction dosage. This has been well-documented using thiobarbiturates and propofol. Both xylazine (Tranquilli 1984) and medetomidine (Raiha 1989b, Scheinin 1988, Ewing

1993, Maze 1991) reduce dosages required for anesthetic induction. Medetomidine is more likely to influence inhalant anesthetic maintenance requirements (Ewing 1993, Maze 1991). Xylazine analgesic effects last about 15 minutes, whereas medetomidine analgesia lasts 40 to 60 minutes at comparable doses. Patient response to an adjustment in inhalant anesthetic vaporizer settings may not be as rapid in medetomidine-treated animals. This is partly due to CNS depression from medetomidine. The uptake of the anesthetic agent in vessel rich tissues also may be altered by medetomidine mediated circulatory changes. However, concentrations needed to maintain anesthesia will be reduced.

As with all sedatives, analgesics and anesthetics, caution is advised when using medetomidine as a pre-anesthetic agent in patients with hepatic and renal disease and in pregnant patients. Studies using medetomidine in animals with diabetes have not been reported but in healthy subjects, insulin levels are reduced and transient hyperglycemia results. This response is also observed with other alpha$_2$-agonists.

Romifidine

Romifidine is also a potent alpha$_2$ adrenergic sedative–analgesic. It is being used in dogs and cats as premedication prior to both inhalant and injectable anesthetics. While dosages of 5-120µ/kg IV have been given in dogs and 100-400µ/kg IM in cats; lower dosages are the more common practice (5-40µ/kg IV or IM in dogs and 100µ/kg IM in cats). It has been shown that effects of 200µ/kg medetomidine is equivalent to 1mg/kg xylazine. Romifidine has about 50% of the potency of medetomidine. Onset of sedation and duration are similar at equivalent dosage. Dosages mediating significant sedation and analgesia are associated with an increase in vascular resistance, increased blood pressure and slowing of heart rate as with other alpha$_2$ medications (Selmi et al. 2004; Sinclair et al. 2003; Muir and Gadawski 2002). Lowering the dosages of romifidine reduce cardiovascular effects (Pypendop and Verstegen 2001). Even though administration of either atropine or glycopyrolate will prevent bradycardia, neither significantly improve other cardiovascular indices (Sinclair et al. 2003).

Romifidine, like other alpha$_2$ agonists reduce anesthetic requirements in both dogs and cats in a dose related rate of 60% or more. It can be used safely and effectively if this is understood (Redondo et al. 1999; England and Hammond 1997; England et al. 1996). Combining romifidine with opioids (i.e. romifidine 120µ/kg IV and butorphanol 0.1mg/kg IV) significantly speeds onset and prolongs duration (England and Watts 1997). Similar side effects including emesis have been observed (Cruz et al. 2000). Changes in ventilation, body temperature and other physiologic functions are characteristic of alpha$_2$ agonists.

Dexmedetomidine

Dexmedetomidine is a highly selective and potent alpha$_2$ adrenergic agonist. The sedative, analgesic and physiologic effects of racemic medetomidine are more widely known. The dosage of dexmedetomidine in µ/kg is basically 50% of the dosage of medetomidine. Clinical effects and pharmacokinetics of dexmedetomidine in dogs at 10 and 20µ/kg IV compared to medetomidine 40mg/kg IV were similar levels of sedation and cardiorespiratory effects. The pharmacokinetics was similar with a half life of 0.94h for medetomidine 40mg/kg and 0.84 and 0.79h for 20 and 100µ/kg dexmedetomidine respectively (Kuusela et al. 2000). Peak sedation was during the first hour following administration but dogs receiving lower doses of dexmedetomidine will recover in shorter total time. Blood pressure increases and slowing of heart rate can be expected following administration of dexmedetomidine.

Dexmedetomidine has a significant dose sparing effect on anesthetic requirements especially if routine doses are used. Anesthetic levels will be profound if concentrations of the combinations are not adjusted. Treatment of dogs with 2-4µ/kg IV as a pre-anesthetic reduces anesthetic requirements and the cardiovascular system has greater stability than when high doses of the alphas agonists are used (Kuusela et al. 2000b). The use of 10μ/kg IM dexmedetomidine has been effective in both propofo infusion and propofol/isoflurane anesthesia (Kuusela et al. 2005). Even though approved dosages of medetomidine and dexmedetomidine have been safely used in many cases, the use of lower doses in combination with other medication has become common practice.

Receptor Antagonists
Opioids
Naloxone HCl
Naloxone, the N allyl derivative of oxymorphone, has no opioid receptor agonist properties and does not produce analgesia or respiratory depression. It is 13 times more potent than nalorphine and its antagonist half life is 12 to 40 minutes. In comparison, the effects of oxymorphone may last 45 to 90 minutes. Administration to reverse the effects of oxymorphone is 0.1mg of naloxone per 1mg of the opioid or 0.04mg/kg (Table 1-9). Depending on the amount of opioid used and duration of effect prior to reversal, an additional dose of naloxone may be needed to antagonize induced respiratory and CNS depression.

Naltrexone
Along with the introduction of mu opioid receptor agonists with characteristics of very high potency ratios, there is a need for opioid antagonists that have a long duration of action. Carfentanyl is 10,031 times more potent than morphine and is primarily used for capture of wild animals (Short 1987b). Naltrexone is a long acting opioid receptor antagonist that is used to reverse effects of long acting opioids such as carfentanyl in capture situations. Opioids currently used for small animals do not have long durations of action and under most circumstances; effects are adequately reversed with naloxone when needed. Therefore, naltrexone does not have much application in small animal anesthesia.

Table 1-9 | Alpha$_2$ Antagonists and Dosages*

Medication	Dosage	Route
Alpha$_2$ Antagonists		
Atipamezole	5 x dose of medetomidine in μ/kg	IM
Yohimbine	10% of xylazine dosage in mg/kg	IV
Opioid Antagonist		
Naloxone	0.04mg/kg	SC, IM, or IV

* It should be understood that reversal of either an opioid or alpha$_2$ agonist not only reverses side effects and sedation associated with the individual medication but also the analgesic benefits. As duration of action of the agonist is extended, less antagonist is expected to be required for reversal.
Source: Compendium of Veterinary Products 5th Edition 1999. Publisher: Adrian J. Bagley

Alpha₂ Adrenergic Receptor Antagonists

Atipamezole

Atipamezole is an effective antagonist of sedation, analgesia, and other physiologic changes in animals receiving medetomidine (Savola 1989, Vainio 1990). It produces dose-dependent increases in the turnover of norepinephrine. Atipamezole is a selective and specific alpha₂ adrenoceptor antagonist (Vainio 1990). In receptor-binding studies, an $\alpha2: \alpha1$ selectivity ratio of 8,526 was obtained for atipamezole, while yohimbine showed a ratio of 40. Atipamezole had about 100 times more affinity for alpha₂ adrenoceptors than did yohimbine. In binding studies and studies with isolated organs, atipamezole had no effect on β_1 and β_2, histamine (H_1 and H_2), serotonin (5-HT_1 and 5-HT), muscarine, dopamine (DA_2), tryptamine, Gabba-aminobutyric acid (GABA), opiate, or benzodiazepine receptors.

The dosage recommended is a 5:1 ratio of atipamezole to medetomidine (Table 1-9) Note that the concentration of the available preparation is 5mg/ml for atipamezole and 1mg/ml for medetomidine. Atipamezole competes with medetomidine at the alpha₂ receptors and is effective in reversing all responses to the alpha₂ receptors including sedation and analgesia. As indicated, it does not reverse the influence of concurrent medications. Dosage requirements for atipamezole can be reduced by 20 to 80% when more than 1 hour has lapsed from medetomidine administration. Dose of yohimbine is 10% of xylazine dosage in mg/kg (Table 1-9).

Neuroleptanalgesia and Neuroleptanesthesia

The state of central nervous system depression and analgesia produced by a neuroleptic tranquilizer and opioid is referred to as *neuroleptanalgesia*. By convention and definition, this term is used when a neuroleptic tranquilizer such as droperidol and an opioid such as fentanyl, are used in combination (Soma 1964). A more modern use of the term would be when any analgesic is combined with a neuroleptic as long as the same effect is achieved. When nitrous oxide, an inhalation or injectable anesthetic is used alone or in combination as part of the neuroleptanalgesic protocol, the state is referred to as *neuroleptanesthesia*. When this concept was first introduced in the 1960's, addition of nitrous oxide to achieve neuroleptanesthesia was considered preferable to barbiturate anesthesia in dogs at risk because of cardiovascular stability and more controllable duration of action (Krahwinkel et al. 1975). Anesthesia protocols have evolved to include inhalants: halothane, isoflurane, or sevoflurane. The neuroleptic/opioid combination along with an inhalation anesthetic offers many advantages, the major effect being more stable cardiovascular dynamics and better control of anesthetic depth (Cornick & Hartsfield 1992). The decreased requirements for potent inhalation agents and provisions for postoperative analgesia are also advantageous.

There are many possible drug combinations, which in a compounded form induce neuroleptanalgesia. Fentanyl, a potent opioid, and droperidol, a butyrophenone tranquilizer, were available to veterinarians in the U.S. in a fixed combination called Innovar-Vet™ but was removed from production in 1998.

One of the major reasons fixed combination of the tranquilizer and opioid lost its popularity was that other neuroleptic tranquilizers could be combined separately with an opioid of choice and used for the same purpose. The ratio of the two drugs could be varied under different clinical situations. This allowed the anesthetist to increase the proportion of the tranquilizer in some situations, e.g., comparatively younger dogs, or to decrease the dose in geriatrics and patients at risk. One might also choose to use pentobarbital or a minor tranquilizer such as diazepam or midazolam along with the opioid to achieve the desired effect. The opioid might then be used throughout the procedure along with low concentrations of a volatile liquid anesthetic, a technique commonly used for high risk patients.

The tranquilizer and opioid may be given independently with the advantage of being able to administer the tranquilizer as pre-anesthetic medication 15 to 30 minutes before induction with the opioid either used alone IV or combined with either a major or minor tranquilizer. When an opioid is given either by infusion or intermittently during the procedure along with an inhalant such as isoflurane or sevoflurane, a very stable anesthetic state, neuroleptanesthesia, is achieved. A local anesthetic may also be used at the incision site to allow lower concentrations of the more depressant anesthetic to be used. Recovery is usually rapid and the effects of the opioid can be either partially or completely reversed with an opioid antagonist.

More widely used combinations of the neuroleptic acepromazine and different opioids are morphine/acepromazine, hydromorphone/acepromazine and butorphanol/acepromazine (Dyson et al. 1992) (Table 1-10). In Europe, the fixed combination of fentanyl/fluanisone is available under the brand name of Hypnorm (Janssen Pharmaceuticals).

Table 1-10

Composition and Dosages of Various Neuroleptanalgesic Combinations Used in Dogs

Drug Combination Neuroleptic and Opioid	Dosage (mg/kg) IM or SC	Dosage (mg/kg) IV
Acetylpromazine and	0.02-0.1	0.005-0.05
Oxymorphone	0.05-0.2	0.05-0.2
Acetylpromazine and	0.02-0.1	0.005-0.05
Meperidine	2.0-5.0	1.0-3.0
Acetlypromazine and	0.02-0.1	0.005-0.05
Butorphanol	0.1-0.2	0.1-0.2
Acetylpromazine and	0.02-0.1	0.005-0.05
Morphine	0.25-0.5	0.1-0.3
Acetylpromazine and	0.02-0.1	0.005-0.05
Hydromorphone	0.05-0.2	0.02-0.1

Pentobarbital as Premedication

Historically, pentobarbital has been used as a general anesthetic at doses approximating 28-30mg/kg IV. However, it may be used in lower doses as a premedicant to induce sedation without the side effects of a phenothiazine tranquilizer. It may be given orally, IM or IV, and greatly reduces the requirements for other anesthetic drugs. There is wide variability in individual responses to pentobarbital, which makes it an unreliable sedative. As a general rule, it may be used as a sedative in geriatric patients and has been recommended as a premedicant at a dose of 5mg/kg to prevent seizures associated with cervical myelograms (Gray et al. 1987). With the advent of more modern drugs, its use as a premedicant has decreased or been eliminated entirely. If used for IM or SC injection, it is recommended to use a pentobarbital product with a concentration of 50mg/ml rather than the veterinary preparation of 64.8mg/ml. The veterinary preparation is irritating to tissues and depending on the volume injected by routes other than IV, it can cause minor to significant tissue reactions.

Nonsteroidal Anti-inflammatory Drugs (NSAIDs)

Often regarded as the less potent option for analgesia, NSAIDs have been used in veterinary therapeutics for many years. However, it is relatively recently that they have been used in conjunction with anesthesia and surgery. Their lack of CNS depressant effects and entirely different mode of action to that of opioids has given them a unique role in perioperative analgesia, both alone and in combination with traditional opioid agonists. Advances in knowledge of the body's enzyme systems affected by the NSAIDs have led to development of safer and more potent NSAIDs for the treatment of pain and inflammation. Depending upon the circumstances and conditions of pain management, NSAIDs may sometimes be a better alternative than opioids alone.

NSAIDs are used in the treatment of fever, inflammation and pain. This originates from centuries of use of extracts of willow bark (*Salix Alba*) to treat fever. Active ingredients, salicylates, were isolated in the 19th century, thus began the quest for new and better therapeutic NSAIDs. A wide range of NSAID compounds has been developed being derived from a number of different molecules. All NSAIDs have the potential for toxic effects as well as therapeutic effects and new developments are always aiming to improve safety and efficacy.

Cyclo-oxygenase Inhibition

NSAIDs' mode of action is to block the enzyme cyclo-oxygenase (COX) activity (Vane, 1971). COX catalyses conversion of arachidonic acid, released from normal cell membrane turnover, to the eicosanoids (Figure 1-8). The eicosanoids include the prostanoids, prostacyclin (PGI_2) and prostaglandin E2 (PGE_2) as well as thromboxanes. Another enzyme, 5-lipoxygenase, catalyses production of further ecoisanoids, the leukotrienes, from arachidonic acid. Leukotrienes are also involved in some inflammatory processes and a few NSAIDs block lipoxygenase as well as COX.

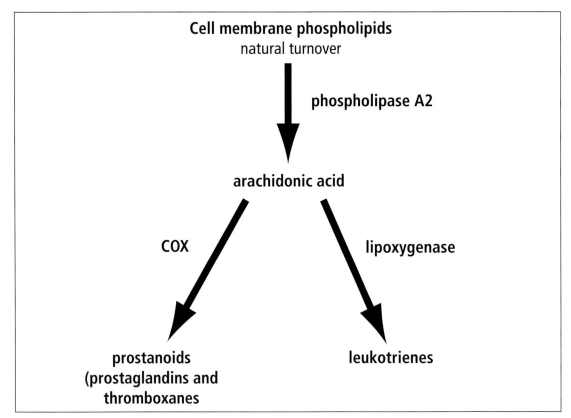

Figure 1-8 Eicosanoid production from arachidonic acid.

Effect on Homeostasis

Prostaglandins and thromboxanes perform a wide range of homeostatic and protective mechanisms in the body (Wilson 1991). Preservation of normal gastric mucosa, renal blood flow and platelet function are particularly significant. Toxic effects of NSAIDs usually result from disruption of one or more of these homeostatic functions. In the stomach, prostanoids thicken the mucous layer and increase bicarbonate secretion, both essential in preventing acid erosion of the mucosal lining. Maintenance of adequate gastric microcirculation is also sustained through PGI_2 mediated vasodilation. Renal blood flow autoregulation ensures normal perfusion in spite of wide variations in systemic blood pressure. Autoregulation is controlled by a number of processes and prostanoids make an important contribution. Dogs appear to be particularly susceptible to pre-renal failure if COX inhibitors upset autoregulation during a period of systemic hypotension, a situation which may develop during anesthesia and surgery. Platelet function depends on a balance between the effects of thromboxane (TX) A_2 and PGI_2. TXA_2 produced by COX in platelets controls platelet aggregation, hence COX inhibition may cause defective clotting. PGI_2 in vascular epithelium down-regulates platelet activity and tends to counteract the TXA_2 effect. PGI_2 is also a potent vasodilator and TX a less potent vasoconstrictor. Since clotting may be affected by small blood vessel dynamics, these characteristics also affect clotting. Thus, the overall effect of NSAIDs on platelet activity is complex but depends on access by the NSAID to COX at each location. Prolonged bleeding time is a potential hazard of NSAIDs but is not normally a clinical problem sufficient to prevent short term perioperative use.

Effect on Inflammation

COX products induce many cardinal signs of inflammation. This process produces large quantities of eicosanoids, particularly PGE_2, that lead to vasodilatation and erythema. Vasodilatation increases local blood flow and augments fluid extravasation caused by bradykinin-induced increases in vascular permeability, producing localized edema. PGE_2 acts synergistically with other inflammatory products causing inflammatory pain. Although it does not itself cause pain, PGE_2 reduces the threshold to stimulation of nerve endings. PGE_2 production is stimulated by interleukin-1 released in bacterial and viral infections and causes pyrexia, thus contributing to fever during systemic infection.

Analgesia

NSAIDs exert their analgesic effects through local inhibition of prostaglandin production and may also produce analgesic effects through other routes. Interference with G-protein mediated signal transduction may form the basis of an analgesic mechanism. Some NSAIDs also disrupt the lipoxygenase pathway, which may contribute to analgesia. In addition, NSAIDs induce a central analgesic action that may result from inhibition of COX activity in the brain. NSAIDs may have other central analgesic effects unrelated to COX inhibition via endogenous opioid peptides, blockade of serotonin release and inhibition of N-methyl-D-aspartate (NMDA) receptor activation.

COX-1 and COX-2

NSAIDs are mainly used in treating inflammation and pain via COX inhibition. However, COX inhibition affects production of homeostatic prostanoids as well as those causing inflammation and pain. This has not prevented the widespread clinical use of NSAIDs, largely because huge quantities of mediators, particularly PGE_2, are produced during the inflammatory process. Therefore, even partial reduction has a therapeutic benefit. Nevertheless, toxic effects of NSAIDs are a cause for concern, particularly when they are used in sick animals or in conjunction with anesthesia and surgery.

Discovery of two isoforms of the COX enzyme has helped develop safer NSAIDs with less effect on homeostatic function. COX-1 is the normal constitutive enzyme produced continuously in small quantities and is responsible for homeostatic prostaglandins and thromboxanes. COX-2, the inducible form, is structurally distinct and produced in large quantities in response to stimuli such as infection. It is largely the products of COX-2 that are responsible for the inflammatory process although COX-1 and COX-2 catalyze the same reactions and produce the same mediators. What differentiates COX-1 and COX-2 is how enzyme production is controlled and the amount of enzyme produced. COX-1 is always available for homeostasis; COX-2 is induced by inflammatory stimuli. COX-1 is available in small quantities whereas COX-2 is present in large amounts. Recently it has been realized that COX-2 also has some constitutive properties in certain tissues such as brain, kidney, and gut.

In view of the differences between COX-1 and COX-2, NSAIDs that block only COX-2 have the potential to treat inflammation and pain without affecting homeostatic prostanoids. A number of COX-2 selective NSAIDs have been developed for clinical use and are proving to have some advantages over older non-selective or COX-1 selective NSAIDs. The relative COX-1 and COX-2 inhibitory action is expressed as a ratio of COX-2/COX-1 activity. This is measured by a number of different techniques that do not always agree. However, most methods used to assess COX-2/COX-1 ratios indicate that aspirin, piroxicam and indomethacin have high ratios (selective COX-1 inhibition). Carprofen is intermediate while nimesulide, meloxicam and eltenac are some of the lowest (high COX-2 selectivity).

Inevitably, COX-2 selectivity is not the perfect answer to NSAID toxicity. In some systems, COX-2 has a regulatory role in normal function and in some cases, most probably in chronic inflammation. COX-1 also plays a role in the inflammatory process. There may be substantial species differences so that a process that may depend largely on COX-1 in humans may depend on COX-2 in dogs.

NSAIDs for Perioperative Analgesia

Numerous NSAIDs are available but a relatively small number of products have been used to provide perioperative analgesia in small animals. The injectable form is most convenient, although not essential, for pre-operative administration to provide preemptive analgesia for elective surgery. Where NSAID therapy is required pre or post operatively to provide immediate analgesia for acute pain, an injectable form is necessary. It is essential that NSAIDs used in association with anesthesia are the least toxic and do not have a history of adverse reactions with anesthetic drugs and adjunct sedatives. Most of the drugs recommended have been subjected to clinical trials and considerable clinical use. In addition, some of these drugs are mentioned for their potential perioperative application in the future.

Carprofen

Carprofen is a unique modern NSAID that has limited COX inhibitory action but retains potent analgesic and anti-inflammatory properties (Strub et al. 1982). The exact mode of action of carprofen is not well understood. There is evidence from ex vivo studies in dogs that it is COX-2 selective (Ricketts et al. 1998). Alternatively, carprofen may have a significant effect on CNS COX activity or perhaps on another iso-enzyme.

In the United Kingdom, carprofen (Rimadyl, Pfizer) has transformed post operative analgesia in dogs and cats (Balmer et al. 1998; Lascelles et al. 1994; Lascelles et al.1995; Nolan and Reid, 1993). Carprofen is a weak COX inhibitor in these species (McKellar et al.1994; Taylor et al.1996), limiting potential adverse effects on kidney function. Renal autoregulation is maintained in the presence of carprofen if hypotension occurs. Carprofen was the first NSAID licensed for preoperative use in the UK. Given preoperatively, it has been widely used with remarkably few problems. The benefits of preoperative analgesia will be discussed further. The value and safety of carprofen given preoperatively have been demonstrated in numerous studies (Welsh et al. 1997; Ko et al. 1999).

In the USA, carprofen was originally available only in oral form for treatment of osteoarthritis in dogs. However, it has recently been licensed as injection for pre-operative use in dogs and will hopefully be as successful in this role as it has been in Europe. Prior to availability of the injectable form in the US, hepatocellular toxicosis was reported in 21 dogs treated with the drug (MacPhail et al. 1998). All of these animals received oral carprofen for a number of days to treat musculoskeletal pain. Similar problems have not been reported in Europe. Whether this is due to a different dosage regimen or to genetic and environmental factors is unknown. There is absolutely no evidence that a single parenteral preoperative administration at the recommended dose of 4mg/kg causes any such problems. As with any NSAID, it is important not to overdose, to ensure normal hydration and not to give the drug longer than necessary. A maximum of 5 days postoperatively is recommended under normal circumstances.

Meloxicam

Meloxicam (Metacam; Merial) has been used for post-operative or chronic use in dogs since 1997. It is a relatively selective COX-2 inhibitor and is expected to be safer than COX-1 inhibitors. A number of investigations into potential renal toxicity, particularly in association with anesthesia during both hypo-and normotensive conditions, have demonstrated its relative safety compared with COX-1 inhibitors (Bostrom & Nyman1998; Poulsen 1999). Analgesia also appears to be good (Cross et al. 1997), suggesting that meloxicam may prove to be one of the most effective and safe NSAIDs for perioperative use. Meloxicam is available as injection and as a honey flavoured syrup and is now licensed for preoperative use in dogs and cats in the UK and for osteoarthritis in dogs in the USA. The syrup is well tolerated in this species and has been widely and successfully used even for long term treatment (Robertson and Taylor 2004).

Ketoprofen

Ketoprofen is a potent COX and lipo-oxygenase inhibitor that provides good postoperative analgesia and in some circumstances, may even be superior to opioids (Pibarot et al. 1997; Grisneaux et al. 1999). Analgesia may also be superior to that of carprofen. However, as a potent COX inhibitor, caution must be taken with preoperative use. In a study by Grisneaux et al. (1999), preoperative administration did not cause clinical evidence of renal disruption but clotting time was prolonged more after ketoprofen than after carprofen or opioids. However, because this study measured the combined effect of ketoprofen with a cephalosporin antibiotic, it was not clear that the small changes in buccal mucosal bleeding time (BMBT) were due only to ketoprofen. Administration of cephalosporin antibiotics before surgery inhibits whole blood platelet aggregation (WBPA) and prolongs BMBT in dogs (Schermerhorn et al. 1994). In contrast, Lemke et al (2002) found that preoperative administration of ketoprofen inhibited WBPA but did not alter bleeding time. These results suggest that ketoprofen can be given before surgery to healthy dogs undergoing elective OHE provided that dogs are screened for potential bleeding problems presurgery and monitored for BMBT postsurgery. Further studies are needed to document whether ketoprofen can be safely used for preemptive analgesia.

Keterolac

Keterolac has been widely used off-label in dogs and appears to provide excellent post operative analgesia for at least 24 hours (Mathews, 1996a; Mathews et al. 1996b; Popiliskis et al.1997). As with other NSAIDs, post-operative analgesia may be as good as and perhaps better than that produced by butorphanol. As a potent COX inhibitor, it can cause renal damage and particularly gastric ulceration, especially in hypotensive and hypovolemic patients. Keterolac is most safely given postoperatively. Where another condition predisposing towards gastric ulceration is relevant, e.g., recent corticosteroid treatment or trauma, sucralfate should be given (dogs 0.5-1.0gm, cats 0.25gm) orally before feeding.

Deracoxib

Deracoxib (Deramaxx, Novartis) is the first coxib-class NSAID in veterinary medicine. It is licensed in America for control of postoperative pain and inflammation associated with orthopedic surgery (up to 3-4mg/kg as needed for a maximum of 7 days) and for the control of pain and inflammation associated with osteoarthritis (1-2mg/kg) in dogs. Deramaxx is available as a chewable tablet which has been shown to be effective under both fed and fasted conditions. For postoperative orthopedic pain, Deramaxx is administered orally prior to surgery. Although the plasma terminal elimination half-life for Deramaxx tablets is approximately 3 hours, a longer duration of clinical effectiveness is observed and the drug is labeled for once per day administration in the dog. In one chemical synovitis model (Millis et al. 2002) deracoxib was shown to be more effective than carprofen. Precautions in the use of deracoxib are similar to other NSAID-class drugs and four years of field use have shown a safe and efficacious profile. By accordance to the label, this drug is approved for perioperative use. Administration of Deramaxx in the cat is not recommended.

Firocoxib
Under the name of Previcox (Merial), this drug also belongs to the coxib class. It is currently available in chewable tablet form for pain relief and inflammation associated with osteoarthritis in dogs. It is unique as there is no significant COX-1 inhibition at therapeutic dosage. Information on clinical use in perioperative analgesia was not available and as with all drugs in this group, GI, renal or hepatic side effects may occur.

Etodolac
Etodolac (Etogesic, Fort Dodge) is available in the USA as an oral preparation and is licensed only for treatment of osteoarthritis. Hence there is again little experience or recommendation for general perioperative use.

Tepoxalin
Tepoxalin (Zubrin, Schering Plough) is a new NSAID now available for use in dogs in Europe and the USA. It is unique in being a dual action NSAID, acting on both COX and lipoxygenase (LOX). Hence it may have superior analgesic and anti-inflammatory properties. Tepoxalin appears to be effective and as well tolerated as any NSAID. However, it is currently available only in an oral preparation and is licensed only for treament of osteoarthritis and there is little experience or recommendation for general perioperative use.

Flunixin
Flunixin has been found to provide postoperative analgesia in dogs and cats, often being superior to opioids (Mathews et al. 1996a; Reid and Nolan, 1991; Fonda, 1996). There were no adverse effects of any significance in these investigations. However, flunixin is a potent COX-1 inhibitor and is most safely given postoperatively. Other NSAIDs are probably safer than flunixin for perioperative use.

If given preoperatively, considerable caution and effort to maintain good cardiovascular function is essential. Flunixin has a reputation for adverse effects in dogs given the drug preoperatively. This is based on two reports (Elwood et al. 1992; McNeil, 1992) where renal failure developed after a single dose of flunixin was given before major surgery. In both cases, anesthesia was prolonged, blood pressure was not monitored and little support provided with fluid therapy. It is likely that any COX-1 inhibitor would lead to renal failure in such cases but flunixin may be the most toxic in dogs. Even in studies conducted under closely controlled conditions during anesthesia, some biochemical evidence of renal disruption by flunixin was observed although clinical signs of disease were not apparent (Mathews et al.1996b). This was not the case with other NSAIDs that have been subjected to similar investigation.

Fewer studies have been conducted in cats compared to dogs. In spite of a reputation for adverse effects of NSAIDs in cats, tolerance and excretion of flunixin was reported to be better than in dogs (Taylor et al. 1994) and clinical studies (Fonda 1996) have demonstrated good analgesia with no adverse effects.

Phenylbutazone

Phenylbutazone has been used successfully for many years in the dog but reports of perioperative use are limited. Although phenylbutazone is widely used in large animals, its potent COX inhibitory action has the potential to cause toxicity in dogs. Other NSAIDs offer better choices for perioperative use in this species. There is remarkably little information available on phenylbutazone in cats, although a number of clinicians use it routinely in this species.

Aspirin

Aspirin has been used for many years and is now widely accepted as being a selective COX-1 NSAID. It is unique in that its binding with COX is irreversible and it retains its effect until a new enzyme is made. Aspirin is most commonly used for its anti-thrombotic activity and is rarely used for perioperative analgesia. Since aspirin is a potent COX-1 inhibitor, if anesthesia and surgery are required for an animal receiving aspirin therapy, every attempt must be made to maintain good hydration and to ensure that arterial hypotension does not occur in order to prevent pre-renal failure.

Role of NSAIDs in Veterinary Anesthesia

NSAIDs are now widely used peri-operatively although it is difficult to quantify their effects during anesthesia. Carprofen failed to reduce anesthetic requirements (MAC) during anesthesia (Alibhai and Clarke, 1996) but it has been shown in dogs to provide a convincing preemptive analgesic effect (Welsh et al.1997). Hence, pre-operative administration of the safer NSAIDs, carprofen and meloxicam, is a logical and effective means to provide perioperative analgesia.

NSAIDs provide excellent pre- and post-operative analgesia. In many instances, they can be as effective as opioids in addition to offering an anti-inflammatory component. They do not contribute to the overall CNS depression induced by sedatives and anesthetics. Toxic effects of NSAIDs, particularly those involving the kidney and gastric mucosa, must be taken into consideration. However, since NSAIDs, opioids and other sedative/analgesic drugs act by entirely different mechanisms, they can safely be used together to provide "balanced analgesia", where a combination of different agents acting by synergistic mechanisms provides the best overall analgesia for the patient (Taylor et al. 1999). In many cases, intense but short duration analgesia from opioids combines well with the longer acting and slower onset of NSAIDs, particularly in the first few hours following surgery.

A well-tested approach to balanced preemptive analgesia is to use a combination of an opioid and a COX-sparing NSAID as premedication. Infusion or incremental doses of a non-cumulative opioid is given during anesthesia with a longer acting opioid given post-operatively if further analgesia is required in the first 12-24 hours. Additional pain management can safely be given with local blocks as well as spinal or epidural analgesia. Dose and frequency of administration are described in Table 1-11.

Table 1-11

NSAID Dosing for Perioperative Use

Drug	Preoperative Use	Post operative Use	Comments
Carprofen (Rimadyl; Pfizer)	4mg/kg SC or IV	Dog: 2mg/kg once or twice daily Cat: no data sheet rec (2mg/kg daily for 2 days probably safe)	Monitor if > 7 days Monitor any post op use
Meloxicam (Metacam; Merial)	Dogs: 0.2mg/kg Cats: 0.3mg/kg	Dogs and cats: 0.1mg/kg daily; monitor for long term use. Cats max 3 days.	Off label long term use is usually well tolerated, but monitor Cats successfully treated off label with as little as 1 drop daily of oral liquid.
Ketoprofen (Ketofen; Merial)	2mg/kg SC, (dogs also IV)	1mg/kg daily injection or orally Max 5 days	Pre-op is off label–watch hydration and BP
Ketorolac (Toradol; Roche)	No recommendation	Dogs: 0.3-0.5mg/kg IV or IM Cats: 0.25mg/kg IM	All off label
Deracoxib (Deramaxx; Novartis)	1-2mg/kg oral	3-4mg/kg/day up to seven days Dogs only, post orthopedic surgery	Not recommended for cats
Etodolac (EtoGesic; Fort Dodge)	No recommendation	10-15mg/kg/day Little experience of post operative use	Not recommended for cats
Tepoxalin (Zubrin; Schering Plough)	No recommendation	10mg/kg per day Not more than 4 consecutive weeks Little experience of post operative use	Not recommended for cats
Flunixin	Not recommended	Dogs: 1-2mg/kg daily for max 3 days Cats: 1mg/kg once	Off label

- See text for Europe/USA differences
- All NSAIDs: watch for apathy, vomiting, any sign of renal or gastro-intestinal disease
- All NSAIDs have similar mode of action–do not use more than one NSAID concurrently
- Do not use NSAIDs with steroids or within at least 24 hr of steroid administration
- Use opioid in premedication and for immediate post operative pain, NSAID will give longer action (12-24 hours)

Pain Management from a Surgeon's Perspective

Many physicians believe that postoperative pain and other chronically painful conditions have been poorly treated in human patients even though very effective agents have been available for many years. Physicians have even been prosecuted because of perceived overuse of opioids in painful patients with doses that are now agreed to have been appropriate. It is clear that doses of analgesics used in the past were inadequate to control severe pain following surgery and for chronic pain of cancer and other conditions. The advent of pain clinics with the sole function to diagnose and treat pain by specialists is testament to this new realization of how poorly pain has been handled in human patients.

This emphasis on pain control has come even later to veterinary medicine. There was a time, in the not too distance past, when noted veterinary surgeons would state that pain is good because it keeps the patient quiet and, therefore, will be less likely to injure surgical repair, ensuring better recovery. It is now evident that this argument has no merit and every surgery produces pain that needs to be addressed in an appropriate fashion.

When tissue is traumatized either by accident or by surgical incision, mechanisms addressed earlier in this chapter are put into motion. If these are not dealt with very early, potential for serious problems are the consequence (see Figure 1-1). Catecholamines released by the conscious sensation of pain upon recovery can contribute to cardiac arrhythmias, vasoconstriction with potentially reduced blood flow to the surgical site, tachycardia, and patient anxiety (D'Agrosa 1977). Poor blood flow can retard healing and pain response can result in excessive licking or other attention to the surgical site by the patient. Animals may be more difficult to handle and even be aggressive to care givers. A patient in pain will likely have a poor appetite and not perform other normal body functions until much later in the course of their recovery, perhaps necessitating use of extensive measures to insure proper fluid and nutrient intake. Protein depletion due to pain-induced anorexia may require the use of plasma infusions which might have been avoided with early high quality food intake following surgery. Pain can restrict depth and frequency of respiration and analgesics will often help breathing when given in proper dosages. Moderating the pain that is causing the animal to not breathe properly will provide great divends.

It is important to be able to recognize pain when it occurs. The body language of the patient speaks volumes. An animal that refuses to lie down following median sternotomy is responding to inadequately controlled pain. Other examples can be given for surgery in various sites on the body, but the basic operating premise must be that: "pain follows surgery and must always be dealt with." Prevention of pain with proper treatment before it is needed (preemptive analgesia) is clearly the best approach. If attempts to control pain are instituted after the animal feels the pain, it is much less effective and higher doses are required. Continued pain management for the days following surgery provides for more rapid return to normal function and a patient that is easier to manage.

It is imperative that veterinarians understand how really detrimental postoperative pain can be to the outcome of their efforts. It is easy to dismiss the fact that animals feel pain because they cannot tell us what they are going through. While it is true in animals as it is in humans that some individuals respond differently to a painful stimulus; the basic assumption must be that it is very important to deal effectively with pain that is known to exist in animals related to trauma, surgery and many disease conditions.

References

Abrahamsson J, Niemand D, Olsson AK, et al. (1983). Buprenorphine (Temgesic) as a peroperative analgesic. A multicenter study. *Anaesthesist* 32:75-79.

Al-Gizawly MM, P-Rude E (2004). Comparison of preoperative carprofen and postoperative butorphanol as postsurgical analgesics in cats undergoing ovariohysterectomy. *Vet Anesth Analg* 31:164-174.

Alibhai HI, Clarke KW (1996). Influence of carprofen on minimum alveolar concentration of halothane in dogs. *J Vet Pharmacol Ther.* 19:320-321.

Baldwin, CH (2002). *Personal communication.* Lebanon Animal Hospital, Lebanon, CT.

Balmer TV, Irvine D, Jones RS, et al.(1998). Comparison of carprofen andethidine as postoperative analgesics in the cat. *J Small Anim Pract* 39:158-164.

Beleslin DB, Krsti'c SK, Topmi'c-Beleslin N (1984). Nicotine-induced salivation in cats: effects of various drugs. *Brain Res Bull* 12:585-587.

Bickel WK, Stitzer ML, Bigelow GE, et al. (1988). A clinical trial of buprenorphine: comparison with methadone in the detoxification of heroin addicts. *Clin Pharm Therap* 43:72-78.

Booth NH (1982). Psychotropic agents. In *Veterinary Pharmacology and Therapeutics.* Ed. By HN Booth and L McDonald. The Iowa State University Press, Ames, pp 321-345.

Bostrom I, Nyman G (1998). Preliminary study of pre-operative meloxicam in dogs - a pharmacological evaluation. *Proc.6th Int Cong Vet Anaes.* 113(Abstract)

Brodbelt DC, Taylor PM, Stanway GW (1997). A comparison of preoperative morphine and buprenorphine for postoperative analgesia for arthrotomy in dogs. *J Vet Pharm Therap* 20:284-289.

Briggs SL, Sneed K, Sawyer DC (1998). Antinociceptive effects of oxymorphone - butorphanol - acepromazine combination in cats. *Vet Surg* 27:466-72.

Bullingham RE, McQuay HJ, Dwyer D, et al. (1981). Sublingual buprenorphine used postoperatively: clinical observations and preliminary pharmacokinetic analysis. *Brit J Clin Pharm* 12:117-122.

Campbell VL, Drobatz KJ, Perkowski SZ (2002). Postoperative arterial blood gases in spay/castration dogs: a comparison of butorphanol versus hydromorphone. *Vet Anaesth Analg* 29: 102. Proceedings abstract of the ACVA 26th Annual meeting, New Orleans.

Capner CA, Lascelles BDX, Waterman-Pearson AE (1999). Current British veterinary attitudes to perioperative analgesia for dogs. *Vet Rec* 145:95-99.

Capogna G, Celleno D, Tagariello V, et al. (1988). Intrathecal buprenorphine for postoperative analgesia in the elderly patient. *Anaesthesia* 43:128-130.

Carroll GL, Howe LB, Peterson KD (2005). Analgesic efficacy of preoperative administration of meloxicam or butorphanol in onychectomized cats. *JAVMA* 226: 913-919.

Caulkett N, Read M, Fowler D, et al. (2003). A comparison of the analgesic effects of butorphanol with those of meloxicam after elective ovariohysterectomy in dogs. *Can Vet J* 44:565-570.

Chan WH, Lin CJ, Sun WZ, et al. (1999). Comparison of subcutaneous hydromorphone with intramuscular meperidine for immediate postoperative analagesia. *Kaohsiung J Med Sci* 15:419-427.

Clarke KW, England GCW (1989a). Medetomidine sedation in the dog: clinical effects and reversal with atipamezole. *Proc WSAVA/BSAVA Congress* 30(3):2,4.

Clarke KW, England GCW (1989b): Medetomidine, a new sedative-analgesic for use in the dog and its reversal with atipamezole. *J Small Anim Pract* 30:343-348.

Coda B, Tanaka A, Jacobson RC, et al. (1997). Hydromorphone analgesia after intravenous bolus administration. *Pain* 71:41-48.

Conrad KA (1981). Effects of atropine on diastolic time. *Circulation* 63:371-377.

Copland VS, Haskins SC (1987). Oxymorphone: cardiovascular, pulmonary, and behavioral effects in dogs. *AJVR* 48:1626-1630.

Cornick JL, Hartsfield SM (1992). Cardiopulmonary and behavioral effects of combinations of acepromazine/butorphanol and acepromazine/oxymorphone in dogs. *JAVMA* 200:1952-1956.

Court MH, Greenblatt DJ (1992). Pharmacokinetics and preliminary observations of behavioural changes following administration of midazolam to dogs. *J Vet Pharm Therap.* 15:343-350.

Cross AR, Budsberg SC and Keefe TJ (1997). Kinetic gait analysis assessment of meloxicam efficacy in a sodium urate-induced synovitis model in dogs. *Am J Vet Res* 58:626-631.

Cruz ML, Luna SP, de Castro GB, et al (2000). A preliminary trial comparison of several anesthetic techniques in cats. *Can Vet J.* 2000 41(6):481-5.

D'Agrosa L S (1977). Cardiac Arrhythmias of Sympathetic Origin in the Dog. *Am J Physiol* 233:H535.

Davenport DJ, Breitschwerdt EB, Carakostas MC (1982). Platelet disorders in the dog and cat. Part I. Physiology and pathogenesis. *Comp Cont Educ* 4:762-776.

Davis LE, Donnelly EJ (1968). Analgesic drugs in the cat. *JAVMA* 153:1161-1167.

Davis LE, Kitchel RL (1983). Species differences in drug disposition as factors in alleviation of pain. In *Animal Pain Perception and Alleviation.* Amer Physiol Soc, Bethesda, MD, pp 161-178.

Dobromylskyj P, Flecknell PA, Lascelles BD, et al. (2000). Management of postoperative and other acute pain. In *Pain Management in Animals.* PA Flecknell and A Waterman-Pearson, Eds. WB Saunders pp. 81-145.

Dodman NH, Seeler DC, Court MH (1984). Aging changes in the geriatric dog and their impact on anesthesia. *Comp Cont Ed Pract Vet* 6:1106-1113.

Dohoo SE, Dohoo IR (1996a). Post-operative use of analgesics in dogs and cats by Canadian veterinarians. *Canad Vet J* 37:546-551.

Dohoo SE, Dohoo IR (1996b). Factors influencing the postoperative use of analgesics in dogs and cats by Canadian veterinarians. *Canad Vet J* 37:552-556.

Dubner R (1987). Research on pain mechanisms in animals. *JAVMA* 191:1273-1276.

Dyson DH, Atilola M (1992). A clinical comparison of oxymorphone-acepromazine and butorphanol-acepromazine sedation in dogs. *Vet Surg* 21:418-421.

Edge WG, Cooper GM, Morgan M (1979). Analgesic effects of sublingual buprenorphine. *Anaesthesia* 34:463-467.

Elwood C, Boswood A, Simpson K, et al. (1992). Renal Failure after flunixin meglumine administration. *Vet Rec* 130:582-583.

England GC, Andrews F, Hammond RA (1996). Romifidine as a premedicant to propofol induction and infusion anesthesia in the dog. *J Small Anim Pract* 37:79-83.

England GC, Hammond R (1997). Dose-sparing effects of romifidine premedication for thiopentone and halothane anesthesia in the dog. *J Small Anim Pract* 38:141-146.

England GC, Watts N (1997). Effect of romifidine and romifidine-butorphanol for sedation in dogs. *J Small Anim Pract* 38:561-564.

Ewing KK, et al (1993). Isoflurane MAC-reduction by medetomidine and its reversal by atipamezole in dogs. *Am J Vet Res* 54:294-299.

Flecknell PA, Waterman-Pearson A (2000). *Pain Management in Animals.* Flecknell PA and A Waterman-Pearson, Eds. WB Saunders pp. 1-184.

Fonda D (1996) Post operative analgesic actions of flunixin in the cat. *J Vet Anaesth* 23:52-55.

Fox S (1995). *Pain-Induced Distress and Its Alleviation Using butorphanol After Ovariohysterectomy of Bitches.* PhD Thesis. Massey University, Palmerston North, New Zealand. Volumes I & II.

Fox SM, Mellor DJ, Stafford KJ, Lowoko CRO (2000). The effects of ovariohysterectomy plus different combinations of halothane anaesthesia and butorphanol analgesia on behavior in the bitch. *Res in Vet Sci* 68:265-274.

Giusti P, Buriani A, Cima L, Lipartiti M (1997). Effect of acute and chronic tramadol on [^{3}H]-5-HT uptake in rat cortical synaptosomes. *Brit J Pharm* 122:302-306.

Gleed RD (1987). Tranquilizers and sedatives. In *Principles and Practice of Veterinary Anesthesia.* Williams & Wilkins, pp 16-27.

Gray PR, Indrieri RJ, Lippert AC (1987). Influence of anesthetic regimen on the frequency of seizures after cervical myelography in the dog. *JAVMA* 190:527-530.

Greene SA, Benson GJ, Hartsfield SM (1993). Thiamylal-sparing effect of midazolam for canine endotracheal intubation. A clinical study of 118 dogs. *Vet Surg* 22:69-72.

Greene SA, (2002). *Veterinary Anesthesia and Pain Management Secrets.* Elsevier

Grisneaux E, Pibarot P, Dupuis J, et al.(1999). Comparison of ketoprofen and carprofen administered prior to orthopedic surgery for control of postoperative pain in dogs. *Am J Vet Res* 215:1105-1110.

Gross ME, Tranquilli WJ, Thurmon JC, et al. (1992). Yohimbine/flumazenil antagonism of hemodynamic alterations induced by a combination of midazolam, xylazine, and butorphanol in dogs. *JAVMA* 201:1887-1890.

Guyton AC (1991). *Basic Neuroscience.* Philadelphia, WB Saunders Co.

Hall LW, Clark KW (1983). *Veterinary Anesthesia, 8th edition.* Bailliere Tindall, London. P 55.

Halder S, Bose PK (2001). Pre-emptive analgesic studies of xylazine and buprenorphine combination via epidural route in dog. *Indian J Ani Health* 40:28-30.

Halpern SH, Arellano R, Preston R, et al. (1996). Epidural morphine vs hydromorphone in post-Caesarean section patients. *Canad J Anaesth* 43:595-598.

Hamlin RL, Bednarski LS (1989). Studies to determine the optimal dose of medetomidine for the dog. *Acta Vet Scand* 85:89

Hansen B (1997). Through a glass darkly: using behavior to assess pain. *Semin Vet Med Surg* 12:61-74.

Heavner JE (1970). Morphine for postsurgical use in cats. *JAVMA* 156:1018-1019.

Hellyer PW, Mama KR, Shafford HL, et al. (2001). Effects of diazepam and flumazenil on minimum alveolar concentrations for dogs anesthetized with isoflurane or a combination of isoflurane and fentanyl. *Am J Vet Res* 62:555-560.

Hellyer PW (2002). Ethical considerations in the treatement of pain. *Vet Forum June:* 38-41.

Hill CS (1995). When will adequate pain treatment be the norm? *JAVMA* 274:1881-1882.

Hobbs WR, Rall TW, Verdoorn TA (1996). Hypnotics and Sedatives; Ethanol. In Goodman & Gilman's *The Pharmacological Basis of Therapeutics, Ninth Ed.* Eds. Hardman JG and Limbird LE. McGraw-Hill, New York, pp 361-396.

Holliday TA (1980). Therapeutics of convulsive states. In *Scientific Foundations of Veterinary Medicine.* Phillipson AT, Hall LW, Pritchard WR, eds. William Heinmann Medical Books, London, pp 201-213.

Houghton KJ, Rech RH, Sawyer DC, et al. (1991). Dose-response of intravenous butorphanol to increase visceral nociceptive threshold in dogs. *Proc Soc Exp Biol Med* 197:290-296.

Hsu WH, Lu ZX, Hembrough FB (1985). Effect of xylazine on heart rate and arterial blood pressure in conscious dogs, as influenced by atropine, 4-aminopyridine, doxapram and yohimbine. *JAVMA* 186:153-156.

Hubbel JAE, Muir WW II (1996). Evaluation of a survey of the diplomates of the American College of Laboratory Medicine on use of analgesic agents in animals used in biomedical research. *JAVMA* 209:918-921.

Ilkiw JE, Pascoe PJ, Tripp LD (2002). Effects of morphine, butorphanol, buprenorphine, and U50488H on the Minimum Alveolar concentration of isoflurane in cats. *Am J Vet Res* 63:1198-1202.

Ilkiw JE, Suter CM, Farver TB, et al. (1996a). The behavior of healthy awake cats following intravenous and intramuscular administration of midazolam. *J Vet Pharm Therap.* 19:205-216.

Ilkiw JE, Suter CM, McNeal D, et al. (1996b). The effect of intravenous administration of variable-dose midazolam after fixed-dose ketamine in healthy awake cats. *J Vet Pharm Therap.* 19:217-224.

Itamoto K, Kikasa Y, Sakoniyu I, et al. (2000). Anaesthetic and cardiopulmonary effects of balanced anaesthesia with medetomidine-midazolam and butorphanol in dogs. *J Vet Med* 47:411-420.

Jaffe JH, Martin WR (1990). Fentanyl, opiate analgesics and antagononists. In: Goodman A, Gilman L, ed. *The pharmacologic basis of therapeutics.* 8th ed. Elmsfordm NY: Pergamon Press Inc, pp 494-534.

Jalanka H (1989).The use of medetomidine, medetomidine-ketamine combinations and atipamezole at Helsinki Zoo - a review of 240 cases. *Acta Vet Scand* 85:193.

Jasinski DR, Pevnick JS, Griffith JD (1978). Human pharmacology and abuse potential of the analgesic buprenorphine: a potential agent for treating narcotic addiction. *Arch Gen Psychiatry* 35:501-516.

Jebeles JA, Reilly JS, Gutierrez JF, et al. (1991). The effect of pre-incisional infiltration of tonsils with bupivacaine on the pain following tonsillectomy under general anesthesia. *Pain* 47:305-308.

Joubert KE (2001). The use of analgesic drugs by South African veterinarians. *J South African Vet Assn* 72:57-60.

Kantilip JP, Alatienne M, Gueroguieu G, Duchene-Marullaz P (1985). Chronotropic and dromatropic effects of atropine and hyoscine methobromide in unanesthetized dogs. *Br J Anaesth* 57:214-219.

Katz J, Kavanagh BP, Sandler AN, et al. (1992). Preemptive analgesia. *Anesthesiology* 77:439-446.

Keegan RD, Greene SA, Moore MP, Gallagher LV (1993). Antagonism by flumazenil of midazolam-induced changes in quantitative electroencephalographic data from isoflurane-anesthetized dogs. *Am J Vet Res* 54:761-765.

Kitchell RL, Erickson HH, Carstens E, Davis LE (1983). *Animal Pain Perception and Alleviation,* Amer Phy Soc, Bethesda, pp 221.

Klein LJ, Trachtenberg AI (1998). *Acupuncture References: a bibliography of 2302 titles,* Jan 1979-Oct 1997. http://www.nlm.nih.gov/pubs/cbm/acupuncture.html

Klide AM, Calderwood HW, Soma LR (1975). Cardiopulmonary effects of xylazine in dogs. *Am J Vet Res* 36:931-935.

Ko JCH, Miyabashi, TK, Mandsager, RE, et al. (1999) Renal effects of carprofen in dogs following general anesthesia. *26th Annual Conference of the Veterinary Orthopaedic Society,* p 6.

Ko JCH, Mandsager RE, Lange DN, Fox SM (2000). Cardiorespiratory responses and plasma cortisol concentrations in dogs treated with medetomidine before undergoing ovariohysterectomy. *JAVMA* 217:509-514.

Krahwinkel DJ, Sawyer DC, Eyster GE, Bender G (1975). Cardiopulmonary effects of fentanyl-droperidol, nitrous oxide, and atropine sulfate in dogs. *Am J Vet Res* 36:1211-1219.

Kuusela E, Raekallio M, Anttila M, et al. (2000a). Clinical effects and pharmacokinetics of medetomidine and its enantiomers in dogs. *J Vet Pharmacol Therap* 23:15-20.

Kuusela E, Raekallio M, Vaisanen, M, et al (2000b). Comparison of medetomidine and dexmedetomidine as premedicants in dogs undergoing propofol/isofluance anesthesia. *AJVR.* 62:1073-1080.

Kuusela E, Vaino O, Short CE (2005). A comparison of propofol infusion and propofol/isoflurane anesthesia in dexmedetomidine premedicated dogs. *J Vet Pharmacol Theory* 26:199-204.

Kyles AE, Papich M, Hardie EM (1996). Disposition of transdermally administered fentanyl in dogs. *Am J Vet Res* 57:715-719.

Kyles AE (1998). Transdermal fentanyl. *Comp Cont Ed Prac Vet* 20:721-726.

Lai J, Ma S, Porreca F, Raffa RB (1996). Tramadol M1 metabolite and enantiomer affinities for cloned human opioid receptors expressed in transfected HN9.10 neuroblastoma cells. *Europ J Pharm* 316:369-372.

Laine E, et al (1986). Structural studies of medetomidine hydrochloride, a new drug substance. *Acta Pharm Fenn* 95(3):119-127.

Lammintausta R (1986). Introduction to adrenoceptor pharmacology. *Acta Vet Scand* 82:11-16.

Lamont LA, Tranquilli WJ, Grimm KA (2000). Physiology of pain. *Vet Clin North Am, Sm Ani Pract* 30:703-728.

Lascelles BDX, Butterworth, SJ, Waterman AE (1994) Postoperative analgesic and sedative effects of carprofen and pethidine in dogs. *Vet Rec* 134:187-191.

Lascelles BDX, Cripps P, Mirchandani S, et al.(1995) Carprofen as an analgesic for postoperative pain in cats: dose titration and assessment of efficacy in comparison to pethidine hydrochloride. *J Small Anim Pract* 36:535-541.

Lascelles BDX, Cripps PJ, Jones A, Waterman-Pearson AE (1998). Efficacy and kinetics of carprofen, administered preoperatively or postoperatively, for the prevention of pain in dogs undergoing ovariohysterectomy. *Vet Surg* 27:568-582.

Lascelles BD, Capner CA, Waterman-Pearson AE (1999). Current British veterinary attitudes to perioperative analgesia for cats and small mammals. *Vet Rec* 145:601-604.

Lascelles BD, Robertson SA (2004a). Use of thermal threshold response to evaluate the antinociceptive effects of butorphanol in cats. *Am J Vet Res* 65:1085-1099.

Lascelles BD, Robertson SA (2004b). Antinociceptive effects of hydromorphone, butorphanol, or the combination in cats. *J Vet Intern Med* 18:190-195.

Lascelles BD, Waterman AE, Cripps PJ et al (1995). Central sensitization as a result of surgical pain: investigation of the preemptive value of pethidine for ovariohysterectomy in the rat. *Pain* 62:201-212.

Lee DD, Papich MS, Hardie E (2000). Comparison of pharmacokinetics of fentanyl after intravenous and transdermal administration in cats. *AJVR* 61:672-677.

Lehmann KA, et al. (1990). Postoperative patient-controlled analgesia with Tramadol: Analgesic efficacy and minimum effective concentrations. *Clin J Pain* 6:212-220.

Leib MS, Wingfield WE, Twedt DC, Williams AR (1985). Gastric emptying of liquids in the dog: Serial test meal and modified emptying-time techniques. *Am J Vet Res* 46:1876-1880.

Lemke KA, Tranquilli WJ, Thurmon JC, et al. (1996). Ability of flumazenil, butorphanol, and naloxone to reverse the anesthetic effects of oxymorphone-diazepam in dogs. 209:776-779.

Lemke KA, Runyon CL, Horney BS (2002). Effects of preoperative administration of ketoprofen on whole blood platelet aggregation, buccal mucosal bleeding time, and hematologic indices in dogs undergoing elective ovariohysterectomy. *JAVMA* 220:1818-1822.

Livingston A, Chambers P (2000). The physiology of pain. In *Pain Management in Animals,* PA Flecknell and A Waterman-Pearson, Eds. WB Saunders pp. 9-19.

Lumb WV and Jones EW (1973). Preanesthetic agents. In *Veterinary Anesthesia.* 2nd ed. Philadelphia, Lea & Febiger, pp 183.

Mastrocinque S, Fantoni DT (2001). Modulation of neuroendocrine response to postoperative pain in dogs. Comparative study between tramadol and morphine. *Clinica Veterinaria, Brazil* 6:25-29.

Maunuksela EL, Korpela R, Olkkola KT (1988). Comparison of buprenorphine with morphine in the treatment of postoperative pain in children. *Anesth Analg* 67:233-239.

MacDonald E, et al. (1988). Behavioral and neurochemical effects of medetomidine, a novel veterinary sedative. *Eur J Pharmacol* 119:11-15.

Machado CEG, Dyson DH (2002). Cardiovascular and subjective evaluations of oxymorphone/diazepam and hydromorphone/diazepam induction in experimentally induced hypovolemic dogs. *Vet Anaesth Analg* 29:100. (Proceedings abstract of the ACVA 26th Annual meeting, New Orleans)

MacPhail CM, Lappin MR, Meyer DJ, et al.(1998). Hepatocellular toxicosis associated with administration of carprofen in 21 dogs. *JAVMA* 212:1895-1901.

Mathews KA (1996a). Nonsteroidal anti-inflammatory analgesics in pain managment in dogs and cats. *Can Vet J* 37:539-545.

Mathews KA, Paley DM, Foster RA, Valliant AE, Young SS (1996b). A comparison of ketorolac with flunixin, butorphanol, and oxymorphone in controlling postoperative pain in dogs. *Can J Vet Res* 37:557-567.

Maze M, Tranquilli W (1991). α2-adrenoceptor agonist, defining the role in clinical anesthesia. *Anesthesiology* 74:581-605.

McIntyre TAJ (1982). Anesthetic management of the canine cesarean section. *The Animal Health Technician.* 3:15-23.

McKellar Q A, Delatour P, Lees P (1994). Stereospecific pharmacodynamics and pharmacokinetics of carprofen in the dog. *J Vet Pharmacol Ther* 17:447-454.

McNeil PE (1992). Acute tubulo-interstitial nephritis in a dog after halothane anaesthesia and administration of flunixin meglumine and trimethoprim-sulphadiazine. *Vet Rec* 131:148-151.

McQuay HJ, Carroll D, Moore RA (1988). Post-operative orthopaedic pain—the effect of opiate premedication and local anaesthetic blocks. *Pain* 33:291-295.

Melzack R, Wall PD (1965). Pain mechanism: a new theory. *Science* 150:971-979.

Meyer CE (1987) Anesthesia for Neonatal and Geriatric Patients. In *Principles & Practice of Veterinary Anesthesia.* C.E. Short, Ed. pp 330-337.

Millis DL, Weigel JP, Moyers T, Buonomo FC (2002). Effect of deracoxib, a new COX-2 inhibitor, on the prevention of lameness induced by chemical synovitis in dogs. *Vet Ther* 3:453-464.

Muir WW III (1978). Effects of atropine on cardiac rates and rhythms in the dog. *JAVMA* 172:917-921.

Muir WW III (1981). Drugs used to produce standing chemical restraint in horses. *Vet Clin N Am* 3:17-44.

Muir WW III, Ford JL, Karpa GE, et al (1999). Effects of intramuscular administration of low doses of medetomidine and medetomidine-butorphanol in middle-aged and old dogs. *JAVMA* 215:1116-1120.

Muir WW III, Gadawski JE (2002). Cardiovascular effects of a high dose of romifidine in propofol - anesthetized cats. *Am J Vet Res* 63:1241-1246.

Muir WW III, Hubbell JAE (1985). Blood pressure response to acetylpromazine and lenperone in halothane anesthetized dogs. *J Am Anim Hosp Assn* 21:285-289.

Muir WW III, Werner LL, Hamlin RL (1975). Effects of xylazine and acetylpromazine upon induced ventricular fibrillation in dogs anesthetized with thiamylal and halothane. *Am J Vet Res* 36:1299-1303.

Mutoh T, Kojima K, Takao K, et al. (2001). Comparison of sevoflurane with isoflurane for rapid mask induction in midazolam and butorphanol sedated dogs. *J Vet Med Series A.* 48:223-230.

Miyabayashi T, Morgan JP (1984). Gastric emptying in the normal dog. *Vet Radiology* 25:187-191.

Nolan A, Reid J (1993). Comparison of the postoperative analgesic and sedative effects of carprofen and papaveretum in the dog. *Vet Rec* 133:240-242.

Nolan AM (2000). Pharmacology of analgesic drugs. *Pain Management in Animals.* Flecknell PA and Waterman-Pearson, Eds. W.B. Saunders pp.21-52.

Nugent M, Artru AA, Michenfelder JD (1982). Cerebral metabolic, vascular and protective effects of midazolam maleate. Comparison to diazepam. *Anesthesiology* 56:172-176.

Pfeffer M, Smyth RD, Pittman KA, et al. (1980). Pharmacokinetics of subcutaneous and intramuscular butorphanol in dogs. *J Pharm Sci* 69:801-803.

Phillips DM (2000). JCAHO pain management standards are unveiled. *J Am Med Assn* 284:428-429.

Pibarot P, Dupuis J, Grisneaux E, et al. (1997). Comparison of ketoprofen, oxymorphone hydrochloride, and butorphanol in the treatment of postoperative pain in dogs. *J Am Vet Med Assoc* 211:438-444.

Popiliskis S, Jordan D, laurent L, et al. (1997) Comparison of keterolac and oxymorphone on postoperative pain relief and neuroendocrine response in dogs. *Proc 6th Int Cong Vet Anaes,* Guelph, Ontario, p 107 (Abstract)

Poulsen Nautrup B, Justus C. (1999) Effects of some veterinary NSAIDs on ex vivo thromboxane production and in vivo output in the dog. *Boehringer Ingelheim Symposium: Recent advances in non-steroidal anti-inflammatory therapy in small animals* 25-33.

Pozzi A, Muir WW II, Traverso F (2006). Prevention of central sensitization and pain by N-methyl-D-aspartate receptor antagonists. *JAVMA* 228:53-59.

Price HL, Ohnishi St (1980). Effects of anesthetics on the heart. *Fed Proc* 39:1575-1579.

Pritchett DB, Sontheimer H, Shivers BD, et al. (1989). Importance of a novel GABA$_A$ receptor subunit for benzodiazepine pharmacology. *Nature* 338:582-585.

Proakis AG, Harris GB (1978). Comparative penetration of glycopyrrolate and atropine across the blood-brain and placental barriers in anesthetized dogs. *Anesthesiology* 48:339-344.

Räihä JE, et al (1989a) Comparison of three different dose regimens of medetomidine in laboratory beagles. *Acta Vet Scand* 85:11115.

Pypendop BH, Verstegen JP (2001). Cardiovascular effects of romifidine in dogs. *Am J. Vet Res* 62:490-495.

Quandt JE, Raffe MR, Robinson EP (1994). Butorphanol does not reduce the minimum alveolar concentration of halothane in dogs. *Vet Surg* 23:156-159.

Räihä MP, et al (1989b). A comparison of xylazine, acepromazine, meperidine, and medetomidine as preanesthetics to halothane anesthesia in dogs. *Acta Vet Scand* 85:97-102.

Räihä JE, et al (1989c). Medetomidine as a preanesthetic prior to ketamine-HCl and halothane anesthesia on laboratory beagles. *Acta Vet Scand* 85:103-110.

Rapp SE, Egan KJ, Ross BK, et al. (1996). A multidimensional comparison of morphine and hydromorphone patient-controlled analgesia. *Anesth Analg* 82:1043-1048.

Reid J, Nolan AM (1991). A comparison of the postoperative analgesic and sedative effects of flunixin and papaveretum in the dog. J Small Anim Pract 32:603-608.

Ricketts AP, Lundy KM, Seibel SB (1998). Evaluation of selective inhibition of canine cyclooxygenase 1 and 2 by carprofen and other non steroidal anti-inflammatory drugs. *Am J Vet Res* 59:1441-1446.

Rigel DF, Lipson D, Katona PG (1984). Excess tachycardia:Heart rate after antimuscarinic agents in conscious dogs. *Am J Physiol* 246:H168-173.

Robertson SA, Taylor PM (2004). Pain management in cats - past, present and future. Part 2. Treatment of pain - clinical pharmacology. *J Feline Med & Surg* (in press).

Robertson SA, Taylor PM (2004). Pain management in cats - past, present and future. Part 2. Treatment of pain - clinical pharmacology. *J Fel Med Surg* 6:321-333.

Robertson SA, Taylor PM, Bloomfield M, Sear JW (2001). Buprenorphine disposition after buccal administration in cats: preliminary observations. *Vet Anaesth Analg* 28:206 (Proceedings Abstract).

Robinson E.P (1983) Anesthesia of pediatric patients. *Comp Cont Ed. Pract Vet* 5:1004-1011.

Robinson EP, Faggella AM, Henry DP, Russell WL (1988). Comparison of histamine release induced by morphine and oxymorphone administration in dogs. *AJVR* 49:1699-1701.

Robinson KJ, Jones RS, Cripps PJ (2001). Effects of meditomidine and buprenorphine administered for sedation in dogs. *J Sm Ani Prac* 42:444-447.

Robinson TM, Kruse-Elliott KT, Markel MD, et al. (1999). A comparison of transdermal fentanyl versus epidural morphine for analgesia in dogs undergoing major orthopaedic surgery. *J Amer Ani Hosp Assn* 35:95-100.

Ronchetti N, Manuela S, Scrollavezza P, Sawyer DC (2002). Tramadol versus butorphanol or carprofen: Comparative study of analgesic efficacy for postoperative pain after abdominal ovariohysterectomy in the dog. *In Prep.*

Ross JN (2005). Tufts University School of Veterinary Medicine. *Personal Communication.*

Roughan JV, Ojeda OB, Flecknell PA (1999). The influence of pre-anaesthetic administration of buprenorphine on the anaesthetic effects of ketamine/medetomidine and pentobarbitone in rats and the consequences of repeated anaesthesia. *Lab Ani* 33:234-242.

Savola JM (1989). Cardiovascular actions of medetomidine and their reversal by atipamezole. *Acta Vet Scand* 85:39.

Sawyer DC (1982). The preanesthetic period. In *The Practice of Small Animal Anesthesia*. W.B. Saunders Co. Philadelphia, pp 1-12.

Sawyer DC (1985). Use of narcotics and analgesics for pain control. *AAHA's 52nd Annual Meeting Proceedings*, pp 7-11.

Sawyer DC, Rech RH (1987). Analgesia and behavioral effects of butorphanol, nalbuphine, and pentazocine in the cat. *J Am Animal Hosp Assn* 23:438-446.

Sawyer, DC, RH Rech, and RA Durham: Effects of Ketamine and Combinations with Acetylpromazine, diazepam, or butorphanol on visceral nociception in the cat. *Status of Ketamine in Anesthesiology*, ed by E.F. Domino, 1990, NPP Books, Ann Arbor, MI pp. 247-259.

Sawyer DC, Rech RH, Durham RA, Adams T, et al. (1991). Dose-response of butorphanol administered subcutaneously to increase visceral nociceptive threshold in dogs. *Am J Vet Res* 52:1826-1830.

Sawyer DC (1992). Controlling Pain in Animals. *AKC Gazette*, October: 75-80.

Sawyer DC, Rech RH, Adams T, et al. (1992). Analgesic and behavioral responses of oxymorphone - acepromazine following methoxyflurane and halothane anesthesia in the dog. *Am J Vet Res*, 53:1361-1368.

Sawyer DC, Rech RH, and Durham RA (1993). Does ketamine provide adequate visceral analgesia when used alone or in combination with acepromazine, diazepam, or butorphanol in cats? *J Am Ani Hosp Assn* 29:257-263.

Sawyer, DC (1998). Pain Control in small-animal patients. *Applied Animal Behaviour Science* 59:135-146.

Scheinin H, et al (1988). Behavioral and neurochemical effects of atipamezole, a novel a_2-adrenoceptor antagonist. *Eur J Pharmacol* 151:35-42.

Schermerhorn T, Barr SC, Stoffregen DA, et al (1994). Whole-blood platelet aggregation, buccal mucosa blooding time, and serum cephalothin concentration in dogs receiving a presurgical antibiotic protocol. *Am J Vet Res* 55:1602-1607.

Schoen AM, ed (1994). *Veterinary Acupuncture: Ancient Art to Modern Medicine*. Mosby, St Louis.

Scrivani PV, Bednarski RM, Myer CW (1998). Effects of acepromazine and butorphanol on positive-contrast upper gastrointestinal tract examination in dogs. *Am J Vet Res* 59:1227-1233.

Sederberg J, Stanley TH, Reddy P, et al. (1981). Hemodynamic effects of butorphanol-oxygen anesthesia in dogs. *Anesth Analg* 60:715-719.

Selmi AL, Barbudo-Selmi GR, Mendes GM, et al. (2004). Sedative, analgesic and cardiorespiratory effects of romifidine in cats. *Vet Anaesth Analg* 31:195-206.

Shafford HL, Lascelles BDX, Hellyer PW (2001). Preemptive analgesia: managing pain before it begins. *Vet Med* 96:478-480.

Short CE, Miller RL (1978). Comparative evaluation of the anticholinergic agent glycopyrrolate as a preanesthetic agent. *Vet Med/Sm An Clin* 5:1269-1272.

Short CE, Martin R, Henry CW Jr (1983a): Clinical comparison of glycopyrrolate and atropine as preanesthetic agents in cats. *Vet Med/Sm An Clin* 10:1447-1460.

Short CE, Martin R, Tracy CH (1983b). Effective dosage levels of glycopyrrolate injectable in cats. *Vet Med/Sm An Clin* 10:1377-1380.

Short CE (1987a). Anticholinergics. In *Principles and Practice of Veterinary Anesthesia*. CE Short ed, Williams & Wilkins, pp 8-15.

Short CE (1987b). Pain, analgesics, and related medications. In *Principles and Practice of Veterinary Anesthesia*. CE Short, ed, Williams & Wilkins, pp 28-46.

Short CE and Van Poznak A (1992a). *Animal Pain*. CE Short & A Van Poznak, eds. Churchill Livingstone, pp 1-587.

Short CE (1992b). The effects of selective a2-adrenoreceptor or agonists on cardiovascular functions and brain wave activity in horses and dogs. Library of Congress #9167510, *Veterinary Practice Publishing Company*, Santa Barbara, CA.

Sinclair MD, O'Grady MR, Kerr CL, et al. (2003). The echocardiographic effects of romifidine in dogs with and without prior or concurrent administration of glycopyrrolate. *Vet Anaesth Analg* 30:211-219.

Smith LJ, Yu JKA, Bjorling DE, Waller K (2001). Effects of hydromorphone or oxymorphone, with or without acepromazine, on preanesthetic sedation, physiologic values, and histamine release in dogs. *JAVMA* 218:1101-1105.

Soma LR and Shields DR (1964). Neuroleptanalgesia produced by fentanyl and droperidol. *JAVMA* 145:897-901.

Stanley TH (1987). New developments in opioid drug research for alleviation of animal pain. *JAVMA* 191:1252-1253.

Stanway GW, Taylor PM, Brodbelt DC (2002). A preliminary investigation comparing pre-operative morphine and buprenorphine for postoperative analgesia and sedation in cats. *Vet Anaesth Analg* 29:29-35.

Strub KM, Aeppli L, Muller RKM (1982). Pharmacological properties of carprofen. *Eur J Rheum and Inflamm* 5:478-487.

Takabashi N, Zipes DP (1983). Vagal modulation of adrenergic effects on canine sinus and atrioventricular nodes. *Am J Physiol* 244:H775-781.

Takeuchi A, Morizane H, Kim H, et al. (1991). The isoflurane sparing effects of midazolam, butorphanol and medetomidine in dogs. *Proc of 4th Int Cong of Vet Anaesth*, Utrecht, Netherlands, 25-31.

Taylor PM, Houlton JEF (1984). Post-operative analgesia in the dog: a comparison of morphine, buprenorphine and pentazocine. *J Sm Ani Prac* 25:437-451.

Taylor PM, Herrtage ME (1986). Evaluation of some drug combinations for sedation in the dog. *J Sm Ani Prac* 27:325-333.

Taylor PM, Winnard JG, Jefferies R (1994). Flunixin in the cat: a pharmacodynamic, pharmacokinetic and toxicological study. *Br Vet J* 150:253-262.

Taylor, P.M., Delatour, P., Landoni, F.M., et al. (1996). Pharmacodynamics and enantioselective pharmacokinetics of carprofen in the cat. *Res Vet Sci* 60:144-151.

Thurmon JC, Tranquilli WJ, Benson GJ eds. (1996). Preanesthetics and adjuncts. *Lumb & Jones' Veterinary Anesthesia*. 3rd ed. Baltimore: Williams & Wilkins Co. pp 196-205

Tranquilli WJ, et al. (1984). Halothane sparing effect of xylazine in dogs and subsequent reversal with tolazoline. *J Vet Pharmacol Ther* 7:23-28.

Tranquilli WJ, Gross ME, Thurmon JC, Benson GJ (1990). Evaluation of three midazolam-xylazine mixtures. Preliminary trials in dogs. Vet Surg 19:168-172.

Tranquilli WJ, Grimm KA, Lamont LA (2004). *Pain Management for the Small Animal Practitioner.* Jackson: Teton New Media.

Turpeinen U, et al. (1988). Crystal structures, thermal behavior, protonation, and mass spectroscopic studies of racemic 4-(1- [2, 3-dimethylphenyl] -ethyl) -1H-imidazole hydrochlorides. *Acta Chem Scand* B42:537-545.

Tverskoy M, Cozacov C, Ayache M, et al. (1990). Postoperative pain after inguinal herniorrhaphy with different types of anesthesia. *Anesth Analg* 70:29-35.

Vähä-Vahe T (1989a). Clinical evaluation of medetomidine, a novel sedative and analgesic drug for dogs and cats. *Acta Vet Scand* 30:267-273.

Vähä-Vahe T (1989b). The clinical efficacy of medetomidine. *Acta Vet Scand* 85:151.

Vainio O, Vähä-Vahe T (1990). Reversal of medetomidine sedation by atipamezole in dogs. *J Vet Pharmacol Ther* 13:15-22.

Vane JR (1971). Inhibition of prostaglandin synthesis as a mechanism of action for aspirin-like drugs. *Nat New Biol* 231:232-235.

Virtanen R (1989). Pharmacological profiles of medetomidine and its antagonist, atipamezole. *Acta Vet Scand* 85:29-37.

Waechter RA (1982). Unusual reaction to acepromazine maleate in the dog. *JAVMA* 180:73-74.

Wagner AE and Hellyer PW (2000). Survey of anesthesia techniques and concerns in private veterinary practive. *JAVMA* 217:1652-1657.

Wall PD (1992). Defining pain in animals. In: *Animal Pain.* CE Short, A Van Poznak, eds. New York, Churchill-Livingstone, 63-79.

Watson ADJ, Nicholson A, Church DB, Pearson MRB (1996). Use of anti-inflammatory and analgesic drugs in dogs and cats. *Aust Vet J* 74:203-210.

Weinger MB, Segal IS, Maze M (1989). Dexmedetomidine, acting through central alpha-2 adrenoceptors, prevents opiate-induced muscle rigidity in the rat. *Anesthesiology* 71:242-249.

Welsh EM, Nolan AM, Reid J (1997) Beneficial effects of administering carprofen before surgery in dogs. *Vet Rec* 141:251-253.

Welsch JA, Wohl JS, Wright JC (2002). Evaluation of postoperative respiratory function by serial blood gas analysis in dogs treated with transdermal fentanyl. *J Vet Emerg & Crit Care* 12:81-87.

Willis W, Chung JM (1987). Central mechanisms of pain. *JAVMA* 191:1987-1202.

Wilson DE (1991). Role of prostaglandins in gastroduodenal mucosal protection. *J Clin Gastroenterol* 13 Suppl 1:S65-71.

Woolf CJ, Chong M (1993). Preemptive analgesia—treating postoperative pain by preventing the establishment of central sensitization. *Anesth Analg* 77:362-79.

Yoxall AT (1978). Pain in small animals—its recognition and control. *J Sm Ani Prac* 19:423-438.

Chapter 2
The Induction Period

Induction to anesthesia can be accomplished by administering a single drug or combinations of drugs by IV, IM, or inhalation routes. Assessment of risk status as discussed in Chapter 1 and proper patient preparation during the pre-anesthetic period is of paramount importance to maximize successful outcome.

IV injection of a single anesthetic or drug combination is a common method of inducing anesthesia in dogs and cats. Dosage is based on body weight usually obtained using a walk-on scale but is given to effect the necessary depth needed for the intended procedure. Guess-estimate of body weight is no longer an accepted practice with the availability of a variety of certified scales for veterinary hospitals. However, obese animals pose a different problem as the anesthetist must be careful not to administer the inducing agent solely on the basis of gross body weight. Fat is not involved with primary uptake of anesthetics so profound cardiac depression is likely to occur because of the potential for an overdose of injected drug that is delivered to body viscera, e.g., myocardium (Eger, 1964). This is accomplished by estimating the weight of the dog as if it were not obese. The animal still should be weighed but the veterinarian must determine the degree of obesity based on normal average weight for animals of similar size, e.g., 10, 20, 30%, etc. This is not as difficult as it might seem and overdose can be potentially avoided. Profound obesity would occur if the body would be double the normal weight. If the intubation dose, rather than the surgical anesthetic dose, is used with these hypnotics, fewer complications will be evident.

IV injection of anesthetic drugs can be done through a needle attached to a syringe inserted directly into a peripheral vein or through a pre-placed catheter. When a syringe is taped in place, it is easy to lose venous access during the procedure subsequent to moving the patient for transport or during positioning on the surgery table. The metal needle will penetrate the vessel wall rendering venous access of no use when needed. Perivascular injection of certain drugs, particularly thiobarbiturates, can be very irritating to tissues and may result in necrosis. Thus for administration of injectable anesthetics, analgesics, adjunctive drugs, and fluids, a plastic catheter is far more reliable. Just from a patient safety standpoint, having a secured catheter in a peripheral vein is essential and may even be lifesaving.

Equipment

IV catheters are classified based on whether they go into the vessel lumen by passing over-the-needle, the "extracath," (Figure 2-1) or through-the-needle, the "intracath" (Figure 2-2).

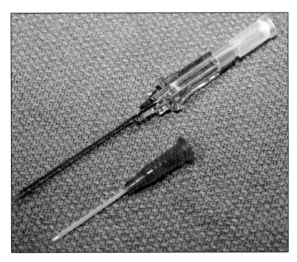

Figure 2-1 Over-needle catheter removed, needle, flash chamber, and plug.
Courtesy of Gail Whiting, photographer.

61

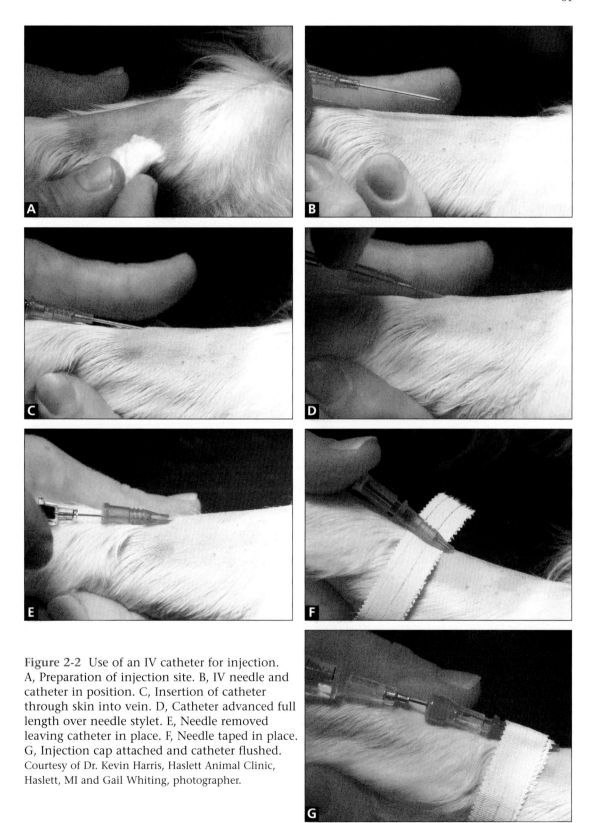

Figure 2-2 Use of an IV catheter for injection.
A, Preparation of injection site. B, IV needle and
catheter in position. C, Insertion of catheter
through skin into vein. D, Catheter advanced full
length over needle stylet. E, Needle removed
leaving catheter in place. F, Needle taped in place.
G, Injection cap attached and catheter flushed.
Courtesy of Dr. Kevin Harris, Haslett Animal Clinic,
Haslett, MI and Gail Whiting, photographer.

Extracaths vary 1 to 5cm in length and are most commonly used in conjunction with anesthesia or for relatively short-term use for repeated or continuous administration of drugs and fluids. The over-the-needle catheter is preferred for peripheral vein cannulation because the bore is larger, there are fewer hazards due to catheter transection by the needle and less bleeding occurs at the site of venipuncture. Intracaths are 12 to 20cm long and are usually placed into a central vein via the Jugular or Cephalic Vein. They are used more in management of intensive care patients. An alternative to this technique is shown in Figure 2-3. Following placement of a needle in the vein, a sterile wire is theaded through the lumen and following withdrawal of the needle, a sheathed vein dilator in inserted over the guide wire. The guide is removed leaving the dilator sheath through which a larger catheter can be inserted.

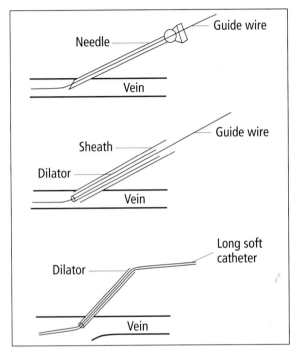

Figure 2-3 Technique for insertion of intracath into a vein by the modified Seldinger technique. Following preparation of the site, vein is first penetrated with a needle through which a sterile guide wire is threaded. Following withdrawal of the needle, a sheathed vein dilator is introduced over the guide wire and dilator. The guide wire is removed leaving the dilator sheath available for insertion of the catheter.
Reprinted with permission. Fig 9-2, page 199. Veterinary Anaesthesia, Tenth Edition 2001. Eds Hall LW, Clarke KW, Trim CM. W.B. Saunders

Sizes of IV catheters are based on needle size and range from 16 to 25ga for small animal patients. Because the plastic catheter must pass over the metal needle, it is obviously larger than the needle. For obtaining access in very small veins or when low venous pressure does not allow good definition of vein location, needle-catheter configuration indentified as a small vein infusion set may be advantageous (Figure 2-4). This is comprised of a thin-walled 0.5 to 1-inch needle attached to flexible tubing at one end with a female opening at the other end to accommodate attachment of IV tubing, syringe or injection cap. Plastic tabs on either side of the needle housing used to aid insertion give the appearance of wings thus this system is often referred to as a "butterfly" catheter. Wings are pinched together with one's fingers to provide a grip for insertion and once the needle is placed into the vessel lumen, wings are flattened against the skin and taped. The flexible tubing closest to the needle is taped in place in such a way to prevent the needle from becoming dislodged. Caution must be taken to avoid penetration of the vessel wall by the indwelling needle. The butterfly needle is available in various sizes over 20-gauge but if a hospital is to stock only one size, the 23-gauge needle would be appropriate for most applications.

The major advantage of the extracath is that once it is secured in position, it remains in place to provide a reliable route for injection of fluids and/or drugs. The major disadvantages include cost and a possibility of phlebitis. Inflammation may be the result of mechanical irritation and likelihood of this problem increases the longer it remains in the vessel. Therefore, IV catheters should be changed or removed within 72 hours. If aseptic procedures are not followed, infection may be a consequence and catheters may need to be changed more frequently.

Figure 2-4 Small vein infusion set. Used mostly in small needle gauge sizes, these "butterfly catheters" have a length of plastic tubing attached to the needle with tabs (that look like butterfly wings) to aid in insertion and fixation to the site. This needle-catheter set is most useful in very small difficult to hit veins and facilitates injection from a syringe or infusion set without causing movement of the needle.

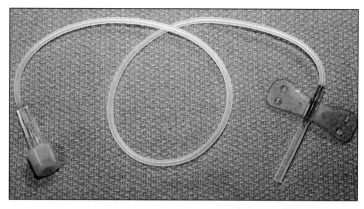

When infusion of large amounts of fluid or blood is needed, placement of two catheters may be most appropriate. The smallest catheter or needle permitting rapid blood administration is 20-gauge. It is well to remember that when high fluid volumes are needed, it is better to increase catheter size rather than raise the height of the infusion bottle. Doubling flow rate occurs when the height of the bottle is doubled. But according to Poiseuille's law, doubling the internal diameter of the catheter increases flow by 16 times. Elastic in-line pump-bulb infusion sets with check valves are available to assist the process of delivering fluids rapidly.

Infusion or drip sets are available in various lengths and the longer tubing is most convenient for use in surgery. Extension catheters are used when added length is needed and when it is advisable to have the injection port of the infusion set located away from the patient rather than close to the catheter. In situations where the catheter is placed in the hind leg and the surgical site is also in the same general area, the IV bag and injection port should be in the front where the anesthetist can more easily monitor fluid administration and have better access to the injection port.

Depending on manufacturer guidelines, IV drip infusion sets are designed to deliver fluids at 15 to 20 drops per ml. Pediatric infusion sets incorporate a 100-ml volume in-line bag or drip chamber permitting 60 drops per ml. These units are useful in patients less than 2kg for more precise measurement of fluid administration. Number of drops per ml is provided with the infusion set.

Placement Technique

For most procedures, the IV catheter is usually placed after pre-anesthetic drugs have taken effect but prior to anesthesia induction. Local anesthetics may be applied to skin prior to venipuncture. A eutectic mixture of lidocaine and prilocaine (EMLA, Astra-Zeneca) is the most widely used formulation for this purpose and is applied under an occlusive dressing for at least 20 minutes prior to catheter placement. Hair should be clipped over the venipuncture site; the skin should be cleaned and aseptically prepared. Alternate iodine and isopropyl alcohol applications are preferred. Before inserting catheters larger than 20ga, intradermal injection through a 25 gauge needle with 0.5% lidocaine or 0.25% bupivicaine at the puncture site can be used to minimize discomfort. Topical anesthetic preparations are also available.

Cephalic veins in the dog and cat are the most accessible sites for venipuncture. Saphenous veins may be used as alternatives (Figure 2-5). A tourniquet may be placed on the leg or the vein may be occluded by an assistant. It is important to have the leg in the extended position to straighten the vein for better definition of location and easier placement. It is best to make the cephalic venipuncture just proximal to the bifurcation of the vein and nearer the carpus in long-legged dogs. In giant breeds, it may be possible to place the catheter distal to the bifurcation. In short legged dogs such as Pugs, Dachshunds, English Bulldogs, and Basset hounds, it may be better to make the venipuncture at the bifurcation. With the skin stretched over the site, the needle is inserted through the skin to one side of the vein. For animals with tough skin, the catheter may be damaged as it enters the hole created by the needle. To prevent damaging the catheter tip, it

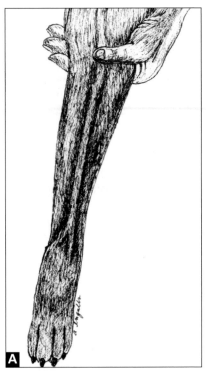

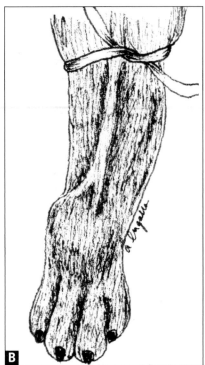

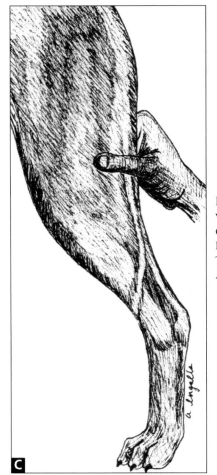

Figure 2-5 Position of cephalic vein (A), bifurcation in short legged dogs (B) and saphenous vein (C). Reprinted with permission. Sawyer, D C, The Practice of Small Animal Anesthesia, W.B. Saunders 1982

may be desirable to cut the skin with the edge of a 20 gauge needle. Insert the bevel of a 20 gauge needle in the skin, rotate the needle vertically and pull up quickly to cut the skin. For others, this is not necessary as the catheter will usually not be damaged as it passes through skin into the vessel lumen. The needle should be directed into the vein with the bevel up until penetration of the vessel wall occurs. When blood is seen in the flash chamber, advance the needle at least 1 to 2mm further to ensure that both the needle and distal part of the catheter are in the vessel lumen. The catheter should then be pushed over the needle to the hub, the needle removed and a syringe or infusion set attached. As an alternative, an injection cap may be connected to the catheter hub and flushed with heparinized saline. Heparinized saline is prepared by adding 0.75ml of 1:1000 heparin sodium solution to a 250ml bag of isotonic NaCl. If an "intracath" is used, the catheter is threaded through the needle, the needle is then removed and secured to the catheter with the protective cover. The catheter is fixed into position by attaching adhesive tape first to the catheter and then to the leg to prevent dislodgement.

Catheter placement must be checked at each step to ensure that proper placement has been made and extravascular infiltration has not occurred. Catheters placed close to the elbow make improper catheterization and infiltration more difficult to verify because of loose skin. Shar-peis can be particularly challenging because of loose skin folds and subcutaneous fat on the limbs. Also, large breeds usually have wide flat veins which make vessel definition and insertion difficult. In apprehensive, aggressive, or vasoconstricted patients, it may be beneficial to accomplish venipuncture following delivery of an inhalation agent such as isofluane or sevoflurane which will produce vasodilation. There is inherent danger in inducing anesthesia without a catheter in place but when restraint or discomfort is the problem in an otherwise healthy patient, performing venipuncture at this time is better than making many unsuccessful attempts pre-induction. However, if hypovolemia is a consideration or in patients in P3, P4, or P5 physical status, establishing IV access before induction is essential for patient safety.

Methods of Induction

Induction of general anesthesia is a transition from the patient being conscious to becoming unconscious. It is the most dangerous period of anesthesia. Body systems are placed immediately in an unstable state and undesirable cardiovascular and respiratory responses may be observed. Recovery from anesthesia can also be an unstable period because of the surgical stresses interposed and the changing status of drug effects.

In general, there are two means of accomplishing anesthetic induction. One is with the same drug that is used for maintenance, e.g., inhalation anesthetics, dissociative agents and various combinations of drugs. The other method is to use a single agent or drug combination that has a rapid onset followed by delivery of an inhalation agent either by mask or through an endotracheal tube. Continuing effects of anesthesia take place during uptake of the inhalant while effects of the injectable agent dissipate. Induction of anesthesia has been achieved when the patient has become unconscious and is not responding to noxious stimuli. Even though the ability to achieve tracheal intubation is often used as a sign induction has been achieved, it does not always mean a surgical level of anesthesia has been reached.

Injectable Anesthetics

The most common injectable agents used for IV induction in the dog and cat are thiopental Na, ketamine/diazepam, ketamine/midazolam, tiletamine/zolazapam and propofol. Thiamylal Na was used in the U.S. for more than 40 years until it was removed from the market in the mid 90's. With any of the injectable drugs and combinations, when one is not familiar with effects and responses because of infrequent use, patient safety may be compromised. For example, if drug X is only used in high risk patients and very few such patients are anesthetized in a practice, that drug might not be used in a proper manner or under the right circumstances. Consultation with an anesthesiologist in advance might pay big dividends should this occur.

Ultrashort Barbiturates

Thiopental Sodium

Thiopental was first introduced during World War II for human patients in field hospitals. Following the war, this drug became widely used in human hospitals essentially because physicians had become familiar with its actions. This was the first time a drug could be administered IV to induce unconsciouness so rapidly and the descriptive term "crash induction" was coined to best describe this response. From mid 1950 into the 1990's, thiopental was not nearly as popular as thiamylal in veterinary practice principally because of a difference in marketing rather than differences between these two drugs. However, once thiamylal was no longer available, transition to thiopental was relatively easy. Thiopental has the same potency as thiamylal and twice that of methohexital (Turner 1990a). Recovery times for thiopental and thiamylal were similar, e.g., 71 and 75 minutes respectively, and twice that for methohexital (34 minutes). Despite the availability of new injectable agents, ultrashort acting thiobarbiturates continue to be popular, at least in the Midwest and Eastern United States, perhaps because of pharmacodynamic properties that have good application in certain situations (Ilkiw 1992a). These include patients with raised intracranial pressure, patients with a history of seizures, patients with corneal lacterations or glaucoma, patients with hyperthyroidism, and patients thought to be susceptible to malignant hyperthermia.

Thiopental sodium is structurally similar to pentobarbital, a long-acting barbiturate, except for the addition of sulfur at the 2nd carbon on the barbituric acid ring (Price, 1960). This shortens the duration of action by increasing lipid solubility of the drug in blood and tissues. Classified as an ultrashort-acting thiobarbiturate, this hypnotic has a rapid onset of action and fast recovery due to redistribution from vessel-rich tissues to muscle and fat (Price 1960) (Figure 2-6). Elimination half-life for thiopental in the dog is anticipated to be 2 to 4 hours (Ilkiw et al 1991a).

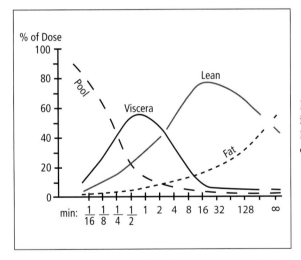

Figure 2-6 Uptake and distribution of an intravenous dose of thiopental.
Reprinted with permission. Sawyer, D C, The Practice of Small Animal Anesthesia, W.B. Saunders 1982

Thiopental, a C-III drug listed by the U.S. DEA, is marketed as a yellow powder contained in a multiple injection bottle. The powder is reconstituted to liquid form by adding sterile water diluent provided in the package yielding a 2.0 or 2.5% concentration depending on the amount of diluent added. For animals less than 5kg it is best to dilute the drug further to a 1% concentration to allow more accurate dosing. Once the diluent has been added, the bottle must be clearly labeled with date and concentration. Reasonably stable at room temperature, the drug will remain in solution without precipitation or deterioration for several days. Because of the decrease in potency with time, the solution should not be used beyond 72 hours following mixing. It should not be used at any time if the solution is cloudy or contains particulates or precipitates.

There is a higher incidence of laryngospasm with thiobarbiturates than with inhalation induction, especially in cats (Lumb and Jones, 1973). Nerve impulse frequency is higher which indicates a greater irritability of the larynx (Rex, 1970). Topical anesthetic spray with 0.2 % lidocaine will help and may be used prior to intubation in the cat. The calculated induction dose necessary to depress the laryngoscopic reflex for endotracheal intubation in non-premedicated dogs was reported to be 19mg/kg in normal healthy dogs (Turner 1990a). However, one third to one half of this dose should be injected as an IV push with the balance administered more slowly to reach the desired anesthetic level. If used alone, recovery may be rough, but this can be avoided if patients are tranquilized or maintained with an inhalation agent.

For obese animals, the anesthetist must be careful not to administer the induction agent solely on the basis of gross body weight. Profound cardiac depression is likely to occur because of the potential for an overdose of injected drug being delivered to body viscera, e.g., myocardium (Eger 1964).

There are dose-related cardiopulmonary changes induced by thiopental in healthy dogs that may be much more severe in patients at risk. Within the first 30 seconds following injection, stroke volume is decreased; heart rate, left atrial pressure, and mean pulmonary arterial pressure increased; with no change in cardiac index, myocardial contractility, and systemic and pulmonary vascular resistances (Turner 1990b). Mean arterial pressure may not change initially but is increased within 30 seconds lasting 5 to 7 minutes (Sawyer et al. 1971). These effects are usually very short lasting in healthy patients (Sawyer 1973) but may persist for almost an hour in patients at risk (Ilkiw et al 1991b). There is also a tendency to produce ventricular arrhythmias, especially bigeminy, that has been associated with hypoventilation, tachycardia, increased total peripheral resistence, and systemic hypertension.

Cardiac rhythm is often altered when surgical anesthetic doses are used. The most frequent dysrhythmia observed is ventricular premature depolarization occurring alternately with sinus beats (bigeminy) (Muir, 1977). This is minimized when lesser doses are used, when given in 1 to 2% concentrations or if the animal is preoxygenated. These changes are of little consequence in P1 patients and usually dissipate within 3-5 minutes. However, this may have profound effects in sick animals. In addition, care must be taken when epinephrine is considered for use with thiobarbiturates (Muir et al. 1975). An alternative method of induction should be used where these compromises cannot be tolerated. In young adult healthy patients, most recover from these arrhythmias and may not even be noticed by the anesthetist. However, if these changes persist, oxygen should be administered by mask or endotracheal tube. In addition, lidocaine can be given IV. Cardiopulmonary effects of thiopental with and without lidocaine were evaluated in 13 dogs anesthetized to surgical levels (Rawlings 1983). Thiopental was given alone at a dose of 22mg/kg IV compared to the combination of thiopental (11mg/kg) and lidocaine (8.8mg/kg). It is not surprising that these data demonstrated that the combination has a shorter duration, produced no arrhythmias, and resulted in less cardiopulmonary depression than the high dose of thiopental alone. In fact, bigeminy developed during 19 of 20 thiopental inductions compared with 0 of 22 thiopental/lidocaine inductions. Administering lidocaine with thiopental may be advantageous in situations where doses of thiopental would not be well tolerated or alternative induction agents are not available for patients ASA class 3 or higher. However, early supplementation with oxygen has great benefit for improved tissue oxygenation in patients at risk. Because of cardiopulmonary changes induced by thiopental, many veterinarians prefer alternative IV drugs such as ketamine/diazepam, propofol, or a balanced opioid/tranquilizer combination.

A period of apnea lasting 30 to 45 seconds may be observed in patients given a bolus surgical anesthetic dose of thiopental (Quandt 1998). Because of the relative lack of analgesia, there is a narrow margin between the dose required to produce unconsciousness and the dose evoking apnea. Spontaneous breathing quickly resumes and following endotracheal intubation with subsequent administration of oxygen, a period of apnea may reappear. This sequence may be a result of hypoxemia initially due to the CNS depressant effects of thiopental leading to resumption of spontaneous breathing of room air. Then arterial PCO_2 may drop below the apneic threshold subsequent to hyperventilation induced by tracheal stimulation during insertion of the tube. In most cases, an inhalation agent will be introduced following induction with thiopental but uptake of the inhalant will obviously not take place if the patient is apneic. Therefore, manual ventilation should be provided at a rate of 6 to 8 breaths per minute for a few minutes. One must avoid hyperventilating the patient by manual or mechanical means if spontaneous breathing is to resume.

Barbiturates can produce any degree of CNS depression, ranging from mild sedation to deep coma. The individual patient's tolerance, physical status, and dose administered all determine the totality of effect. The mode of action is thought to be depression of the short synaptic pathways in the central reticular core of the medulla with sparing of direct spinolemniscothalamic pathways. Thiobarbiturates are poor analgesics and recognition of these differences is essential for the rational use of such agents for general anesthesia. Certain patients may require higher doses for adequate anesthesia. Often the degree of anesthesia appears adequate but subsequent to surgical stimulation, movement or struggling may occur, indicating insufficient afferent blockade. Thiobarbiturates also sensitize vagal nerve endings which may lead to laryngospasm–again evidence that the afferent pathways are not blocked. Under these circumstances, administration of additional doses must be done carefully.

With thiopental, 20mg/kg IV, surgical anesthesia may be provided for 15 minutes in dogs. Additional injections may be given to prolong the effect with the objective of keeping drug levels in plasma and brain sufficient for anesthesia maintenance. The rate of metabolic removal is 10 to 15% per hour; thus the more drug that is given, the longer will be recovery. Primary indications for the use of the thiobarbiturates for anesthesia maintenance are: relatively short diagnostic procedures such as cerebral spinal fluid tap, radiographic examination, proctoscopy, and bronchoscopy and minor surgical procedures such as repair of lacerations and removal of orthopedic devices.

Because of a direct effect on the control centers in the medulla, respiration may be depressed immediately following injection. Apnea may occur and to avoid further problems, controlled breathing of 4 to 6 breaths/minute should be given until spontaneous breathing resumes. The central stimulatory response to CO_2 is depressed at all levels of anesthesia and may be eliminated at deeper levels. The normal response to increased PCO_2 is an increase in tidal volume. During anesthesia, tidal volume is depressed with rate of breathing increased. Therefore, respiratory acidosis is a common sequel to barbiturate anesthesia that can be avoided if breathing is adequately controlled.

Myocardial contractility is reduced resulting in decreases in stroke volume and cardiac output of 30 to 50% (Sawyer et al. 1971. Mean arterial pressure is increased because barbiturates induce peripheral vasoconstriction through enhanced vascular tone. Heart rate is also increased 10 to 20%. Baroreceptor reflexes, conduction in autonomic nerves, and sympathetic ganglion transmission are not appreciably depressed.

Extravascular injection of the alkaline thiobarbiturates may result in vasospasm with eventual ulceration of the affected area. Careful observation of the site of injection can avoid this unnecessary complication. The best method is to place an intravascular catheter first and assure proper placement before administering the drug. Either a balanced electrolyte drip is started and the drug is given concurrently or an injection cap is attached to the catheter to permit intermittent injection of the anesthetic.

If extravasation occurs, treatment consists of injecting 0.5% lidocaine into the involved area to dilute and neutralize the barbiturate and to increase blood flow to the area by sympathetic blockade of capillary vessels and subsequent vasodilation.

Intra-arterial injection is highly unlikely in the dog or cat but it can take place if the artery and vein are in proximity such as in the femoral area or where the artery is superficial. Chemical endarteritis destroys the endothelial and subendothelial layers of the vessel wall and may result in diffuse thrombosis. The injury is immediate and appears to be due to the drug itself and its alkalinity. If extensive arterial thrombosis occurs, amputation may be necessary. Some human patients have recovered from the thrombosed artery without treatment whereas others have developed gangrene in spite of therapy. Treatment consists of intra-arterial injection of 2 to 10ml of 1% procaine or lidocaine. Local heparinization may be helpful and local injection of an alpha-adrenergic blocker such as phentolamine may be justified. General anesthesia with an inhalation anesthetic may be helpful because of peripheral vasodilation and increased blood flow to the affected site.

Benign ventricular arrhythmias may persist into the anesthetic period with thiobarbiturates. A transient bigeminal rhythm can be observed following injection of thiopental and unless pulse rate is below 70 and continuing to decrease, treatment is unnecessary. Muir and associates have found that ventricular bigeminy is directly correlated to the increase in tension imposed on the myocardium by increased arterial blood pressure (Muir et al. 1975). Transiently decreasing venous return by holding end-inspiratory pressure at 20 to 25cm H_2O for 15 to 30 seconds may remove the dysrhythmia. Should more frequent and more severe ventricular dysrhythmias occur, appropriate treatment is lidocaine, 0.5 to 3mg/kg, IV in the dog.

It is apparent that sight hounds such as Greyhounds, Whippets, and Afghans, may have prolonged recovery from thiobarbiturates. Mean recovery times from recombency to standing were 3 to 4 times longer for Greyhounds anesthetized with thiopental or thiamylal than for mixed-breed dogs with recovery times for some Greyhounds lasting more than 8 hours (Robinson et al 1986b). Studies in Greyhounds demonstrated that thiobarbiturates were metabolized differently and the metabolic products were pharmacologically active leading to longer recoveries compared that in other breeds (Sams et al 1985; Robinson et al 1986b). Prolonged recoveries have also been attributed to a lower ratio of body fat to muscle resulting in a slower rate of redistribution from muscle to fat. Hematological differences such as a higher packed cell volume and lower serum protein and impaired hepatic biotransformation of drugs contribute to problems of anesthetic management of these dogs (Court 1999a; Court et al, 1999b). This does not mean that thiopental should never be used in this species but to recognize the possibility of an undesirable response if a member drug in this class is used. Proper anesthetic management includes sedative premedication and appropriate use of preemptive analgesia. Propofol, ketamine/diazepam combination or methohexital are advised as useful alternatives.

The potential for deep anesthesia exists when thiopental is used in conjunction with myelography. Protein-bound thiopental may be displaced by the contrast agent, thus deepening anesthesia (Bonhaus et al., 1981). Acidosis from any cause will deepen barbiturate anesthesia because of a change in ionization of the drug, making more available for entry into the CNS.

Thiamylal Sodium
Thiamylal is a thio-analog of secobarbital sodium. It differs slightly in structure from thiopental but has essentially the same pharmacological action. Publications on the use of this anesthetic first appeared in 1950's and subsequently it became the most commonly used ultra short-acting injectable anesthetic for small animals. However, because of a problem in the manufacturing process, availability of the base product was discontinued in the late 1990's subsequent to withdrawal of prior approval by the Center of Veterinary Medicine (CVM) of the U.S. Food and Drug Administration (FDA). Existing supplies were available for a few years thereafter but expiration dates have long since passed.

Methohexital

Methohexital is an ultrashort acting oxybarbiturate and is unique in that it does not contain sulfur and is highly soluble in blood. Therefore, it has similar characteristics to those of the thiobarbiturates, e.g., rapid induction and recovery. It has an allyl group, a long chained methyl-pentyl group at carbon 5 and a methyl group at nitrogen 3 which markedly increases its solubility in lipid membranes. This confers a short duration of action which is due not only to high solubility but also to rapid biotransformation rather than redistribution. The dry powder is reconstituted with sterile water to provide a clear solution of 2.5% concentration. Onset of action and recovery are very rapid. A problem to be avoided is violent movement and excitement that occurs during recovery in both cats and dogs when this drug is used alone. If it is used only for induction preceding inhalation anesthesia or with tranquilization, this problem can be avoided. Because of its rapid metabolism, methohexital can be used for anesthesia in sight hounds. If used only by the IV route, 11mg/kg provides light anesthesia sufficient for intubation and the duration of effect is 5 to 10 min.

Non-Barbiturates

Propofol

Ultra short-acting barbiturates have been in common use for more than 50 years. However, because of their adverse effects on the cardiovascular system, they have limitations especially for use in geriatric and high risk patients. Propofol is a unique sedative-hypnotic that has increased in popularity for small animals since it was first introduced (Glen 1980; Watkins 1987). Although the anesthetic profile was similar to that of thiopental, differences included rapid induction, rapid recovery even following repeated administrations, no tissue damage from perivascular or intra-arterial injection, and greater reflex depression with more profound EEG changes produced at equipotent doses. It was also found to be compatible with a wide range of drugs used for pre-anesthetic medication, inhalation anesthesia, and neuromuscular blocking drugs. Following recovery from propofol anesthesia, there was no evidence of any central anticholinergic or anticonvulsant affects (Glen et al 1985). The arrhythmic threshold to epinephrine was greater in animals anesthetized with propofol compared to halothane (Kamibayashi et al 1991). Bronchomotor tone and gastrointestinal motility were unaffected by propofol (Glen et al 1985). The clinical efficacy and safety of propofol was evaluated for use in dogs and cats and it was found to be useful as an induction agent prior to delivery of inhalation anesthetics (Brearley et al 1988; Morgan 1989; Weaver 1990). The mean induction doses of propofol for unpremedicated dogs and cats were 6.6 and 8.0 mg/kg, respectively. Another study reported the induction dose to be 4.7 ± 1.3mg/kg in dogs (Watney 1992). There were no reported differences between sexes. There was a low incidence of side effects and no incompatibility was observed between propofol and various premedicants. Propofol was found to be especially useful for outpatient surgery because of its rapid, smooth, and complete recovery (Ilkiw 1992a). The veterinary product is approved for use in small animals in the United Kingdom, most European countries, Australia, and Canada. In the U.S., it received CVM-FDA approval for use in dogs in November 1996 and is not classified by the US DEA as a controlled substance.

Propofol is a 2,6-diisopropylphenol of low molecular weight (178.3) prepared as a 1% isotonic oil-in-water emulsion containing soybean oil, glycerol, and purified egg lecithin. This anesthetic appears milk-white, contains 10mg/ml of propofol and is supplied in 20ml single dose ampules or fliptop vials. Propofol is a CNS depressant similar to ultra short acting barbiturates with rapid onset after bolus injection. It has a strong association with formed elements in blood with a high protein-binding component (96-98%). The pharmacokinetics of propofol have been described by a three-compartment open "mammillary" model (Cockshott 1992). It is distributed into vessel rich tissues and then is quickly redistributed to less vascular tissue, e.g., muscle and skin. Studies in laboratory animals including rat, pig, rabbit and cat after a single IV injection indicated that half-life of the distribution phase was extremely short (1-6 min) and terminal half-life was 16-55 min (Adam et al 1980). Recovery following propofol is very rapid in most dogs and cats because of its high metabolic clearance (Zoran 1993). However, slower recovery times may be observed (Reid and Nolan 1992). Studies in Greyhound dogs demonstrated that recovery times were 55 to 72% longer than in non-greyhounds (Robertson et al 1992). Pharmacokinetic studies confirmed that metabolic clearance of the drug is slower in greyhounds (Court et al 1999b). Biotransformation of propofol is initiated by a specific hepatic cytochrome P-450 (CYP) isoenzyme. Hay Krause et al. (2000) assayed microsomes from Greyhound, Beagle, and mixed breed dogs. Their results suggested that propofol hydroxylation was primarily mediated by CYP2B11 and that breed and possibly gender differences in recovery rate may be due to lower hepatic levels of this CYP.

Propofol is an effective induction agent in healthy adult dogs prior to maintenance with an inhalant anesthetic. Propofol can also be used for maintenance of anesthesia either by continuous rate infusion (CRI) or intermittent injection. A number of studies have provided cardiopulmonary and neurological evidence of the efficacy and safety when used as an induction agent under normal and impaired conditions in the dog. Although propofol has proven to be a valuable adjuvant during short ambulatory procedures, its use for maintenance of general anesthesia has been questioned for procedures lasting more than 60 minutes. This is primarily because of increased cost and marginal differences in recovery times compared with those of standard inhalant or balanced anesthetic techniques. However, a continuous propofol infusion is an acceptable alternative to inhalation anesthesia to facilitate radiographic imaging or similar procedures (Keegan 1993). Because of the potential for propofol to produce apnea and cyanosis at anesthetic levels, it is advisable to provide supplemental oxygen and ventilation if needed. To determine if propofol produces cardiovascular changes by direct actions or by indirect actions secondary to depression of the CNS, investigators concluded that propofol anesthesia may be accompanied by decreased cardiac output secondary to reduction of preload due to a direct venodilator effect (Goodchild 1989). Cardiac output and arterial pressure were preserved at normal anesthetic levels as long as preload was maintained. Effects on myocardial function as a cause of propofol induced arterial hypotension have been evaluated. At anesthetic levels, propofol caused direct depression of myocardial contractility (Pagel 1993). Thus, the significant decrease in systolic blood pressure that may be observed during propofol CRI anesthesia in dogs is likely due to direct negative inotropic actions of the drug along with its direct effects on arterial and venous vascular tone. However, when systemic vascular effects during propofol anesthesia were compared to those induced by isoflurane, propofol better preserved aortic pressure and increased aortic compliance therefore improving the energy transmission from the left ventricle to the arterial system (Deryck et al. 1996). When propofol is used for maintenance of anesthesia in combination with a sedative/analgesic, the quality of anesthesia is improved as well as the ease with which the anesthetist can titrate propofol. However, propofol should be used with caution in cardiac compromised or hypovolemic patients (Ilkiw et al 1992b). Three minutes after 6mg/kg of propofol was given IV to dogs with experimentally induced hypovolemia, pulmonary vascular indices increased while mean arterial pressure and arterial pH decreased. All of these changes returned to baseline values by 30 minutes.

Respiratory depression can be a problem when using propofol. In a study conducted to determine adverse effects of propofol with various preanesthetic regimens, 40 dogs were given propofol by IV push prior to isoflurane anesthesia following 1) no preanesthetic medication; 2) 0.1mg acepromazine/kg IM; 3) 0.2mg diazepam/kg IV; or acepromazine/butorphanol, 0.02/0.4mg/kg IM, respectively (Smith et al 1993). With no preanesthetic drugs, a variable period of apnea occurred in 34 of 40 dogs with cyanosis observed in 2 dogs. They found that adverse cardiopulmonary effects did occur but could be minimized by preanesthetic medication. When propofol was first tested and used clinically, it was administered by IV push usually within less than 10 seconds. There was a significant incidence of apnea associated with this process that has been reported to be as high as 85%. Cardiorespiratory effects of 8 mg propofol/kg of body weight were compared to 19mg thiopental/kg administered to mixed-breed dogs (Quandt et al 1998). In this study, they found that respiratory depression and an incidence of 50% apnea were major adverse effects produced by either anesthetic. However, as would be anticipated, recovery from propofol induced changes was faster than recovery after thiopental. When propofol became available in the U.S., it appeared that a slower rate of injection might be advantageous to avoid some of its adverse respiratory effects. To determine whether the drug should be given by IV push or as a 60 second bolus, investigators administered 4mg propofol/kg IV either rapidly or slowly to dogs premedicated with acepromazine and morphine (Murison 2001). Apnea was observed with both rates of administration but time to first breath was longer with the slower rate of propofol injection, e.g., 19.5 seconds following rapid injection and 28.8 seconds for slow rate of injection. Although this was only about 10 seconds longer, an important guideline is that the dose of propofol should be carefully titrated against the needs and responses of the individual patient as there is considerable variability in anesthetic reqirements among patients. Thus the 60 second bolus is recommended to minimize the depressant cardiac and respiratory effects seen after rapid bolus administration (Glowaski 1999). The cardiovascular effects of propofol are well tolerated in healthy animals but these effects may be more problematic in high-risk patients with intrinsic cardiac disease as well as in those with systemic disease. These data are important considerations for judicious use of propofol for anesthesia in all patients including seniors and geriatrics. Use of appropriate preanesthetic medication will allow lower doses of propofol to be used for intended purposes. Comparisons of effects of propofol in dogs and cats are listed in Table 2-1.

Table 2-1 Comparison of Propofol Administered to Dogs and Cats

Variable	Dog	Cat
Induction dose (unpremedicated)	5.5-7.0	8.0-13
Duration of effect	5-7 min	5-12 min
Time to standing recovery	10-20 min	30-45 min
Ease of ET intubation	Similar to barbiturates	Similar to barbiturates (Requires deeper level of anesthesia)
Lower maintenance dose; Duration of its effect	1.1mg/kg Effect lasts 2-6 min	1.1mg/kg Effect lasts 5-7 min
Higher maintenance dose; Duration of its effect	3.3mg/kg Effect lasts 6-10 min	4.4mg/kg Effect lasts 12-18 min
Effect of repeated maintenance doses on full recovery time	Minimal	Slight increase
Incidence of induction apnea	< 20%	< 2%
Primary side effect	Respiratory depression w/wo apnea	Paddling during recovery
Effect of consecutive day treatments	No adverse effects	Possible Heinz body anemia
Used with preanesthetics?	Induction dose decreased	Induction dose decreased Avoid using with ketamine
Use for induction prior to inhalation anesthesia	Because of quick recovery, need to increase initial recovery, concentration of inhalant	Because of quick need to increase initial concentration of inhalant

Prepared courtesy of CE Short.

Requirements for safe and prompt induction of anesthesia prior to inhalant anesthesia with and without surgery have been determined (Short 1999). When coupled with subjective responses to painful stimuli, EEG responses during propofol anesthesia provided clear evidence that satisfactory anesthesia could be achieved in experimental dogs. When propofol was used as the only anesthetic agent, a higher dose was required to induce an equipotent level of CNS depression than in premedicated dogs. Propofol induction dose requirements should be appropriately decreased by 20 to 80% when propofol is administered in combination with sedative or analgesic agents as part of a balanced technique as well as in elderly and debilitated patients (Morgan 1989; Geel 1991; Bufalari et al 1996). Because propofol does not have marked analgesic effects, use of local anesthetics, NSAIDs and opioids to provide postoperative analgesia improve the quality of surgical recovery after propofol anesthesia. When propofol was included in a comparative study to select an alternative regimen for cats with cardiomyopathy, it was found to be less preferable than a balanced technique with acepromazine, buprenorphine and etomidate (Akkerdass et al 2001). However, it is not uncommon for propofol to be given to cats with undiagnosed cardiomyopathy without incident.

On rare occasion particularly in smaller patients, pain on injection may be observed following IV push administration (Smith et al 1993, Weaver 1990). Excitatory or muscle tremors during or after infusion have been reported (Robertson et al 1992; Smedile et al 1996). Human patients report various sensations from a feeling of being warm or cold at the injection site to a severe burning feeling. Animals do not seem to be as sensitive but small dogs and cats may exhibit behavior that indicates an uncomfortable sensation. Giving propofol slowly as indicated by the instructions will eliminate most problems. Another method that may be used for small cats is to dilute the propofol concentration to 5mg/ml. From a survey to evaluate perioperative risk factors affecting neonatal survival after cesarean section, data from 807 cesearean-delivered litters (3908 puppies) were collected from 109 practices (Moon et al 2000). The most common methods of inducing and maintaining anesthesia were mask induction and maintenance with isoflurane (34%) and IV propofol for induction followed by isoflurane for maintenance (30%).

Propofol is a lipid-based emulsion capable of supporting microbial growth. As a result, guidelines for using this drug include wiping the neck of ampules or top of flip-top vials with alcohol before opening and being careful not to contaminate contents when loading syringes (Zacher et al 1991). Although it may appear safe to keep unused propofol for 2 days or longer, manufacturer guidelines suggest that the drug should be used the same day, preferably within 6 hours of opening the container (Downs et al 1991). The only reason to keep unused propofol overnight is based on cost. There is a potential risk of iatrogenic injury to patients given the drug that is kept beyond manufacturer guidelines and no benefits to patients who are given a tainted drug. A reasonable guideline is to not keep unused propofol overnight to be used the following day unless quality control measures have been established and followed. Stock supplies of propofol should not be kept in a temperature environment lower than 5°C or higher than 29°C. Thus, caution should be taken when storing propofol in a refrigerator or when kept in an enclosed area with an outside wall that would possibly allow temperatures to exceed the recommended limits. High or low temperatures will cause breakdown of the product and decrease efficacy of the drug.

Propofol should not be used in patients that may potentially be septic, e.g., tissue abscess, pyometritis, infected wound, etc. To determine if propofol could contribute to postoperative infection of clean surgical wounds, a retrospective study was conducted surveying 863 dogs and cats undergoing clean surgical procedures (Heldmann et al 1999). Investigators found that out of the total number of animals with clean wounds, 46 animals (13%) receiving propofol developed postoperative wound infections. This compared to an infection rate of 4% in animals not receiving propofol. In this study, animals receiving propofol were 3.8 times more likely to develop postoperative wound infections compared to animals not given propofol. However, this was a very small sample size and there were many factors that could have influenced these results. Based on the thousands of animal and human patients that have been given this drug, if infection of clean wounds was a significant risk factor with the use of propofol, it would have become evident a long time ago. However, this emphasizes that aseptic techniques be followed in opening containers of propofol to curtail the potential for extrinsic contamination.

One of the useful applications of propofol anesthesia in veterinary patients is for procedures that might need to be performed on consecutive days such as wound dressing changes. To determine effects of consecutive day anesthesia, 6 cats were given 6mg propofol/kg IV with anesthesia maintained for 30 min with 0.2-0.3mg/kg CRI propofol (Andress et al 1995). The initial protocol was designed such that each cat would be anesthetized for 30 min with propofol on 10 consecutive days. Following the 3rd day of propofol anesthesia, there was a significant increase from baseline in the mean percentage of Heinz bodies. However, hemolysis was not detected in any cat. In addition, recovery time significantly increased after the second day and five of the six cats developed generalized malaise, anorexia, and diarrhea on day 5, 6, or 7. Two cats developed facial edema. Because of these occurrences, the initial protocol was aborted as none of the cats were anesthetized on more than 7 consecutive days. Thus, caution should be taken when propofol is used for consecutive day anesthesia, especially in cats, and if adverse side-effects are observed, an alternative protocol should be selected. For a non-anesthetic application, 0.5 to 3.0mg propofol/kg was reported to have an appetite stimulating effect in dogs during the initial 15 minutes following injection (Long, 2000).

In summary, propofol causes brief dose-dependent cardiovascular and respiratory depression. It can be used as a traditional induction agent with maintenance of surgical anesthesia provided by an inhalation agent, e.g., halothane, isoflurane, or sevoflurane. It provides poor analgesia except at deep anesthetic levels. Propofol is considered to be an appropriate anesthetic in sighthounds but recovery from anesthesia might be expected to be somewhat longer than non-sighthounds (Robertson et al 1992; Court 1999b). As with certain injectable anesthetics, caution must be taken in patients with severe hepatic disease since biotransformation will be slower. This drug must only be given IV either using a single 60 second bolus, intermittent injection, or by CRI. The suggested dose-range for anesthesia induction in dogs is 5-7mg/kg and 8-13mg/kg for cats. If given following preanesthetic medication with a tranquilizer, opioid or alpha$_2$-adrenergic agonist, doses may be reduced as much as 80% (Bufalari 1996; Short 1999). Maintenance of anesthesia may be sustained using CRI at the rate of 0.4mg propofol/kg/min or by giving multiple 1mg/kg injections as needed (Hall 1987). Anesthesia can also be maintained following propofol with an inhalation anesthetic. The favorable recovery profile associated with propofol offers advantages over traditional anesthetics in clinical situations in which rapid recovery is important. Also, propofol compatibility with a large variety of preanesthetics has been an important criterion for its use as a safe and reliable IV anesthetic for induction and maintenance of general anesthesia and sedation in small animal veterinary practice. Recovery will usually be relatively quick, e.g., within 15 min, with little or no ataxia evident after 30 min.

Propofol / Thiopental

There are reports of compounding thiopental and propofol as a 1:1 by volume mixture for anesthesia induction: propofol (10mg/ml) and thiopental 25mg/ml). The dosage by volume of the mixture would be 0.45ml/kg or dosed at 1mg/lb (0.45mg/kg) as if the concentration in the bottle was 10mg/ml (Evans 2003). Given slowly to effect over 60 seconds, induction occurs rapidly and recoveries are usually without consequence: slower than with propofol alone but faster than with thiopental alone. No difference in recovery time should occur if an inhalation agent is used for maintenance. Echocardiographic evaluation of this combination was made in healthy dogs (Evans et al 2004). An initial dose of 5mg propofol/kg, 13mg thiopental/kg, or the mixture of 2mg/kg propofol with 6mg/kg thiopental was given and titrated until animals were intubated. There was no significant effect between treatments on systolic or diastolic ventricular wall thickness, left atrial diameter or systolic left ventricular diameter. NIBP decreased over time with each treatment and none of the changes was considered to be of clinical significance. It was concluded that a 1:1 mixture of propofol and thiopental could be used for induction as an alternative to either propofol alone or thiopental alone. Anesthetic and cardiorespiratory effects of this combination appear to be of similar quality to those of propofol alone but better than those of thiopental alone (Ko et al. 1999). Stability studies on this mixture have not been conducted so it would be best to discard any unused drug at the end of the day.

Propofol / Ketamine
Combining propofol and ketamine has been suggested as a possible alternative to using propofol alone. The combination was found to be about the same as propofol alone but not necessarily an advantage (Lerche et al. 2000). In this study, authors compared effects of these two treatments for anesthetic induction. Dogs were premedicated with acepromazine and meperidine followed by propofol, 4mg/kg alone, or with ketamine at 2mg/kg each, given IV with anesthesia maintained with halothane delivered in oxygen and nitrous oxide (1:2). Various cardiorespiratory variables were measured over a 30 minute period. Post-induction apnea, higher heart rates but not at tachycardic levels and muscle twitching were more common in the ketamine group but recovery times were similar. In another study, cardiovascular effects of equipotent maintenance anesthetic doses of propofol and propofol/ketamine were evaluated in cats (Ilkiw and Pascoe 2002). A loading dose of propofol 6.6mg/kg was followed by infusion of 0.22mg/kg/minute. After 60 minutes, the propofol infusion was decreased to 0.14mg/kg/minute and ketamine (loading dose 2mg/kg, infusion 23µg/kg/min) was administered. Response to a noxious stimulus with propofol was not changed by the addition of ketamine. They further concluded that propofol alone provided cardiopulmonary stability but the addition of ketamine did not offer any advantage. These results would suggest that this combination will not become a common protocol for use in dogs or cats.

Etomidate
Etomidate is a pure hypnotic first synthesized in 1965 and it has no analgesic properties. It was first evaluated in 1972 as an IV anesthetic induction agent for use in humans and was approved in 1983 for this purpose in the United States (Giese 1983). It is an imidazole prepared in vials containing 20mg of the white powder dissolved in a 10ml mixture of 35% propylene glycol and 65% water. It is 76% protein bound with pharmacokinetics in dogs being very similar to those of thiopental (Meuldermans 1976). Based on pharmacokinetics determined in cats, distribution half-life was 3 min with redistribution requiring 21 min (Wertz et al 1989). The elimination half-life was 2.9 hours. Its metabolic profile includes rapid hydrolysis by the liver and plasma that yields inactive byproducts. It has 11 times the potency of thiopental and there is a high incidence of spontaneous involuntary muscle movement, tremor, and hypertonus following IV injection in unsedated dogs (Kissin et al 1983). The associated muscle movements are not associated with epileptogenic or convulsant activity.

Initial studies regarding the sparing effects of etomidate on myocardial contractility indicated that this drug produced a dose-dependent depressant effect in dogs but at equianesthetic doses, was less than that produced by thiopental (Kissin et al 1983). However, studies in hypovolemic dogs demonstrated that minimal changes in cardiopulmonary function were produced by 1mg/kg etomidate suggesting that it would have good application for patients at risk (Pascoe et al 1992). Etomidate was shown to be part of a preferred anesthetic protocol in the Netherlands for cats with cardiomyopathy (Akkerdass et al 2001). In addition, a survey was conducted to review the use of selected sedatives and anesthetics in dogs and cats with cardiovascular diseases referred to a center in Switzerland for diagnostic, therapeutic, and surgical interventions (Skarda et al, 1995). They concluded that etomidate or thiopental was used in 30% of cases for IV induction followed by isoflurane for maintenance in the majority of procedures.

Studies in dogs indicated that etomidate can induce a variety of side effects including excitement, myoclonus, pain at site of injection, vomiting, hemolysis, and apnea (Muir 1989; Ko et al. 1993). Frequency of these undersirable effects was dose related and could be markedly attenuated or eliminated by diazepam, acepromazine, or morphine prior to etomidate administration. Pain following injection may be lessened if the drug is administered into a large vein. Etomidate inhibits increased plasma cortisol levels and aldosterone concentrations associated with surgical stress. Thus, one can anticipate that the drug will suppress adrenocortical function for 2 hours or more following administration in surgical patients (Kruse-Elliott 1987), an effect that would be advantageous in geriatric or high risk patients. This drug is more commonly used by veterinarians in European countries, especially for patients at risk and is often combined with an opioid. It has never achieved a sufficient level of popularity in the U.S. probably because of increased cost and undesirable side-effects including injection pain and muscle movements.

Opioids
Use of opioids, with or without a tranquilizer, by IV injection offers a useful alternative to more rapid inductions accomplished with an ultrashort acting barbiturate, ketamine combinations or propofol. There are minimal depressant effects on the circulatory system with some vasodilation in the coronary and peripheral circulation. Most opioids are considered to be respiratory depressants; therefore, attention should be given to supporting ventilation when necessary. Use of opioids as a technique for anesthetic management is confined to use in dogs, and as a general rule canine patients are not as prone to respiratory depression from opioids as are human patients. Cats may have bizarre reactions to opioids, which is very much dose-related. Low doses of opioids are appropriate for pain management in cats, but when high doses are needed, behavioral problems will follow. Further, use of opioids for anesthetic induction appears to have its best application in sick and depressed canine patients. It is best to administer an opioid slowly over a 2 to 4-min period to avoid severe hypotension due to vasodilation. If given too rapidly, stimulation of the central nervous system may induce seizures. Atropine is advised to avoid drug induced bradycardia.

Meperidine
Analgesic effects of meperidine are 9 times less than those of morphine, the drug has a spasmolytic effect similar to atropine and decreases salivary and respiratory secretions. Atropine should be given as premedication to help prevent bradycardia but tachycardia may be produced if the opioid is given IV too rapidly. The meperidine dose is 1 to 2mg/kg IV; 2 to 4mg/kg IM and for induction, meperidine is usually combined with a neuroleptic tranquilizer. However, this drug is used fairly infrequently for this purpose.

Oxymorphone
This semi-synthetic opioid analgesic has 70 to 130 times the potency of morphine and produces less sedation in the dog than morphine or meperidine. Depression of ventilation is less and the analgesic effect lasts longer because of its longer half-life. The induction dose is 0.05 to 0.2mg/kg IV or IM. With or without prior tranquilization, animals will respond to noise or movement; therefore, induction should be done in a quiet area. An IV drip is established at the onset and the opioid is injected as the fluids are delivered. An alternative is to administer the opioid directly through the catheter instead of into the drip set. If the calculated dose does not induce sufficient CNS depression, isoflurane or sevoflurane can be given by mask to supplement the opioid in order to reach a level sufficient to permit tracheal intubation. It must be emphasized that when opioids are used for premedication or anesthesia induction prior to maintenance with inhalation anesthetics, dose-dependent depression of spontaneous breathing may occur. This may affect both respiratory rate and tidal volume. If profound, it is advisable to control ventilation either mechanically or manually. Also, since all of the opioid effects can be reversed with an antagonist such as naloxone, depression of ventilation can be reversed to allow effective spontaneous breathing to resume. However, animals that fit this technique best are usually sick (physical status P3, P4, or P5) and ventilation should be controlled to prevent or correct respiratory acidosis. Reversal of the sedative effects from opioids with naloxone will usually reverse analgesic effects as well.

Neuroleptanesthesia / Balanced Anesthesia

It may be that common use of a neuroleptic tranquilizer with an opioid that produces a state of central nervous system (CNS) depression called neuroleptanalgesia is nearly extinct. In the 70's, 80's and most of the 90's, this was one of the most common methods of providing sedation and analgesia in canine patients for minor procedures. It was also used for induction for patients at risk. If nitrous oxide or a volatile liquid anesthetic was added with the neuroleptic and opioid, neuroleptanesthesia was achieved (Short 1987a). Balanced anesthesia usually described the circumstance when muscle relaxants or neuromuscular blocking agents were also used. Because of the common practice of using various analgesics and tranquilizers (not just neuroleptics) together with inhalants and/or injectable agents, neuroleptanalgesia/anesthesia is not the best description for modern anesthetic practice (Bissonnette 1999). Conscious or unconscious sedation and analgesia with drug combinations such as alpha$_2$ agonists, benzodiazepines, propofol, ketamine and opioids with diverse effects offer advantages without some of the undesirable side effects.

There are many possible drug combinations, which in a compounded form induce neuroleptanalgesia. This allows the anesthetist to increase the proportion of the tranquilizer in some situations, e.g., comparatively younger dogs or to decrease the dosage for patients at risk. One might also choose combinations of a barbiturate, minor tranquilizer such as diazepam or midazolam, ketamine, tiletamine/zolazapam, xylazine, medetomidine, along with an opioid agonist or mixed agonist to achieve the desired effect. The opioid might then be used throughout the procedure along with low concentrations of an inhalant anesthetic and/or ketamine by constant rate infusion (CRI), techniques that are used more commonly, especially for high risk patients.

The tranquilizer and opioid may be given independently with the advantage of giving the tranquilizer as premedication 15 to 30 minutes before induction with the opioid either used alone IV or combined with either a major or minor tranquilizer. When an opioid is given either continuously or intermittently during the procedure along with an inhalant such as isoflurane or sevoflurane, a very stable neuroleptanesthesia/balanced anesthetic state can be achieved. A local anesthetic may also be used at the incision site to allow lower concentrations of the more depressant anesthetic to be used. Recovery is usually rapid and the effects of the opioid can be either partially or completely reversed with an opioid antagonist such as naloxone. Combinations of a neuroleptic and opioid in addition to fentanyl and droperidol are meperidine/acepromazine, oxymorphone/acepromazine, butorphanol/acepromazine and are listed in Table 1-9.

Meperidine / Acepromazine

This combination in equal volumes (50mg/ml meperidine / 10mg/ml acepromazine) can be mixed and given for restraint and minor surgery to provide neuroleptananalgesia. If given IM or SQ, 0.5ml is used for small dogs 7 to 16kg and up to 1ml for larger patients. With the addition of atropine, this has been referred to as "Premix" in Canada. It is still used this way but not as often because of the availability of combinations with different opioids.

Oxymorphone / Acepromazine

Dogs and cats can be sedated with 0.02-0.1mg/kg of acepromazine and 0.01mg/kg atropine, 15 min pre-anesthesia. For dogs, 0.05 to 0.2mg/kg oxymorphone can be given IV to affect the desired depth of analgesia. These drugs can be combined and given IM but greater control of depth is achieved when administered separately. In cats, opioid dose should not exceed 0.1mg/kg. In dogs at risk (P3, P4, or P5) acepromazine is generally not included and is substituded with a benzodiazepine. Supplementation with isoflurane or sevoflurane may be advantageous to provide neuroleptanesthesia.

Oxymorphone or Hydromorphone / Diazepam or Midazolam

Diazepam (5mg/ml), at a dose of 0.2mg/kg given IV to effect, is advantageous in high-risk patients when used in combination with opioids. Midazolam is water soluble and can be used as an alternative to diazepam. This process is initiated by loading each drug in separate syringes, since diazepam cannot be mixed with the opioid. By inserting the needles of each syringe into the injection port of an IV catheter or drip set, diazepam is given simultaneously with oxymorphone (10mg/ml) with the induction process conducted over a 2 to 3-min period. Starting with oxymorphone, 0.25ml of each drug is given alternately at 15-s intervals until the desired level is reached. Dogs will respond to sound and movement thus this procedure should be conducted in a quiet area with no abrupt movements of the patient. This induction technique is very useful in P3, P4 and P5 canine patients. With slow deliberate positioning of the head and mouth, endotracheal intubation can be accomplished with the patient having a relatively strong palpebral reflex. Hydromorphone can be used at the same doses listed for oxymorphone.

Clinical Management and Antagonists

If profound sedation induced by the opioid is observed post-anesthesia, naloxone (0.1 to 0.4mg) or nalbuphine (0.5mg/kg) may be given IV 5 to 10 min after an inhalant is discontinued. Additional doses of the antagonist can be given as needed, which will depend upon the amount of the opioid given and duration of the procedure. As a general rule, up to 0.4mg of naloxone is sufficient to reverse respiratory depressant effects of the opioid. However, antagonists are often not needed because of the desired analgesia provided for surgical recovery.

Neuroleptanesthesia is of great value in geriatric and high-risk canine cases because of the minimal depressant effects to the cardiovascular system (Krahwinkel, 1975). The cardiovascular system remains stable as long as adequate fluids are given to prevent hypotension. As mentioned, opioids may depress spontaneous breathing but this is easily compensated with manual or mechanically controlled ventilation.

Alpha$_2$ Adrenergic Receptor Agonists
Use in Dogs

Even though dosages of 5 to 100mg/kg have been used in dogs, medetomidine at a median range of 30 to 40µg/kg IV can produce profound sedation, analgesia and recumbency lasting 40 to 60 minutes (Niffors 1989, Vainio 1989). IM dosages of 10 to 20µg/kg result in milder sedation, making it easier to handle and examine active patients. The response to IV administration is more predictable than for IM injection and requires approximately 75% of the IM dosage (England 1989). Once moderate dosages are administered (30 to 40µg/kg IV), supplemental medetomidine extends the duration of effects but does not result in significant increases in the depth of sedation and analgesia. In research trials with dogs, best results were obtained when medetomidine dosage was calculated on a body surface basis. This helps prevent varying responses often observed between small and large breed dogs. However, since calculating body surface is impractical in clinical practice, the package insert for medetomidine will provide an injection volume per weight guide based on a dose of 750µg IV or 1,000µg IM per square meter of body surface. It can be assumed that smaller, more high-strung breeds will require higher dosages than larger, calmer breeds. Large aggressive dogs will also require higher dosages.

Diagnostic or minor procedures can be completed following medetomidine administration. For example, minor dental procedures can be completed with the injection of medetomidine (30 to 40µg/kg IV or IM) and use of a mouth speculum. Care should be taken, since medetomidine is not an anesthetic and the dog can still bite down on anything in its mouth. The scope of minor surgical procedures in which medetomidine can be considered is increased by the use of local or regional nerve blocks.

When medetomidine is inadequate for more involved diagnostic and surgical procedures, general anesthesia must be considered. Even though many agents have been used to provide general anesthesia in conjunction with alpha$_2$-agonists, one should be advised that medetomidine will significantly reduce the dosage requirements for anesthetic agents in dogs (Tranquilli 1984; Räihä 1989a; Räihä 1989b; Räihä 1989c; Maze 1991; Ewing 1993). Even doses of 5 to 10µg/kg IV or IM will reduce requirements for anesthetia induction by 25 to 50%.

Use in Cats

Medetomidine has been administered for a wide range of procedures in cats (Vainio 1986, Young 1990). In Europe, dosages have ranged from 20 to 140µg/kg IM. A dose range of 80 to 100µg/kg IM has often been used to induce profound sedation and analgesia for diagnostic and minor surgical procedures. Profound relaxation and depression ensue. Clinical experience indicates that dosages exceeding 60µg/kg IM are not needed in the cat. A tendency toward bradycardia is present in the cat but does not appear to be as significant as in the dog. Lower doses of medetomidine (10 to 20µg/kg IM or IV) can effectively be used for preanesthetic medication in cats. With increasing medetomidine dosages, a corresponding reduction of up to 90% of anesthetic requirements should be expected.

Medetomidine/Ketamine Combinations

Numerous combinations of dissociative anesthetics with tranquilizers and sedatives are used in companion animal practice. Doses of medetomidine in the range of 5-15µg/kg would be considered a preanesthetic dose. Higher doses would be full sedative/analgesic level (Otto 2004). When xylazine is administered instead of medetomidine, xylazine dosages will range from 0.1-0.5mg/kg IM. Alpha$_2$ agonists have been shown to have an important role in sedation and analgesia when used alone or as a preanesthetic. Medetomidine (5µg/kg IV) combined with ketamine/diazepam has been shown to be useful for IV anesthesia induction in dogs (Ko et al. 1998). When used as a preanesthetic, dosages are usually reduced by 25-90% that of the alpha$_2$ agonist used as a sole medication. Likewise it should be recognized that even low dosages of alpha$_2$ agonists result in significant reduction in anesthetic dose requirements.

The combination of alpha$_2$ agonists with ketamine provides improved muscle relaxation and quality of anesthesia compared to ketamine alone (Table 2-2). Likewise heart rate does not slow with the combinations so much as when alpha$_2$ agonists are used as a sole medication. Butorphanol has a similar influence on anesthetic requirements as found with acepromazine. It does, however, have analgesic properties whereas acepromazine does not. When combined with medetomidine, the response is similar to that seen if dose is doubled, and duration lasts up to three times as long. Thus 5ug/kg medetomidine plus 0.2mg/kg butorphonol is equivalent to approximately 10ug/kg medetomidine. The combination of medetomidine with butorphanol produced more reliable and uniform sedation in dogs than did medetomidine alone (Ko et al. 2000). Medetomidine-Butorphanol combinations are listed in Table 2-3.

Table 2-2 — Medetomidine-Ketamine Combinations*

	Medetomidine (µg/kg IM)	Ketamine (mg/kg)
Dog	5-15	5-10 IV
	20	5-10 IV
	30	3 IM
	40	2.5-7.5 IM
	50	2.5 IM
Cat	5-20	15-20 IM
	50	7.5-10 IM
	80	5-7 IM

*Otto (2004)

Table 2-3   Medetomidine-Butorphanol Combinations*

	Medetomidine (µg/kg IM)	Butorphanol (mg/kg IM)
Dog	5-10	0.1-0.2
	20	0.1
	22	0.22
	30	0.2
	35	0.1

*Otto (2004)

Medetomidine-Propofol Combinations

When medetomidine is used as premedication prior to other injectable anesthetics such as propofol, lower dosage requirements of propofol can be used. Alpha$_2$-agonist / anesthetic combination may be used for induction, short surgical procedures with/without regional nerve blocks or in combination with inhalant anesthetics. Various dose combinations of propofol following medetomidine are listed in Table 2-4. The response to IV administration will be observed in 1-4 minutes whereas the responses after IM administration may take up to 6-10 min to reach maximum levels.

Table 2-4   Medetomidine-Propofol Combinations*

	Medetomidine (µg/kg IM)	Propofol (mg/kg IV)
Dogs	10	5-6
	20	4
	30	2
	40	1

*Otto (2004)

Anesthesia lasts 10-30 minutes following low dose alpha$_2$ agonists prior to IV propofol or IV ketamine whereas following ketamine given IM, effects may last up to two hours. Route of administration, dosage levels and number of repeat doses all increase duration. After anticipated levels of anesthesia are achieved, additional doses of alpha$_2$-agonists or ketamine are more likely to extend duration than to provide more profound levels of anesthesia. Expected responses from medetomidine in addition to sedation include: significant reduction in neurologic responses to noxious stimuli; an increase in vascular resistance with corresponding increase in blood pressure and decrease in heart rate; transient reduction in respiratory responses; transient reduction in insulin levels with increase in blood glucose.

Recoveries after alpha$_2$ agonist/anesthetic combinations are expected to be smooth. Recovery can be hastened by reversal with an appropriate antagonist. Atipamezole reverses sedation and analgesia and also side effects by competitive action at the receptor sites. Reversal following medetomidine or xylazine/proprofol results in smooth recovery whereas reversal following medetomidine or xylazine/ketamine may result in muscle rigor in dogs and cats or even seizure-like activity in dogs if the concurrent tissue level of ketamine is high.

Adverse effects of the combinations include emesis and vomiting, salivation, muscle fasciculation and limb paddling. On rare occasions, pulmonary edema has been observed. More profound respiratory depression, more frequent cardiac arrhythmia and hypertension may be associated with higher doses of the drug combination. The concurrent usage of anticholinergics, especially atropine at 0.04mg/kg IM or IV, is more likely to be associated with prolonged hypertension than when an anticholinergic drug is not used.

Role of Diazepam

The addition of diazepam to the protocol is to achieve smooth inductions. The duration of diazepam influence on the quality of analgesia and anesthesia is limited to a period of approximately 30 minutes following injection.

Role of Other Opiods

Most of the available opiods have been administered in combination with xylazine or medetomidine. The combined effect of 5-10ug/kg medetomidine IM added to 0.5-1.0mg/kg morphine IM or 0.2mg/kg hydromorphone IM can produce profound sedation/analgesia. Anesthetic dose requirements will be significantly reduced compared to many other preanesthetic medications or combinations.

Additional Considerations and Patient Monitoring with Alpha$_2$ Agonists (Figure 2-7)

Medetomidine mediates an increase in systemic blood pressure, a corresponding decrease in heart rate and reduction in cardiac output. Experience has shown that these physiologic changes are well endured in exercise-tolerant dogs and cats. Pretreatment with atropine or glycopyrrolate more than 5 minutes before administration of medetomidine will usually prevent bradycardia. Anticholinergic use, however, also will prolong duration of the hypertension. The increased myocardial work is tolerated well in young healthy P1 dogs and cats but may be detrimental in geriatric patients or animals with myocardial disease. Concurrent administration of anticholinergic agents following medetomidine-induced bradycardia can result in transient dysrhythmias as the anticholinergic action is initiated. Even though higher heart rates are observed with concurrent usage of anticholinergics and alpha$_2$ agonists, this does not assure improvement in cardiac output.

Caution should be taken with the use of an anticholinergic to treat the induced slow heart rate. Giving routine anticholinergic treatment for medetomidine-induced bradycardia is not recommended. Once the cardiovascular changes mediated by medetomidine are evident, respiratory effects may concurrently be observed. As a result, it has been shown that premedication with glycopyrrolate or atropine sulfate protects against severe bradycardia and is safer for this purpose than if used as a therapeutic measure.

Respiration can be depressed at higher medetomidine dosage levels. Mucous membrane color is not as effective an index for assessing adequate ventilation during medetomidine sedation as it is with injectable anesthetics. The cyanotic appearance is partly due to changes in peripheral perfusion mediated by medetomidine. Measurements of oxygen saturation or arterial blood gases provided supportive data that ventilation was adequate in healthy animals receiving an appropriate dose of medetomidine. Animals with preexisting heart or lung diseases are more likely to be compromised by alpha$_2$ agonist medication.

Direct arterial blood pressure, arterial blood gas, and pH measurements accurately reflect medetomidine's influence on cardiopulmonary function. Because these measurements are not currently practical in small animal practice, noninvasive blood pressure monitoring is encouraged. In medetomidine affected animals, noninvasive blood pressure monitors must be able to measure blood pressures at heart rates below 60 beats per min. Persistent cardiac dysrrhythmias will make NIBP measurements difficult to obtain as well. The influence of alpha$_2$ agonists on peripheral vasoconstriction affects pulse quality so NIBP measurements may be difficult to obtain in very small patients.

Monitoring of patients often includes use of pulse oximetry. The tongue is the most common site for placement of the sensor. Because of changes in perfusion during medetomidine sedation, accuracy of oxygen saturation readings is compromised. Pulse oximeters with excellent sensitivity and fast calibration are more likely to be effective in determining oxygen saturation. Oxygen saturation values determined from arterial blood samples have been higher than those determined by pulse oximeters. In clinical practice, when there is concern that ventilation is inadequate after any sedative/anesthetic administration, oxygen is the treatment of choice. Reversal of medetomidine by atipamezole should correct cardiopulmonary changes.

Schematic Response to Medetomidine Administration

↓

Injection Dose Per Package Insert

IV	IM
1.0 Full response within 2-5 minutes	**1.2.0 Full response within 10-15 minutes**
1.1 Sedation and analgesia	2.1 Sedation and analgesia
1.2 Vasoconstriction	2.2 Vasoconstriction
1.3 ↑ blood pressure	2.3 ↑ blood pressure
1.4 ↓ heart rate (potential A-V block)	2.4 ↓ heart rate (potential A-V block)
1.5 Recumbency/muscle relaxation	2.5 Recumbency/muscle relaxation
1.6 Slight depression of respiration	2.6 Slight depression of respiration
1.7 ↓ in insulin levels	2.7 ↓ in insulin levels
1.8 ↑ in blood glucose	2.8 ↑ in blood glucose
1.9 ↑ in urine production	2.9 ↑ in urine production
2.1.0 Duration	**2.2.0 Duration**
1.1 Diagnostic and minor surgical procedures	2.1 Diagnostic and minor surgical procedures
1.2 Recovery without atipamezole	2.2 Recovery without atipamezole
1.3 Recovery with atipamezole	2.3 Recovery with atipamezole
1.4 Post-procedural sedation and analgesia	2.4 Post-procedural sedation and analgesia
3.1.0 Side effects	**3.2.0 Side effects**
1.1 Bradycardia (pretreatment with anticholinergics)	2.1 Bradycardia (pretreatment with anticholinergics)
1.2 Hypertension (transient: use of concurrent medications)	2.2 Hypertension (transient: use of concurrent medications)
1.3 Excessive depression of respiration (when to use oxygen)	2.3 Excessive depression of respiration (when to use oxygen)
1.4 Inadequate muscle relaxation (when to add anesthetic)	2.4 Inadequate muscle relaxation (when to add anesthetic)
1.5 Prolonged effect (use of atipamezole)	2.5 Prolonged effect (use of atipamezole)
4.1.0 Inadequate sedation/analgesia	**4.2.0 Inadequate sedation/analgesia**
1.1 Dosage incorrect	2.1 Incorrect or injection in fat or SQ
1.2 Predose excitement	2.2 Predose excitement
1.3 Procedure too painful or involved	2.3 Procedure too painful or involved
1.4 Need to add other medication	2.4 Need to add other medication
5.1.0 Concurrent use of tranquilizers and analgesics	**5.2.0 Concurrent use of tranquilizers and analgesics**
1.1 Tranquilizers (e.g., acepromazine)	2.2 Tranquilizers (e.g., acepromazine)
1.2 Opioid agonist/antagonists (e.g., butorphanol)	2.2 Opioid agonist/antagonists (e.g., butorphanol)
1.3 Opioid agonists (e.g., morphine, oxymorphone)	2.3 Opioid agonists (e.g., morphine, oxymorphone)
1.4 Regional nerve blocks	2.4 Regional nerve blocks

6.1.0	**Anesthetic induction**	6.2.0	**Anesthetic induction**
1.1	Ketamine	2.1	Ketamine
1.2	Thiobarbiturate	2.2	Thiobarbiturate
1.3	Propofol	2.3	Propofol
1.4	Inhalants	2.4	Inhalants
7.1.0	**Complications**	7.2.0	**Complications**
1.1	Heart block	2.1	Heart block
1.2	"Blue gums"	2.2	"Blue gums"
1.3	Hypertension	2.3	Hypertension
1.4	Post-procedural analgesia	2.4	Post-procedural analgesia
1.5	"Can't do procedure"	2.5	"Can't do procedure"
1.6	Inadequate sedation	2.6	Inadequate sedation
1.7	Poor recovery	2.7	Poor recovery
1.8	Excessive central nervous system depression with/without anesthetic	2.8	Excessive central nervous system depression with/without anesthetic
1.9	Contributing factors which could cause death	1.9	Contributing factors which could cause death
8.1.0	**Resuscitation**	8.2.0	**Resuscitation**
1.1	Oxygen (airway/breathing/massage, if arrested)	2.1	Oxygen (airway/breathing/massage, if arrested)
1.2	Reversal (atipamezole)	2.2	Reversal (atipamezole)
1.3	Supportive therapy	2.3	Supportive therapy

Figure 2-7 Schematic Response to Medetomidine Administration.

Reversal of Medetomidine's Effects

Medetomidine's central and peripheral effects are reversible with the alpha$_2$ antagonist atipamezole (Laine 1986, Scheinin 1988, Savola 1989, Vainio 1990, Vaha-Vahe 1990). The dosage recommended is a 5:1 ratio of atipamezole to medetomidine. Note that concentration of the preparation is 5mg/ml for atipamezole and 1mg/ml for medetomidine. Atipamezole competes with medetomidine at alpha$_2$ receptors. It can be effective in reversing all responses to alpha$_2$ receptors including sedation and analgesia. It does not reverse the effects of other medications. Dosage requirements for atipamezole can be reduced by 20 to 80% if more than 1 hour has lapsed since medetomidine administration. Use of other alpha$_2$ adrenergic antagonists to reverse medetomidine has not been thoroughly investigated.

Summary

Alpha$_2$ agonists induce predictable dose-dependent levels of sedation in both dogs and cats. Many studies support the safe and effective use of medetomidine in veterinary practice. Medetomidine is more potent than xylazine and the intensity and duration of effect are dose-dependent. Even though there are hemodynamic changes, medetomidine has proven to be a useful drug when used appropriately in P1 and P2 patients. It can be reversed by the alpha$_2$ antagonist antipamezole. Alpha$_2$ agonists are effective premedication agents when used before both injectable and inhalant anesthesia. Results indicating that subjects lack responsiveness to noxious stimuli support the classification of alpha$_2$ agonists both as sedatives and analgesics.

Dissociative Anesthesia

Dissociative anesthetics were introduced in the 1960's for use in man and animals. This was a new group of drugs that did not appear to be receptor oriented, producing CNS effects quite different from those induced by opioids, barbiturates and inhalation anesthetics. Phencyclidine was the most widely used dissociative anesthetic in primates and was capable of producing an anesthetic-like state that seemed to separate or dissociate patients from the environment. This dissociation was caused by interruption of CNS impulses and differential depression of various areas in brain. Animals appeared to be awake with active ocular, oral, laryngeal and swallowing reflexes. Eyelids remained open with pupils dilated and instead of relaxation; muscle tone might even be increased. Some patients even had extensor rigidity, tonic spasticity and evidence of CNS stimulation including apparent convulsive activity. Clinicians were concerned because animals appeared to be observing activities in the operating room.

Ketamine HCl

Ketamine is chemically related to phencyclidine and cyclohexamine. It is a dissociative agent that has acquired a unique place in clinical veterinary practice. Since its development in 1963 and the first report in humans by Domino and later by Corssen et al in 1969, a much better understanding of its anesthetic, sedative and analgesic properties has been gained from extensive clinical experience and research. Amnesia is known to occur in human patients but only can be speculated to occur in animals. One of the first clinical reports on ketamine appeared in 1970 relating experiences in cats (Commons 1970). Onset of surgical anesthesia seemed to be induced in one to eight minutes following IM injection. Tonic-clonic spasms occurred along with active palpebral and pedal reflexes, eye lids remained open and recovery took as long as 5 hours. This was encouraging news and other authors followed over the next 2 years with articles on the use of ketamine in primates, cats and dogs (Beck 1971; Humphrey 1971; Kaplan 1972; Amend et al. 1972; Beck 1972; Bree et al. 1972; DeYoung et al. 1972). Birth of the ketamine era happened about the same time as halothane and methoxyflurane were making a big impact on veterinary anesthesia. Most practitioners had been using pentobarbital so this seemed like a major step with the advantage that ketamine could be given IM. Simple but dangerous was a label placed on ketamine. Experience when the drug was used alone at high doses led to recognition of undesirable rough emergence reactions, prolonged recoveries, undesirable renal and cardiovascular effects and suspected lack of visceral analgesia (Short, 1987b). Prolonged duration of effect occurred in healthy patients owing to probable abnormal metabolites. Some of the metabolites of ketamine have analgesic effects and contribute to the anesthetic action of the parent compound (Heavner and Bloedow, 1979). Even with these side effects, some practitioners were adamant about ketamine filling a void that was long overdue even calling it an excellent anesthetic without research to support this contention (Myers 1973). Caution was given early in its development that ketamine should not be used alone in dogs (Bree et al 1972). Because of its questionable ability to ablate abdominal visceral pain, ketamine was advised not to be used alone for ovariohysterectomy or other abdominal surgical procedures (Haskins et al., 1975).

Attempts to gain FDA veterinary approval for use of ketamine as an anesthetic in dogs was abandoned primarily because of numerous undesirable side effects including seizure-like activity, muscle tremors and poor skeletal muscle relaxation. Subsequently, cardiopulmonary consequences and clinical characteristics of 10mg/kg ketamine given IV were evaluated in dogs (Haskins et al 1985). In this study, ketamine was found to produce unsatisfactory anesthesia for surgical purposes. Muscle tone was extreme and exuberant spontaneous movement was virtually continuous. Core temperature was also increased. In more recent years, ketamine has been considered to be more of a chemical immobilizer than an anesthetic (Taylor 1999, Robertson 2002a) but it has regained viability as an effective drug when administered by constant rate infusion (CRI) especially with opioids (Reboso-Morales 1999).

Ketamine had its primary application when used alone in primates, exotics, and cats. Its effects are characterized by providing somatic analgesia, weak or no visceral analgesia (Sawyer et al. 1990 and 1993), near normal pharyngeal and laryngeal reflexes, skeletal muscle tone, cardiovascular stimulation with hypertension and tachycardia and an increase in cerebral spinal fluid pressure. Severe respiratory depression and airway obstruction can occur in animals given ketamine alone or in combination with other drugs. Respiratory rate is usually rapid and shallow shortly after administration but may or may not return to normal during maintenance. The pattern of respiration is also changed by ketamine as the pause occurs at the end of inspiration rather than at the end of expiration (inspiratory pause or apneustic breathing).

Not all of these characteristics are desirable but ketamine can be a very useful drug with proper patient selection. Although cats given ketamine may maintain protective laryngeal reflexes, endotracheal intubation is advised but it must be understood that this does not guarantee an airway (Haskins et al 1975). Studies using radiopaque contrast medium and radiography demonstrated competency of the laryngeal closure reflexes of cats with ketamine doses between 12 and 48mg/kg (Robinson 1986a). However, incidence of aspiration is significantly increased when ketamine is given with sedatives and analgesics. One reason is the increased salivation that occurs with ketamine use. Laryngeal adductor responses to afferent stimulation play an important role in airway protection. Laryngospasm is a common consequence in cats and this may occur from repeated attempts for tracheal intubation. Studies to determine the role of NMDA receptors in modulating these responses demonstrated that ketamine would have an effect in long latency laryngeal responses to afferent stimulation (Ambalavanar et al. 2002). As a result, it behooves one to be patient and not attempt to intubate cats until reflex responses are sufficiently suppressed with ketamine. Exposure of the larynx is improved and laryngospasm lessened by use of an appropriate topical local anesthetic. Tracheal intubation in cats is less difficult if ketamine is combined with a benzodiazapine or an alpha$_2$ agonist.

Severe respiratory depression and airway obstruction can occur with ketamine alone or in combination with other drugs. Immobilization from ketamine may cause respiratory obstruction due to the patient becoming wedged in the corner of a cage or against an object. As a result, animals given ketamine or any other similar CNS depressant should never be left unattended since they cannot always protect their airway. Besides, it is just good anesthetic practice.

The Changing Role of Ketamine

Ketamine's role in clinical anesthesia has changed as a result of evolving concepts of its mechanism of action, advantages of alternative routes of administration and a better understanding of how to use the drug with sedatives, hypnotics and analgesics. Supplementation with drugs including opioids, benzodiazepinies and alpha$_2$ receptor agonists were found to reduce many undesirable side effects and because of this, ketamine has found many useful applications in veterinary practice. There have been a number of reviews on ketamine including White et al. in 1982 and those published at the time of its 25th anniversary (Reich 1989, Domino 1990). A current review of the literature illustrated that ketamine is used in many different ways but not as a sole anesthetic.

Ketamine has a molecular weight of 238 and a pKa of 7.5. It is water-soluble and the lipid solubility is 10 times greater than that of thiopental. The molecular structure is that of a cyclohexanoane and contains a chiral center at the C-2 carbon so that two enantiomers of the molecule exist: (S)-ketamine and (R)-ketamine (Adams 1998). *Enantiomers are chemical compounds whose molecular structures have a mirror-image relationship to each other.* Racemic ketamine, known commonly as ketamine HCl under many different brand names, contains equal concentrations of the two enantiomers. Analgesic and anesthetic potency of (S)-ketamine is about 3 times greater than that of (R)-ketamine and the pharmacologic profile of the racemic mixture is comparable to that of the (S)-enantiomer alone. The enantiomer alone had faster elimination and allowed improved control of the anesthetic state with reduced drug load. Cardiopulmonary and chemical restraining effects of racemic ketamine and its enantiomers was evaluated in dogs (Muir and Hubbel, 1988). No significant differences were found between ketamine and its enantionmers. To evaluate the effects of (S)-ketamine (6mg/kg) for anesthesia induction in dogs, 0.5mg/kg diazepam or 0.2mg/kg of midazolam were combined with the enantiomer (Riviera 2002). Dogs were premedicated 20 minutes before induction with 0.1mg/kg acepromazine and 5mg fentanyl/kg. No statistical differences were found in all variables although time to intubation was about 20 seconds faster with the midazolam combination. Based on these data, it would appear that ketamine enantionmers do not have much if any advantage over racemic ketamine.

As noted, the "anesthetic" state of ketamine is associated with adverse effects of hypersalivation, hallucinations (suspected but not proven in animals) and marked sympathomimetic reactions. The analgesic, anesthetic and sympathomimetic effects are mediated by different sites of action. NMDA receptor antagonism is the most important neuropharmacological mechanism for the analgesic effects of ketamine (Adams 1998; Olivar and Laird 1999; Castroman and Ness 2002). The same mechanism may be involved in neuroprotective potency of the drug. Effects on opioid receptors may also contribute to the analgesic effects and dysphoric reactions associated with ketamine. Ketamine's affinity for opioid receptors is not completely understood but there is some evidence to support this concept (Baker et al 2002, Mikkelsen et al 1999, Yamakura et al 1999). Naloxone has been shown to reverse part but not all of the adverse behavioral effects thought to be due to stimulation of sigma opioid receptors.

Oral Ketamine
Oral ketamine is now being effectively used for preanesthetic sedation in young children. Intraoral or mucusal administration of ketamine has also been used as a means of chemical restraint of very mean cats. If the only target the animal will provide is an open mouth while charging the front of the cage (door closed) and hissing, squirting ketamine into the mouth of the charging cat can be very effective for chemical restraint. Generally, there is only one chance of giving ketamine by this method probably because of the bitter taste and the insult. After being squirted, cats usually register their complaints with their mouth closed. Once physically restrained, anesthesia induction can be continued with an inhalation anesthetic.

Wetzel and Ramsey (1998) compared four regimens for sedating cats by intraoral administration prior to euthanasia: medetomidine (0.5mg/kg); ketamine (5mg/kg); medetomidine (0.5mg/kg) and ketamine (5mg/kg); and medetomidine (0.5mg/kg) and ketamine (10mg/kg). Cats were evaluated for degree of sedation at 3-minute intervals for 60 minutes. The most effective and reliable method was found when 0.5mg/kg detomidine was combined with 10mg/kg ketamine. Most of these drugs will be absorbed through the mucus membranes but some will be lost in the saliva and from head shaking.

Nonmedical Use of Ketamine
Ketamine became a controlled substance (C-III) in 1998 by U.S. Drug Enforcement Administration (DEA). Although ketamine was known for its substance abuse potential early on, it took more than 30 years for it to be listed by the DEA. Veterinary hospitals were targeted for break-ins by addicts because of the stock supplies of ketamine and these still occur. In addition, there are many instances of employees being drawn to its addictive properties (Shomer 1992). Ketamine users can become dependent on the drug with craving and high tolerance but no evidence of physiological withdrawal syndrome (Jansen 2001). Ketamine dependence is linked to effects that are not only common to cocaine and amphetamine but also to opioids, alcohol and cannabis. The psychological attractions of its distinctive psychedelic properties are well known. Ketamine produces effects of a psychological nature that usually last about 30 minutes, depending on route of administration: oral, buccal or parenteral injection (Quail et al 2001). The psychotropic effects of ketamine range from the expected dissociation and depersonalization to psychotic experiences that include a sensation of feeling light, body distortion, absence of sense of time, novel experiences of cosmic oneness and out-of-body experiences (Pal et al 2002). In a clinical setting while in the process of attempting to administer an IM injection of 80mg ketamine to a cat, the animal struggled at the precise moment of injection (Sawyer & Hoogstraten 1980). It was estimated that the person administering the drug had inadvertently self injected 30mg ketamine IM into thumb muscle. Within 3 minutes, as the subject described following recovery, symptoms of blurred vision, leg

weakness and sensation of walking down the hall many feet in front of the body were felt. About 15 minutes later, both hands felt much larger than the head and the subject was inwardly apprehensive and frightened about being left alone even though she was never left unattended. The subject was incapable of expressing this very unpleasant experience even though she said that she felt fine. These effects lasted about 45 minutes. From reports in humans, it can take as little as 3mg in an adult to induce a "ketamine trip" (Johnstone 1973). Abuse of telazol which contains tiletamine, a drug similar to ketamine, can also occur even to the point of it being used for suicide (Quail et al 2001, Cording et al 1999).

Veterinary hospital owners and managers must be aware that there are warning signs of ketamine addiction including changes in behavioral characteristics of individuals (Dillman 1998). Finding small syringes in unusual places and diminished effects of the drug in veterinary patients should not be ignored. Small amounts of the drug removed from a ketamine vial for non-medical purposes will usually be replaced with water or saline so a change in volume will not be noticed. Stock supplies should be kept in a well secured location with limited access. Even though ketamine is a C-III drug, it should be treated as if it were classified as a C II substance, same as narcotics and barbiturates.

Clinical Management

Induction with ketamine can be accomplished by either IM or IV injection. If 10 to 20mg/kg is given IM, onset of effect will be noted within the first 1 to 2 minutes. If given IV, 1 to 2mg/kg will result in a more rapid onset but duration of action will be shorter than if given IM. It can be used for procedures lasting less than 30 min but a 2 to 6-h recovery period may follow. It can also be used for induction either IM or IV to facilitate intubation and maintenance provided with an inhalation agent but this is usually done in combination with other sedatives. Caution must be taken to avoid severe respiratory depression by using light levels of inhalation anesthesia early, and as ketamine is metabolized and excreted, anesthesia can be maintained by increasing the levels of inhalation anesthesia.

An increase in intraocular pressure produced by ketamine is a result of increased tone in extraocular muscles and this limits its use for surgery of the eye. It should not be used alone in cats with heart disease, severe tacycardia, hyperthyroidism, renal disease or chronic urinary obstruction. Animals should be allowed to recover from ketamine with skillful neglect. That is, they should be allowed to recover in a cage under observation, undisturbed and unstimulated. This will promote a smoother and more peaceful recovery. Ketamine is a hallucinogenic drug in adult humans and it appears to produce similar effects in cats. Cats occasionally may dig at their mouth as if a bone was lodged between the upper arcade or look at the floor with wild back and forth eye and head motions as if watching an imagined tennis match. It is difficult to know if cats hallucinate, but if their recovery is accompanied by wild emergence delirium, 0.05 to 0.1mg/kg of acepromazine may be beneficial. A darkened room may also help to smooth recovery from ketamine.

An anticholinergic should be given as premedication to reduce salivary secretions. Induction via the IV route offers more control of depth and a shorter recovery period. Additional doses should be 30 to 50% of the induction dose. Indications for additional drug are based on the response to stimulation and lack of visceral analgesia.

Drug Combinations with Ketamine

To minimize side effects of ketamine, various drug combinations were found to be effective. The most common of these included acepromazine, diazepam, midazolam, oxymorphone, butorphanol, xylazine or medetomidine. These drugs also allowed doses of ketamine to be reduced as much as 25%, improved muscle relaxation, and produced fewer side effects (Reid & Frank 1972; Short & Paddleford 1976; Manziano & Manziano 1978). A key finding in studies to evaluate these combinations is that they should only be used for chemical restraint, anesthesia induction or minor surgery. It is also recognized that ketamine provides different levels of analgesia, e.g., better somatic analgesia but little or no visceral analgesia. Although ketamine produces profound sedation, it does little to block visceral pain (Sawyer et al, 1990 and 1993). These studies demonstrated that ketamine is a weak visceral analgesic, that diazepam and acepromazine do not enhance this effect and that 0.1mg/kg butorphanol produces long lasting analgesia alone and in combination with ketamine in cats. Consequently, ketamine should not be used alone for intra-abdominal or intrathoracic procedures unless supplemented with an inhalation anesthetic or appropriate opioid analgesic (Sawyer 1987). Clinical evidence of this differential effect is demonstrated during an OHE in cats where a complete absence of response is observed during skin incision (Short 1987b). However, when the ovarian pedicle is manipulated, animals will respond physiologically with movement and if not intubated, may vocalize. In general, a standard dose of atropine or gycopyrrolate should be used with any of these combinations.

Ketamine / Acepromazine

Acepromazine / ketamine does not provide effective surgical anesthesia and analgesia for deep abdominal procedures, fracture repair, decompression laminectomy, and cesarean section even though it was reported by Manziano & Manziano in 1978. Considerable advances in knowledge have been made over the past 25 years regarding the effects of ketamine and combinations. Acepromazine is not an analgesic and it is now known that ketamine is better at augmenting analgesic effects of other drugs rather than providing profound visceral analgesia by itself. Usually acepromazine/ketamine is given IM as an induction agent for cats, preceding an inhalation anesthetic by mask to allow endotracheal intubation and maintenance of anesthesia with an inhalant agent. Others may give acepromazine (0.05-0.1mg/kg) as preanesthetic medication 30 to 60 minutes before ketamine (10-30mg/kg). Butorphanol (0.1mg/kg) is often added to this combination to provide effective visceral analgesia but there are better ways of providing surgical anesthesia in a clinical setting for major surgery, including OHE. Regarding procedures for mass sterilization of feral female cats, see comments below.

Ketamine / Diazepam

The combination of ketamine and diazepam, referred to as ket/val by many, has been found to be most advantageous for IV anesthesia induction in cats. It all started when it became known that diazepam, that is not water soluble, could be mixed with ketamine and safely given IV. The low dose of ketamine allowed patients to not have much of a hangover effect and the diazepam given simultaneously with ketamine seemed to blunt the sympathomimetic effects of ketamine (Haskins et al. 1986, Chen et al. 1989). In some practices, ket/val is the only IV induction agent used for dogs and cats. Ketamine-diazepam when combined with nitrous oxide has also been promoted as a circulatory system-sparing type of anesthesia for experimental surgery in animals, especially when used with opioids to provide adequate analgesia (Lesser et al. 1993). It is also reported to be of practical use in dogs with acute cardiac tamponade (Chen et al 1989). Ket/val is usually given in a 50-50 by volume mixture of ketamine (100mg/ml) and diazepam (5mg/ml). It can be mixed in a syringe or a multiple dose vial. Anecdotal reports indicate that some generic brands of diazepam that are of a different concentration and with a different solvent may not be compatible with ketamine. It is a matter of convenience to mix ketamine and diazepam in a multiple dose vial. However, the issue of physical compatibility and stability over time is another matter. Studies by Lechner and Kreuscher (1989) indicated that when ketamine was mixed with isotonic infusion solutions of 5% fructose, 5% glucose or 0.9% NaCl, all were physically true homogenous solutions with no change over a 24 hour period. Beyond that time, small amounts of dissolved particles were found. Information on stability and efficacy of the mixture is not known. Again, anecdotal reports suggest that the ketamine-diazepam mixture can be used within 7 days but there is nothing in the literature to support this recommendation. Therefore, it would be prudent not to use ketamine-diazepam more than 24 hours after mixing.

Recommended IV dosage is 0.1ml/kg (1ml / 20lbs). An additional 0.1ml is usually added to the syringe to assure adequate dosage for induction. The best way to administer ket/val is not by IV push but rather over a period of 1-2 minutes. Because tissue uptake of diazepam is slower than ketamine, a longer injection process allows the effects of the tranquilizer to take effect along with that of ketamine (Klotz et al 1976). Thus 25% of the calculated dose should be given initially and then followed by the same rate at 15 to 30 second intervals until the desired level is reached or the calculated dose has been given. Although commonly used in cats, many veterinarians also use this drug combination in dogs for anesthesia induction or minor procedures. Based on a study comparing thiopental, propofol and ketamine-diazepam for evaluation of laryngeal function in dogs, it was determined that ketamine-diazepam was not as effective as the other two agents (Gross et al. 2002). Because of cardiovascular stability in patients with cardiac disease, ketamine-diazepam may be preferable to thiopental and propofol depending upon the risk category of the patient (Kolata 1986). However, one must be cautious when using ketamine-diazepam for induction of anesthesia which will be maintained with isoflurane or sevoflurane. The inhalant should be introduced gradually at low vaporizer settings in order to avoid severe cardiac depression as the affects of the induction agent dissipate.

Ketamine / Midazolam

In the continuing search for better drug combinations with ketamine, the benzodiazepine midazolam seemed to have great potential due its water-soluble characteristics and greater potency compared to diazepam. Midazolam has also been shown to be compatible in solution with ketamine for up to 24 hours (Lectner and Kreuscher 1989). An additional advantage with this combination is that it can be given IM or IV. The dosage of 10mg/kg ketamine-midazolam 0.2mg/kg given IM produced reliable sedation in aged cats that was adequate for radiography or minor procedures (Chambers and Dobson 1989). Ketamine-diazepam and ketamine-midazolam (K 5.5mg/kg–D or M 0.28mg/kg) were evaluated in greyhounds, presumably as an alternative to thiobarbiturates (Hellyer et al. 1991). Time to intubation was significantly shorter with ketamine-midazolam but all other variables were not different between these two induction methods. In fact, they offered that there was little advantage over ketamine-diazepam. Ilkiw et al (1996 and 1998) evaluated variable doses of midazolam with 3mg/kg ketamine in cats. The purpose of these studies was to determine beneficial and/or detrimental effects of a range of midazolam doses from 0.0 to 5.0mg/kg. All doses of midazolam produced adverse effects that were almost entirely due to the tranquilizer rather than to ketamine. Although it was not the intent of this study to evaluate the effective dose of ketamine-midazolam, it does illustrate the importance of using a high enough dose of ketamine when combined with the benzodiazipine.

The best utility of the midazolam-ketamine combination would be that it would have minimal cardiorespiratory effects. It would also help to know the best method of IV administration, e.g., by bolus injection or infusion. Cardiovascular and cardiorespiratory effects of ketamine-midazolam given by IV bolus and infusion, alone and during isoflurane anesthesia, were evaluated in dogs (Jacobson and Hartsfield, 1993a and 1993b). The experimental protocol included administering a mixture in the same syringe of 10mg/kg ketamine and 0.5mg/kg midazolam as a bolus over a 30 second period. They also administered this same mixture as an infusion over 15 minutes. For infusions, 5ml of ketamine (100mg/ml), 5ml of midazolam (5mg/ml), and 90 ml of 0.9% NaCl were mixed in a sterile plastic container just prior to administration. A dosage of 2ml/kg was then delivered by infusion pump over 15 minutes. Rates of administration were 0.667mg/kg/minute for ketamine and 0.033mg/kg/minute for midazolam. In the first study, ketamine-midazolam was given for induction of anesthesia (1993a) while the second paper presented data from the two methods of administration in isoflurane anesthetized dogs (1993b). Bolus or infusion of the solution induced minimal cardiorespiratory effects with the exception of a significant increase in heart rate. However, based on data when ketamine-midazolam was given with isoflurane, the combination should be used with great caution. Isoflurane blocked cardiostimulatory effects of ketamine-midazolam leading to decreases in various cardiovascular variables and there were differences between bolus and infusion administrations. This appeared to be dose dependent as ketamine-midazolam given by bolus injection produced greater decreases in mean arterial pressure and cardiac index than when given by infusion. In fact, one dog died after the solution was given by bolus indicating the severity of effect during isoflurane anesthesia. Administration during isoflurane anesthesia is not the customary method of using ketamine-midazolam and it would not be advisable to use the combination as a means of increasing anesthetic depth (a topping off effect). Since ketamine-midazolam is used as a method of inducing anesthesia prior to isoflurane maintenance, one should deliver the inhalant at lower concentrations at the onset while the effects of the injectable combination moderate over the ensuing 5 to 10 minute period. Otherwise, severe cardiovascular depression may be the consequence.

Telazol®-Ketamine-Xylazine (TKX); Medetomidine-Ketamine-Buprenorphine (MKB); and Medetomidine-Ketamine-Butorphanol (MKBu)
The TKX combination has been proposed for situations where inhalation anesthesia is not available or when injectable techniques are appropriate for short surgical procedures that do not take longer than 30 minutes (Benson 2004). TKX is compounded by dissolving 500 mg (1 vial) of Telazol powder in 4ml (400mg) of ketamine and 1ml of LA xylazine (100 mg). Dosage in the cat is 0.03ml/kg with the dose of individual components being 3mg/kg Telazol, 2.4mg/kg ketamine and 0.6mg/kg xylazine. A comparative study with TKX was conducted to evaluate the combination of medetomidine-ketamine-buprenorphine (MKB) given IM for mass sterilization of feral female cats (Cistola et al. 2002). Dosage for the MKB combination was medetomidine 40mg/kg, ketamine 15mg/kg and buprenorphine 10mg/kg. Although TKX has been used with apparently good success, results of this study suggested that MKB may be more suitable most likely because of better visceral analgesia, improved muscle relaxation and sedation and cardiovascular stability (lack of change of mean arterial pressure subsequent to surgical stimulation). In addition, recovery was faster after 0.5mg/cat of yohimbine IV given to achieve sternal recumbency. An alternative for better recoveries and seemingly improved analgesia is a slightly different combination of medetomidine 80mg/kg, ketamine 5mg/kg and butorphanol 0.2mg/kg as a single IM injection (Ko 2002). This provides fairly uniform anesthesia with adequate analgesia for about 30 minutes. Recovery takes about 2 hours but effects of medetomidine can be reversed with antipamazol (Antisedan). Because of the lower dose of ketamine, it is unlikely to have much of a hangover effect if the alpha$_2$ agonist is reversed.

Role of Ketamine in Pain Management
Ketamine alone, especially at anesthetic doses, is associated with many undesirable side effects. It is well documented that it provides little or no visceral analgesia, but even early in its development investigators found that it provided good somatic analgesia. However, at subanesthetic doses, the story is quite different. As more experience is gained in managing painful episodes in small animals patients, the hemodynamic stability and lack of respiratory depressant properties with low dose ketamine offer certain advantages (McArdie 1999). Even ketamine given orally at 10mg/kg qid was found to be a very useful adjunct in providing analgesia for dogs with burn-wound injuries (Joubert 1998).

With the increasing trend of using ketamine with opioids to minimize acute postoperative pain, having these two drugs premixed in the same solution offers certain advantages. Consequently, the stability of morphine sulfate and racemic ketamine solution in saline at pH 5.5-7.5 was evaluated over a 4-day period (Schmid et al. 2002). They found that this mixture at clinically relevant concentrations was stable at room temperature for at least 4 days. It is not known if this would be true with a mixture of ketamine and other opioids.

Is there a place for ketamine in what has been referred to as "balanced anesthesia and analgesia?" The wish list is fairly large with ketamine being administered in almost every way possible: epidural, intrathecal, local, oral and even intra-articular that was not effective (Huang et al. 2000). The balanced technique implies that ketamine would be used with other anesthetic and analgesic drugs usually by bolus injection and/or constant rate infusion (CRI). This takes advantage of its NMDA antagonistic and opioid agonist properties at low doses. Cruz et al. (2000) investigated use of ketamine with various combinations of atropine, xylazine, romifidine, methotrimeprazine, midazolam or fentanyl for short term anesthesia in cats. Each had advantages and disadvantages but none should be considered for major surgery alone. In a study with human patients undergoing rectal surgery, patients were given an epidural bolus followed by infusion of a bupivacaine/sufentanil/clonidine mixture (De-Kock et al. 2001). Patients were then given ketamine epidurally or IV by CRI. In recovery, frequency of use of a morphine patient-contolled analgesia (PCA) device connected to their IV line was used to evaluate the effectiveness of ketamine. Observations supported that subanesthetic doses of IV ketamine (0.5mg/kg bolus followed by 0.25mg/kg per hour) was a useful adjuvant in perioperative balanced analgesia. In another study, intraoperative ketamine, even at a dose of only 0.15mg/kg IV, was found to be a useful adjuvant to perioperative analgesic management of human patients undergoing anterior cruciate ligament repair (Menigaux et al. 2000). Postoperative pain and behavior were evaluated in dogs given low-dose ketamine added to a standard perioperative anesthetic protocol (Wagner et al. 2002). Twenty-seven dogs undergoing forelimb amputation were anesthetized with glycopyrrolate, morphine, propofol and isoflurane. Dogs were then given saline or ketamine and also received an infusion of fentanyl for the first 18 hours after surgery. They found that adding ketamine to a standard anesthetic protocol using a 0.5mg/kg bolus given before surgery, 10μ/kg/min CRI during surgery and 2μ/kg/min CRI for 18 hours after surgery was advantageous. Patients had significantly lower pain scores and were more active in the recovery period. Thus CRI ketamine seems to augment analgesic effects of opioids and to have a beneficial effect especially for procedures that are known to be very painful including amputations and spinal surgeries. It is clear that CRI ketamine can be used as the sole analgesic but the suitability of using low dose or CRI ketamine for critically ill patients remains to be validated. This is especially true in patients with compensated renal function. However, there is insufficient evidence that low dose ketamine, e.g., 2mg/kg, can be effective in managing severe postoperative pain in cats (Robertson et al. 2002a). Prolonged use of CRI ketamine beyond the effective duration of concurrent medications to reduce behavioral changes still needs further investigation.

Using a pain model in mice, the combination of ketamine and tramadol was evaluated to determine antinociceptive effects (Chen et al. 2002). They found that the net effect with the thermal component was additive but with chemical induced stimulation, the combination produced synergistic antinociception. It is uncertain if this combination would be effective in small animals but the possibility exists.

Epidural analgesia has become a very useful component in managing severe pain for dogs and cats (Jones 2001). Opioids produce their effects in the spinal cord by two mechanisms: by direct action on the neural transmission at the spinal cord dorsal horn and by an indirect effect exerted through action on the supraspinal pain inhibition system. However, there is a lack of direct suppression of pain transmission provided by ketamine at the spinal dorsal horn. Although intrathecal ketamine was shown to be analgesic in a rat formalin model, it did not provide preemptive analgesia (Lee 2001). Even when ketamine was given concurrently with morphine by epidural injection in human patients, no clinically relevant reduction in postoperative pain relief was achieved (Subramaniam et al. 2001). Chemically induced synovitis was used to evaluate the effects of 2mg ketamine/kg given epidurally in dogs (Hamilton et al, 2002). They concluded that this use of ketamine was not effective in providing significant analgesia. The possibility of inducing undesirable behavioral effects along with minimal or short duration of action seems to preclude the effective use of epidural ketamine in dogs and cats. As a result, there does not appear to be much scientific evidence to support the use of epidural or intraththecal ketamine for this purpose.

Telazol (tiletamine / zolazepam)
This agent was developed for anesthesia and / or chemical restraint in a variety of animals. Tiletamine is a cyclohexanone similar to ketamine. It is combined with zolazepam to reduce convulsive and clonic muscle reactions and to improve the degree of muscle relaxation. Although classified as a general anesthetic, it appears to be a weak visceral analgesic as with other dissociative agents and should not be used as a sole agent for abdominal surgery.

Telazol is effective when given IM or IV. Dose range is 5 to 20mg/kg in the cat and dog (Hellyer et al. 1988; Hellyer et al. 1989). Most commonly, the dose is 4 to 5mg/kg with lower doses given IV. The desired response to IM injection will usually be reached within 5 to 7 min. It can be used in normal healthy cats for anesthesia induction prior to intubation and maintenance with a volatile anesthetic. Recovery will be 1 to 2 hours depending on dose and route of administration. Even though tiletamine is combined with zolazepam, results have been improved with the addition of other medications to improve muscle relaxation and/or behavioral responses.

Effects on the Heart and Circulation

Although barbiturates have a depressant effect on the myocardium similar to inhalation agents, their influence on the peripheral circulation is different. Increased arterial pressure and total peripheral resistance probably results from increased sympathetic tone (Conway, 1969). Heart rate is also increased. Short-acting agents are used most commonly to induce anesthesia and, consequently, the depressant effects are usually transient. Cardiac output is reduced and may or may not be accompanied by a compensatory increase in peripheral vascular resistance.

It appears that equivalent doses of ultrashort-acting barbiturates produce similar degrees of cardiovascular depression. These agents also cause reduction in tone of systemic capacitance vessels leading to pooling of blood in these sites in preference to pooling in the capacitance vessels of the lung. The shift of blood reduces left ventricular diastolic filling and stroke volume. Rapid injection may lead to decreased arterial pressure whereas slow infusion may or may not increase blood pressure. Rapid injection of surgical anesthetic doses of these drugs may lead to profound myocardial depression and circulatory collapse particularly in high-risk patients. Extreme caution must be taken when injectable anesthetics are used in hypovolemic patients and consequences may be lethal. With light doses sufficient to permit tracheal intubation, depression will usually be minimal. The decrease in cardiac output and arterial pressure is antagonized by increased sympathetic outflow due to stimulation of baroreceptors reflexes. As the drug leaves the myocardium, sympathetic outflow may antagonize the depression and cause increased cardiac output, arterial pressure, tachycardia and ventricular arrhythmias such as bigeminal rhythm. Arrhythmias are relatively minor and transient when doses of 6 to 8mg/kg are used but persist for longer periods if higher doses are injected.

The effects of analgesics such as fentanyl, meperidine, morphine, oxymorphone and hydromorphone on the cardiovascular system are minimal. Mean arterial pressure and heart rate may decrease slightly but cardiac output should remain within normal limits. Since total peripheral resistance may decrease, it is imperative to provide adequate support with balanced electrolyte solutions.

Ketamine is an unusual agent since it selectively depresses areas of the CNS while simultaneously stimulating others. As a result, the agent affects the cardiovascular system in several ways. Arterial pressure, heart rate and cardiac output are significantly increased, whereas total peripheral resistance remains unchanged. Some studies have shown no direct myocardial depression with the agent except at high doses. However, others have demonstrated evidence of myocardial depression. It also has been shown that ketamine either directly or indirectly stimulates the sympathetic nervous system or may improve adverse responses to epinephrine. With the exception of tachycardia, ketamine does not significantly alter cardiac rhythm. Antiarrhythmic activity has even been demonstrated.

Propofol has become a common means of accomplishing rapid IV induction and recovery. The rapid, smooth and complete recovery even following repeated propofol administration, gives this agent a unique place in veterinary practice for both in-patient and outpatient anesthesia. The cardiovascular depressant properties of propofol at deep anesthetic levels of anesthesia are similar to or greater than those of thiopental. Direct myocardial depression, peripheral vasodilation and venodilation have been reported to cause arterial hypotension (Goodchild, 1989). The cardiovascular changes can be minimized by titrating the dose to a suitable end-point. Propofol should be used with caution in hypovolemic patients or in those with impaired left ventricular function (Ilkiw, 1992b).

Inhalation Induction

Patient preparation, as discussed in Chapter 1, is important especially for inhalation induction. Equipment for delivery of inhalants is dealt with in Chapter 3 as are the principles and pharmacology of inhalation anesthesia. Important considerations of the inhalation method are not to obstruct breathing in the process of delivery. Therefore, the mechanical dimensions of a mask, for example, must be as small as possible to minimize dead space, which is defined by the amount of carbon dioxide rebreathed. If CO_2 is exhaled into an infinite space, as occurs in a room with adequate ventilation, little or no CO_2 will be rebreathed. However, if a tight-fitting mask is applied to the face without the use of valves for fresh gas inflow, the inspiration of air may be restricted, and elimination of CO_2 may be severely compromised.

Historically, open-drop mask induction with diethyl ether was very popular prior to 1970 and was used for general anesthesia in humans and animals for more than 100 years. In the 1950's and 60's, ether was the choice for C-section and in small patients in which venous access for barbiturates would be difficult. Ether's flammable and explosive properties are well-known and documented. Back then, it would not be uncommon to find a can of ether in the refrigerator (nobody paid any attention to having explosion proof devices) or just sitting on the shelf with electric clippers running. One thing was certain when a veterinarian used open-drop ether for a procedure; the family knew what had been done when doctor came home from the practice with clothing permeating the smell of ether–for days! Open-drop as described involves placing cotton in a mask or cone open at both ends, dripping ether into the material and placing the mask over the face. When air was drawn through the absorbent material soaked with liquid ether, volatilized liquid was delivered to the patient. Levels could be adjusted by changing the position of the cone to the face allowing air to bypass the ether-containing cone or adding more liquid to the cotton. This had to be a very unpleasant experience for veterinary patients if human experiences can be used for comparison. Receiving ether for tonsillectomy as a child and when as a teenager, open-drop ether was given to reset a green-stick fracture of a metacarpal bone, without sedative premedication of course. Thankfully, it is rarely if ever used anymore with the availability of potent inhalants delivered from precision vaporizers. This technique has the greatest potential for producing hypoxia and hypercarbia during induction. If supplemental oxygen is not used or if the patient is not allowed to breathe room air frequently without the mask, hypoxia will result. Diethyl ether has a vapor pressure of 444mm/Hg at 20°C. If the gas vehicle is fully saturated, inspired ether concentration would be greater than 50%. In this example, oxygen concentration in room air would be reduced by 50% thus providing only 10% O_2. Increased resistance to breathing caused by gauze or cotton containing the liquid anesthetic provides impairment to inspiration and expiration. This must be avoided.

Mask Induction

Two techniques of inhalation induction will be described: mask alone and chamber plus mask. For induction with any inhalant, it is important that the area used for induction be quiet and that a second person be available to assist with restraint. Because of limitations associated with the open-drop technique and anesthetic waste gas risk, this method should be avoided if modern techniques are available. If necessary, detailed descriptions of the open-drop technique can be found in other sources. The volatile liquid anesthetics, i.e., halothane, isoflurane and sevoflurane should be delivered from calibrated vaporizers capable of delivering large amounts of anesthetic vapor in predictable concentrations. If a glass vaporizer is used, vaporization of the liquid anesthetic with the high flow rates necessary for mask induction will cause a drop in vapor pressure because of loss of heat of vaporization. This heat loss makes the vaporizer much less efficient. The inhalation agent delivered in oxygen alone or oxygen plus nitrous oxide can be delivered either through a mask or, in the case of very small animals, by means of an endotracheal tube adapter or syringe barrel. The mask technique is best suited for cats, dogs and other species weighing less than 8kg. However, there are situations in which the mask technique is most advantageous for larger animals. The only precaution is to deliver a total gas flow equal to or approaching the inspiratory flow rate of the patient's tidal volume (Table 2-5). The animal is placed in a comfortable position; if a struggle does not appear imminent, a sitting or prone position may be naturally assumed by the animal. Try first to place the mask over the muzzle or face without anything attached. If the animal objects too much, place the mask to the side of the face to allow gas to pass across the nose. The total gas flow is started and the anesthetic vapor is introduced, starting at a low vaporizer setting.

Table 2-5

Method of Calculating Inspiratory Flow Rate

Patient	Feline 5kg
Estimated Tidal Volume	50ml (10 ml/kg)
Respiratory Rate	20 BPM
Total Flow from anesthetic machine	3L/min

Assume 1-sec inspiratory time, 1-sec expiratory time, and 1-sec pause.
Inspiratory flow rate calculated as follows:

$$\frac{\text{Total flow}}{60 \text{ sec/min}} = \text{Inspiratory flow rate}$$

$$\frac{3000}{60} = 50 \text{ ml/sec}$$

Total flow would need to increase if tidal volume increases.

An animal tends to hold its breath while inhaling a pungent vapor odor. Halothane and isoflurane have noticeable characteristic odors but when either is started at a concentration of 0.5%, animals usually will not object to the odor, thus will not breathhold and induction will be much smoother. Breath-holding is not a problem with sevoflurane.

In the case of the cat or dog, it is well to talk to the patient in a soft reassuring tone, which induces a hypnotic-like state as the animal begins to breathe the vapor. Gently scratching ears and stroking the back will also provide comfort and reassurance. At intervals of 10 to 20 sec, the anesthetic concentration is increased at 0.5% increments up to 4% halothane, 3% isoflurane or 5% sevoflurane. As the patient loses consciousness, the mask is moved over the nose increasing the inspired concentration (some room air is breathed when the mask is not directly on the face). When sufficient depth is achieved, intubation of the trachea should be attempted. The reason the mask is not initially placed over the nose is because it is alarming to the patient and if the mask is large enough, it may not allow the animal to see its surroundings. It is best to fit the mask below the eyes and also to put ointment in them to prevent drying of corneas. Without being able to use scavenging systems, mask induction is associated with exposure to breathing anesthetic gases intended for patients. As a result, risk of exposure should be explained to hospital personnel and mask induction must not be used when pregnant women are in the working area (details provided in Chapter 3).

An anticholinergic should be given to control salivation and preanesthesia sedation with a tranquilizer will instill a "non-caring" attitude in the patient, which will be most helpful in these circumstances. Close monitoring is necessary to prevent excessive anesthetic depth and care must be taken to not allow the patient to breathe high concentrations of the induction agent after intubation. Intubation reduces the anatomical space by at least 50% and if anesthesia is deep enough to permit intubation, the addition of excessive anesthetic levels may lead to profound CV depression. One should adjust the concentration before connecting the breathing circuit to the endotracheal tube. A few breaths of 4% halothane, isoflurane or sevoflurane with the patient intubated may lead to myocardial depression and possible cardiac arrest. Maintaining an adequate flow rate is most important to prevent dilution of the inspired anesthetic concentration with room air (Table 2-5). Nitrous oxide (60-80%) is advantageous not only because of its analgesic effects but also because it increases the rate at which the alveolar concentration of an inhalation anesthetic rises (De Young 1980). If tidal volume increases during induction volume delivered from the flow meter will remain the same, but if, for example, tidal volume doubles, 4% halothane in 50ml/sec will be 2% the inhalant at the same flow rate because of inspiration of air around the mask. This would obviously slow induction. This is the reason why 5L/min is used as total flow for animals up to 7kg and why total flow must be increased accordingly for large patients. Limitations of total flow for larger animals are the upper limits of the flow meters. Oxygen flow meters on most veterinary units usually only deliver a maximum of 5L/min. If one wishes to use 80% N_2O and the maximum output from each flow meter is 8L/min, then the total flow possible would be 10L/min, 8L/min N_2O, 2L/min O_2. Higher total flow could be achieved by reducing the N_2O concentration to 66 per cent (8L/min N_2O and 4L/min O_2). For a dog weighing 30kg with an estimated tidal volume of 300 ml and an inspiratory flow rate of 300 ml/sec, the flow delivered from the flow meters at 10L/min would be only 166ml/sec. One might anticipate that although 4% of the volatile liquid anesthetic may be delivered at the mask, only 2% may be inspired because the flow delivered would be only about 50% of the tidal volume, assuming that volume is inspired in 1 second. It may be desirable to induce a 30kg stoic, 14-year-old dog for a short procedure by mask rather than by an injectable technique and this dilutional factor may serve only to make induction a little slower and safer depending on the health status of the animal.

A comparative study was conducted to evaluate different methods of inducing anesthesia in cats (Sawyer 1975). Animals were induced with isoflurane by mask with and without acepromazine premedication (0.05mg/kg IM) either increasing vaporizer concentration over time (Gradual) or with 4% isoflurane during the entire period (Abrupt). The gradual method is advantageous as the rise in delivered anesthetic concentration tends to avoid breath holding. Cats were much more cooperative to the procedure as well. Adding acepromazine obviously is an advantage, rendering the patient in a more tranquil state. This method eliminates adverse effects of thiobarbiturate induction in puppies and cats. It provides more control because the depth of inhalation anesthesia can be rapidly reversed on a breath by breath process. If one uses sevoflurane instead of isoflurane, the lack of an objectionable pungent odor will offer distinct advantages over isoflurane. Recovery from mask induction anesthesia is more rapid since residual drug effects are not present.

Mask induction is much more complex and may not be as safe as with some injectable methods. Severe myocardial depression is possible when delivering high vaporizer concentrations with a tight fitting mask. Mask induction can be more expensive depending on agent costs and it requires special equipment, i.e., mask, vaporizer and anesthetic system. Exposure of personnel to excess anesthetic vapor is difficult to control. This method is most applicable with anesthetic agents of high potency such as halothane, isoflurane and especially sevoflurane with its lack of pungency and rapid uptake.

Chamber Induction

Use of boxes, bags, or chambers for anesthesia induction of small animals is not a new or uncommon practice. It has its greatest applications for puppies, small adult dogs, birds (not always) and various species of rodents and lagomorphs. A bell jar may be used with a cotton pledget soaked with volatile liquid anesthetic placed in the jar with the patient until induction of anesthesia is accomplished. Diethyl ether and methoxyflurane were most commonly used for this procedure. Anesthetics of high potency and vapor pressure should never be used this way unless careful calculations have been made relative to chamber volume and amount of volatile liquid anesthetic added to the chamber.

In 1927, Hardenberg and Mann described a technique of etherizing small dogs and cats in a cabinet. Stiles (1959) reported inducing ether anesthesia in cats using a clear plastic box with L/min of oxygen delivered as the carrier for diethyl ether vaporized from a nebulizer adjacent to the box. Others have described similar systems for halothane induction in rabbits.

Clinical use of the chamber was reported in using a 5.5-gallon fish tank, 40cm x 23cm x 20.5cm, with a plexiglass top (Sawyer 1975). This unit had an 18.5-liter volume. Similar chambers are commercially available (Figure 2-8). With delivery of 4% halothane to the 18-liter chamber, a predictable rate of rise in halothane concentration will occur (Figures 2-9 and 2-10). The same rate of rise would be anticipated with 4% isoflurane or sevoflurane. In a study comparing the mask and chamber induction techniques, halothane-oxygen provided an induction time with the chamber of 4.7 ± 0.5 minutes for halothane alone 3.5 ± 0.5 minutes for halothane with 80% N_2O (Sawyer 1975). If total flow rates are used for different compartment sizes (Table 2-6), induction times will be roughly the same.

For chamber induction, the animal is placed in the chamber, the lid secured and the delivery hose inserted through a hole in the lid cover or side away from the animal's head. Total flow for the appropriate compartment size is then selected along with 4% halothane, 4 % isoflurane or 5% sevoflurane. When the animal reaches unconsciousness and does not respond to noise or chamber movement, it should be removed with anesthesia continued by mask for 1 to 3 minutes to achieve the desired depth to allow endotracheal intubation. During this induction period by mask, surgical preparation could begin. Appropriate flow rates will prevent significant rebreathing of CO_2 while the patient is in the chamber.

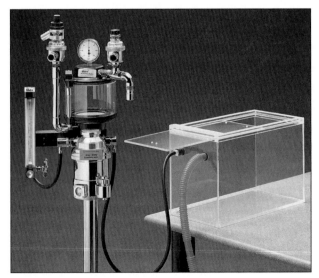

Figure 2-8 Induction Chamber. Outlet tube from the vaporizer is shown connected to the chamber. The corrugated 22mm tubing is shown connected to the chamber carrying excess gases to the scavenging system (not shown). The lid can be moved in groves at the top to close and open as needed. Different sizes are available.
Courtesy of Matrx, Orchard Park, NY

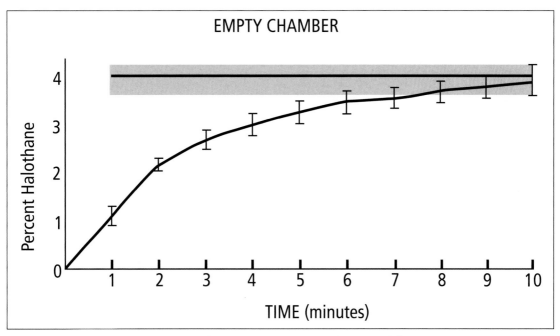

Figure 2-9 Halothane tension rate of rise in an 18 liter chamber. Five different calibrated vaporizers were used with concentrations measured by gas chromatography. Total flow = 5L/min oxygen. X ± SD. (Reprinted by permission from Sawyer DC: Comparative effects of halothane-nitrous oxide induction: face mask versus induction chamber. 25th Gaines Symposium. October 23, 1975. White Plains, NY. Gaines Dog Reseach Center.

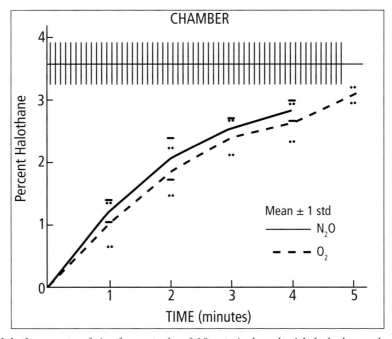

Figure 2-10 Halothane rate of rise from study of 10 cats induced with halothane alone of halothane plus 80% nitrious oxide. Total flow = 5L/min in an 18 liter chamber.
(Reprinted by permission from Sawyer DC: Comparative effects of halothane-nitrous oxide induction: face mask versus induction chamber. 25th Gaines Symposium. October 23, 1975. White Plains, NY. Gaines Dog Reseach Center.

Table 2-6

Flow Rate Requirements for Chambers of Various Sizes

Compartment Internal Volume (L)	Total Flow Rate (L/min)	1 Time Constant* (min)
18	5.0	3.6
14	4.0	3.5
10	3.0	3.3
7	2.0	3.5
3	0.8	3.7

*63% of the delivered anesthetic concentration from vaporizer will be achieved in 1 time constant. If 4% vapor is delivered, expected concentration in the chamber in 3.5 min would be 2.5%.

The chamber technique is very useful. It is not usually associated with hypoxemia or hypercapnia and from the standpoint of simplicity; it is superior to mask induction alone in certain small patients. When the anesthetist is presented with a provoked, anxious domestic feline skilled in the art of inflicting injury, the chamber can be placed over the animal in a cage or the owner can place the cat directly in the chamber to be promptly anesthetized. Hard to handle animals are usually covered by a towel, removed from the transport cage and placed in the chamber with little resistance. Puppies less than 6kg can best be induced the same way and mean adult toy breeds of dogs are induced much more easily and safely than with the "snatch, struggle, and inject" procedure. Another advantage of the chamber is that the animal does not hold its breath, as might occur with the mask technique because it is not initially confronted with the inhalants pungent odor. At the onset, anesthetic concentrations start at 0 and rises to about 2% over a 2.5 minute period (Figure 2-10). It then continues to rise over the next 2 minutes to roughly 2.7%, at which time induction to light anesthesia has been accomplished.

Chamber induction simplifies management, negates requirement of physical restraint, maximizes patient comfort, minimizes stress and prevents injury to the animal handler and the anesthetist. It also may provide better management of anesthesia induction in patients at risk depending upon one's ability to provide physical restraint.

Special equipment is needed, which increases the cost of the procedure. Another disadvantage is that the anesthetist is not in direct contact with the animal being anesthetized which is especially important in patients at risk. Neglect by the anesthetist may result in deep anesthesia if the patient remains in the chamber too long. If the patient is removed from the chamber too soon, breathholding may occur after application of the mask and thus prolong induction. Unless the gases discharged from the chamber are scavenged, anesthetic pollution of the room atmosphere will occur. If proper cleaning of the chamber between uses is not accomplished, spread of disease is enhanced. Placing a towel over the chamber during induction and leaving a small area for viewing sometimes calms those occasional animals that fight and struggle inside the chamber.

Laryngoscopy and Endotracheal Intubation

When the animal reaches unconsciousness sufficient to permit the mouth to be held open and tongue extended, the trachea can usually be intubated. Depth of anesthesia must be sufficient to eliminate chewing movements and prevent excessive movement of the tongue. One must be careful not to produce deep anesthesia that would cause severe cardiovascular depression at a time when oxygenation may be compromised owing to respiratory depression. In addition, bradycardia may occur because of laryngeal stimulation and this, combined with myocardial depression produced by deep anesthesia, may lead to undesirable complications, the worst being cardiac arrest. For some high-risk cases, it is advisable to provide oxygen by mask prior to induction and intubation to avoid hypoxemia.

Intubation of the trachea assures, but does not guarantee, a patent airway. In brachycephalic breeds, respiratory obstruction often occurs when anesthesia is induced and tracheal intubation must be accomplished without delay. Endotracheal intubation decreases anatomic dead space by at least 50%. Controlled breathing by manual or mechanical means is facilitated with the cuff inflated to prevent partial loss of the intended tidal volume. Secretions can be removed by suction and the patient can be placed in any position with less chance of compromising the airway. In addition, the anesthetist can be situated away from the patient's head and still maintain control of the airway via the anesthetic circuit. If regurgitation of stomach contents should occur, tracheal aspiration will be prevented as long as proper procedures have been followed, e.g., proper fit of the ET tube and cuff inflated. For these reasons, there are very few circumstances that would justify not intubating the trachea.

Equipment
Laryngoscopes
Most dogs can be intubated without the aid of a laryngoscope. However, this instrument is a valuable asset to the novice developing skills of tracheal intubation. It is also advantageous to the experienced anesthetist for use in cats, rabbits and rodents as well as certain canine breeds such as the Pug, English Bulldog and Saint Bernard. Most laryngoscopes have detachable blades that can be used interchangeably on a battery-containing handle. A hook-on connection between the handle and blade is most common although one-piece handles and blades are available. One end of the handle is fitted with a hinge pin that fits a slot on the base of the blade for easy attachment and detachment. Handles come in various sizes to accommodate different sizes and types of batteries and some handles are available with a recharable battery. Small handles, available for AA batteries, are easier to manipulate but battery life will be shorter.

Most laryngoscopes are made for use in humans with the patient lying on their back. For a right-handed anesthetist, the handle is held with the left hand such that the bottom of the handle is pointed upward. For both cats and dogs, the most convenient position is for the patient to be in sternal recumbency. In this situation, the handle is held in the left hand with the bottom pointed downward (Figure 2-11).

Blades may be either straight or curved and are available in many different shapes and sizes. The base of the blade attaches to the handle and has a slot that engages the hinge pin of the handle. The heel of the blade is at the other end. The tongue or spatula is the main shaft where a bulb or fiberoptic bundle is located to transmit light. For most blades, the socket is located near the tip but off to one side so as not to obstruct visibility of laryngeal structures. The tip is positioned either ventral to the epiglottis pulling it downward to expose the glottis (opening) or in larger patients, directly on the epiglottis itself (Figure 2-11). Touching the epiglottis of cats will promote laryngospasm.

On most blades made for use in human patients, there is a flange positioned on the side of the main shaft and is used to deflect the tongue. The Macintosh blade has a very prominent flange. The most common position for intubation of small animals is sternal recumbency. As a result, when the laryngoscope blade is positioned upright (handle pointed downward), the tongue deflector is in the way of visualizing laryngeal stuctures especially in sizes for smaller patients. For this reason, blades such as the Miller that has a smaller flange or Bizarri-Guiffrida with the flange removed, have definite advantages in small patients. The latter is available in three sizes: child (110mm), medium adult (130mm) and large adult (158mm). Seward and Robert Shaw blades have smaller or reversed flanges. Sizes of Miller blades range from #0 (75mm) to #4 (205mm) and this range will accommodate most all situations in small animal practice. MRI compatible laryngoscopes are now available (Figure 2-12).

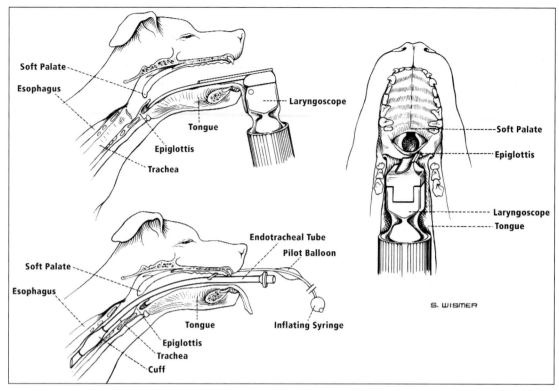

Figure 2-11 Tracheal intubation of the dog.
Reprinted with permission from Sawyer DC.: Inhalation anesthesia using halothane. NY, Ayerst Laboratories, 1979.

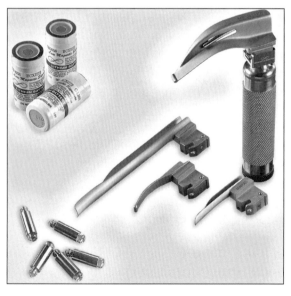

Figure 2-12 Various laryngoscope blades, handle, bulbs and rechargeable batteries. Equipment shown is MRI Compatible.
Courtesy of Minrad Inc, Buffalo, NY

Endotracheal Tubes

Endotracheal (ET) tubes are made of rubber or plastic. Special armored tubes reinforced with coiled wire or heavy nylon thread can be used to prevent collapse or kinking. Since the head and trachea of animals are for the most part in straight alignment, plastic tubes are usually stiff enough to preclude kinking. Tubes are chosen for durability, thin walls and maximum internal diameter to assure minimal resistance to breathing, lack of compressibility and ease of cleaning. The most common types are the Magill and the Murphy. The eye position opposite to the bevel distinguishes Murphy from the Magill. The eye is designed to prevent complete obstruction in the event that the bevel of the catheter is situated against the tracheal wall. Tubes are designated by internal diameter (ID), with low number sizes used for cats and small puppies and higher number tubes according to patient size. This ID designation has been accepted as the American standard by the American Society of Anesthesiologists; it is also the British standard. Comparison of the Magill ID number to the French scale, i.e. the Davol number, can be made but for an approximate conversion from the French scale to ID, the French scale number may be divided by 4.

ET tubes are usually longer than needed when received from the manufacturer and, except for the large sizes, i.e., greater than 11mm ID, they are the same as those used for human patients. They must be cut to appropriate lengths to lessen the possibility of bronchial intubation. Because of variations among breeds, a reliable guide for size selection of endotracheal tubes for small animals is not available. A rough estimate of size can be made by palpating the trachea and estimating the appropriate number of tube to be used. The length should allow the tube to extend from the incisor teeth to the distal third of the trachea, proximal to the thoracic inlet.

A plastic connector with a standard 15-mm adaptor for connection to the breathing circuit must fit snugly to the proximal end of the tube to prevent inadvertent disconnection. This adaptor must be thin-walled and as large as possible to minimize turbulence and resistance to gas flow. This is particularly important with tubes of less than 5mm ID. Most ET tubes are packaged with the adapter included.

A stylet of malleable wire or plastic is useful to keep the tube straight or curved as desired. However, one must be sure that the stylet does not protrude beyond the distal end to prevent puncture or abrasion to tracheal structures.

Whenever possible a cuffed tube should be used because the inflated cuff allows a sealed connection between the animal and the anesthetic circuit. It also permits easy control of breathing, prevents dilution of anesthetic gases by inspiration of room air and reduces the possibility of passage of foreign material into lungs. Cuffs are of high or low pressure design. The low-pressure cuff is very compliant and prevents high pressure from being exerted against the tracheal wall if the cuff is overinflated. Most tubes are obtained with the cuff permanently affixed to the distal end, a pilot balloon incorporated to indicate inflation of the cuff and a valve inflation syringe adapter.

Straight tubes are also available without cuffs but in order to have a complete airway connection, a tube of perfect fit is needed. The Cole tube is uncuffed but the distal end is tapered; the smaller portion is inserted into the trachea with the barrel portion located in the pharynx. The sloping shoulder located at the junction is designed to fit against the arytenoid cartilage and function somewhat as a cuff. This is very useful for small patients since the cuff and pilot balloon on other tubes reduce the size of tube that can be used. Cole tubes are available in 1.5 to 4.0mm ID and also in 10, 12, and 14mm ID for dogs larger than 40kg. Cuffed tubes are available in these small sizes as well.

A clean tracheal tube of appropriate diameter and length should be selected. It is best to have several selections available since the most appropriate size can best be determined when observing the glottis. The tube must be examined beforehand to ensure patency and the cuff must be inflated to check for leakage. Inflating the cuff during equipment set-up and checking it after a few minutes will provide assurance of a non-leaking cuff. Too rapid an inspection may miss a very slow leak. An underwater check of the cuff is also an effective method, especially if done during cleaning.

For reuse of endotracheal tubes, proper handing and cleaning is very important. Once the tube has been removed, it should be placed in a container of water so that mucous and debris does not dry before the cleaning process can be done. An underwater leak check of the cuff and pilot balloon should be made prior to cleaning and the tube discarded if indicated. A soft brush is then used to gently scrub both the outside and inside of the tube with a surgical soap followed by a thorough water rinse. Tubes are then soaked in a suitable chemical solution for the recommended interval, rinsed again with water, patted on a towel and hung on a rack to dry. ET tubes should be stored in a convenient location and protected so that disinfectant aerosols, air fresheners, or other chemicals cannot contaminate them. This might be in a drawer or covered wall cabinet.

The dog is best intubated when sternally recumbent with the help of an assistant. The head is held by the mandible and lips with the head extended in straight alignment with the neck. The assistant can also extend the tongue with the other hand, thus moving the epiglottis forward (Figure 2-13). The laryngoscope blade or tip of the endotracheal tube is placed at the base of the epiglottis. When the mouth is opened and glottis brought into view, the tip of the epiglottis may be above the soft palate. It must be brought into view in order to expose the dorsal surface of the epiglottis, glottis, and arytenoid cartilages. The tube may be lubricated with water or water-soluble jelly and, under direct vision, passed through the glottis. Once through the glottis, the tip should be moved dorsally to avoid the laryngeal diverticulum; keeping the tube straight with a stylet is the best way to avoid this part of the anatomy. The distal end of the tube must be located proximal to the thoracic inlet and the connector end should be located at the level of the incisor teeth. Palpation of the esophagus and trachea will ensure proper location. If two tubes are palpated, determination of esophageal intubation has been made indicating the necessity of repeating the process correctly. Immediately following intubation, the tube is connected to the inhalation system and secured with 1 inch gauze wrap or other suitable material. Then the gauze

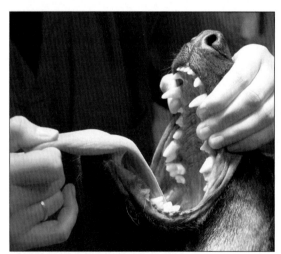

Figure 2-13 Assistant holding head and extending tongue in position for intubation. Courtesy of Dr. Kevin Harris, Haslett Animal Clinic, Haslett, MI and Gail Whiting, photographer.

is passed around the upper or lower jaw or behind the ears and tied (Figure 2-14). It must be tight enough to prevent dislodging, which may otherwise occur when the animal is moved or as a result of slippage if the gauze gets wet. Care must be taken not to cinch the tie around the muzzle too tightly to avoid tissue damage or swelling. Other methods, such as a heavy rubber band or adhesive tape to secure the tube are effective. Regardless of method used to secure the tube, it is important to provide ease of extubation at the time of arousal following anesthesia. Recovery can be so rapid following propofol or sevoflurane that in some cases, caution is needed to avoid injury to the hands during extubation.

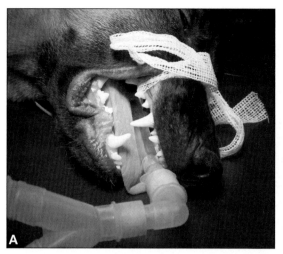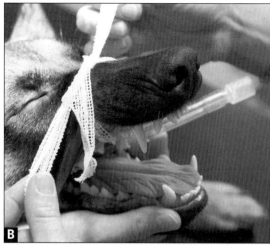

Figure 2-14 Use of 1 inch rolled gauze tied to endotracheal tube (A) and in place around muzzle (B). Courtesy of Dr. Kevin Harris, Haslett Animal Clinic, Haslett, MI and Gail Whiting, photographer.

For the experienced anesthetist, this process can be accomplished without a laryngoscope. The fingers are placed behind the upper and lower incisor teeth and the tongue can be extended with the same hand. The tube is used to depress the epiglottis and is then inserted. Available light must be used in order to view the laryngeal structures. Blind intubation with or without palpation is not advised. Reflex jaw muscle contraction can result in closure of the mouth, which may result in a bite or crushing wound to the anesthetist's hand. Dogs can also be intubated in the lateral position but either the table should be elevated or the procedure should be done with the anesthetist in a kneeling position.

To test the fit of the tube, the reservoir bag is compressed while listening for escape of air at the mouth. An inflation of 12 to 20cm H_2O without a leak is indicative of a good fit. If this does not occur, inflate the cuff with the proper amount of air while simultaneously compressing the bag to the pressure indicated. For thoracotomy procedures or ventilation of a lung with low compliance, higher inflation pressures are needed so cuff inflation must be adjusted accordingly.

Most often, the fit of the tracheal tube is acceptable at the onset but after 5 to 10 minutes, the cuff might require additional air volume. This is due to tracheal dilation or relaxation of muscles surrounding the trachea during anesthesia. If N_2O is used as part of the anesthetic protocol, the cuff may increase in volume as a result of N_2O diffusing through the cuff wall. In practicality, this may be a potential problem only for procedures longer than 60 minutes. Over-pressure and potential damage to the tracheal endothelium can be prevented by periodically deflating the tube, moving the tube slightly, and reinflating the cuff.

Occasionally, the cuff will develop a leak during a procedure and replacement of the tube is not feasible. In this situation, a pharyngeal pack around the tube with rolled gauze may be used to create a seal if reintubation is not possible during surgery.

Cats are much more difficult to intubate than dogs because of their small pharynx and extreme sensitivity to laryngospasm, especially if a thiobarbiturate has been used for induction. Laryngospasm will also occur if the epiglottis is touched by the blade of the laryngoscope. The arytenoid cartilages do not relax as much in cats compared to dogs, which provides a very small opening for intubation. The cat is best positioned in sternal recumbency with the tongue extended and the glottis visualized (Figure 2-15). Frequency of breathing with cartilage movement can be observed and during inspiration, the tube can be inserted with the bevel of the tube in the vertical position. A short stylet is very helpful to keep the tube straight during the intubation

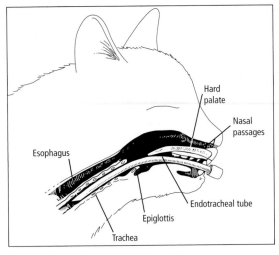

Figure 2-15 Endotracheal intubation of a cat with anatomy.
Reprinted with permission. Fig 2-4, pg 65. Veterinary Anesthesia and Analgesia, Third Edition 2003. Eds McKelvey D, Hollingshead KW. Mosby

process. For a cat weighing 5kg, a 3.0 to 3.5mm ID tube should be adequate. The tube is secured with gauze and tied behind the ears (Figure 2-16). The key to successful intubation of the domestic feline is adequate depth of anesthesia. Problems with intubation of felines are almost always related to attempting intubation when the patient is too light. If laryngospasm should occur, laryngeal reflexes can be depressed with a topical anesthetic such as 0.05% lidocaine or 0.25% mepivicaine.

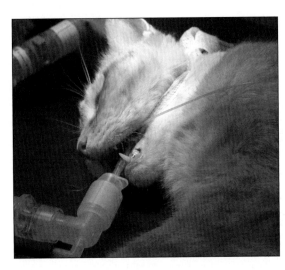

Figure 2-16 Cat intubated and breathing apparatus connected with tube secured behind ears.
Courtesy of Dr. Kevin Harris, Haslett Animal Clinic, Haslett, MI and Gail Whiting, photographer.

For the cat or dog in which deep anesthesia cannot be tolerated, a depolarizing muscle relaxant can be given to facilitate intubation. Following anesthesia induction and unconsciousness, succinylcholine, 0.1 to 0.2mg/kg can be given IV to produce muscle relaxation sufficient to permit intubation. Of course, apnea occurs following the blockade of respiratory musculature; therefore, controlled ventilation must be provided immediately following intubation. To prevent hypoxemia, the patient must be adequately oxygenated, because 30 to 45 seconds may pass before muscle fasciculations subside and masseter muscles relax to permit intubation. Cats often become severely bradycardia from succinylcholine and an anticholinergic IV just before the succinylcholine will prevent this adverse reaction.

Induction and Intubation of the Unfasted Dog or Cat

Emergency procedures may necessitate anesthesia of the unfasted patient. Therefore intubation must be accomplished with the anticipation of vomiting and possible aspiration. Whenever the possibility exists, induction of anesthesia must be deep enough to depress pharyngeal reflexes sufficiently to preclude emesis before intubation has been completed. In general, deeper anesthesia prior to intubation is needed than in the conventional technique. If emesis and aspiration occur, tracheal lavage with saline should be done following intubation removing as much material as possible, preferably with suction. A large syringe and catheter can be used if a power suction unit is not available. The patient should receive antibiotic therapy for several days. For recovery of the anesthetized patient with a full stomach, the animal should be awake as much as possible before extubation. Should vomiting occur, the patient must have its reflexes returned in order to protect the airway. If regurgitation occurs with the patient intubated, the mouth should be lavaged to remove as much vomitus as possible. When the trachea is extubated, the cuff should be left partially inflated to remove contents trapped between cuff and trachea.

Tracheostomy and Intubation by Pharyngotomy

These are two special intubation procedures used to facilitate repair of mandibular and maxillary fractures or for oral and facial surgery (Hartsfield 1977). Either procedure can be used depending on the duration needed for postanesthesia maintenance of the airway. For a recovery of short duration, a pharyngotomy is used to keep the ET tube out of the way during the surgical procedure. It is accomplished following conventional intubation and surgical preparation of the lateral aspect of the head and neck. An index finger is inserted into the piriform fossa, caudal to the base of the tongue and lateral to the hyoid apparatus producing a bulge to indicate the area for skin incision. Following surgical preparation, a small incision is made to permit passage of forceps by blunt dissection from the external surface into the pharynx (Figure 2-17). The tube adapter is removed from the pre-placed tube, the cuff is deflated and the tube advanced into the mouth to allow it to be grasped at the adapter end with the forceps that have been inserted into the pharynx through the incision (Figure 2-18). The tube's distal end is then inserted into the

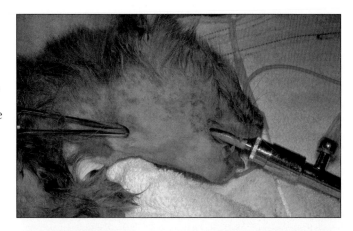

Figure 2-17 Pharangotomy–cat. Forceps are inserted through incision. Tracheal tube is inserted down the trachea with system detached and the distal end of the tube is brought through the incision. The anesthetic system is then reattached.

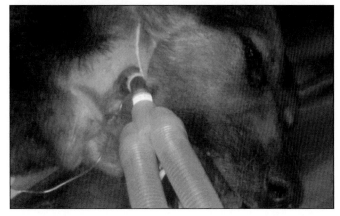

Figure 2-18 Pharangotomy–dog. Endotracheal tube has been inserted through incision to provide better access and assessment of repair for fractured mandible. A reinforced endotracheal tube is useful to avoid kinking as it turns 108° within the pharynx.

trachea and the tube is advanced to its proper position with the adapter end exiting the incision on the neck. It is then secured with tape and skin sutures (Figure 2-19) and connected to the anesthetic circuit. The ET tube must be removed from the pharyngotomy incision prior to anesthesia recovery in the reverse order of placement. If control of the airway is to be maintained postanesthesia, tracheostomy should be used instead of tracheal pharyngotomy. Either of these procedures will be very helpful for repair of jaw fractures and for major procedures involving the mouth.

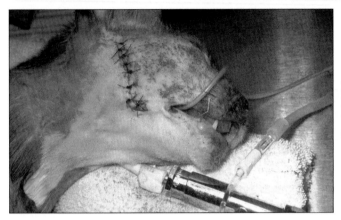

Figure 2-19 Pharangotomy–cat. Incision for surgical repair is shown with endotracheal tube on opposite side and pilot balloon catheter visible.

References

Adams HA (1998). Mechanisms of action of ketamine. *Anaesthesiol Reanim* 23:60-63.

Adam HK, Glen JB, Hoyle PA (1980). Pharmacokinetics in laboratory animals of ICI 35 868, a new i.v. anaesthetic agent.*Br J Anaesth* 52:743-746.

Akkerdaas LC, Mioch P, Sap R, Hellebrekers LJ (2001). Cardiopulmonary effects of three different anaesthesia protocols in cats. *Vet Q* 23:182-186.

Ambalavanar R, Purcell L, Miranda M, et al. (2002). Selective suppression of late laryngeal adductor responses by N-methyl-D-aspartate receptor blockade in the cat. *J Neurophysiol* 87:1252-1262.

Amend JF, Kiavano PA, Stone EC (1972). Premedication with xylazine to eliminate muscular hypertonicity in cats during ketamine anesthesia. *Vet Med/ Sm Ani Clin* 67:1305-1307.

Andress JL, Day TK, Day D (1995). The effects of consecutive day propofol anesthesia on feline red blood cells. *Vet Surg* 24:277-282.

Baker AK, Hoffmann VL, Meert TF (2002). Interactions of NMDA antagonists and an alpha 2 agonist with mu, delta and kappa opioids in an acute nociception assay. *Acta Anaesthesiol Belg* 53:203-212.

Beck CC, Coppock RW, Ott BS (1971). Evaluation of Vetalar (ketamine HCl). A unique feline anesthetic. *Vet Med Small Anim Clin* 66:993-996.

Beck CC, Dresner AJ (1972). Vetalar (ketamine HCl) a cataleptoid anesthetic agent for primate species. *Vet Med Small Anim Clin* 67:1082-1084.

Benson J (2004). University of Illinois-Champaign/Urbana, IL.

Bissonnette B, Swan H, Ravussiin P, Un V (1999). Neuroleptanesthesia: current status. *Can J Anaesth* 46:154-168.

Bonhaus DW, Sawyer DC, and Hook JB (1981). Displacement of protein-bound thiopental by sodium methiodal (Skiodan) may contribute to anesthetic complications during canine myelography. *Amer J Vet Res* 42:1612-1614.

Brearley JC, Kellagher REB, Hall LW (1988). Propofol anaesthesia in cats. *J Small Anim Pract* 29:315-322.

Bree MM, Cohen BJ, Rowe SE (1972). Dissociative anesthesia in dogs and primates: clinical evaluation of CI 744. *Lab Ani Sci* 22:878-881.

Bufalari A, Short CE, Giannoni C, Vainio O (1996). Comparative responses to propofol anaesthesia alone and with alpha 2-adrenergic medications in a canine model. *Acta Vet Scand* 37:187-201.

Castroman PJ and Ness TJ (2002). Ketamine, an N-methyl-D-aspartate receptor antagonist, inhibits the reflex responses to distension of the rat urinary bladder. *Anesthesiology* 96:1401-1409.

Chambers JP, Dobson JM (1989). A midazolam and ketamine combination as a sedative in cats. *J Ass Vet Anaesth* 16:53-54.

Chen TL, Huang FY, Lin SY, Chao CC (1989). Hemodynamic response to ketamine and diazepam in dogs with acute cardiac tamponade. *Anaesthesiologica Sinica* 27:19-25.

Cistola AM, Golder FJ, Levy AM, et al. (2002). Comparison of two injectable anesthetic regimes in feral cats at a large volume spay clinic. *Proc Ann Mtg Am Coll Vet Anes,* Orlando, P 43.

Cockshott ID, Douglas EJ, Plummer GF, Simons PJ (1992). The pharmacokinetics of propofol in laboratory animals. *Xenobiotica* 22:369-375.

Commons M (1970). Clinical experiences with KETAMINE HYDROCHLORIDE as an intramuscular general anesthetic in the cat. *Vet Med/Sm Ani Clin* 65:1151-1152.

Conway CM, Ellis DB (1969). The hemodynamic effects of short-acting barbiturates. *Br J Anaesth* 41:534-542.

Cording CJ, DeLuca R, Camporese T, Spratt E (1999). A fatality related to the veterinary anesthetic telazol. *J Anal Toxicol* 23:552-555.

Corssen G, Domino EF, Bree RL (1969). Electroencephalographic effects of ketamine anesthesia in children. *Anesth Analg* 48:141-147.

Court MH (1999a). Anesthesia of the sighthound. *Clin Tech Small Anim Pract* 14:38-43.

Court MH, Hay-Kraus BL, Hill DW, et al (1999b). Propofol hydroxylation by dog liver microsomes: assay development and dog breed differences. *Drug Metab Dispos* 27:1293-1299.

Cruz ML, Luna SP, de Castro, et al. (2000). A preliminary trial comparison of several anesthetic techniques in cats. *Can Vet J* 41:481-485.

De Kock M, Levand'homme P, Waterloos H (2001). "Balanced analgesia" in the perioperative period: is there a place for ketamine? *Pain* 92:373-380.

Domino EF (1990). *Status of ketamine in Anesthesiology:* NPP Books, Ann Arbor.

Deryck-Yvon LJM, Brimioulle-Serge A, Maggiorini-Marco, et al (1996). Systemic vascular effects of isoflurane versus propofol anesthesia in dogs. *Anesth Analg* 83:958-964.

DeYoung, DJ and Sawyer DC. Anesthetic potency of nitrous oxide during halothane anesthesia in the dog. *J Amer Anim Hosp Assn* 16:125-128, 1980.

DeYoung DW, Paddleford RR, Short CE (1972). Dissociative anesthetics in the cat and dog. *JAVMA* 161:1442-1445.

Dillmann J (1998). Ketamine abuse-a new edge. *Todays Surg Nurse* 20:37-39.

Dodam JR, Kruse-Elliott KT, Aucoin DP, Swanson CR (1990). Duration of etomidate-induced adrenocortical suppression during surgery in dogs. *Am J Vet Res* 51:786-788.

Downs GJ, Haley PR, Parent JB (1991). Propofol: Can a single ampule be used for multiple patients? (Correspondence) *Anesthesiology* 74:1156.

Eger EI, II (1964): Respiratory and circulatory factors in uptake and distribution of volatile anaesthetic agents. *Brit J Anaesth* 36:155-171.

England GCW and Clarke LW (1989): The effect of route of administration upon the efficacy of medetomidine. *J Assoc Vet Anaesth* 16:32-34.

Ewing KK (1993). Isoflurane MAC-reduction by medetomidine and its reversal by antipamezole in dogs. *Am J Vet Res* 54:294-299.

Evans AT (2002). Personal communication. Michigan State University, E. Lansing, MI.

Evans AT (2004). Echocardiographic evaluation of propofol–thiopental combination in healthy dogs. In prep, Michigan State University, E. Lansing, MI.

Geel JK (1991). The effect of premedication on the induction dose of propofol in dogs and cats. *J S Afr Vet Assoc* 62:118-123.

Giese JL, Stanley TH (1983). Etomidate: a new intravenous anesthetic induction agent. *Pharmacotherapy* 3:251-258.

Glen JB (1980). Animal studies of the anaesthetic activity of ICI 35 868. *Br J Anaesth* 52:731-742.

Glen JB, Hunter SC, Blackburn TP, Wood P (1985). Interaction studies and other investigations of the pharmacology of propofol ("Diprivan"). *Postgrad Med J* 61 Suppl 3:7-14.

Glowaski MM, Wetmore LA (1999). Propofol: applicationin veterinary sedation and anesthesia. *Clin Tech Small Anim Pract* 14:1-9.

Goodchild CS, Serrao JM (1989). Cardiovascular effects of propofol in the anaesthetized dog. *Br J Anaesth* 63:87-92.

Gross ME, Dodam JR, Pope ER, Jones BD (2002). A comparison of thiopental, propofol, and diazepam-ketamine anesthesia for evaluation of laryngeal function in dogs premedicated with butorphanol-glycopyrrolate. *JAAHA* 38:503-506.

Hall LW, Chambers JP (1987). A clinical trial of propofol infusion anesthesia in dogs. *J Sm Anim Prac* 28:623-638.

Hamilton SM, Broadstone RV, Johnston SA (2002). The evaluation of analgesia provided by epidural ketamine in dogs with chemically induced synovitis. *Proc Ann Mtg Am Coll Vet Anes*, Orlando, P 19.

Hardenkergh JG, Mann FC (1927). The auto-inhalation method of anesthesia in canine surgery. *J Amer Vet Med Assn* 71:493.

Hartsfield SM, Gendreau CL, Smith CW, et al (1977). Endotracheal intubation by pharyngotomy. *J Amer Anim Hosp Assn* 13:71-74.

Haskins SC, Farver TB, Patz JD (1985). Ketamine in dogs. *Am J Vet Res* 46:1855-1860.

Haskins SC, Farver TB, Patz JD (1986). Cardiovascular changes in dogs given diazepam and diazepam-ketamine. *Am J Vet Res* 47:795-798.

Haskins SC, Peiffer RL, Stowe CM (1975). A clinical comparison of CT 1341, ketamine, and xylazine in cats. *Am J Vet Res* 36, 1537-1543.

Hatch RC (1966): The effect of glucose, sodium lactate, and epinephrine on thiopental anesthesia in dogs. *J Am Vet Med Assn* 148:135-143.

Hay Kraus BL, Greenblatt DJ, Venkatakrishnan K, Court MH (2000). Evidence for propofol hydroxylation by cytochrome P4502B11 in canine liver microsomes: breed and gender differences. *Xenobiotica* 30:575-588.

Heavner JE, Bloedow DC (1979). Ketamine pharmacokinetics in domestic cats. *Vet Anesth* 6:16-19.

Heldmann E, Brown DC, Shofer F (1999). The association of propofol usage with postoperative wound infection rate in clean wounds: a retrospective study. *Vet Surg* 28:256-259.

Hellyer PW, Freeman PW, Hubbell JA (1991). Induction of anesthesia with diazepam-ketamine and midazolam-ketamine in greyhounds. *Vet Surg* 20:143-147.

Hellyer PW, Muir WW 3rd, Hubbell JA, Sally J (1988). Cardiorespiratory effects of the intravenous administration of tiletamine-zolazepam to cats. *Vet Surg* 17:105-110.

Hellyer PW, WW 3rd, Hubbell JA, Sally J (1989). Cardiorespiratory effects of the intravenous administration of tiletamine-zolazepam to dogs. *Vet Surg* 18:160-165.

Huang GS, Yeh CC, Kiong SS, et al. (2000). Intra-articular ketamine for pain control following arthroscopic knee surgery. *Acta Anaesthesiol Sin* 38:131-136.

Humphrey WJ (1971). Ketamine HCl as a general anesthetic in dogs. Mod Vet Pract 6:38-39.

Ilkiw JE, Benthuysen JA, Ebling WF, McNeal D (1991a). A comparative study of the pharmacokinetics of thiopental in the rabbit, sheep and dog. *J Vet Pharmacol Ther* 14:134-140.

Ilkiw JE, Haskins SC, Patz JD (1991b). Cardiovascular and respiratory effects of thiopental administration in hypovolemic dogs. *Am J Vet Res* 52:576-580.

Ilkiw JE (1992a). Advantages and guidelines for using ultrashort barbiturates for induction of anesthesia. *Vet Clin North Am Small Anim Pract* 22:261-264.

Ilkiw JE (1992b). Other potentially useful new injectable anesthetic agents. *Vet Clin North Am Small Anim Pract* 22:281-289.

Ilkiw JE, Pascoe PJ (2002). Cardiovascular effects of propofol alone and in combination with ketamine for total intravenous anesthesia in healthy cats. Proc Ann Mtg Am Coll Vet Anes, Orlando, P 45.

Ilkiw JE, Pascoe PJ, Haskins SC, Patz JD (1992b). Cardiovascular and respiratory effects of propofol administration in hypovolemic dogs. *Am J Vet Res* 53:2323-2327.

Ilkiw JE, Suter CM, McNeal D, et al. (1996). The effect of intravenous administration of variable-dose midazolam after fixed-dose ketamine in healthy awake cats. *J Vet Pharmacol and Ther* 19:217-224.

Ilkiw JE, Suter C, McNeal D, et al. (1998). The optimal intravenous dose of midazolam after intravenous ketamine in healthy awake cats. *J Vet Pharmacol and Ther* 21:54-61.

Jacobson JD and Hartsfield SM (1993a). Cardiorespiratory effects of intravenous bolus administration and infusion of ketamine-midazolam in dogs. *Am J Vet Res* 54:1710-1714.

Jacobson JD and Hartsfield SM (1993b). Cardiovascular effects of intravenous bolus administration and infusion of ketamine-midazolam in isoflurane-anesthetized dogs. *Am J Vet Res* 54:1715-20.

Jansen KL, Darracot-Cankovic R (2001). The nonmedical use of ketamine, part two: A review of problem use and dependence. *J Psychoactive Drugs* 33:151-158.

Johnstone RE (1973). A ketamine trip. *Anesthesiology* 39:460-461.

Jones RS (2001). Epidural analgesia in the dog and cat. *Vet J* 161:123-131.

Joubert K (1998). Ketamine hydrochloride-an adjunct for analgesia in dogs with burn wounds. *J S Afr Vet Assoc* 69:95-97.

Kamibayashi T, Hayashi Y, Sumikawa K, et al (1991). Enhancement by propofol of epinephrine-induced arrhythmias in dogs. *Anesthesiology* 75:1935-1040.

Kaplan B (1972). Ketamine HCl anesthesia in dogs: observation of 327 cases. *Vet Med/Sm Ani Clin* 67:631-634.

Keegan RD, Green SA (1993). Cardiovascular effects of a continuous two-hour propofol infusion in dogs. Comparison with isoflurane anesthesia. *Vet Surg* 22:537-543.

Kissin I, Motomura S, Aultman DF, et al (1983). Inotropic and anesthetic potencies of etomidate and thiopental in dogs. *Anesth Analg* 62:961-965.

Klotz U, Antonin KH, Bieck PR (1976). Pharmacokinetics and plasma binding of diazepam in man, dog, rabbit, guinea pig and rat. *J Pharmacol Exp Ther* 199:67-73.

Ko JC (2002). Feral cat anesthesia. Personal communication. University of Florida, Gainsville, FL.

Ko JC, Fox SM, Mandsager RE (2000). Sedative and cardiorespiratrory effects of medetomidine, medetomidine-butorphanol, and medetomidine-ketamine in dogs. *JAVMA* 216:1578-1583.

Ko JC, Golder FJ, Mandsager RE, et al. (1999). Anesthetic and cardiorespiratory effects of a 1:1 mixture of propofol and thiopental sodium in dogs. *JAVMA* 215:1292-1296.

Ko JC, Thurmon JC, Benson GJ, et al (1993). Acute haemolysis associated with etomidate-propylene glycol infusion in dogs. *J Vet Anaesth* 20:92-94.

Ko JC, Nicklin CF, Melendaz M, et al (1998). Effects of a microdose on diazepam-ketamine induced anesthesia in dogs. *J Am Vet Med Assoc* 213:215-219.

Kolata RJ (1986). Induction of anesthesia using diazepam/ketamine in dogs with complete heart block: A preliminary report. *Vet Surg* 15:339-341.

Krahwinkel DJ, Sawyer DC, Eyster, GE, Bender G (1975). Cardiopulmonary effects of fentanyl-droperidol, nitrous oxide, and atropine sulfate in dogs. *Am J Vet Res* 36:1211-1219.

Kruse-Elliott KT, Swanson CR, Aucoin DP (1987). Effects of etomidate on adrenocortical function in canine surgical patients. *Am J Vet Res* 48:1098-1100.

Laine E, et al: Structural studies of medetomidine hydrochloride, a new drug substance. *Acta Pharm Fenn* 95(3): 119-127, 1986.

Lerche P, Nolan AM, Reid J (2000). Comparative study of propofol or propofol and ketamine for the induction of anaesthesia in dogs. *Vet Rec* 146:571-574.

Lechner MD, Kreuscher H (1989). The physical compatibility of ketamine and diazepam in infusion solutions. *Anaesthesist* 38:418-420.

Lee IO, Lee IH (2001). Systemic, but not intrathecal, ketamine produces preemptive analgesia in the rat formalin model. *Acta Anaesth Sin* 39:123-127.

Lesser T, Ebner E, Zwiener U (1993). Ketamine-diazepam N20 combination anesthesia-a new "circulatory-system-sparing" type of anesthetic in experimental surgery. *Res Exp Med* 193:207-211.

Long JP, Greco SC (2000). The effect of propofol administered intravenously on appetite stimulation in dogs. *Contemp Top Lab Anim Sci* 39:43-46.

Lumb WV (1963):The barbiturates and thiobarbiturates. In *Small Animal Anesthesia*, Lea & Febiger, Philadelphia. pp 170-197.

Lumb WV and Jones EW (1973): The barbiturates. In *Veterinary Anesthesia*. Lea & Febiger, Philadelphia.

Manziano CF, Manzaino JR (1978). The combination of ketamine HCl and acepromazine maleate as a general anesthetic in dogs. *Vet Med SAC* June: 727-730.

Maze M, Tranquilli W (1991). Alpha $_2$-adrenoceptor agonist, defining the role in clinical anesthesia. *Anesthesiology* 74(3):581-605.

McArdle P (1999). Intravenous analgesia. *Crit Care Clin* 15:89-104.

Menigaux C, Fletcher D, Dupont X, et al. (2000). The benefits of intraoperative small-dose ketamine on postoperative pain after anterior cruciate ligament repair. *Anesth Analg* 90:129-135.

Meuldermans WE, Heykants JJ (1976). The plasma protein binding and distribution of etomidate in dog, rat and human blood. *Arch Int Pharmacodyn Ther* 221:150-162.

Mikkelsen S, Likjaer S, Brennum, Borgbjerg FM (1999). The effect of naloxone on ketamine-induced effects on hyperalgesia and ketamine-induced side effects in humans. *Anesthesiology* 90:1539-1545.

Moon PE, Erb HN, Ludders JW, et al (2000). Perioperative risk factors for puppies delivered by cesarean section in the United States and Canada. *J Am Anim Hosp Assoc* 36:359-368.

Morgan DW, Legge K (1989). Clinical evaluation of propofol as an intravenous anaesthetic agent in cats and dogs. *Vet Rec* 124:31-33.

Muir WW III, Werner LL, Hamilton RL (1975). Arrhythmias in dogs associated with epinephrine and thiamylal anesthesia. *Am J Vet Res* 36:1291-1297.

Muir WW III (1977). Electrocardiographic interpretation of thiobarbiturate-induced dysrhythmias in dogs. *J Amer Vet Med Assn* 170:1419-1424.

Muir WW III and Hubbell JA (1988). Cardiopulmonary and anesthetic effects of ketamine and its enantiomers in dogs. *Am J Vet Res* 49:530-534.

Muir WW III, Mason DE (1989). Side effects of etomidate in dogs. *J Amer Vet Med Assn* 194:1430-1434.

Murison PJ (2001). Effect of propofol at two injection rates or thiopentone on post-intubation apnoea in the dog. *J Small Anim Pract* 42:71-74.

Myers RA (1973). More on Ketamine Evaluation (Letters to Editor). *JAVMA* 163:694.

Niffors L, et al. (1989): Sedative and analgesic effects of medetomidine in dogs-an open clinical study. *Acta Vet Scand* 85:155.

Olivar T and Laird JM (1999). Differential effects of N-methyl-D-aspartate receptor blockade on nociceptive somatic and visceral reflexes. *Pain* 79:67-73.

Otto K (2004). Personal communication. Institut für Versuchstierkunde und Zentrales Tierlaboratorium Medizinische Hochschule Hannover. Carl-Neuberg-Str. 1,D-30625 Hannover, Germany.

Pagel PS, Waritier DC (1993). Negative inotropic effects of propofol as evaluated by the regional preload recruitable stroke work relationship in chronically instrumented dogs. *Anesthesiology-Hagerstown* 78:100-108.

Pal HR, Berry N, Kumar R, Ray R (2002). Ketamine dependence. *Anaesth Intensive Care* 30:382-384.

Pascoe PJ, Ilkiw JE, Haskins SC, Patz JD (1992). Cardiopulmonary effects of etomidate in hypovolemic dogs. *Am J Vet Res* 53:2178-2182.

Price HL, Kovnat BS, Conner EH, Price ML (1960). The uptake of thiopental by body tissues and its relation to the duration of narcosis. *Clin Pharmacol Ther* 1:16-23.

Quail MT, Weimersheimer P, Woolf AD, Magnani B (2001). Abuse of telazol: an animal tranquilizer. *J Toxicol Clin Toxicol* 39:399-402.

Quandt JE, Robinson EP, Rivers WJ, Raffe MR (1998). Cardiorespiratory and anesthetic effects of propofol and thiopental in dogs. *Am J Vet Res* 59:1137-1143.

Räihä MP, et al. (1989a): A comparison of xylazine, acepromazine, meperidine, and medetomidine as preanesthetics to halothane anesthesia in dogs. *Acta Vet Scand* 85:97-102.

Räihä JE, et al. (1989b). Medetomidine as a preanesthetic prior to ketamine-HCl and halothane anesthesia on laboratory beagles. *Acta Vet Scand* 85:103-110.

Räihä MP, et al. (1989c). Comparison of three different dose regimens of medetomidine in laboratory beagles. *Acta Vet Scand* 85:111.

Rawlings CA and Kolata RJ (1983). Cardiopulmonary effects of thiopental/lidocaine combination during anesthetic induction in the dog. *Am J Vet Res* 44:144-149.

Reboso-Morales JA, Gonzalez-Miranda F (1999). *Rev Esp Anestesiol Reanim* 46:111-122.

Reich DL, Silvay G (1989). Ketamine: an update on the first twenty-five years of clinical experience. *Can J Anaesth* 36:186-197.

Reid J, Nolan AM (1992). Prolonged recovery following propofol infusion in a dog: a case report. *J Vet Anaesth* 29:61-64.

Reid JS, Frank RJ (1972). Prevention of undersirable side reactions of ketamine anesthesia in cats. *JAAHA* 8:115-119.

Rex MEA (1970). A review of the structural and functional basis of laryngospasm and a discussion of the nerve pathways involved in the reflex and its clinical significance in man and animals. *Br. J. Anaesth*. 42:891.

Riviera FB, Pires JS (2002). Comparison between S(+) ketamine-diazepam and S(+) ketamine-midazolam on anesthetic induction and recovery in dogs. *Proc Ann Mtg Am Coll Vet Anes*, Orlando, P 38.

Robertson SA (2001). Analgesia and analgesic techniques. *Vet Clin North Am Exot Anim Pract* 4:1-18.

Robertson SA, Johnston S, Beensterboer J (1992). Cardiopulmonary, anesthetic, and postanesthetic effects of intravenous infusions of propofol in greyhounds and non-greyhounds. *Am J Vet Res* 53:1027-1032.

Robertson SA, Lascelles BDX, Taylor PM (2002a). Effect of low dose ketamine on thermal thresholds in cats. *Proc Ann Mtg Am Coll Vet Anes*, Orlando, P 39.

Robertson SA, Lascelles BDX, Taylor PM (2002b). Effect of 0.1, 0.2, 0.4 and 0.8 mg/kg of intravenous butorphanol on thermal antinociception in cats. *Proc Ann Mtg Am Coll Vet Anes*, Orlando, P 29.

Robinson EP, Johnston GR (1986a). Radiographic assessment of laryngeal reflexes in ketamine-anesthetized cats. *Am J Vet Res* 47:1569-1572.

Robinson EP, Sams RA, Muir WW (1986b). Barbiturate anesthesia in greyhound and mixed-breed dogs: comparative cardiopulmonary effects, anesthetic effects, and recovery rates. *Am J Vet Res* 47:2105-2112.

Sams RA, Muir WW, Detra RL, et al. (1985). Comparative pharmacokinetics and anesthetic effects of methohexital, pentobarbital, thiamylal, and thiopental in greyhound dogs and non-greyhound, mixed breed dogs. *Am J Vet Res* 46:1677-1683.

Savola JM (1989). Cardiovascular actions of medetomidine and their reversal by atipamezole. *Acta Vet Scand* 85:39.

Sawyer DC, Lumb WV, and Stone HL (1971). Cardiovascular effects of halothane, methoxyflurane, pentobarbital, and thiamylal. *J Appl Physiol* 30:36-43.

Sawyer DC (1973). Effect of anesthetic agents on cardiovascular function and cardiac rhythm. *Vet Clin North Am* 3:25-31.

Sawyer DC (1975). Comparative effects of halothane-nitrous oxide induction: Face-mask versus induction chamber. *25th Gaines Symposium*, October 23rd.

Sawyer DC, Hoogstraten S (1980). A ketamine experience: Unintentional injection of ketamine HCl into a human. *JAAHA* 8:123.

Sawyer DC, Rech RH (1987). Analgesia and behavioral effects of butorphanol, nalbuphine, and pentazocine in the cat. *J Am Anim Hosp Assoc* 23,438-446.

Sawyer DC, Rech RH, Durham RA (1990). Effects of ketamine and combination with acetylpromazine, diazepam, or butorphanol on visceral nociception in the cat, In *Status of ketamine in Anesthesiology*: Domino EF (Ed), NPP Books. pp. 247-259.

Sawyer DC, Rech RH, Durham RA (1993). Does ketamine provide adequate visceral analgesia when used alone or in combination with acepromazine, diazepam, or butorphanol in cats? *JAAHA* 29:257-263.

Scheinin H, et al (1988). Behavioral and neurochemical effects of atipamezole, a novel alpha$_2$-adrenoceptor antagonist. *Eur J Pharmacol* 151:35-42.

Schmid R, Koren G, Klein J, Katz J (2002). The stability of a ketamine-morphine solution. *Anesth Analg* 94:898-900.

Shomer RR (1992). Misuse of ketamine (Letters to Editor). *JAVMA* 200:256-257.

Short CE (1987a). Neuroleptananalgesia and alpha-adrenergic receptor analgesia. In: Short, C.E. (Ed.), *Principles and Practice of Veterinary Anesthesia*. Williams and Wilkins, Baltimore, pp. 47-49.

Short CE (1987b). Dissociative Anesthesia. In: Short, C.E. (Ed.), *Principles and Practice of Veterinary Anesthesia*. Williams and Wilkins, Baltimore, p. 165.

Short CE, Bufalari A (1999). Propofol anesthesia. *Vet Clin North Am Small Anim Pract* 29:747-778.

Short CE, Paddleford RR (1976). The use of dissociative tranquilizer combinations for anesthesia in the dog. *26th Gaines Symp*, Oct 27, Columbus. pp. 7-11.

Skarda RT, Bednarski RM, Muir WW, et al (1995). Sedation and anesthesia in dogs and cats with cardiovascular diseases. I. Anesthesia plan considering risk assessment, hemodynamic effects of drugs and monitoring. *Schweiz Arch Tierheilkd* 137:312-321.

Smedile LE, Duke T, Taylor SM (1996). Excitatory movements in a dog following propofol anesthesia. *J Am Anim Hosp Assoc* 32:365-368.

Smith JA, Gaynor JS, Bednarski RM, Muir WW (1993). Adverse effects of administration of propofol with various preanesthetic regimens in dogs. J Am Vet Med Assoc 202:1111-1115.

Stiles SW (1959). Induction of ether anesthesia in cats. *J Am Vet Med Assoc* 134:275.

Subramaniam B, Subramaniam K, Pawar DK, et al. (2001). Preoperative epidural ketamine in combination with morphine does not have a clinically relevant intra- and postoperative opioid-sparing effect. *Anesth Analg* 93:1321-1326.

Taylor PM (1999). Newer analgesics. Nonsteroid anti-inflammatory drugs, opioids, and combinations. *Vet Clin North Am Small Anim Pract* 29:719-735.

Tranquilli WJ, et al (1984). Halothane sparing effect of xylazine in dogs and subsequent reversal with tolazoline. *J Vet Pharmacol Ther* 7:23-28.

Turner DM, Ilkiw JE (1990a). Potency of rapidly acting barbiturates in dogs, using inhibition of the laryngeal reflex as the end point. *Am J Vet Res* 51:595-597.

Turner DM, Ilkiw JE (1990b). Cardiovascular and respiratory effects of three rapidly acting barbiturates in dogs. *Am J Vet Res* 51:598-604.

Vähä-Vahe T (1990). The clinical effectiveness of atipamezole as a medetomidine antagonist in the dog. *J Vet Pharmacol Ther* 13:198-205.

Vainio O, et al. (1986). Medetomidine: a new sedative and analgesic drug for dogs and cats. *J Assoc Vet Anaesth Great Britain Ireland* 7(14):53.

Vainio O, et al (1989). Sedative and analgesic effects of medetomidine in dogs. *J Vet Pharmacol Ther* 12:225-231.

Vainio O, Vähä-Vahe T (1990). Reversal of medetomidine sedation by atipamezole in dogs. *J Vet Pharmacol Ther* 13:15-22.

Wagner AE, Walton JA, Hellyer PW, et al. (2002). Use of low doses of ketamine administered by constant rate infusion as an adjunct for post-operative analgesia in dogs. *JAVMA* 221:72-75.

Watkins SB and Hall LW (1987). Propofol as an intravenous anesthetic agent in dogs. *Vet Rec* 120:326-329.

Watney GCG, Pablo LS (1992). Median effective dosage of propofol for induction of anesthesia in dogs. *Am J Vet Res* 53:2320-2322.

Weaver BM, Raptopoulos D (1990). Induction of anaesthesia in dogs and cats with propofol. *Vet Rec* 126:617-620.

Wertz EM, Benson GJ, Thurmon JC, et al (1990). Pharmacokinetics of etomidate in cats. *Am J Vet Res* 51:281-284.

Wetzel RW, Ramsay EC (1998). Comparison of four regimens for intraoral administration of medication to induce sedation in cats prior to euthanasia. *JAVMA* 213:243-245.

White PF, Way WL, Trevor AJ (1982). Ketamine-Its pharmacology and therapeutic uses. *Anesthesiology* 56:119-136.

Wright M (1982). Pharmacologic effects of ketamine and its use in veterinary medicine. *JAVMA* 180:1462-1471.

Yamakura T, Sakimura K, Shimoji K (1999). Direct inhibition of the N-methyl-D-aspartate receptor channel by high concentrations of opioids. *Anesthesiology* 91:1053-1063.

Young LE and Jones RS (1990): Clinical observations on medetomidine/ketamine anesthesia and its antagonism by atipamezole in the cat. *J Small Anim Pract* 31:221-224.

Zacher AN, Zornow MH, Evans G (1991). Drug contamination from opening glass ampules. *Anesthesiology* 75:893-895.

Zoran DL, Riedesel DH, Dyer DC (1993). Pharmacokinetics of propofol in mixed-breed dogs and Greyhounds. *Am J Vet Res* 54:755-760.

Chapter 3
The Anesthetic Period

Anesthetic Machines

Although veterinarians were using anesthetic machines for delivery of diethyl ether for small animals in the late 40's and early 50's, these were units that had been used for human patients with names like Ohio, Heidbrink, Foregger, and McKesson. Machines specifically designed for small animals were not introduced until methoxyflurane and halothane were approved for use in veterinary patients. Two names were most familiar in the early 60's: Pitman-Moore and Fraser Sweatman. Later, Dupaco, Foregger, and North American Drager made their entrance into the veterinary market. At of the beginning of the 21st century, there were more than 15 different manufacturers of veterinary machines for small animals.

Human anesthetic machines were governed for 10 years by a standard first published in 1979 by the American National Standards Institute (ANSI). The ANSI standard was superseded by a standard prepared under the auspices of the American Society for Testing and Materials (ASTM 1988). This defined basic design, performance and safety requirements for human machines made in the 1990's. Manufacturers of veterinary machines are not mandated to follow the ASTM standards but there are some companies that do this on a voluntary basis. A large number of pre-owned human anesthetic machines can be found in veterinary hospitals and there are a few companies that market used human machines to veterinarians. Some of these older machines can still be serviced but owners of machines from companies that are no longer in business or who have discontinued manufacturing veterinary anesthesia units, may find it difficult to have these serviced because of the unavailability of parts.

Anesthetic machines have two basic components: the gas delivery system and a breathing circuit. The delivery system is the same for semi-open, semi-closed or closed circuits. It contains sources of compressed gases, cylinder yokes, cylinder valves, pressure gauges, pressure-reducing valves, flow meters, flow meter controls, flush valve and vaporizers for volatile liquid anesthetics. For a circle CO_2 absorption system, additional components are: carbon dioxide absorber, inspiratory and expiratory valves, APL valve, reservoir bag, connecting hoses, breathing conduits, Y-piece and low pressure manometer (Figure 3-1).

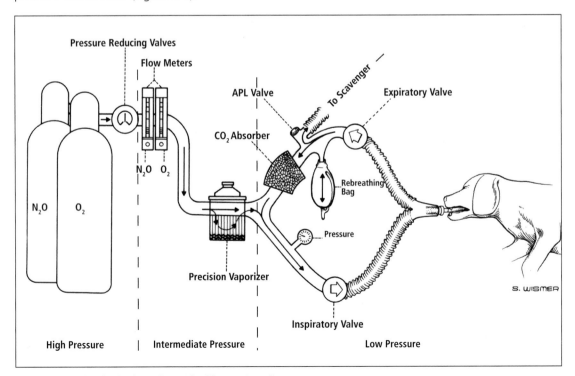

Figure 3-1 Circle Carbon Dioxide Absorption System.

To better understand the operation of an anesthesia machine, it is helpful to consider the system as three separate units in one. The <u>high pressure system</u> receives gases at cylinder pressure, e.g., oxygen and nitrous oxide. The pressure is then reduced to a constant 50-55psi by the regulator before entering the <u>intermediate pressure system.</u> Gases are received from the regulator or hospital pipeline and delivered to flow control valves (flow meters) and the oxygen flush. <u>The low-pressure system</u> receives gases from the flow control valve(s) and delivers them to the common gas outlet which then is connected to flow inlet of the breathing circuit and to patient.

High Pressure System

The high-pressure system consists of those parts of the machine that receive gas at cylinder pressure. These components include the hanger yoke by which a cylinder is connected to the machine, the cylinder pressure gauge and regulator that converts a high variable pressure to a lower constant pressure. The hanger yoke has several parts including body, retaining screw to hold the cylinder in place, nipple through which gas enters the machine, index pins, washer to provide a seal between the cylinder and yoke, filter to remove dirt from gas in the cylinder and check valve assembly that prevents gas flowing from another cylinder or pipe line system (Figure 3-2). Many older machines lack check valves so the possibility of accidentally transfilling E tanks can happen. Transfilling of cylinders can lead to rapid expansion and compression of gases which may result in an explosion. Of course, this can occur only if both tanks are open or if a small tank is opened with the central supply connected.

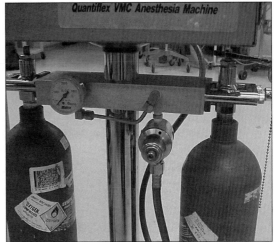

Figure 3-2 Veterinary Anesthesia Machine with two size E oxygen tanks.

Each yoke assembly must be identified with name and color code for the specific gas. To hold the cylinder in place, the conical point of the retaining screw must fit the conical depression of the cylinder valve. Pins of the Pin Index Safety System (PISS) are mounted into holes just below the nipple on the valve (Figure 3-3A). This is used on size D and E cylinders. Two pins project from the yolk and are positioned to fit into two corresponding holes in the valve mounted at the top end of the cylinder. If pins and holes are not aligned properly, the tank cannot be tightly fitted against the yoke washer. Positioning of pins and holes is different for each gas: oxygen, nitrous oxide, air, nitrogen, helium and various mixtures of oxygen and CO_2. To maintain patient safety, it is essential that pins on the yoke not be removed that would allow mounting the wrong gas containing cylinder on the machine.

Compressed Gases

Compressed Gases for anesthetic machines are available in aluminum or steel cylinders of different sizes designated by a letter code (Table 3-1). Letters D and E are used for smaller tanks and G or H for large tanks. Color is used to designate gas content of a cylinder and there are differences

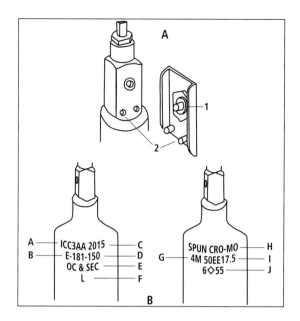

Figure 3-3A & B Features of Various Gas Cylinders

between United States and International standards (Table 3-2). For cylinders containing a single gas, they are covered entirely with a water-insoluble paint. The color code for the United States identifies oxygen as green and blue for nitrous oxide. Several countries including Canada have adopted an international code for oxygen which is white. Blue for nitrous oxide is used for both codes.

Compressed gases may be supplied from one or more large cylinders (G or H) usually from a bank-manifold system in a separate part of the hospital (Figure 3-4) or from small cylinders mounted on the unit (E-tanks, Figure 3-2). There are indications and precautions to follow for both systems. Because a central supply may fail, it is a safety precaution to keep small tanks (D or E cylinders) on the anesthesia unit for use in an emergency or when transporting an anesthetized patient. For intermediate needs, an M or F tank may used on the anesthesia machine but this requires a special bracket and mounting frame (Figure 3-5). For economic reasons, it is far better to use compressed gases from large cylinders as the primary source because they contain eight to ten times more gas than small tanks for approximately the same cost.

Table 3-1 Steel Medical Gas Cylinders*

Cylinder Size	Dimensions OD X Length (inches)	Weight of empty cylinder (lbs)	Capacity and pressure @ 70°F	Oxygen	Nitrous Oxide	Air
D	4½ x 17	11	liters	400	940	375
			psig	1,900	745	1,900
E	4¼ x 26	14	liters	660	1590	625
			psig	1,900	745	1,900
M / F**	7 x 43	63	liters	3,450	7,570	2,850
			psig	2,200	745	1,900
G	8½ x 51	97	liters	5,299	13,800	5,050
			psig	2,200	745	1,900
H	9¼ x 51	119	liters	6,900	15,800	6,550
			psig	2,200	745	2,200

Modified from Dorsch & Dorsch, Understanding Anesthesia Equipment, Williams & Wilkins, 1994.
*Aluminum cylinders are shorter and have a larger diameter than steel cylinders.
**F is the international designation

Table 3-2

Medical Gases

Gas	United States Color	International Color	Condition in Cylinder
Oxygen	Green	White	Gas
Carbon Dioxide	Gray*	Gray	Liquified below 88°F
Nitrous Oxide	Blue	Blue	Liquified below 98°F
Air	Yellow	White & Black	Gas

* Oxygen – Carbon Dioxide mixtures have both green and gray colors on the cylinder. If CO_2 content is less than 7%, predominant color is green with gray at the top; if greater than 7%, predominant color is gray.

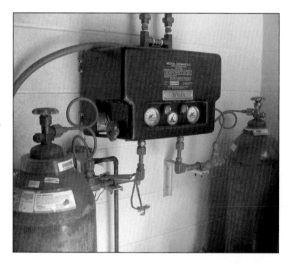

Figure 3-4 Bank of 2 oxygen tanks connected to manifold for central supply. One tank is open to system with the other tank in reserve.

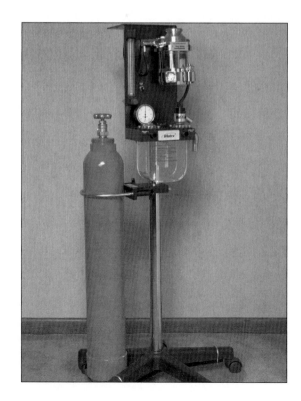

Figure 3-5 Size F oxygen tank mounted on anesthesia machine.
Courtesy of Matrx, Orchard Park, NY

Compression to a liquid state is the most economical way to store gas in the smallest volume. Nevertheless, compressed oxygen is most commonly supplied as a gas because the critical temperature for liquefaction is below environmental temperature. As oxygen in medical gas cylinders is used, there is a decrease in pressure and contents of the tank can be judged by change on the high pressure regulator. At a given temperature, if the original pressure is reduced from a full tank at 2200 to 1100psig, the cylinder would be judged to be half full. With N_2O however, until all of the liquid nitrous oxide is used, cylinder pressure will remain constant at approximately 750psig at 20°C. This pressure will change as ambient temperature changes. Pressure in a nitrous oxide tank does not indicate the amount of gas remaining until it drops below the vapor pressure. When that occurs, liquid is depleted and pressure will continue to drop in the same manner as with compressed oxygen. Nitrous oxide tanks can be weighed for determination of content but that is impractical in a veterinary hospital. A timetable for exhaustion is available using cylinder pressure as a guide (Haskins et al. 1975). Vaporization of liquid requires heat, which is extracted from the metal cylinder. Water vapor condenses or freezes on cylinders when large gas flows are used and will be more prevalent when the ambient humidity is high.

The Food and Drug Administration supervise the United States specification for identity and purity of medical gases. Safe practice for manufacture, packaging, handling and storing of gases is established by the Interstate Commerce Commission (ICC), Compressed Gas Association (CGA), and the National Fire Protection Association (NFPA). These organizations determine safety devices, markings on cylinders, valve thread uniformity on large tanks and a pin-indexing system for post-type valves on D and E cylinders (Figure 3-3A&B). Manufacturers and distributors of medical gases are responsible for maintaining cylinders in good condition, insuring purity and identity of the gas and retesting of cylinders at high pressure every 5 years.

Compressed gases must be handled and stored to avoid the risk of fire or explosion. D and E tanks should be carried by the head with the bottom of the tank a few inches from the floor. In the event the tank should drop when carried in this manner, the bottom of the tank will hit the floor first. If the head should be damaged when dropped sufficiently to allow escape of gas, the tank can become a lethal missile. Tanks must not be stored with flammable materials and kept at temperatures below 52°C (126°F). Cylinders must be either chained to a wall or secured in a way that will prevent them from being knocked over and damaged. Detailed specifications are provided in "Standard for the Use of Inhalation Anesthetics" and "Nonflammable Medical Gas Systems," published by the NFPA, and in publications of the CGA.

A few precautions will be helpful. Oil, grease, or combustible material should never be allowed to come in contact with cylinders, valves, regulators, gauges, or fittings. Petroleum products react with oxygen and nitrous oxide with explosive violence. Cylinder valves open in a counter-clockwise manner and should <u>always</u> be opened slowly. It is best to open the valve two turns beyond the point where pressure is registered on the gauge. If this is not done, the valve could automatically close subsequent to rapid flow of gas through the valve. The flow control valve of the flow meter on the anesthesia machine must be closed prior to opening the cylinder valve. If the flow control valve is in the open position when the cylinder valve is opened, the bobbin may rise with a force sufficient to lodge it at the top and possibly damage the flow meter unit.

Cylinder Pressure Gauge
The gauge will be clearly marked with the name of the gas and each yoke on the machine will have a separate gauge. Each gauge displays the pressure of cylinder-supplied gas.

Pressure Regulator
The regulator is an essential component of the high-pressure system to maintain constant flow rates with changing supply pressure. This device is usually not visible on the machine. Other names for this device are pressure reducing valve, reducing regulator, and regulator valve. The

high and variable pressure in a cylinder is changed to a lower constant pressure, usually 50-55 pounds per square inch (psig). Regulators on anesthesia machines are preset at the factory and must not be altered. If the machine is connected to a central supply, cylinder valves on the machine must be closed. The machine will always use the gas from the source with the highest pressure. Therefore, if pipeline pressure drops below that of the cylinder regulator and the valve is open, some gas will be withdrawn from the cylinder, ultimately leading to depletion of the cylinder. For machines that incorporate delivery systems for both oxygen and nitrous oxide, fail-safe devices are included on modern anesthesia machines to preclude the possibility of administering nitrous oxide alone in the presence of failure in the oxygen supply system. These devices are pressure-regulated. As oxygen pressure falls, flow decreases and nitrous oxide flow automatically decreases. An audible signal is provided on some units and the valve opens to allow ambient air to be drawn into the circuit to provide at least a minimal oxygen supply for the patient until the problem can be corrected.

Intermediate Pressure System

Components of the anesthetic machine that receive oxygen and nitrous oxide at reduced pressures are incorporated in this system. These include pipeline inlet connections, pipeline pressure gauges, piping, oxygen pressure failure devices with or without alarms, oxygen flush, and flow control valves (flow meters).

Pipeline Connections

A pipeline connection is any system that supply gases from cylinders not mounted on yokes attached to the anesthesia machine. Most veterinary machines do not include pipeline connections as standard equipment and must be added at the time of purchase. Pipeline inlets are equipped with a check valve to prevent transfer of gas from the piping system to tanks on the machine.

Central Oxygen Supply

Oxygen may be supplied to an anesthesia machine through a hose connected to a single G or H cylinder. A bank of 2 or more cylinders might be placed in the same location and properly secured. Cylinder(s) may be kept in a separate room used only for this purpose with access restricted to those familiar with and trained to manage the system. If the central supply is located outdoors, it must be in an area to protect the control panel from cold weather. Ideally, the central supply of cylinders should be located in a separate room attached to the hospital with easy access for supply trucks. If oxygen use is great enough, a bank of multiple tanks may be used as a central supply. Each tank must have its own pressure regulator connected to a common manifold (Figure 3-4) and a check valve must be included to prevent loss of gas from the manifold should there be a leak in one of the tanks. Usually this type of system has a primary supply in use with a secondary supply set up in reserve. When the primary system nears the low pressure limit, the secondary or stand-by supply is automatically switched to become the primary source. This is accomplished by a pressure-sensitive device to make the change-over. Empty cylinders must be replaced to continue the system in full operation.

Liquid oxygen is commonly used as a central supply in large veterinary centers. This form of oxygen supply is only economical under circumstances of high demand as significant losses will occur if the system is only used intermittently. The size of the liquid oxygen container will vary depending on the amount used and frequency needed for refilling from a supply truck. Liquid oxygen is stored in vacuum-insulated containers under low pressure and at temperatures below $^-150$ to $^-160°C$. Location must be outside where the possibility of ignition is minimal and there is ready access for refilling by the gas supplier.

Medical Oxygen Generators

In situations where delivery of compressed or liquid oxygen is unreliable or uneconomical, an oxygen concentrating device (OCD) is an alternative (Figure 3-6). Air, which contains 21% oxygen,

78% nitrogen, and 1% other gases, can be compressed and passed through a regenerative adsorbent material. The OCD uses two vessels filled with a molecular sieve adsorber. As compressed air passes through one of the adsorbers, nitrogen and impurities are removed. Before the adsorber becomes saturated with nitrogen, flow is switched to the second adsorber allowing the first adsorber to regenerate. This process is then repeated. Under normal operating conditions, the molecular sieve material does not have to be replaced and will last indefinitely. Oxygen exits the adsorber into a surge tank. Expected concentration of oxygen is 95-90% and can be withdrawn from the tank at flow rates up to 8 liters per minute at 50-55psig. Oxygen concentrators use standard 115V electricity to operate and automatically shut off when oxygen is not being used. To avoid problems with oxygen supply during power outages, equipment failure, or peak demands above 8 liters/min, a back-up of compressed oxygen must be part of this system. Oxygen concentrators are available in various sizes to meet different needs of a veterinary facility. Smaller units designed for human patient home use deliver a continuous flow at low pressures. This may not be adequate to power flow meters of anesthesia machines and certainly will not power pneumatically driven ventilators.

Quality assurance is important when considering use of OCDs in a veterinary hospital. In contrast to commercial suppliers who are responsible for certifying quality and purity of medical oxygen in compressed cylinders, veterinarians share part and perhaps all of the liability for monitoring quality and safety of delivered gas from an OCD (Steffey et al. 1984). Periodic or continuous testing of concentration and line pressure must be a component of implementing oxygen concentrator use in a veterinary practice.

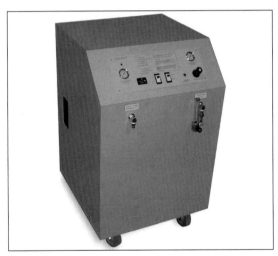

Figure 3-6 PSA Oxygen Concentrator. Reliant MK 164-1.
Courtesy of the AirSep Corporation.

Terminal Units

The point at which connection of the anesthesia machine is made to the piping system from a central supply is called the terminal unit. This may be in the form of a wall outlet, ceiling hose, or rigid column mounted on the ceiling. Each terminal unit is fitted with a gas-specific connector that is unique for the manufacturer (Figure 3-7). The male component is attached to the anesthesia machine or to a flexible hose leading to the unit. The female component is referred to as the socket or outlet connector. The male component is called the plug or inlet connector. Each is coded by color and name of the gas being delivered. Quick connectors are most commonly used to provide a threadless means of accessing the machine to the central supply (Figure 3-8A). The Diameter Index Safety System (DISS) is designed to provide a non-interchangeable connector for medical gas lines at pressures of 200psig or less. Each quick connector or DISS connection must be equipped with a backflow check valve to prevent flow of gas from the anesthesia machine into the piping system. Manufacturers of pipeline systems have individualized outlets and DISS connectors that are not interchangable from one company to another. Thus, within a hospital it is necessary that all machines be equipped with the common DISS connector in order to fit the wall or ceiling outlet.

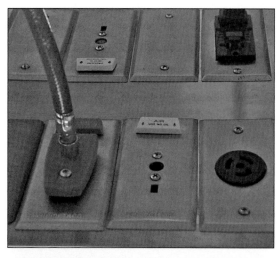

Figure 3-7 Terminal Fresh Gas Pressure Outlets with oxygen line connected.
Veterinary Teaching Hospital, Michigan State University.

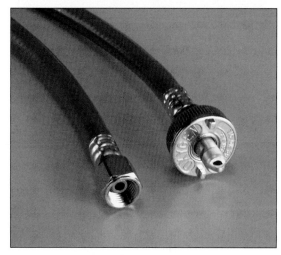

Figure 3-8A Fresh gas outlet connections: threaded and quick connects.
Courtesy of Matrx, Orchard Park, NY

Wall Outlets vs Ceiling Hoses

Wall outlets are appropriate in a small area where the anesthesia machine can be connected with a short hose. The hose should be off the floor and not in the way of mobile equipment within the room or tripped over by people walking in the room. For large operating rooms, two sets of outlets may be desirable. Height from the floor must be sufficient to avoid being damaged by equipment or tables but not too high that it makes it difficult for people to push the DISS connector into the outlet. In areas where it is not possible to install wall outlets in a convenient location, a rigid column with built-in outlets or hoses connected to the ceiling provide a good alternative (Figure 3-8B). Again, height is an important consideration since placing it beyond the reach for short people will make it difficult to make connections. To avoid head knocking of connectors, retractable hoses or hose reels may be advantageous. Periodic cleaning of these components is desirable to reduce build up of dust and possible contamination of surgical sites.

Hoses

Hoses are used to connect anesthesia machines or other assemblies such as ventilators to the gas outlet. Hoses must be kept away from any heat source to avoid rupture. It is best to keep them off the floor to prevent a tripping hazard and getting in the way of other equipment in the room. At least once a year, hoses should be checked for leaks, damage from normal use, and to assure that the normal curvature is maintained to avoid kinking.

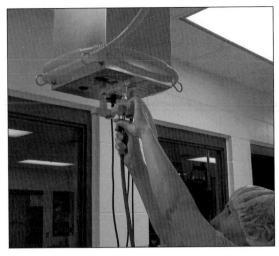

Figure 3-8B Rigid Ceiling column with Fresh Gas Pressure Outlets.
Veterinary Teaching Hospital, Michigan State University

Oxygen Flush Valve

This device is found on all anesthesia machines either as a self-closing toggle or push button. The purpose is to deliver unmetered oxygen flow to the common gas outlet of the unit at flows of 35-75L/min. The switch should never be in a position on the machine to allow accidental activation. It can be used to fill the system with oxygen to start a procedure or more commonly, to flush other gases or a volatile liquid anesthetic from the circle system. It should never be used in a semi-open system, e.g. a Bain Circuit with patient connected, to avoid inducing pulmonary damage.

Activation of the flush valve should minimize pressure fluctuations on the vaporizer that may produce a pumping effect. Some units incorporate a check valve to prevent output from the vaporizer during oxygen flush and to prevent any effect on flow meter readings. In no situation should the flush valve be placed in such a position that oxygen can flow through a vaporizer outside the circle, and if an in-the-circle vaporizer is used, it must be in the off position.

Flow Control Valve

Also called the needle valve or flow adjustment control, this valve regulates the rate of gas flow from the flow meter by manual adjustment (Figure 3-9). This is a dual process with an on-off function as well as finite control of gas flow. Components of the flow control valve are the body, stem and seat, and control knob. The stem and seat allow gas to pass through the valve to the flow meter as it is turned outward in a counterclockwise direction. Some valves have stops that prevent stripping of the valve in a closed position. If there is not a stop, the valve should only be closed finger tight.

Control Knob

The control knob is attached to the stem of the flow control valve. Knobs must be marked with the name or chemical formula of the gas it controls. Before 1979, knobs were the same size and shape. Thereafter, the oxygen flow control knob was mandated by ASTM to have a fluted profile (Figure 3-9) and be larger than knobs for other gases. All other knobs must be round and have fine groves. This touch-coded profile was implemented to reduce the possibility of operator error with different knobs on the machine. Knobs are turned counterclockwise to increase flow and clockwise to decrease flow. Knobs must move smoothly, be easy to adjust, but not too loose to allow inadvertent changes by accidentally touching or brushing the knob.

When a machine is not in use, compressed gas supply should be disconnected or turned off. The knob must be closed as well. If for any reason the knob is opened widely, which may occur when the machine is being cleaned or moved, the flow meter may become damaged when the gas supply is attached. The indicator may rise all the way to the top, not be visible, and even become lodged within the tube. It is possible that the sudden rise of the indicator could affect flow meter accuracy by damaging the tube. The set-screw holding the knob on the valve stem may become stripped allowing the knob to loosen. It is important to replace the damaged knob should this occur.

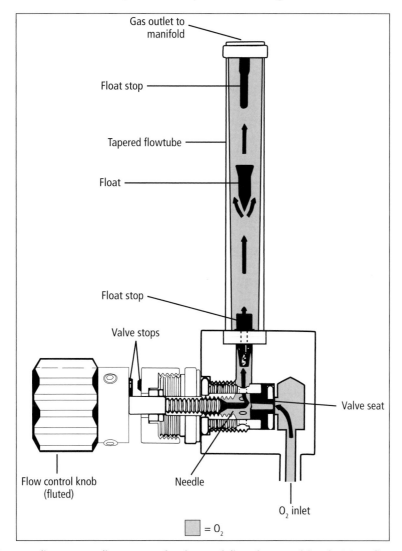

Figure 3-9 Oxygen flowmeter, flow control valve and fluted control knob. Most flowmeters have an unbreakable shield to protect the flowtube (not shown in diagram).
Reprinted with permission. Principles and Practice of Anesthesiology, Second Edition 1998. Eds Longnecker DE, Tinker JH, Morgan GE. Mosby. Fig 48-3, pg 1016.

Low Pressure System
Once gases move downstream from the flow control valve, they are at pressures only slightly above atmospheric. In this part of the anesthesia machine, components include flow meter(s), vaporizer(s), back pressure safety devices, and the fresh gas outlet. From that point, the system is connected to the fresh gas inlet of breathing systems and then to patient.

Flow Meters
The flow meter assembly consists of a glass tube, float indicator, a stop at the top of the tube, and scale. The assembly is housed in a metal or hard plastic block with the front covered by a protective clear plastic shield (Figure 3-9). The glass tube of the flow meter has a variable orifice. The inside diameter of the tube is narrower at the bottom compared to the top and is often

identified as a Thorpe tube (Figure 3-10). Each tube contains an indicator that moves upward as the flow control valve is opened. Float or bobbin indicators freely move within the tube which must be vertical. Gas passes through the annular opening between indicator and tube to the outflow at the top. As the tube becomes wider, more gas passes through the annular space. Smooth glass tubes contain non-rotating floats or rotameters while ribbed tubes are used for ball floats. Ribs are thickened bars that are evenly spaced on the inside circumference to keep the ball in the center of the tube. Some but not all flow meters on veterinary machines indicate the point of reference for reading the indicator. As a general rule, the line for bobbin-type floats is the upper rim, whereas, the reading for a ball float is taken at the indicator's center (Figure 3-10). Rotating bobbins have an upper rim that is larger than the body. Slanted groves are cut into the rim of the float to make the bobbin rotate as gas passes by it. These bobbins are usually marked with different colors so that the rotations can be easily seen, verifying gas flow around it. Ball floats may rotate and often have two colors to make them more visible. Each flow meter contains a stop at the top to keep the float visible and to prevent the flow indicator from plugging the outlet. If there is a break in the stop or if the tube becomes dirty or damaged, the indicator will not rotate or move up the tube correctly. This is an indication that the unit must be serviced by a certified medical repair technician. When this happens, a new flow meter assembly will be installed to replace the broken one.

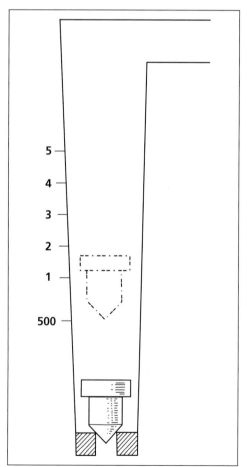

Figure 3-10 Variable orifice flowmeter. Gas flow is zero with float at bottom of flowtube. Gas enters at the base and flows through the annular opening around the float. The area of this annular space increases with the height of the indicator. The height of the float, read as the top of the bobbin in this diagram or center of a ball float, is a measure of gas flow through the tube.
Reprinted with permission. Veterinary Anaesthesia, Tenth Edition 2001. Eds Hall LW, Clarke KW, Trim CM. W.B. Saunders. Fig 9.7, page 203.

Scale

Flow meters are calibrated in L/min except for flow rates below 1L/min. Lower flows may be marked either in ml/min or decimal fractions per minute. Scale may be marked either on the tube or next to it on the right side as viewed from the front. On some flow meters, scale will be printed in the color code for the indicated gas. Flow meters are calibrated at 760mmHg and 20°C. Line pressures for anesthesia machines are normally set at 50-55psig. Modern flow meters are designed so that pressure is not critical for operation or calibration. If that is not the case, they must be pressure compensated and have tolerance limits of line pressure for proper operation. Room temperature will not vary much in a small animal practice so there will be little effect on calibration. In areas where barometric pressure is decreased such as occurs at higher altitudes, the actual flow rate will be higher than the scale indicates.

Changes in Float Position

Flow meters on veterinary anesthesia machines are usually not equipped with devices to prevent backpressure transmitted from the breathing system or oxygen flush. Pressure will increase from the rapid flow of oxygen from the flush valve or from positive pressure ventilation thus causing gas within the flow meter tube above the float to be compressed. The float will temporally drop during inspiration to a lower position but return to the former position at the end of the inspiratory cycle.

Should the supply pressure of a compressed gas drop below 50psig, the float will begin to drop as the pressure decreases until it reaches zero. Frequent observation of the indicator will identify this problem so that the oxygen supply can be re-established before an emergency develops.

Arrangement of Flow Meter Tubes

Anesthetic machines may have a single flow meter for oxygen, two oxygen flow meters, and/or a flow meter for nitrous oxide. US standards require that the oxygen flow meter be located on the right side of a flow meter bank as one looks at the unit front. Gas moves from left to right through a manifold at the top allowing oxygen to be the last gas to enter the manifold on the right side. By placing oxygen nearest the outlet, a leak upstream from the oxygen flow meter results in a loss of nitrous oxide rather than oxygen (Eger et al 1963). In many countries, the oxygen flow meter is located on the left side but the safety arrangement in this situation is reversed with gas flowing from right to left in the manifold.

Two oxygen flow meters may be found on some machines with one used for flows of 1L/min or less, the other for higher flows. In this situation, tubes may be arranged either in parallel or in series. If they are in parallel, two separate flow meter assemblies will be present with knobs and flow control valves for each. They may flow into a manifold at the top of the assembly or flow directly to the common gas outlet. In series, there will be only one assembly but two tubes. Oxygen flows through the lower flow tube first, passing into the second tube calibrated for higher flows. The total flow is shown on the tube with higher flow which starts at 1L/min. The lower volume flow tube may either be on the right or left on veterinary machines. On older human units, the lower flow tube will usually be on the right.

Fresh Gas Outlet

Also called the common gas outlet, this can be identified as a black rubber tube downstream from other tubes on the machine. On cabinet units, the FGO is a 15-mm female slip-joint connection. Because this is a frequent source of leaks, machines may be equipped with a device to prevent the FGO from being accidentally loosened or dislodged.

Fresh Gas Inlet

The point of connection from the FGO is the fresh gas inlet (FGI) on the absorber assembly (Figure 3-11). This inlet will also be found as the point of connection for non-rebreathing and semi-open systems. This port or nipple should have an inside diameter of 4.0mm and the delivery hose, usually black rubber, should have an inside diameter of at least 6mm. The FGI is most commonly located on the inspired side of the absorber assembly between the unidirectional valve and CO_2 absorber. During exhalation and expiratory pause, fresh gas will flow back through the absorber and out the APL valve once the reservoir bag is full. Other locations are downstream of the inspired directional valve, upstream from the absorber and on either side of the expired valve. Positioning of the FGI is at the discretion of the manufacturer. Advantages and disadvantages may be found in other sources (Eger 1968, Berry 1972, Shanks 1974).

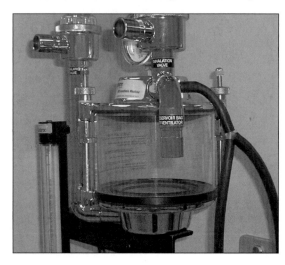

Figure 3-11 Fresh gas inlet on carbon dioxide absorber housing.

Vaporizers

Three factors are fundamental in the design of modern vaporizers: temperature dependence of vaporizing liquid anesthetics; latent heat of vaporization; and surface area for the gas-liquid contact. Vapor phase of the liquid is in direct proportion to temperature. Temperature of the liquid will decrease as it vaporizes; thus heat must be returned to the liquid to prevent changes in vapor pressure. For this reason, copper is used to provide high heat capacity and good conductivity which also increases vaporizer weight. For a liquid to vaporize, it must be in contact with a gas above it and the interface must be large enough to yield efficient vaporization. To provide linearity over a wide-range of flow rates in a vaporizer, a large gas-liquid interface is used.

Until 1958, vaporizers were rather simple devices used to deliver diethyl ether. Ohio Either 8 vaporizers were made of glass and a wick provided a greater surface area from which to vaporize the liquid. The discovery of halothane, an agent of relatively high potency and vapor pressure, created the need to develop vaporizers not only to change the inhalation anesthetic from liquid to vapor but also to control the amount of vapor added to the fresh gas flow delivered to the anesthesia system. Over a period of more than 45 years, only 4 inhalation anesthetics have been approved for use in small animals in the US with only 3 in current use: halothane, isoflurane and sevoflurane. Physical properties are listed in Table 3-3.

Vapor Pressure

In a closed container containing a volatile liquid, molecules in the vapor phase above the liquid will create a pressure as they impact the wall of the container. When the air above the liquid is fully saturated and at equilibrium for the specific temperature, vapor pressure of the specific agent is described. Vapor pressure is temperature dependent but not affected by normal changes in barometric pressure.

Partial Pressure and Concentration

Concentration of a gas can be expressed as partial pressure or in volumes percent. Using a mixture of gases in a closed container again as an example, that part of the total pressure caused by any one gas is called the partial pressure. Total pressure is the sum of partial pressures of all

Table 3-3

Physical Properties of Inhalation Agents

Form	Agent	Vapor Pressure (mm Hg @ 20°C)	Blood / Gas Partition Coefficient	Oil / Gas Partition Coefficient	MAC (volume %)	Percent Metabolized
Gas	Nitrous Oxide	Gas	0.5	1.4	> 100	< 1
Volatile Liquid	Desflurane	664	0.4	92	6.0	0.02
	Sevoflurane	160	0.7	95	2.4-2.6	2.0
	Isoflurane	238	1.5	99	1.3-1.6	0.2
	Enflurane	175	2.0	98	1.7	2.5-10
	Halothane	243	2.5	224	0.9	> 20
	Methoxyflurane	23	15.0	970	0.3	> 50

Modified from Steffey EP. Inhalation Anesthetics. In *Lumb & Jones' Veterinary Anesthesia, 3rd ed.* Williams & Wilkins, 1996.

gases in a mixture and as it pertains to anesthetic vaporizers, is equal to atmospheric pressure. The partial pressure is only affected by temperature and is not influenced by the pressure above the liquid. The highest partial pressure of a gas is the vapor pressure at a given temperature. Concentration expressed in percent is the ratio within a volume of gas molecules in a mixture to the total pressure: partial pressure/total pressure = volumes percent / 100. Using the figures provided in Table 3-3 for isoflurane as an example, the concentration in the gas phase above the liquid at equilibrium at 20°C would be 31.3 volumes percent: 238 / 760 x 100. Concentrations used for anesthesia range from 1.5 to 3.0% so agent specific vaporizers are necessary for exquisite control.

Heat of Vaporization

Heat of vaporization becomes very important in the delivery of volatile liquid anesthetics. As molecules are removed from the liquid, temperature decreases. The temperature lost is then replaced from the environment surrounding the liquid. When rate of vaporization is at its greatest, the temperature gradient between the liquid and area around it will be high. For delivery of anesthetic vapors, carrier gas(s) pass through the container, a.k.a., the vaporizer sump, thus removing molecules of vapor. The higher carrier gas flow, e.g., oxygen, the more vapor will be removed and the greater will be heat loss from the liquid. As temperature drops, so does vapor pressure and ultimately, the concentration of anesthetic vapor in the carrier gas. To replace heat of vaporization, materials must be used to allow rapid replacement of heat lost. Most agent-specific calibrated vaporizers and measured flow vaporizers use copper, which has a high degree of thermal conductivity, to surround the vaporizing chamber. The alternative is to supply heat to the chamber which is the method used in Tec 6-type vaporizers provided on human anesthesia work stations.

Classification of Vaporizers

Measured-Flow Vaporizers

Before more sophisticated vaporizers were developed, measured-flow devices were used to deliver volatile liquid anesthetics. These are better known as kettle-type, flow metered, flow meter-controlled, bubble, or saturation vaporizers (Dorsch & Dorsch 1994). To operate this unit, a measured flow of oxygen is delivered to the vaporizer to carry fully saturated anesthetic vapor to the common outlet. The flow meter is calibrated either for the flow of oxygen to the vaporizer or for the vapor flow at 20°C. Bubble vaporizers were made of glass and may be found on early model human machines. Later designs of these vaporizers were made of copper. Saturation vaporizers such as the Copper Kettle* (Foregger) and Vernitrol* (Ohio Heidbrink) had a separately metered flow of oxygen with an on-off switch that controlled delivery of the metered flow of oxygen to the vaporizer. These vaporizers consisted of a body (sump) that held the liquid, a window to view the liquid level, and a thermometer to indicate temperature of liquid inside the vaporizer. Oxygen was dispensed as fine bubbles through the liquid and was nearly saturated with the anesthetic vapor as it left the vaporizer. Saturated gas was mixed with the carrier gas as it flowed toward the common outlet where anesthetic vapor was reduced to the desired concentration. A slide rule type of device was used to facilitate calculation of the gas flow needed for the vaporizer output at a given temperature. Without the calculator, the operator would use the following method to calculate the needed flow: concentration is equal to its vapor pressure at that temperature divided by the atmospheric pressure.:

1. $$\text{Percent vapor} = \frac{\text{vapor pressure x 100}}{\text{atmospheric pressure}}$$

To calculate the amount of metered oxygen that was to be delivered to the vaporizer in order to yield the desired concentration, the total gas flow and desired concentration must be determined:

2. $$\text{Solving: ml vapor} = \frac{\text{\% anesthetic x total flow}}{100}$$

Using equation (1) and (2), the desired figures could be rapidly calculated. For halothane, the vapor pressure (P_{vap}) is 243 at 20°C. If barometric pressure is close to 760mm Hg, 243 divided by 760 is about 32% halothane or one third of an atmosphere. Therefore, one third of the gas exiting the common outlet will be halothane and two thirds will be the carrier gas(s), oxygen alone or oxygen/nitrous oxide. That is, if 1% halothane is desired in 3L/min oxygen, 1% of 3000ml/min is 30ml/min of halothane vapor. The flow meter to the vaporizer would be set at 60ml/min in order to carry the 30ml/min of halothane vapor needed in 3L/min oxygen for 1% halothane delivered to the patient. In actuality, the total flow would be 3090ml/min but because of the small influence on the total, the 90ml/min (60ml oxygen plus 30ml halothane vapor) need not be considered. This would not be the case when using anesthetics with a higher vapor pressure and less potency, such as diethyl ether which has a P_{vap} of 450mm Hg at 20°C. The oxygen flowing through the vaporizer would be considered as part of the total flow. Output of these vaporizers is greatly influenced by environmental temperature because vapor pressure increases as liquid temperature increases.

Measured flow vaporizers can be quite dangerous. Mistakes in calculation or using a lower total flow than that used in the calculation could lead to lethal concentrations of volatile liquid anesthetics. Therefore, it is essential that anesthetists are careful and deliberate in using this type of vaporizer.

Calibrated Vaporizers

Concentration-calibrated, precision, or Tec-type are common names for these vaporizers which are designed to allow the anesthetist to dial-in a desired concentration without hazards of temperature changes or variability in flow rate. With this device, total gas flow is delivered to the inlet port of the vaporizer (Figure 3-12). Some of that flow is diverted into the sump containing liquid anesthetic with the remainder passing to the vaporizer outlet and then to the fresh gas outlet of the anesthesia machine. Concentration is controlled in volumes percent by a spindle at the top that opens in a counterclockwise direction. This turning direction is standard on all calibrated vaporizers. The ratio of bypass gas to gas going to the sump is called the splitting ratio and is controlled by the ratio of resistances in the two pathways. There is an adjustable orifice that may either be in the inlet to the sump or as is the case for most currently manufactured models, at the outlet. The splitting ratio also depends on the total flow delivered to the vaporizer. The importance of this design will be discussed later in the section on inhalation agents. It should be noted that Tec-type vaporizers are calibrated using oxygen but there is little difference if air is used as the carrier gas.

Effects of variability in ambient temperature are negligible at commonly used dial settings. Tec-type vaporizers are constructed and calibrated for specific agents to provide relatively constant

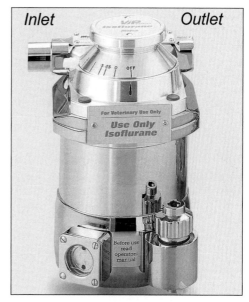

Figure 3-12 VIP 3000 Isoflurane Vaporizer with inlet and outlet ports identified.
Courtesy of Matrx, Orchard Park, NY

concentrations over wide variations in temperature and flow rate. Modern designed units* respond very slowly to changes in ambient temperature and as a safety feature, a temperature sensitive valve does not respond to temperatures below 12-15°C (53-59°F). This prevents the valve from closing completely at low temperatures but concentrations will be lower than that indicated on the dial control. At temperatures above the range indicated on performance curves supplied with vaporizers, output may be unpredictably high. Although there are differences between manufacturers and models, delivered concentrations can be considered linear with accuracy of ± 10% between temperatures of 62 and 85°F (17-29°C) and flow rates between 150ml/min and 10L/min. However, settings on the dial are linear only within the temperature and flow rate limits specified by manufacturers. *Matrx VIP 3000, Orchard Park, NY.*

Filler Receptacle
When Tec-type vaporizers were first developed, halothane was the only highly potent anesthetic being used so there wasn't a hazard of filling the vaporizer with the wrong agent. Enflurane, isoflurane and sevoflurane were subsequently introduced so agent-specific filling systems were developed. Dark amber bottles containing the liquid are color coded and fitted with a collar with two projections (Figure 3-13). This is designed to mate with the corresponding indentation on the bottle adaptor (Figure 3-14A) in a system similar to that for pin indexing of gas cylinders. The

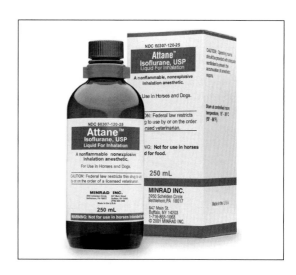

Figure 3-13 Isoflurane bottle clearly showing knobs at top.
Courtesy of Minrad Inc, Buffalo, NY

agent specific male adaptor at the opposite end of the tube is designed to fit into the filler receptacle or block (Figure 3-14B). The screw on the block allows the male adaptor to be secured and sealed to preclude spilling while the liquid is poured into the sump. There is also a valve attached to the block that controls the opening into the vaporizer. This process is reversed when emptying the sump.

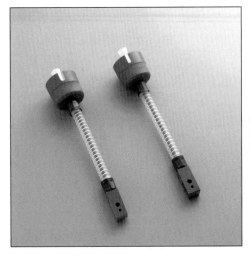

Figure 3-14A Key Fill Adaptors. In addition to color coding, caps on fill spouts are designed to accept knobs specific for each inhalation anesthetic.
Courtesy of Matrx, Orchard Park, NY

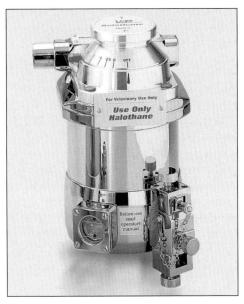

Figure 3-14B Key Fill Receptacle is mounted on the vaporizer to specifically accept the Key Fill Adaptor. The chain is attached to the plug that is removed to accept the adaptor.
Courtesy of Matrx, Orchard Park, NY

Vaporizers without agent-specific filling devices have a plug that is screwed into the fill spout to seal the filler opening (Figure 3-15). This plug has a depression on the top that fits onto a lug inside the filler receptacle. This is used to open the drain to remove liquid from the sump. If the filler plug is not replaced or not tightly secured, liquid anesthetic will be blown out through the filler receptacle when the spindle knob of the vaporizer is opened concurrent with gas flowing into the system. Cross threading by careless replacement of the filler plug can occur and this can lead to loss of liquid anesthetic.

The glass window (Figure 3-15) next to the filler receptacle is used to identify liquid level in the vaporizer sump. It has an etched line near the bottom to indicate when it is empty and another at the top above which the liquid cannot be added. Liquid anesthetic will spill from the receptacle

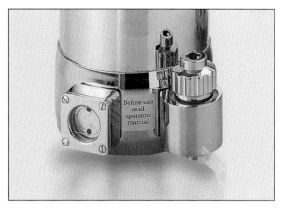

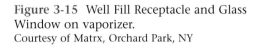

Figure 3-15 Well Fill Receptacle and Glass
Window on vaporizer.
Courtesy of Matrx, Orchard Park, NY

since over-filling the sump is prevented by the position of the filler on the vaporizer housing. To help avoid spillage of liquid anesthetics during filling of vaporizers equipped with the standard receptacle, a bottle adaptor with a plastic beveled end is available (Figure 3-16). This device is color coded for each specific agent to avoid filling the vaporizer with the wrong agent: red (halothane); purple (isoflurane); yellow (sevoflurane).

Another precaution is to make sure the filler receptacle is clean of dirt and debris before pouring liquid anesthetic into the sump. Blood, dirt and other debris can collect in the receptacle and be washed into the sump during filling. This is a sure way to cause the vaporizer to malfunction and will damage internal mechanisms. Foreign substances including hair, toe nails, blood, peroxide, bleach, water and even vomit have been found in vaporizers sent in for service. Some have even been found with the wick missing presumably having been removed by the customer in the process of attempting to perform unqualified self service. Wiping the receptacle clean before filling will avoid the need for unexpected service and repair.

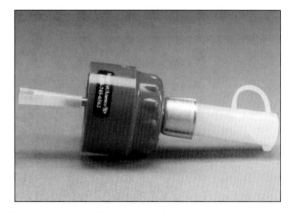

Figure 3-16 Vapofil adaptor. With this device
attached to the bottle, liquid anesthetic can be
easily poured into the well fill receptacle of the
vaporizer.
Courtesy of Matrx, Orchard Park, NY

Brand names such as Fluotec Mark 2, Fluotec Mark 3, Pentec Mark 3, Fluomatic, Drager Vapor, Drager Vapor 19.1, and Ohio Medical Product / Ohmeda vaporizers are no longer manufactured but may be obtained from equipment dealers. However, one must be cautious in purchasing pre-owned units to make sure vaporizers have appropriate mounting brackets for veterinary anesthesia machines and to assure that parts are still available for service. For example, manufacturers of the Fluotec Mark 2 (Cyprane) and Drager Vapor (North American Drager) no longer provide parts for these units. The only Tec-type vaporizers presently manufactured for veterinary anesthesia machines are Matrx VIP 3000, Penlon UK and Bickford Vapomatic (Figures 3-12, 3-17, and 3-18). The Ohio series calibrated vaporizer is being remanufactured and serviced by Surgivet (Figure 3-19). Tec 4, Tec 5 and Tec 6 type vaporizers are designed for use in human anesthesia work stations in such a manner that the mounting brackets may not conform to veterinary anesthesia machines unless modifications are made. These units are more expensive and the Tec 6 vaporizer is equipped with a sump heater.

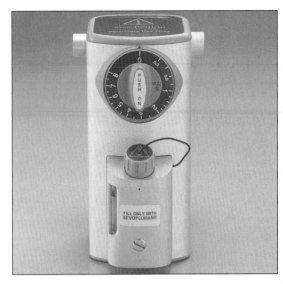

Figure 3-17 Calibrated Vaporizer by Penlon.
Courtesy of Matrx, Orchard Park, NY

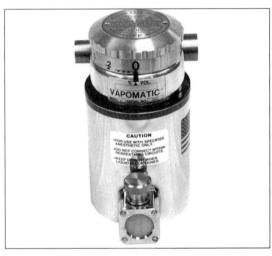

Figure 3-18 Vapomatic vaporizer.
Courtesy of A.M. Bickford Inc, Wales Center, NY.

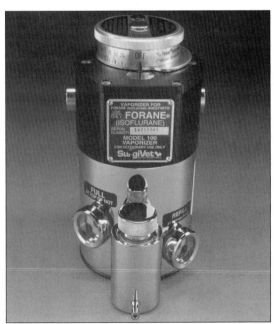

Figure 3-19 Ohio 100 series calibrated vaporizer.
Courtesy of SurgiVet, Inc. Waukesha, WI

Flow-Over Vaporizers

Vaporizers placed in the circle (VIC) are defined as wick, surface or draw over vaporizers (Figure 3-20). They are made of glass and the wick in contact with liquid at the bottom serves to increase gas-liquid interface. Output of these vaporizers is greatly influenced by ambient temperature, fresh gas flow and patient minute ventilation. Vapor pressure changes in the same direction as temperature and because heat of vaporization is lost, efficiency is decreased. In the same respect, as total gas flow is increased, more vapors are needed for a given setting, causing vapor pressure to drop. For any given vaporizer setting, the larger minute ventilation, the higher the output. Controlled ventilation is usually associated with increased tidal volume. Therefore, lower settings must be used with controlled breathing than with spontaneous breathing because of a larger gas flow through the vaporizer. Location of the VIC is found on either the inspiratory or the expiratory side of the breathing circuit. However, the preferable location is on the inspiratory side to minimize condensation of water inside the sump. These vaporizers do not have many working parts, are not agent specific and cannot be calibrated. Periodic cleaning is required to remove water and preservatives from the wick. Settings on the vaporizer only indicate the degree the unit is open or closed; therefore, concentration being delivered cannot be determined from the dial setting. These vaporizers were used to deliver diethyl ether and subsequently, methoxyflurane. However, with these agents no longer available in the U.S. and most other countries for clinical use, these vaporizers have become obsolete. Halothane, isoflurane and sevoflurane are not recommended for delivery with this type of vaporizer but published reports provide methodology for their use (Bednarski 1991; Bednarski 1993). Veterinarians are more accustomed to delivering these anesthetics with agent specific vaporizers and agent specific vaporizer delivery is also specified by anesthetic and vaporizer providers. In addition, there are anesthetic machines such as Komesaroff and Stevens units equipped with VIC for delivery of these highly potent inhalation anesthetics (Laredo et al 1997; 1998; 2000). A complicating factor is the accumulation of water in an in-circle vaporizer contaminating the anesthetic, especially after long procedures (Harrison 2000). Veterinarians should be aware that this methodology is possible should delivery with calibrated vaporizers not be available.

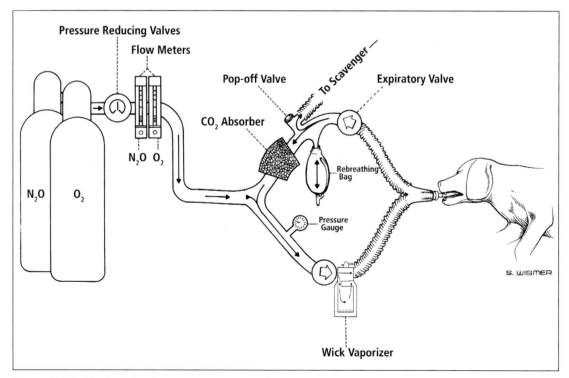

Figure 3-20 Circle-CO_2 absorption system with vaporizer inside circle (VIC).
Reprinted with permission. Sawyer, D C, The Practice of Small Animal Anesthesia, W.B. Saunders 1982

Hazards

When different agent specific vaporizers are present in a hospital setting, there is always the possibility of accidentally filling units with the wrong agent. However, there are ways this can be avoided with keyed filling devices (see Filler Receptacle Section). The bottle adaptor filling device is helpful to prevent errors but not as fool-proof as the keyed device. Placing isoflurane in a halothane vaporizer can result in isoflurane concentrations as much as 50% more than expected (Shih and Wu 1981). In contrast, adding halothane to a vaporizer intended for isoflurane will result in lower than expected concentrations. The same would be true if agent specific vaporizers are available for isoflurane and sevoflurane. Vapor pressures are quite different for these two agents and variable mixtures will occur depending upon the amount of each anesthetic in the sump. Concentrations would likely be higher if isoflurane were to be placed in a vaporizer calibrated for sevoflurane and vaporizer settings would normally be set higher because anesthetic requirements for sevoflurane are higher. Without keyed filling devices, hazard of incorrect filling is enhanced so considerable caution is needed to prevent problems. When multiple vaporizers are placed side-by-side on an anesthesia machine, an interlocking device may be added that allows only one vaporizer to be opened at a time.

Calibrated vaporizers manufactured for veterinary anesthesia machines and some older units are not designed to protect units against tipping. Vaporizers filled with liquid anesthetic must be kept upright during handling and be securely mounted to a bracket or machine. This is done to prevent liquid anesthetic from getting into the bypass or outlet. If vaporizers are tipped, extremely high and dangerous concentrations may be delivered. If a vaporizer is to be moved, it should be drained first and then refilled after it has been remounted. Should a vaporizer containing liquid anesthetic be tipped, it should be connected to an anesthesia machine at high flows with the dial at a low setting until high concentrations can no longer be detected.

Sevoflurane has minimum purity of 99.97%. However, it is susceptible to chemical degradation in certain precision vaporizers resulting in production of hexafluoroisopropanol (HFIP). This slight instability is not a problem unless the vaporizer contains elements such as boron or aluminum. Sevoflurane products stored in Penlon Sigma Delta vaporizers were shown to be degraded extensively, resulting in substantial increases in fluoride and reduced pH (Kharasch et al 2007). In this model of Penlon vaporizer manufactured before October 1, 2006, etching of the sight glass that gives it a yellow appearance and degradation of the metal filler shoe and internal mechanism makes the liquid level in the sight glass difficult to see and with time will likely affect perform-ance. It is possible for sevoflurane to be left unused in vaporizers on anesthesia machines for extended periods of time. This is more likely to occur when sevoflurane is used less frequently such as in veterinary hospitals in which isoflurane is the primary anesthetic. Typically, vaporizers are refilled when partially empty. Except for scheduled maintenance, it is uncommon for a vaporizer to be completely emptied of liquid anesthetic. The degradation process will be longer in develop-ment with Penlon Sigma Delta vaporizers that are replenished because of more frequent use or when sevoflurane is the sole inhalation agent in the practice. Vaporizers that do not contain such elements of aluminum appear not to have a problem with stored sevoflurane.

Calibration should be verified periodically or the vaporizer should be sent to a certified service company. For large hospitals, gas indicators for each specific anesthetic can be obtained to verify vaporizer settings.* As a general rule, calibrated vaporizers should be serviced and recalibrated every 1 to 2 years. Need for service may be signified by either lower or higher concentrations being delivered than expected by the dial setting. If calibration is off at the low end, it may become difficult to maintain anesthesia at expected concentrations. However, faulty vaporizers may deliver a higher concentration than indicated, increasing risk of lethal anesthetic concentra-tions. One of the more common problems associated with the need for recalibration is accumulation of the nonvolatile preservative in halothane. Thymol does not vaporize and will concentrate over time unless the vaporizer is drained and washed with anesthetic, effluent discarded, and vaporizer refilled. A yellow color will appear in the indicator window of the vaporizer as thymol becomes concentrated. It is best to drain the vaporizer every 1 to 2 months when the liquid volume is low. This will not prevent the need for recalibration but may extend the interval between service times. Isoflurane and sevoflurane do not contain preservatives but mechanical parts should be periodically checked and vaporizers serviced every 1 to 2 years. Care should be taken when filling vaporizers without a key-fill device. This should be done in a well ventilated area if at all possible with extreme care to avoid spillage and room contamination.

* Riken Gas Indicator, AM Bickford, Wales Center, NY

Breathing Systems

What is a closed system? What is an open system? And when is it semiopen or semiclosed? There have been many attempts to develop an easy to understand system for describing anesthesia breathing systems. There are at least eleven different definitions, the first being that of McMahon in 1951 who used rebreathing as a basis to differentiate open, semi-closed, and closed systems. Two years later, a nomenclature was offered based on whether a reservoir bag was included and if rebreathing CO_2 was a component (Moyers 1953) (Table 3-4). Using these guidelines, an open system was one that had no reservoir and no rebreathing. A semi-open system included a reservoir bag but no rebreathing. The semi-closed system had a reservoir bag and partial rebreathing and the closed system included the bag and total rebreathing. This simplified definition appeared to be very straightforward but one must fully understand what was meant by rebreathing and the function of a reservoir bag. During the process of considerable debate among anesthesiologists (Adriani 1962; Collins 1966; Hall1966; Dripps 1968; Conway 1970; Baraka 1977), a method was proposed to just describe the equipment used, provide patient weight and flow rates of compressed gases instead of using terms that could be confusing (Hamilton 1964). Because terms *open, semi-open, semi-closed,* and *closed* are used, these will be described in more detail.

Table 3-4

Nomenclature for Inhalation Anesthesia Systems

System	Reservoir	Rebreathing
Open	No	No
Semiopen	Yes	No (slight)
Semiclosed	Yes	Yes (partial)
Closed	Yes	Yes (complete)

Modified from Moyers J (1953). A nomenclature for methods of inhalation anesthesia. *Anesthesiology* 14: 609-611.

System
Open Systems

These are relatively simple systems that have no reservoir tubing or bag and no rebreathing (Table 3-4). Some open systems have directional valves, such as Fink or Stephen-Slater valves, but most do not (Table 3-5). The open drop method is the simplest of open systems and requires the least amount of equipment. It was very common to use this technique with diethyl ether or methoxyflurane. The anesthetic was dripped on gauze stretched over a mask held over the patient's nose and mouth. If the gauze was not too thick, resistance to breathing was minimal. Dead space could be minimized by having a tight fitting mask with the opening close to the nose and mouth. Room air was breathed which resulted in hypoxia at anesthetic levels. This could be prevented or minimized by flowing oxygen into the mask.

A volatile liquid anesthetic cools as it vaporizes, thus lowering vapor pressure and slowing induction. Also, water vapor can condense on the gauze and impede vaporization. This technique is seldom used anymore because of the difficulty in obtaining these ethers.

Table 3-5

Inhalation Anesthesia Breathing Systems

System	Reservoir Bag	Rebreathing CO_2	Chemical Absorption of CO_2	Directional Valves
Open				
(nonrebreathing)	No	No	No	No
Fink, Stephen-Slater valves				
Open drop	No	No	No	No
Ayres-T	No	No	No	No
Norman Mask Elbow	Yes	No	No	No
Semiopen				
Bain Circuit	Yes	Slight	No	No
Magill	Yes	Slight	No	No
Semiclosed				
Circle	Yes	Partial	Yes	Two
To-and-Fro	Yes	Partial	Yes	No
Closed				
Circle	Yes	Complete	Yes	Two

Ayres-T was first introduced as a delivery system for human infants because of the great difficulty small patients had in moving metal disks in unidirectional valves of very early circle systems. These disks were much heavier than modern leaflets and were responsible for morbidity and mortality of infants in the early days of inhalation anesthesia (Ayre 1937). The T-piece was just as the name implies with connection of the inflow tube to one end of the "T" and patient connection at the other end with the outflow located at the base of the "T". Various modifications followed this very simple system by adding tubing at the outflow and a 15mm adaptor attached at the patient end to permit attachment of a mask. The Mapleson F system is called the Jackson-Rees modification of the Ayres T piece (Rees 1950). The Norman Mask Elbow modification placed the inflow tube at the patient end in the middle of the 15mm female connection and provided an outside diameter of 22mm for use with a face mask (Figure 3-21). This allowed fresh gas from the anesthesia machine to be connected directly to the elbow. Once the patient was induced, the inside fitting of the elbow was connected to the tracheal tube. This system had a bag attached at the end of a corrugated tube and a hole either in the bag-tail or side for venting expired and excess gases. For manual ventilation, the bag tail could be pinched to allow accumulation of gases in the bag with subsequent compression of the bag. With the hole in the side of the bag, a finger placed over the hole would occlude escape with the same hand used to compress the bag. Capture devices for scavenging gases fit either in the bag tail or over the side hole. Open systems are intended not to permit rebreathing of expired gases so are correctly called nonrebreathing systems.

These devices can be very dangerous with potential of producing pulmonary barotrauma and death if the outflow would become occluded (Manning 1994; McMurphy 1995; Evans 1998). High flow rates of 1 to 3L/min (2-3 times minute ventilation) were typically used with this system to ensure sufficient flushing of expired CO_2. That yields a flow rate of 17 to 50ml/sec which means that a 500ml bag would fill in 10 to 30 seconds leaving very little time to respond to the problem if the anesthetist is involved in other matters of patient care.

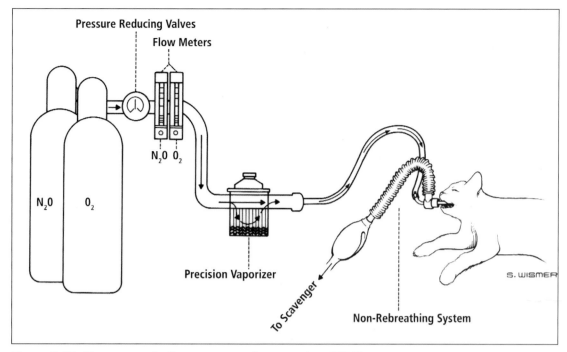

Figure 3-21 Norman mask elbow connected to vaporizer (VOC).
Reprinted with permission, Sawyer, D C, The Practice of Small Animal Anesthesia, WB Saunders, 1982

Masks

As indicated, a face mask or cone is often a part of an open system. A universal mask is not available for dogs or cats but cone-shaped masks made of hard plastic and a soft rubber gasket are most common (Figure 3-22). These can also be fabricated from empty liquid cartons. Usually an absolute tight fit is not possible because of differences in anatomy in dogs and cats. For most circumstances, the mask is used to direct gases as they flow across the nose for inhalation. If it is possible for the mask to fit tightly, it can be connected to a breathing circuit. The malleable rubber ring on the mask can be molded to the face of most patients and is preferred. A human anesthesia face mask, in adult or pediatric sizes, can be used for some brachcephalic breeds. Mask induction with isoflurane or sevoflurane offer definite advantages that can be delivered from vaporizers at dialed concentrations carried by gas mixtures with oxygen tensions higher than air. Care should be taken not to damage the corneas with the edge of the mask, especially on those breeds with protruding eyes.

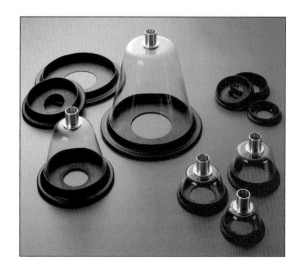

Figure 3-22 Face masks with rubber gaskets.
Courtesy of Matrx, Orchard Park, NY

Semi-open

Using the Moyer definition, a semi-open system has a reservoir bag but permits no rebreathing (Table 3-4). However, this system has been mistakenly called a nonrebreathing system. Depending on total gas flow, a portion of exhaled gases may or may not be rebreathed. For the same reasons as open systems, semi-open devices are used principally on patients less than 7kg. It may be difficult for small patients to make unidirectional valves of a circle system function properly. The animal's small tidal volume may not be adequate to close one valve and open the other, especially since valves are prone to stick when wet. Therefore, an added resistance to breathing may occur. To test this possibility, three inhalation delivery systems were compared in cats and kittens during and following 60 minutes of isoflurane anesthesia: Bain breathing circuit, a double canister absorber with adult breathing hoses and a double canister absorber with pediatric breathing hoses (Sawyer et al. 1991). Respiratory rate, indirect blood pressure, pulse rate, inspired and expired anesthetic concentrations and end-expired CO_2 were recorded during each anesthetic period. No clear differences were found in comparing the three inhalation delivery systems. At least based on these findings, recommendation is that low resistance modern circle systems with minimal dead space can be safely used on small patients with provision that semi-open systems might be preferable for animals less than 3kg. Although there seems to be consensus that semi-open / nonrebreathing systems are advised for patients less than 3-5kg, clinical judgment must be considered as well. Obesity is associated with decreased lung compliance and lower tidal volumes. Therefore, an obese patient with a body weight of 10kg that should only weigh 5kg would likely do better with a semi-open system than with a circle rebreathing system.

Semi-open systems are designed to permit inspiration of inflow gases and some of the expired gases in the reservoir tubing. Traditionally, high gas flows were recommended for open systems and this recommendation initially applied to semi-open systems. This high flow resulted in loss of water vapor and body heat and a higher incidence of hypothermia.

Most semi-open devices are patterned after Mapleson breathing systems that are characterized by the absence of valves that direct gas flow and have no means for absorption of CO_2. Classified as A through F, components of Mapleson systems include reservoir bag, corrugated tubing, APL valve, fresh gas inlet and patient connection. Mapleson A is configured with the fresh gas inflow coming through or next to the reservoir bag, corrugated tubing, an APL valve at the patient end and 15mm connection. Mapleson A is also called the Magill system and has been much more popular in the United Kingdom than in North America (Lerche 2000b). Flowrates of 100 to 150ml/kg were recommended indicating that it could be used for dogs up to 60kg assuming the capacity of the flow meters was sufficiently high.

The Lack modification of Mapleson A or Magill system placed the APL valve at the opposite end of the patient connection just proximal to the fresh gas inflow and reservoir bag. This also included a coaxial version that placed the expiratory tubing inside the corrugated inspiratory tubing (Lack 1976; Robinson and Lack 1985). This system was evaluated in small animal patients during spontaneous breathing to determine optimal flow rates to prevent significant rebreathing as determined by capnography (Waterman 1986). These were found to be 130 ± 31ml/min/kg for dogs 10-15kg and 96 ± 13ml/min/kg for patients > 15kg. The other finding for the Magill system was significant rebreathing of CO_2 at flow rates less than 120ml/kg/min. Mapleson D had the inflow tubing attached outside the expiratory limb with a scavenging line connected to the APL valve. Bain modified the Mapleson D system by placing the fresh gas tubing inside the corrugated tubing which not only simplified applications with one tube instead of two but inflow gases could be warmed to some degree by expired gases (Figure 3-23) (Bain 1972). Dr. Bain performed anesthesia for ophthalmologic procedures in infants and children and needed to provide space for abundant equipment typically used by surgeons. Therefore, initial Bain Circuits were 60-inches in length. Coaxial tubing could be connected to a metal adaptor on the anesthesia machine or table

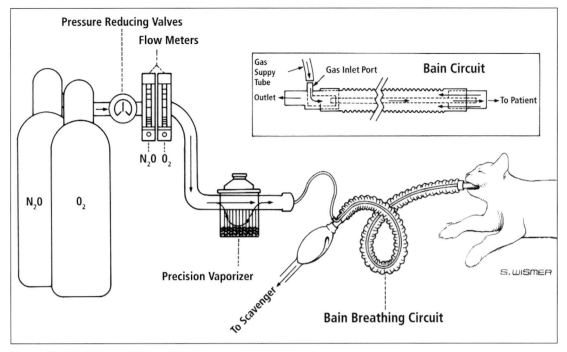

Figure 3-23 Bain breathing circuit.
Reprinted with permission. Sawyer, D C, The Practice of Small Animal Anesthesia, W.B. Saunders, 1982

that provided a 15mm attachment for the corrugated tubing, a reservoir bag, pressure manometer, and APL valve (Figure 3-24). It also made it more convenient to make adjustments to the APL valve just like the Lack system. Without the adaptor and with the outflow opening at the bag tail connected to the scavenging system, this system is more dangerous to use. The tail can twist which effectively closes the outflow. This is not nearly as convenient as the fixed mount that incorporates the APL valve. Subsequently, an 18-inch version of the Bain Circuit was provided which presently is a popular length for use in cats, small dogs, puppies and kittens. Units intended for humans are disposable for liability reasons but can be reused many times in animals before needing to be discarded.

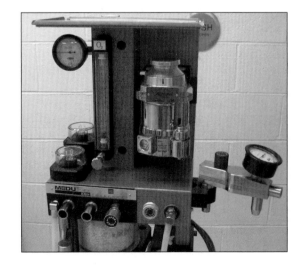

Figure 3-24 Bain adaptor mounted on bracket attached to Dispomed anesthetic machine. Components include APL Valve, Pressure Manometer, Reservoir Bag attachment, and attachment for Bain breathing system.

The Humphrey ADE System is a combination of Mapleson adaptations for use in patients either during spontaneous or contolled ventilation. By moving one or both levers in different up or down positions, the anesthetist could have any of three systems, Mapleson A, Maple D which resembles the Bain modification, or Mapleson E (T-piece, Humphrey 1983). This unit is not very popular and may not even be available.

Flow Rates

The Bain system was initially recommended for use with fresh gas inflows of 200ml/kg/min in spontaneously breathing small animal patients less than 5-7kg (Sawyer 1979). Others suggested a flow rate of 100ml/kg/min (Manley 1979a). Then in a 6-month clinical trial using dogs, cats, birds and piglets, it was demonstrated using capnography to detect rebreathing of CO_2 that 100 ml/kg/min proved adequate when patients were ventilated and up to 130ml/kg/min was adequate during spontaneous ventilation (Manley 1979b). Thus, flowrates of 130 to 150ml/kg/min with the Bain system will be sufficient to prevent elevations of $PaCO_2$ during spontaneous or controlled breathing with normal rates of 15 to 20 breaths/min. Inflow rates of 200ml/kg/min will virtually eliminate all rebreathing of CO_2 assuming that the inflow will be greater than patient inspiratory flowrate (Table 3-6).

Table 3-6

Flow Rates for Various Anesthesia Breathing Systems

System	Body Weight	Flow rate
18-liter Chamber	under 7kg	5.0 LPM
Mask Induction	under 7kg	3-5 LPM
	over 7kg	5-8 LPM
Open system Ayres-T or Norman Elbow 3 x minute ventilation	under 7kg	3.0 LPM
Semi-open Bain Circuit and Magill	under 7kg	0.5-1.0 LPM
	8-14kg	1.0-2.0 LPM
	5-25kg	2.0-4.0 LPM
Semi-closed Circle system	7-18kg	500ml/min
	19-45kg	750-1000ml/min

LPM = liters per minute

During conditions of increased minute ventilation, e.g., high respiratory rate and/or increased tidal volume, inflow rate should be increased. Total flow rates for these systems range 500-2000ml/min for patients less than 7kg. The Bain system is adaptable to patients of any size but is preferable for small patients because of the low resistance to breathing. Because of the length of the circuits (7cm or 24cm) and its light weight at the patient connection, the Bain system especially with the mounting bracket and pressure manometer is useful for a wide variety of applications. The reservoir bag can be used for controlled or assisted breathing and the APL valve easily facilitates scavenging of anesthetic gases.

Semi-closed and Closed Circle Systems

Semi-closed and closed circle systems have the same equipment with the only difference being the degree of rebreathing. Differences include the addition of breathing tubes, valves that direct circuit gas flow, and CO_2 absorber assembly including pressure manometer. Circle systems also incorporate an APL valve and reservoir bag. Gases flow in a circular pathway controlled by two unidirectional valves. The principal reason for using circle systems is based on economy as lower fresh gas flow rates can be used. For example, maintenance oxygen flow for a 25kg dog using a semi-open system would be as much as 5 liters/min compared to 500ml/min in a semi-closed system. Oxygen flow meters on some veterinary units do not go above 4L/m.

Circle systems can be adapted for use in large or small patients by changing certain components such as the reservoir bag and breathing circuit. Disadvantages of circle systems are that they have more moving parts which must be serviced and maintained. They occupy more space with some cabinet and rail models being more bulky than others. Wall mounted units are available to offset this disadvantage.

Partial rebreathing occurs with the semi-closed system and can be a little or a lot, depending on the total flow rate of fresh gases. As a general rule, total gas flow rates at or above 20ml/kg/min are used for a semi-closed system. Excess gases escape through the APL valve into the scavenging system.

Complete rebreathing of expired gases occurs in a closed system with virtually all of the CO_2 being chemically absorbed (Wagner 1992). Sufficient oxygen is added to equal tissue uptake of anesthetic gases and oxygen and the system must be devoid of significant leaks. Between 6 and 10ml/kg/min will usually provide a closed system with little or no excess gas escaping through the APL valve. For low flow systems, oxygen flow will be 10-15ml/min/kg which lessens the amount of rebreathing but increases escape of excess gases. APL valve should be left in the open position except when partially or completely closed for assisted or controlled breathing. As a practical matter, the lower limits of most flow meters at rates below 300ml/min are not easily observed from a distance and precision vaporizers have their low limits of linearity close to this figure. Nitrous oxide should not be used in a closed system unless inspired oxygen can be monitored (Haskins 1982).

In a closed system, a rough estimate of adequate oxygen flow is made by changes in the degree of distension of the reservoir bag. If the amount of gas in the bag decreases, uptake of oxygen will likely to have increased thus necessitating increased oxygen flow. Because most of the anesthetic gases are confined to the circuit, waste anesthetic gas discharged into the room from an unscavenged anesthesia machine will be much less than in a semi-closed system. However, using closed system anesthesia is not an excuse for not having a scavenging system. Because anesthetic concentrations will increase with time in a closed system, more intense and constant monitoring of anesthetic depth are required, especially with agents of high vapor pressure and low solubility (Wagner 1992).

Circle Rebreathing System

The breathing system is that part of the anesthetic machine interposed between the fresh gas outlet and patient. For sake of definition, classification of breathing systems for inhalation anesthesia are identified according to the presence or absence of: (1) rebreathing previously breathed gases, (2) a reservoir bag in the breathing circuit, (3) an absorber for removal of expired CO_2 and (4) valves to control the directional flow of the gases in the system (Table 3-5). Three additional low pressure components of an anesthesia machine are the APL valve, pressure manometer/gauge and breathing tubes.

Rebreathing

Rebreathing includes inhalation of expired gases from which CO_2 may or may not have been removed. A mistaken concept is that rebreathing is primarily defined by inclusion of CO_2. Rebreathing low levels of CO_2 is often desirable but excessive amounts can be harmful. The amount of rebreathing is controlled by the fresh gas flow, mechanical dead space and design of the breathing system. In situations where the fresh gas flow is high, there will be little or no rebreathing. However, if the total volume of gas delivered per minute is less than the minute volume of the patient, rebreathing must occur to make up the difference.

Mechanical dead space is that component within a breathing system occupied by gases that are rebreathed. Composition of dead space gas is not influenced by inflow of fresh gases, removal of CO_2 or changes in anesthetic concentration. The degree of rebreathing is in direct proportion to the volume of dead space. The bigger the mechanical dead space, the more rebreathing of expired gases will occur. Expired gases are composed of anatomical dead space gas (conducting airways without CO_2) and alveolar gas (containing CO_2). Anatomical gas is essentially the same as inspired gas except that it is saturated with water vapor and will be at a higher temperature. Mechanical dead space gas contains CO_2, therefore, it is important to keep this as low as possible especially for very small patients. When inspired gas is the same as that of fresh gas inflow, fresh gas inflow must be relatively high and equal to or higher than patient minute volume. With partial or complete rebreathing, composition of inspired gas is partly fresh gas and partly expired gas. As mentioned, exhaled gases are warmer than inspired gases and are nearly fully saturated with water vapor. Therefore, rebreathing reduces patient heat and water loss.

Reservoir Bag

Various terms used to describe this component of a breathing system are reservoir bag, breathing bag, respiratory bag and rebreathing bag (see Figure 3-1). There are other purposes of the *bag* besides breathing so the inclusion of it being a reservoir is most appropriate. Most bags are made of rubber with the neck having a 22mm opening. The tail usually has a loop to make it easy to hang after cleaning for re-use.

For closed and semi-closed systems, the reservoir bag is needed to compensate for changes in respiratory demand. During inspiration, flow rate is greatest and gas supply is obtained from flow meter inflow and from the reservoir. If gases were available only from flow meters, flow rate would need to be very high. For example, a 20-kg dog with a tidal volume of 200ml may take a breath in 1 second. This provides a rate of 200ml per second or 12L/min. If 600ml/min was provided from an oxygen flow meter, 10ml of the tidal volume would be supplied from the fresh gas inflow and 190ml from the reservoir bag. During expiration and pause, gas inflow from flow meters accumulates in the bag and gas is available for each breath. Thus, the bag should be full to truly function as a reservoir of gases.

The reservoir bag also provides a means of manually assisting or controlling breathing and can serve to facilitate monitoring in the presence or absence of spontaneous breathing. Movement of the bag during anesthesia is not an accurate index of ventilation; it can, however, be used as a rough guide to estimate tidal volume and it is used to indicate frequency.

Because the bag is a reservoir, it should be full when in use. A mistaken concept is that the bag must only be partially full so that there is no pressure imparted to the breathing system. During spontaneous breathing with the APL valve in the open position, pressure on the system is 1.5 to 3cm H_2O. This is required to keep the bag full with creases at the top of the bag still evident. This pressure is innocuous since resistance to breathing through the nose is about 5cm H_2O. Therefore, it is not necessary and may be potentially harmful to keep the bag only partially full.

The bag is essentially the only part of the breathing system that can be distended which then acts as a short-term protective device for the patient. ASTM standard for reservoir bags l.5 liters or smaller requires that pressure shall not exceed 50cm H_2O when the bag is distended to four times its size. For larger bags, that limit is 60cm H_2O when expanded to four times its capacity. This process provides a little time to react to a closed APL valve before damage is imparted to pulmonary alveoli. For example, in a system with a 1 liter bag and 1L/min O_2 flow, an empty bag will fill in 1 minute. The pressure will build during the next minute and another 4 minutes might pass before the pressure would exceed 50cm H_2O. Of course, blood flow is diminished during this period because of increased intrathoracic pressure so it is imperative that the anesthetist be attentive to the overdistended bag. The more compliant the bag, the better protection will be provided. Reservoir bags are less compliant when new so it is a good practice to overinflate and stretch them several times when first attached and before connecting patients to the system.

Bag size is important and is governed by the system used, patient size and operator preference. The bag must be large enough to deliver a good tidal volume (inspiratory capacity) but small enough to allow the anesthetist to comfortably squeeze the bag and "feel" lung compliance. It is easier to squeeze a small bag (1-liter) with one hand compared to a large bag (3-liter) and a small patient's tidal volume is easier to monitor in a small bag compared to a large one. If the bag is too small for the patient, there would be less safety protection from over inflation and possibly an inadequate reservoir. Since semi-open systems are primarily used for small patients, a 500-ml or 1-liter bag is appropriate. For semi-closed systems, a general guide is that the reservoir bag should not be less in size than 6 times the patient's tidal volume. Using an estimated guide for tidal volume of 2.5ml/kg multiplied by 6, 15ml/lb would be needed to fully inflate a lung. Using this as a guide, a 1-liter bag is appropriate for patients up to 16kg (35 lbs); 2 liter bag for 17-32kg (36-70 lbs); and 3 liter bag for 33-45 kg (71-100 lbs). More simply, 1, 2, and 3 liter reservoir bags are used for small, medium, and big dogs, respectively. Reservoir bags are available in sizes ranging from 0.5 to 5 liters. Usually 1, 2, and 3 liter bags will be sufficient for a small animal practice with the one liter bag used most often. Reservoir bags will deteriorate with use and leaks will develop at the most inappropriate time. Therefore, as a precaution, it is good practice to have a backup supply of reservoir bags for anesthetic systems.

CO$_2$ Absorber

The CO$_2$ absorber assembly is usually of metal construction with three ports for connection of breathing tubes and reservoir bag, inspiratory and expiratory unidirectional valves, APL valve, and pressure gauge (Figure 3-25). Disposable plastic absorber assemblies are available.

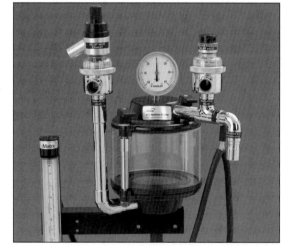

Figure 3-25 Carbon Dioxide Absorber Assembly. Looking at this illustration, inspired directional valve is located on the left, expired valve is on the right.
Courtesy of Matrx, Orchard Park, NY

Absorbers may include one or two canisters. Stacked chambers are especially useful for large dogs and long procedures. Canister sidewalls are made of clear plastic and a screen at the bottom helps contain absorbent. Absorbers made entirely of metal are not recommended because depleted absorbent cannot be easily observed and monitored. Canisters vary in size but larger units are preferable over smaller ones because of better utilization of absorbent and longer intervals between changes. The larger cross-sectional area provides slower flow through the unit and lower resistance. Patient exposure to absorbent dust is also minimized. Absorbents placed in CO$_2$ canisters come in two forms: 1) loose granules available in bags or buckets or disposable pre-pack canister inserts. Pre-packs are made of plastic that are usually placed inside the canister (Figure 3-26A). It is essential to remove the clear plastic seal over both openings before use. These machine packed canisters are more efficient than hand packed units and they are of a standard size. Therefore, pre-packs may not fit smaller size or non-conventional shaped absorbers on some veterinary anesthesia machines.

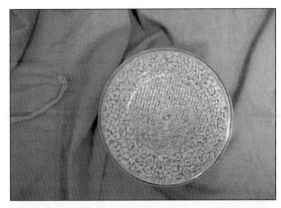

Figure 3-26A Disposable prefilled containers are sealed during the manufacturing process in a foil lined bag. This Soda Lime insert has had the plastic wrap and both the top and bottom label removed before being placed in the canister.
Courtesy of Dr. A.T. Evans, Michigan State University.

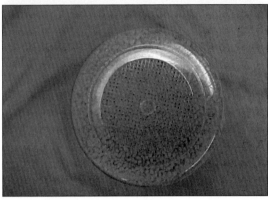

Figure 3-26B Channeling is shown in this prefilled container demonstrating that absorbent has become exhausted except on the sides where the color change is not visible.
Courtesy of Dr. A.T. Evans, Michigan State University.

Gaskets are used to seal metal junctions at the top and bottom of the absorber housing. Depending upon the machine, two methods are used to lower and raise the absorber base when the absorbent is to be changed. Older human machines and some veterinary units have a wing-nut or screw device that is not convenient to use nor quick to operate. Some modern machines have a lever-actuated cam to lower or raise the bottom of the absorber (Figure 3-27). This allows the canister to be quickly changed, especially during an anesthetic procedure and makes it less likely to have gasket junctions close unevenly, creating leaks. A water and dust trap at the bottom of the absorber assembly is a common feature found on most anesthesia machines.

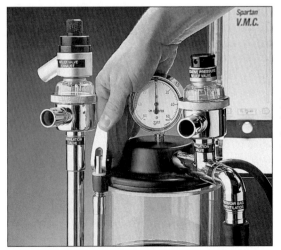

Figure 3-27 Lever-Cam on CO_2 absorber is used to facilitates changing of absorbent or prepack canister replacement.
Courtesy of Matrx, Orchard Park, NY

In the canister, CO_2 is removed by chemical reaction with sodium, calcium, and barium hydroxides. The two most common absorbents are as follows:
1. Soda lime: 4 % NaOH, 1% KOH, 14-19% H_2O and 76-81% Ca $(OH)_2$ (white).
2. Barium hydroxide lime: 20% Ba $(OH)_2$ $8H_2O$, 0.5-1% KOH and 79% Ca $(OH)_2$ (pink or white).

Soda lime has water added to constitute 14 to 19% of the total prepackaged weight and should be kept in a sealed container between uses to prevent loss of water content. Water loss from evaporation is less likely to occur with baralyme because water it is incorporated in the barium hydroxide molecule. The first step in the soda lime reaction is for CO_2 to combine with water to form H_2CO_3. This weakly dissociates as do NaOH, Ca(OH)$_2$ and KOH. The resulting chemical reaction is as follows: $2NaOH + 2H_2CO_3 + Ca(OH)_2 = CaCO_3 + Na_2CO_3 + 4H_2O$. A small amount of potassium carbonate is formed along with heat. Reactions between barium and CO_2 yield barium carbonate, calcium carbonate, potassium carbonate and water.

Both absorbents contain an indicator that changes to a bluish gray or purple as the neutralization reaction occurs. Ethyl violet changes from white to purple and phenolphthalein changes from white to pink. Color change can be used as a guide but is not completely reliable. If the absorbent is too dry, this chemical reaction will not occur. Color may revert back to pre-exhaustion color and thus give a false reading. Channeling can also occur more toward the center of the canister thus not exposing visible granules on the sides (Figure 3-26B). Heat is liberated during this reaction and can be detected even before changes in the color indicator. Thus, as CO_2 is absorbed the canister becomes warm or hot to touch. It will be too hot to touch in patients with malignant hyperthermia.

One may note that depleted soda lime may revert almost to its original color when the absorber rests overnight. This phenomenon is referred to as *regeneration or peaking* (Foregger 1948). The absorption capacity of the regenerated soda lime is low and the depleted indicator color will quickly reappear with only a brief exposure to CO_2. After repeated periods of CO_2 absorption, terminal exhaustion of the absorbent occurs and granules should be replaced. CO_2 absorbent should remain in the canister and not be removed to dry for reuse. If soda lime is without moisture, CO_2 can pass through the absorbent into inspired gases. Depleted absorber granules are hard to the touch and not easily crushed when pressed between the fingers compared to unexposed absorbent.

The greater the surface area of granules, the more rapid and efficient will be the neutralization reaction. Soda lime is supplied in 4 to 8 mesh irregularly shaped granules with silica added for hardness. Baralyme particles are more uniform and about the same size as sodalime. As a general rule, non-depleted absorbent of a completely filled canister should be at least 1.5 times the tidal volume at the start of a procedure. When the flow of expired gases stops in the canister at the end of expiration, CO_2 will have time to be absorbed into granules. As the neutralization reaction continues, the amount of absorbent available decreases with time but canisters are usually big enough to keep the absorbent within efficiency limits. CO_2 absorbers should be changed when half the granules are depleted depending on size of the canister. To maximize CO_2 absorption fresh absorbent should be used for patients in which the canister is less than one tidal volume in size. A good estimate of tidal volume is 10ml/kg. A means of partially eliminating CO_2 through the APL valve and for conserving absorbent is to increase total fresh gas flows in the circle system.

When obstruction to gas flow through the absorber of a CO_2 canister occurs, channeling of gases may result. This can happen when the absorbent granules become caked, hardened, saturated with water, or too loosely packed. Gas will follow the path of least resistance and will continue to contact depleted absorbent. Baffles are used to disperse gases and two canisters may be "stacked" with each canister used to compensate for the inadequate absorption of the other unit or to provide proper absorption for large animals. Both baralyme and soda lime are strongly alkaline and corrosive. If these granules are allowed to contact tissue for any length of time, a chemical burn will occur. Caution should be used to prevent breathing of absorber dust when replenishing canisters.

Carbon Monoxide

Concentrations of carbon monoxide are possible from breakdown of hemoglobin in closed circle system anesthesia (Middleton et al. 1965). However, these levels are not likely sufficient to cause significant clinical effects. Elevated CO levels may also be possible with absorbers that have not been used for a few days, especially at low flows. A few deaths in dogs have occurred in association with the use of isoflurane. This appears to occur when isoflurane vapor has been allowed to remain in the canister for a period of days and the absorbent loses water. Carbon monoxide formation is greater with drier absorbents and more with barium hydroxide than soda lime. Difluoromethylethyl ethers, e.g., isoflurane, form CO but not sevoflurane (monofluoromethyl ether), methoxyflurane (methyl-ethyl ether) or halothane (alkane) (Baxter et al. 1998). A later study confirmed that CO production occurred with isoflurane, desflurane and enflurane but also found a smaller but significant formation in infants (Wissing et al. 2001). CO formation from interaction between CO_2 absorbents and volatile liquid anesthetics seems to be self-limiting but it would be wise to replace absorbents rather frequently. As a precaution, a good practice to follow is to discard and replace absorbent after a period of 3-5 days of not being used. Start Monday with a fresh canister if not used over the weekend and change every 2-3 days during the week.

Absorbents absorb volatile anesthetics which may be most noticeable with the first patient of the day. With higher flow as recommended later in this chapter during induction compared to maintenance, this problem will be avoided. However, if one vaporizer on a machine is switched with a different one used on a previous patient, e.g., halothane to isoflurane, it is advisable to replace the absorbent as well.

Reaction Products with Inhalation Agents

Concerns about compound A, a reaction product between sevoflurane and absorbents containing NaOH and KOH, have not been realized over years of clinical use. Halothane and isoflurane are also degraded by conventional CO_2 absorbents but the by-products have never been of any consequence. Only absorbents free of both KOH and NaOH have been shown not to produce compound A during closed-system sevoflurane (Versichelen et al. 2001). One such product is Superia that was compared to Nofnolime during minimal-flow sevoflurane anesthesia in adult human patients (Bouche et al. 2002). Amsorb and Dragersorb Free have been shown to minimize production of Compound A but there are significant differences between conventional absorbents (Stabernack et al. 2000; Kobayashi et al. 2003). Although production of Compound A with use of sevoflurane is a concern, no clinical or laboratory signs of renal impairment were observed in human surgical patients (Baum and Woehick 2003). It is possible that levels of compound A could be found with the use of sevoflurane in animals during close system anesthesia. The rate of breakdown with sevoflurane appears to be very small and no reports of toxicity from compound A have been found in clinical veterinary anesthesia patients. In addition, most veterinarians use semi-closed circle CO_2 absorption systems with flow rates that are sufficiently high (0.5 to 2.0L/min) to minimize accumulation of reaction products.

Unidirectional Valves

Also referred to as one-way valves, check valves, dome valves, flutter valves or flapper valves, two valves are used in a circle system to ensure that gases flow in one direction. They are part of the absorber assembly with a 22-mm male connection to the inspiratory and expiratory valves (Figure 3-25). Either the name *inspiration or expiration* printed on or next to the valve housing or arrows indicating the direction of flow should be visible to the user. A thin disc or leaflet is held in place by a guide mechanism or cage to keep it in position over the opening. A clear plastic dome covers the assembly so that movement of the discs can be observed during the breathing cycle. Gas flows from the bottom of the valve causing the disc to rise off the seat. Gas flowing in the opposite direction will cause the disc or flapper to contact the seat thus preventing retrograde flow of gases. For upright valves, it is essential that both valve assemblies be vertical so that the disc can seat properly. In some units, the valve may be in a horizontal orientation in which case a flapper valve is used instead of a wafer (Figure 3-28). Moisture, especially on the expired valve, may cause the disc to stick in the open position. Valves have been known to jam or become lodged in the cage mechanism. The anesthetist must be observant to make sure valves are operating properly and periodically clean residue moisture from the valve.

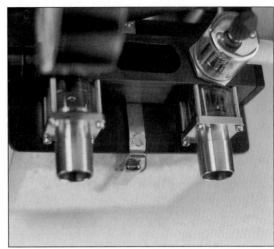

Figure 3-28 Horizontal unidirectional valves in front of absorber assembly.
Courtesy A.M. Bickford, Wales Center, NY

Adjustable Pressure Limiting (APL) Valve

A means for escape of excess gases from a breathing system is a must. A valve is provided for this purpose on anesthesia machines and is referred to as the APL valve, pop-off valve, overspill valve, release valve or simply the escape valve. The APL valve is part of a semi-closed or closed circle breathing system but also is a component with some semi-open systems such as the Bain circuit. The valve is most commonly placed on the CO_2 canister mounted either on the patient side or the absorber side of the exhalation valve. It may also be mounted on top of the clear plastic dome directional valve housing (Figure 3-29). From the standpoint of CO_2 elimination before expired gases reach the absorber, location of the APL valve on the Y piece is more economical but is most inconvenient at this location (Eger, 1968). This configuration is historical and is not used on modern anesthetic systems because it does not provide a means of scavenging waste gases from the machine and provides added weight to the ET tube when attached. The best alternative in absorber economy design is to have the APL valve located between the expiration directional valve and absorber canister, with the fresh gas inflow located between the patient and the inspired directional valve (Figure 3-30).

The APL valve is user controlled that opens in a counterclockwise direction and closes clockwise. It functions to release gases to atmosphere or a scavenging system and to allow assisted or controlled manual ventilation of the patient when partially or completely closed. It must be in a closed position during mechanical ventilation. Valves are made of metal and most use a disc held onto a seat by a coiled spring. A threaded screw cap over the spring allows variable tension to be exerted. When the spring is fully tightened, tension on the disc will prevent escape of gas from the system. When the cap is loosened, the tension on the spring is reduced. To allow the reservoir bag to function as designed, even when there is little or no tension on the spring, the weight of the disc will be sufficient to allow the bag to fill before the disc rises from the seat. The pressure within the system when the APL valve is open will be 1.5-3.0cm H_2O. Design of modern veterinary APL valves is to keep the system pressure below 2cm H_2O for benefit of smaller patients.

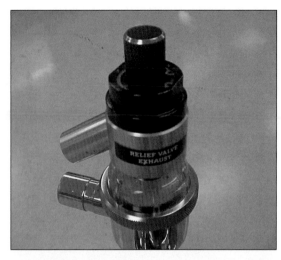

Figure 3-29 APL valve mounted on exhaust dome valve.
Courtesy of Matrx, Orchard Park, NY

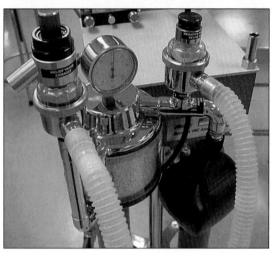

Figure 3-30 Anesthtic machine with APL valve mounted on dome valve positioned between the exhaust (expiratory) valve and CO_2 absorber.
Courtesy of Matrx, Orchard Park, NY

It is advantageous to occasionally provide a breath, often referred to as a sigh, that is 2-3 times the normal tidal volume. Instead of having to close and open the APL valve each time, an Occlusion Valve can be installed that allows the anesthetist to provide a breath of this nature. The valve is closed when the activation button is pressed and opened when it is released. This Occlusion Valve is mounted between the APL valve attachment on the machine and the APL valve.

Valves can malfunction or "stick" and should be cleaned periodically. Water vapor may accumulate causing a residue to form and thus would require increased pressure to open the valve. This could lead to hypercapnia due to decreased respiratory exchange. The APL valve must never be left closed and unattended with a patient spontaneously breathing. Excessive pressure will quickly develop leading to alveolar damage and possible death.

Exhaust port size of APL valves through which gases are discharged are either 19 or 30mm. Most modern valves are smaller than the inspiratory and expiratory ports of the circle absorption system to prevent inappropriate connection of a breathing hose to the system.

Pressure Manometer

Circle CO_2 absorption systems and semi-open circuits should have a manometer located in a position to be conveniently seen by the anesthetist (Figure 3-31). It is usually positioned on the absorber assembly of circle systems between unidirectional valves. It is located on the machine mount of semi-open systems. The pressure gauge may be calibrated in mm Hg, cm H_2O or both.

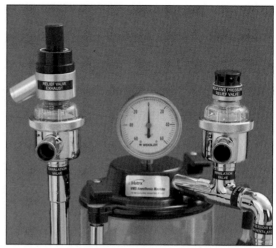

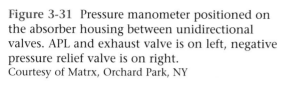

Figure 3-31 Pressure manometer positioned on the absorber housing between unidirectional valves. APL and exhaust valve is on left, negative pressure relief valve is on right.
Courtesy of Matrx, Orchard Park, NY

Pressure within the system is transmitted to the manometer moving the pointer to the indicated position. It is an essential component of the system as a warning device for high pressures due to occlusion, obstruction or closure of the APL valve. It is also useful during manual or mechanical ventilation to avoid high inspiratory pressures.

Breathing Tubes

Wide-bore conducting tubes carry gases from the anesthetic unit to the patient and are essential components of circle systems. They are made of plastic or rubber. Corrugations prevent kinking and provide flexibility. Plastic tubes are light weight but less compliant than conductive black rubber tubes. Most vendors supply a set of plastic breathing tubes with each new machine. They also serve as a reservoir in most systems. Black or clear plastic and black rubber tubing with a 22-mm male and 15-mm female coaxial fitting are most commonly used. Clear or opaque nonconductive materials can be used as long as flammable agents are avoided. Clear plastic tubes provide visibility of the inside and place less weight on the patient connector (Y-piece, mask, or tracheal tube). Breathing tubes can be obtained as disposable or non-disposable units. The former are relatively inexpensive and are obtained in sterile sets containing 2 breathing tubes, 1 Y-connector and either a 1-L or 3-L reservoir bag in conductive or nonconductive plastic.

A coaxial Mera F breathing system is an alternative to the conventional double breathing tubes and Y piece (McIntyre 1986). Now called the Universal F circuit, two separate tubes connect the system to the inspired and expired ports of the absorber assembly. The inspired tube is smooth and located inside the corrugated expired tube. To some extent, inspired gases are warmed by expired gases. It is useful for procedures around the front part of the body as only one tube is connected to the tracheal tube adaptor instead of the Y-piece. However, there are disadvantages such as kinking of the inner tube, misassembly that may result in obstruction of the outer tube and reverse attachment to the absorber.

Corrugated tubes are available in adult human and pediatric sizes (Figures 3-32A and B). Both are used with a standard absorber assembly of the circle system. Pediatric tubes are preferable for cats and dogs less than 20kg since the tubes are shorter and have an internal volume two thirds less than the adult size.

Y-Piece

The Y piece is the device that connects two breathing tubes to the patient via the endotracheal tube or face mask. Two of the openings on the Y-piece are 22-mm male ports for breathing tube connections. The patient port is a 15-mm female opening for attachment to the tracheal tube adaptor. It usually has a 22-mm external diameter to accommodate some mask designs.

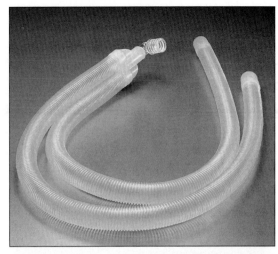

Figure 3-32A Adult breathing tubes. These disposable PVC tubes are manufactured for use in human patients. They can be reused for many months in veterinary patients if cleaned properly. Courtesy of Matrx, Orchard Park, NY

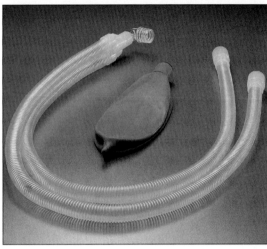

Figure 3-32B Pediatric breathing tubes have a smaller diameter but can be reused if cleaned properly. This set has a 1-liter bag included. Courtesy of Matrx, Orchard Park, NY

Historically, the first Y pieces were made of metal, incorporated the APL valve on top and were bulky. Now Y-pieces are made of lightweight plastic and have a septum at the patient port to decrease dead space.

To and Fro Rebreathing System

This system incorporates a CO_2 canister, reservoir bag, single breathing tube, fresh gas inlet, and APL valve. The canister is positioned horizontally between the reservoir bag and patient with the APL valve and fresh gas inlet located at the patient end. It was originally introduced as an alternative to circle systems but never gained the same popularity (Waters 1936). It is rarely found in veterinary hospitals in the U.S. but has been used in clinical anesthesia by veterinarians in other countries (Hall and Clarke 1991). Although this is a rather simple and inexpensive rebreathing system, it has many disadvantages. It is cumbersome to use because the system with the absorber and APL valve must be close to the patient. Mechanical dead space increases with time as CO_2 absorption occurs further and further into the absorber. Inspired gases can become undesirably hot as the chemical reaction takes place. In addition, channeling of gases can occur in the canister if the absorbent is not tightly packed. There is also the possibility of absorbent dust entering the circuit. If proper precautions are followed, the To and Fro system can be used for specific veterinary anesthesia applications (Hughes 1998; Lerche et al. 2000b).

Assessment of Anesthetic Systems

Typically, high flow rates are used in circle systems during initial stages of inhalation induction for two reasons: (1) to minimize rebreathing of expired gases, which contain low anesthetic concentrations because of rapid uptake of anesthetic gases and (2) to compensate for absorption of gases in rubber and plastic. Lower flows are used during maintenance but must be adequate to meet or exceed metabolic needs. Nitrous oxide is effective only at high concentrations, i.e., 66 to 75 per cent. Therefore, a high flow rate is needed initially to wash out residual nitrogen in the lung in order to replace it with the anesthetic mixture. Two or three times maintenance flow may be used. At the conclusion of anesthesia, higher flows of oxygen may be used to eliminate the more soluble anesthetic agents and hasten recovery. Nitrous oxide, however, must be turned off 2 to 3 minutes before the patient is allowed to breathe room air. This will avoid diffusion hypoxia as long as adequate spontaneous breathing exists or ventilation can be provided for a few minutes following N_2O anesthesia (Roesch, 1972). The practice of allowing the patient to spontaneously breathe room air while still anesthetized will produce various degrees of hypoxia and in the event of airway obstruction following extubation, severe hypoxemia can occur in less than 60 seconds. If oxygen alone is breathed prior to tracheal extubation and airway obstruction occurs, there will be more time to correct the problem, i.e. 3 to 5 minutes. Premature extubation does not permit scavenging allowing anesthetic vapors to be discharged into the ambient air unnecessarily exposing people in the work environment to unnecessary hazards.

Protocol for Machine Check Pre-anesthesia

Using a standard protocol for checking a machine before use will yield great benefits. The worst thing to happen at any time during an anesthetic procedure, especially during induction, is when a patient is in trouble concurrent with improper function of the anesthetic machine. Sometimes, it may not be clear whether it is the patient in trouble or the machine but if a pre-function machine check has been performed, focus of attention initially can be directed to the patient considering that the machine is likely not the source of the problem. One must not assume that just because a machine functioned well the day before or even on the previous patient, that it will function the same way the next day or for the next patient. Breathing hoses and the reservoir bag are likely to be different and a pre-function machine check usually only requires less than a minute to perform. Maintaining a leak-proof anesthetic system is also important to avoid discharge of gases into the working environment instead of into the scavenging system. Pollution may come from leaky circuits, loose connections and high-pressure or low-pressure gas lines. A suggested protocol is as follows:

1. Connect fresh gas supply lines or open the cylinder valve of the compressed gas tank. Check the pressure level to assure adequate quantity is available for the procedure.

2. Connect breathing tubes and reservoir bag.

3. Observe that both discs are present and in proper location inside the unidirectional valves and that domes are secure.

4. Assure that any vaporizer is in the off position and check the level of liquid in the sump. Replenish if necessary. Verify that inflow and outflow connections on the vaporizer are secure.

5. Assure freshness of the CO_2 absorber in the canister and that undepleted quantity is appropriate for the intended patient, e.g. absorbent volume equal to or greater than one tidal volume.

6. Turn the oxygen flow meter knob counterclockwise and observe the float to assure that it moves up the tube as the knob is opened.

7. Establish zero flow on each flow meter.

8. To initiate a pressure check, the APL valve must be closed and the patient port of the breathing circuit occluded by placing a thumb over the opening. Pressurize the system by filling it using the oxygen flush to a pressure of 30cm H_2O. If that pressure is sustained for 10 seconds, one can be assured that there are no leaks in the breathing circuit. If the pressure in the system drops, a leak is evident. To quantify the leak, open an oxygen flow meter sufficient to maintain the pressure at 30cm H_2O. That flow rate will equal the leak. The standard requires that this flow should not exceed 300ml/min (ASTM 1989). Unofficial veterinary sources suggest a maximum leak of 1L/min. Regardless of the magnitude of leak, the anesthetist must assure that the system will function

properly when connected to a patient. Therefore, all tubing connections should be checked as well as the reservoir bag and breathing tubes. To detect location of a leak, the system should be pressurized as described before and starting at the patient port of the Y-Piece, move one's hand over the expired side of the breathing circuit, over all connections of the absorber including the reservoir bag, and then over the inspired breathing hose back to the Y-piece. Be sure to check the water drain on the bottom of the CO_2 canister which is not an obvious location but may not be completely closed. For difficult to find leaks, using a soapy solution painted over all connections will be very helpful. The unit should not be used until all leaks are fixed.

9. To check the integrity of a Bain coaxial circuit, a different set of procedures should be followed (Ghani 1984; Heath 1991). First, the outer tubing is checked for cracks or tears. To test for leaks, connect the fresh gas outflow to the inlet of the Bain system. Close the APL valve or bag tail and occlude patient port connection. Using the flush valve, pressurize to 30cm H_2O and hold for 10 seconds. If a leak is detected by a drop in pressure, quantify the leak with a flow meter in the same manner used to check circle systems. To test the integrity of the inner tubing of a Bain system, establish an oxygen flow of 2L/min. Place a plunger from a small disposable syringe or finger into the opening of the inner fresh gas delivery tubing at the patient end of the system. Hold for a few seconds and observe the flow meter float. If there are no leaks in the delivery tubing, the float will drop somewhat below the 2L mark. If the float does not drop, this would indicate that there is a leak in the delivery tubing. A new Bain system should be attached to the machine and the pressure check repeated.

10. With the desired breathing circuit connected, check that the APL valve is in the open position and the vaporizer dial set at 0. The anesthetic machine is now ready for use.

Cleaning and Maintenance
After use, breathing circuits and reservoir bag should be removed from the machine, washed with a mild soap solution, rinsed with tap water and hung to dry. Care should be taken to clean the Y-piece with special attention given to remove mucous and secretions at the patient port. If properly cared for, disposable units can be used many months before holes in the bags or cracks in the tubing occur.

Exposed rubber tubing that carry fresh gas from flow meters to the vaporizer and then to the common gas outlet can develop leaks and should be replaced as needed. On all machines, the black rubber delivery hose that carry gases from the common gas outlet to the breathing circuit should be periodically checked as well. The common gas outlet is a frequent location for a leak or disconnection and on some machines there is a retaining device to hold tubing in place. Machines should be checked routinely for leaks, sticking or cracked flow meters and dome valves, defective needle valves, loose or worn components and other signs of wear and tear. Unless a staff member is skilled in maintenance and repair of machines, all but minor repairs should be made by a trained technician. It is good policy to have anesthetic machines serviced by a professional on a regular basis once or twice each year depending on use. Service companies are available to provide preventative maintenance to keep units operating in good order for the protection of people and pets.

Flow Rates for Circle Anesthetic Systems
Several factors dictate the rate of gas flow during inhalation anesthesia: (1) patient metabolic requirements, (2) demands of the anesthetic system to prevent rebreathing without CO_2 absorption, (3) function as a vehicle for volatile liquid anesthetics, (4) requirements to achieve and maintain alveolar anesthetic concentration, (5) limits of linearity of vaporizers, (6) dilution or elimination of gases from the breathing circuit and lungs, and (7) matters of economy. Recommended flow rates are listed in Table 3-6. As a guide, minimum maintenance flow for a semi-closed circle system should be 500ml/min for patients up to 50lbs (25kg). Then for each additional 10lbs (5kg) body weight, 100ml/min should be added. Flow rates for closed systems are

also listed in Table 3-6. However, when delivering an inhalation agent following IV induction, flow rates should be higher than maintenance levels. As a general rule, calculated maintenance flow should be 1 to 3L/min during the induction period. As an example, for a semi-closed system in a 25kg dog, induction flow would be 1L/min or greater until the patient reaches maintenance anesthetic level at which time flow rate can be reduced to 500ml/min. It would not be harmful to continue the higher flow rate but consumption of volatile liquid anesthetic would be half at the recommended maintenance flow. The volume of a circle system will blunt the rate of rise of anesthetic concentrations to the patient. The slower the flow rate of carrier gases, the slower will be the displacement of gases in the system (possibly 3 to 5 liters or more). This can be offset by delivering higher inflow rates during induction when higher concentrations are needed to reach anesthetic levels. Similarly, if there is a need to rapidly change anesthetic levels during maintenance, changes in vaporizer settings should be made along with increased carrier gas flow rates.

Scavenging Systems for Waste Anesthetic Gases

Until the late 1960's and into the 1970's, little concern was given to discharging waste gases from anesthesia machines into a working environment of hospitals. Anesthetic gases were considered biologically stable and scavenging systems did not exist as they were not considered essential equipment at the time. It was common practice to discharge excess gases through the APL valve into room air in close proximity to the anesthetist, surgeon and assistants without regard to potential detrimental effects. Ventilation and air exchange in the working environment were considered effective means of removing these gases. Personnel were exposed to low levels of anesthetics even five to six feet off the floor. With gases being heavier than air, some mistakenly thought if gases were discharged below table top that they would not be at a level to be breathed. At that time, nitrous oxide, methoxyflurane and halothane were in common use in human and veterinary hospitals. Numerous survey studies were conducted in anesthesiologists and nurses to demonstrate possible harmful effects, especially in pregnant women exposed to waste anesthetic gases. It was also demonstrated that hepatic metabolism of inhalation anesthetics and their metabolites were most likely doing harm on a long-term basis rather than the anesthetics themselves (Van Dyke 1965, Sawyer et al 1971, Bruce 1974). Studies demonstrated that metabolites were produced predominately at subanesthetic concentrations which made it more likely that operating room personnel were at more risk than anesthetized patients.

Occupational Exposure to Waste Anesthetic Gases

Trace concentrations of anesthetic gases in humans have been declared a health hazard as defined in the National Institute of Occupational Safety and Health criteria document (U.S. Dept of Health, Education and Welfare 1977). The two major consequences appear to be a high risk of spontaneous abortion in females working in operating rooms and an increased incidence of congenital abnormalities in offspring from either males or females working where trace gases are present. However, a review of the subject suggested that data published from human surveys and animal studies do not provide significant criteria to warrant the NIOSH recommendations on health hazards (Ferstandig 1978, Ferstandig 1979). In addition, assessment of occupational exposure to waste anesthetic gases to increase genotoxic risk was found to be inconclusive (Bozkurt et al. 2002). Veterinarians and their hospital personnel have been implicated in all of these studies even though surveys of associated health hazards have not been done.

Although there may not be sufficient evidence in the literature to suggest that breathing trace amounts of anesthetic gases in veterinary operating rooms is harmful, it still may constitute a health hazard (Whitcher 1976, Sawyer 1976, Best 1977, Manley 1980, Wingfield et al. 1981). Certainly one can argue the subject but no evidence has been presented that it is good for humans to be exposed to trace amounts of anesthetic gases over time. There may be a greater problem with people working daily in the operating room for many hours at a time but a dose relationship has not been shown. Fatigue, impairment in cognitive and motor skill and headaches are important possible consequences but a cause–effect relationship has been difficult to verify

(Bruce et al. 1974, Bruce 1976). Subjective observation would indicate that fatigue is more prevalent in unscavenged operating rooms than in those that have been scavenged. Since breathing trace amounts of these gases has not been shown to be beneficial and in fact may be harmful, it is prudent to scavenge waste anesthetic gases from the working environment.

For personnel in veterinary hospitals, it is clear that breathing trace gases cannot be a good practice so choosing not to use scavenging systems cannot be justified. The U.S. National Institute for Occupational Safety and Health (NIOSH) recommended in 1977 that occupational exposure to waste gases from anesthetic procedures be controlled by adherence to standards of scavenging. The standard applies to all workers, including students and volunteers regardless of status, who are exposed to inhalation anesthetics that escape into locations associated with the administration of, or recovery from, anesthesia. This document was designed to protect the health, safety and welfare of workers in locations where exposure to waste anesthetic gases and vapors occur. Trace levels of inhalation agents are considerably below that needed for clinical anesthesia and cannot be detected by smell. Levels are expressed in parts per million (ppm); 0.1% is 1000 ppm. Although no detailed studies have been conducted on a wide scale in veterinary hospitals, levels reported for halothane and nitrous oxide in unscavenged operating rooms in veterinary hospitals commonly exceed 50 ppm. The NIOSH standard indicates that occupational exposure to halogenated anesthetic agents shall be controlled so that no worker is exposed to concentrations greater than 2 ppm of any halogenated agent based on a Time-Weighted Average (TWA) of one hour. The TWA for nitrous oxide is 25 ppm. Anesthetic delivery systems are now equipped with an effective scavenging device on the APL valve that facilitates collection of waste anesthetic gases. These gases must be conveyed to disposal sites in such a manner that occupational re-exposure does not occur and such disposal methods must comply with existing local or federal environmental pollution control regulations. It was found that in some hospitals, scavenged gases were discharged into an employee break room or hospital waiting area so attention must be given to avoid these situations.

The published lower limits of waste gases have not been tested by controlled studies to verify that they are safe but were shown to be attainable using scavenging systems in clinical settings. Studies in nurses and dental assistants failed to demonstrate impairment of skilled performance in exposed personnel to waste anesthetic gases. Non-solicited reports from veterinary students and faculty working in live animal teaching laboratories at veterinary institutions suggest a major difference existed between scavenged and non-scavenged environments. In a teaching laboratory with 10 to 15 anesthetic units discharging 1 to 2% halothane and/or isoflurane into the room at the rate of 1L/min for 4 hours will test a person's stamina and preclude students from being able to study the same evening. Veterinary operating room personnel reported great improvement in their degree of activity following implementation of scavenging, especially for those who may spend many hours per day in an exposed environment.

Because there is a possibility of risk, scavenging of waste anesthetic gases has become the standard of practice in veterinary hospitals when using inhalation agents (Sawyer 1976, Manley 1980, Wingfield 1981). Although there is not a single agency in the veterinary profession that provides standards for animal hospitals, the American Animal Hospital Association includes scavenging as a required standard for its member hospitals that complies with federal, state, provincial and local regulations, e.g., NIOSH standards. Testing measures are not used to confirm that scavenging systems are used in all cases nor that waste gas disposal practices are effective in eliminating gases to appropriate levels to comply with NIOSH standards.

The Occupational Safety and Health Administration (OSHA) is an agency of the U.S. government that is concerned with discharge of waste anesthetic gases in veterinary hospitals. Standards used by OSHA are those published by NIOSH 1977 which can be obtained on their respective web sites.

Scavenging systems are designed as either active or passive. Excess or waste anesthetic gases must be eliminated from anesthetic systems without imposing danger to patients. Two major problems must be avoided:

1. Obstruction of the outflow from a scavenging system would be the same as closing the APL valve. By restricting or closing the escape route from the anesthetic unit, resistance or obstruction to breathing is increased. Severe consequences may result from decreased cardiac output, alveolar rupture and death if the problem is not discovered quickly.

2. If a vacuum or suction system is used for actively eliminating waste gases, care must be taken to avoid placing negative pressure on the anesthetic circuit, thus evacuating the reservoir bag.

For patient safety, an interface is placed between the capture device and the disposal site (Figure 3-33). For positive flow disposal, only a positive relief valve is needed. However, for suction disposal, both positive and negative relief valves are required. Non-valve interface systems are available as well.

Disposal of waste gases can be made with passive flow to the air return vent of nonrecirculating room ventilation systems. That is not an appropriate method with an air recirculation system. For an active system, gases can be drawn into the surgical suction system or removed with a vacuum pump dedicated only for active scavenging. If, as in many veterinary hospitals, neither of these methods is available, gases should be vented directly outside the building. This can be done if operating and preparation rooms have an outside wall (Figure 3-33). If not, gases can be vented using proper precautions through large bore tubing placed in a false ceiling or along a wall. Tubing must be at least one inch in internal diameter, with no restrictions at corners or bends and the outlet must be protected from obstructions. If a distance greater than 50ft is imposed between the capture device and disposal outlet, gas flow should be assisted with a positive flow device. Scavenging systems have been adapted for open, semi-open, and circle techniques. The scavenger valve, tubing and system must accommodate maximal flows used. In addition, exhaust tubing must be protected from kinking or occlusion. In cold climates, water vapor may freeze at the outlet which could eventually result in total occlusion. Thus, a failsafe protective device must be incorporated as part of the system.

Charcoal canisters can be used when active or passive scavenging systems are not possible. This may be an effective means of scavenging halogenated anesthetics in the short term, perhaps for a few days. These absorptive devices can be depleted of their effectiveness without any indication or warning, thus allowing unabsorbed waste gases to be discharged into the room. Perhaps there will be warning sensors developed to attach to the outlet of the canister to warn of unacceptable waste gas levels being discharged.

Figure 3-33 Schematic of scavenging interface with passive exit of waste gases through an outside wall of an operating room. Most often, the exit port is protected on the outside of a building with a screened vent.
Reprinted with permission. Sawyer, D C, The Practice of Small Animal Anesthesia, W.B. Saunders 1982.

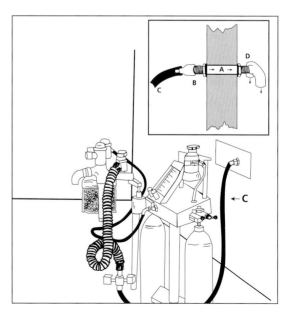

Hazards of Anesthetic Machines

There is always potential hazard with an anesthetic machine but the dangers are primarily those of mishandling of compressed gases, flammable liquids and the CO_2 absorber. The patient is most subject to these dangers since hypoxia or anesthetic overdose may result from improper use or malfunction of equipment. Hypoxia may result from an empty oxygen cylinder, failure to open the supply valve or to turn on the flow meter, loose line connections or malfunctioning flow meters. Steps have been taken to eliminate certain hazards, such as the use of the pin index safety system designed to prevent incorrect installation of oxygen tanks on machine yokes and fail-safe systems on flow meters of newer machines. All machines have color-coded flow meter assemblies, scales and distinctively shaped needle valve knobs to reduce the possibility of human error. However, proper use of the machine rests with the anesthetist; there is no substitute for vigilance.

General Principles of Inhalation Anesthesia

Inhalation anesthetics are compounds that exist either as gases or as liquids that volatilize to a gaseous state. They have certain features that make them different from injectable anesthetics. This relates to their entry into the body and to factors which influence uptake and distribution, metabolism and elimination and mechanisms of anesthetic action (Eger 1974). Search for new anesthetics has been focused on inhalants which have characteristics of an ideal anesthetic, e.g., rapid onset, precise control of anesthetic depth, good muscle relaxation, rapid emergence and safety.

Routes of Administration

Drugs for general anesthesia may be given IV, IM, rectally, by mouth (buccal) or by inhalation. They vary in controllability but the primary objective is to achieve a moment-by-moment regulation of anesthetic depth. This is accomplished by producing a partial pressure or concentration of anesthetic that can be decreased or increased promptly as the situation demands. Blood levels of IV or inhalation agents are achieved more or less in the same manner. With IV agents, injection is made directly into the circulation, whereas, inhalation agents gain entry into the circulation through the tremendously large absorptive surface area of the lung. Although most volatile liquid anesthetics are metabolized, their biotransformation does not have any significant influence on clinical recovery. However, injectable agents are inactivated in the body in varying degrees by oxidation, reduction, hydrolysis and conjugation and safety (controllability) of these agents depends on biotransformation by body systems. Drugs must be carefully titrated to achieve the desired anesthetic depth since once these drugs enter the circulation, there is no prompt method of removal. In the case of opioid and alpha-$_2$ agonists, their effects can be reversed with a specific receptor antagonist but hepatic metabolism and renal excretion, which may be slow and unpredictable, must still be relied on for removal of drugs from the body. Since inhalation agents enter and leave primarily via the pulmonary system, they provide the most controllable method of producing general anesthesia.

The effect of anesthetics varies according to their concentration in brain tissue. Concentration is the product of solubility and partial pressure of the agent in that tissue. Solubility is a constant for each tissue so levels change according to the partial pressure. Thus, concentration of a gas in a mixture is proportional to its partial pressure. These two terms are used interchangeably to describe dosages of inhaled anesthetics. The term "tension" is also used and is synonymous with partial pressure in both gas mixtures and tissues.

Pharmacokinetics of Inhaled Anesthetics

The gas law that describes behavior of gases in solution and in tissues of the body is Henry's Law. Anesthetic gases do not interact chemically with nervous tissue but rather, in theory, they produce anesthesia by a physical effect on cell membranes in brain tissue. Numerous theories propose mechanisms by which certain agents produce general anesthesia. A specific macroscopic site of action has not been identified but the most likely sites are in the cortical area of brain and in the reticular formation of the medulla and spinal cord. The synapse is most probably the cellular site of action but it is not known whether the nerve terminal, the synaptic membrane or another site is primarily affected. It is clearly recognized that the brain is ultimately involved but the specific mechanism is not completely understood.

Understanding Henry's law is important in knowing how anesthetics are delivered to tissues and how equilibrium is achieved. Henry's Law is the relationship between the volume of dissolved gas in a liquid and its partial pressure in the gas phase in equilibrium. The concept of partial pressure or tension of a gas is defined as the individual pressure exerted by a gas in a mixture of gases. For example, partial pressure of oxygen in arterial blood (PaO_2) in a patient breathing 20% oxygen in air is about 100mm Hg. When a liquid (arterial blood) is exposed to a gas in pulmonary alveoli, partial pressure equilibrium will eventually be achieved between the two phases. As blood transports dissolved gases, partial pressure equilibriums are established between brain and other tissues in the body.

Solubility

One of the most important factors that regulate transport of inhalation anesthetics across membranes is its relative solubility. The blood:gas (B/G) partition coefficient relates the amount of inhalant dissolved in fluid (blood) to the amount of that agent in the gas phase (alveolus). This defines the affinity of an agent for blood as compared to air or oxygen. Partition coefficients for the most common agents are given in Table 3-3. A B/G value of 10 would indicate that the agent is 10 times more soluble in the blood phase than the gaseous phase. Conversely, a B/G value of 0.5 means that the agent has only one-half the solubility in blood as in gas. This expression is applied to any two phases, such as tissue/blood or oil/gas ratio. Note that it is important to express both the phases and the phase ratio. In common usage, blood solubility is used interchangeably with blood/gas partition coefficient and tissue solubility with tissue/blood partition coefficient. With the exception of diethyl ether, the trend is for agents of low solubility in blood to also be relatively more insoluble in tissues (Table 3-7).

Table 3-7 Partition Coefficients of Inhalation Anesthetics at 37° C*

Anesthetic	Blood	Brain	Liver	Kidney	Muscle	Fat
Desflurane	0.4	1.3	1.3	1.0	2.0	27.0
Sevoflurane	0.7	1.7	1.8	1.2	3.1	48.0
Isoflurane	1.5	1.6	1.8	1.2	2.9	45.0
Enflurane	2.0	2.7	3.7	1.9	2.2	83.0
Halothane	2.5	1.9	2.1	1.0	3.4	51.0
Diethyl Ether	12.1	1.1	1.0	1.1	1.0	3.7
Methoxyflurane	15.0	20.0	29.0	11.0	16.0	902.0

* Solvent/Gas

Data obtained in part from Steffey EP. Inhalation Anesthetics. In *Lumb & Jones' Veterinary Anesthesia, 3rd ed.* Williams & Wilkins, 1996.

Uptake of Anesthetic Gases

Inhalation anesthetics are in constant movement between alveoli and blood with rate of transport dependent upon solubility. In the case of agents of relatively low solubility such as nitrous oxide, desflurane and sevoflurane, alveolar concentration builds very rapidly. This is because only a small fraction of the drug is transported into blood, leaving a large part of it in the alveoli. Since agents are also relatively insoluble in tissues, tissues take up only small fractions of the gas from blood. Thus, because of their relatively low solubility, equilibrium between arterial blood and pulmonary alveoli is reached very rapidly.

In contrast, more soluble agents such as halothane require a much longer period for equilibrium. At the beginning of the uptake process, the largest part of the more soluble agents is transferred to blood during each breath with very little of the anesthetic remaining in alveoli. Prior to the next breath, concentration in the alveoli falls because of uptake by blood. Because of the higher solubility time required to equilibrate in body tissues is much longer. The alveolar anesthetic concentration and that in the arterioles begin to rise only as blood returning from body tissues to lungs carries more and more anesthetic. Initially, the gradient between alveolar and blood anesthetic partial pressure is high and is also influenced by the inspired anesthetic concentration and minute ventilation. Movement of gas from the alveoli is influenced not only by the gradient but also by the solubility characteristics of the anesthetic. Cardiac output and the alveolar-to-mixed venous anesthetic partial pressure difference also determine uptake. The faster alveolar exchange or wash-in of gases occurs in the alveoli, the faster will be the uptake of anesthetics by blood. Once an anesthetic reaches the alveoli, uptake of that agent by blood begins, thus slowing the alveolar rate of rise of the anesthetic partial pressure. As more anesthetic is absorbed into blood and tissues, slightly less is removed from alveoli with each breath, e.g., the gradient across the alveolar capillary membrane becomes smaller and gradually the alveolar partial pressure rises closer to the inspired level. Therefore, with agents of relatively high solubility, uptake and onset of anesthesia as well as elimination or recovery is slow compared to agents of low solubility.

Distribution of Anesthetic Agents

Factors influencing tissue uptake are the same as those for lung, that is, solubility, arterial-to-tissue anesthetic partial pressure difference and tissue blood flow. Arterial blood transports anesthetic drugs to all parts of the body. Even though general anesthesia is achieved by action of these agents on certain parts of the brain, anesthetics are delivered to all tissues. Extent of distribution is directly determined by perfusion of particular tissues. Tissues are designated as vessel-rich group (VRG), muscle group (MG), vessel-poor group (VPG), and fat group (FG) (Eger 1974). The VRG includes brain, heart, intestines, kidney, liver, spleen and endocrine glands. It constitutes about 9% of the body mass but receives 75% of the cardiac output. Because of the high blood flow per unit volume, these tissues equilibrate with arterial anesthetic partial pressures in 5 to 15 minutes and further uptake becomes negligible. The MG includes both skin and skeletal muscle and although it constitutes more than 50% of body mass, it gets less than 20% of the cardiac output. Equilibrium between blood and MG would proceed at a slower rate and uptake continues over a period of hours. The VPG includes bones, ligaments, cartilage and tendons. Although it comprises about 20% of body mass, it receives less than 2% of the cardiac output and therefore has virtually no influence on the effect of anesthetic uptake. FG tissues receive roughly 3% of the blood supply and constitute about 20% of body mass. Anesthetics are more soluble in fat compared to other tissues but blood supply to FG limits its uptake. This group plays a more important role in recovery from anesthesia after long procedures but for pragmatic reasons, the VRG and MG play much more important roles in the uptake, distribution and elimination of inhalation anesthetics.

Factors Affecting Induction

From a clinical standpoint, a number of factors affect the rate at which inhalation agents achieve anesthesia. Ventilation is a primary factor because it is the process by which these agents are brought to pulmonary capillaries. As alveolar ventilation increases, more anesthetic molecules are presented to blood resulting in more rapid equilibration of alveolar-to-inspired concentration ratio. If, for example, apnea occurs following injection of an anesthetic such as thiopental or propofol, breathing should be controlled not only to provide oxygen and eliminate CO_2 but also to deliver anesthetic vapors to alveoli to facilitate induction. The same applies to an animal with hypopnea or tachypnea. If a small tidal volume occurs during either a slow or rapid rate of breathing, dead space ventilation may predominate at the expense of alveolar ventilation and induction by inhalation anesthesia will be delayed. Partial recovery from the injectable agent may occur before an adequate concentration of the inhalation agent has been reached so the patient may appear light or nearly awake. By initially increasing inspired concentration to two to three times maintenance levels, a larger alveolar-to-arterial gradient will force large numbers of anesthetic molecules into blood and then to tissues, resulting in faster induction. This process is called *over-pressure*. Care must be taken not to make this gradient too high in order to avoid severe depression of cardiac and respiratory function. To avoid *overshoot*, levels above 3 MAC for halothane should not be used. The lower solubility coefficients of isoflurane and sevoflurane, 1.4 and 0.6 respectively, permit a more rapid rise in alveolar concentration so initial settings usually do not need to be set above 2 MAC levels. For example, 2.5.0% isoflurane is adequate for 3 to 5 minutes to provide a large enough gradient for a reasonable induction with the patient intubated. When administered by mask for inhalation induction alone, 4% isoflurane is needed because of the anatomical and physiological dead space buffer imposed by the mouth and upper airway. In very small patients, isoflurane vaporizer concentration should not exceed 3%.

Ventilation-perfusion abnormalities may be present in disease states or may be produced if one bronchus is intubated. If one lung is perfused but not ventilated, an agent of relatively high solubility, e.g., halothane, will allow induction to proceed at about a normal rate compared to less soluble agents such as isoflurane or sevoflurane. Ventilation in the intubated lung will increase and coupled with the higher solubility of halothane, will somewhat compensate for the lack of uptake in the nonventilated but perfused lung. When delayed induction is observed with agents of low solubility, one must first suspect that the endotracheal tube is beyond the thoracic inlet and into one bronchus. Delayed induction might also occur in a patient with a diaphragmatic hernia or space occupying lesion compromising lung volume.

Cardiac Output
The second factor that determines anesthetic uptake from the alveoli is blood flow. It is understood that the greater the blood flow through lungs, the more anesthetic will be removed (taken up by blood). The effect of cardiac output is one factor the anesthetist cannot control but also one that must be recognized. With higher than normal cardiac output, induction using agents with high solubility will be slower than induction using less soluble agents. That is, the less soluble the agent, the smaller will be the influence of changes in blood flow on alveolar concentration (Eger, 1974). However, it is very important to consider the influence of cardiac output on uptake. A 30% change in cardiac will produce a measurable change in end-tidal anesthetic concentration (Kennedy 2001). With highly soluble agents and depressed cardiac output, as blood flows slowly through the lung, uptake by blood will be rapid and thus high concentrations will be delivered almost in a "bolus" to brain, heart, and other VRG tissues. The resulting effects may be sudden induction and likely depression of vital functions. If one provides hyperventilation, vasoconstriction as a result of lowering of CO_2 may occur. In addition, cardiac output may decrease because of the physical effects induced by controlled breathing.

Initially, anesthetic partial pressure in venous blood will almost be zero because tissues will remove most of the anesthetic from arterial blood. However, as uptake by tissues proceeds, gradients between tissue and blood decrease. As uptake by tissue decreases, anesthetic concentration in venous blood increases. This lessens alveolar-to-venous blood anesthetic concentration difference and allows alveolar anesthetic concentration to rise. This is the most important concept to understand in the relationship between alveolar concentration, tissue (brain) partial pressures and anesthetic depth. The mixed venous blood anesthetic concentration reflects the anesthetic concentration in tissues. The higher the concentration in venous blood, the slower the uptake and faster will be the rise in alveolar anesthetic concentration. When anesthetic concentration in all tissues is in equilibrium with that of blood supplying them, uptake from the lung will be zero and the anesthetic concentration in alveoli will equal that inspired. This condition rarely occurs during clinical anesthesia but will be closer with agents of very low solubility such as sevoflurane. It would take days or weeks for this to occur with an agent of high solubility.

Elimination of Inhalation Anesthetics
Recovery from inhalation anesthesia is the inverse of induction and the major route of elimination is through the lungs. In a similar manner, agents of higher solubility are eliminated more slowly than those of low solubility. Recovery should be considerably faster with sevoflurane than with

halothane or isoflurane. Until 1965, it was assumed that the only way anesthetic gases were removed from the body was by pulmonary ventilation. However, as discussed in the section on metabolism of inhalation anesthetics, in the late 1960's and into the 1970's, it was shown that most all of these agents were metabolized to varying degrees by the liver. Since it was found that this occurs primarily at subanesthetic concentrations, from a clinical recovery standpoint pulmonary ventilation is still the route of elimination for anesthesia recovery.

Minimum Alveolar Concentration (MAC)

The power or potency of injectable drugs has long been expressed by the LD_{50} (lethal dose in 50% of a test population) or ED50 (effective dose in 50% of a test population). In order to express something other than the LD_{50} for inhalation anesthetics, it was necessary for anesthesiologists to have a means of expressing potency without having a close association with death since the state of anesthesia should be a reversible process. The concept of MAC developed by Eger fulfills this need and is defined as the lowest anesthetic concentration in the alveoli at 1 atmosphere that produces immobility in 50% of those humans or animals exposed to a somatic noxious stimulus (Eger et al. 1965a). In practicality, it is a measure of anesthetic potency defined by the level needed to prevent gross muscular movement in response to a gross painful stimulus. For animals, one such stimulus is produced by clamping the tail with a large hemostat. If raising the head is defined as gross somatic response, then other actions such as movement of the head, torso, legs, coughing and hyperventilation are not considered movement. Other tests that have been proposed are toe pinch (MAC-pinch), passing a weak electrical current through subcutaneous electrodes (MAC-tetanus) or airway occlusion response (MAC-AOR) (Ide et al. 1998). The response to skin incision also provides a useful stimulus but is limited to only one observation per patient. Bispectral index (BIS) was attempted as a MAC determination for sevoflurane in cats but was determined not to be effective (Lamont et al. 2004). Since amnesia and analgesia are needed in addition to abolition of movement, they are also included in the criteria for MAC. It is a useful standard by which inhalation anesthetics may be compared and equals the partial pressure in per cent of 1 atmosphere at the anesthetic site of action. To achieve surgical anesthesia, alveolar anesthetic concentration must be above MAC. MAC is not surgical anesthesia but multiples of MAC are used as a guide for surgical levels of anesthesia, usually between 1.2 and 1.5 MAC. For isoflurane, this would be 1.6-2.0% with vaporizer setting being 2.0-2.5%. MAC is an extremely valuable measure and has been used widely to evaluate factors that influence anesthetic requirements. Variability of MAC in a single species is small and even between species is relatively narrow (Table 3-8). It is especially useful when one is required to anesthetize an unusual pet, such as a skunk, raccoon or bird in which MAC levels are not available. This is a definite advantage with inhalation anesthetics since the variability of injectable agents may be quite large.

Table 3-8 MAC Values* for Anesthetics in Various Species and Classes

Agent	Dog	Cat	Monkey	Rabbit	Rat	AG Parrot	Hawk	Toad	Goldfish
Desflurane	7.2	9.8		8.9	6.6				
Sevoflurane	2.2	2.6	2.3	3.7	2.4				
Isoflurane	1.3	1.6	1.4	2.0	1.4	1.9	1.4		
Enflurane	2.1	2.4	2.0	2.9	2.2				
Halothane	0.9	1.0	1.0	1.1	1.1			0.7	0.8
Diethyl Ether	3.2	2.1			3.2			1.6	2.2
Methoxyflurane	0.3	0.2		0.3				0.2	0.1

*Percent of 1 Atmosphere
Data obtained in part from Steffey EP. Inhalation Anesthetics. In *Lumb & Jones' Veterinary Anesthesia, 3rd ed.* Williams & Wilkins, 1996.

Factors that have little effect on MAC include: gender, duration of anesthesia, circadian rhythms, hyperthyroidism or hypothyroidism, arterial Pco_2 up to 90mm Hg, hyperventilation to a Pco_2 of 10mm Hg, severe metabolic acidosis or alkalosis, arterial Po_2 from 40 to 500mm Hg, anemia to a hematocrit of 10%, phenylephrine-induced hypertension and atropine or gyclopyrrolate (Eger, 1974). Reductions in MAC are found if $PaCO_2$ is above 90mm Hg, PaO_2 is less than 40mm Hg or hematocrit is less than 10%. Increasing age reduces MAC as does hypothermia but elevation in body temperature increases MAC. Clinically, a puppy or kitten will have a higher MAC than a geriatric; thus, care must be taken not to over anesthetize the older patient. Since solubility of anesthetics increases during hypothermia, in addition to the lowering of MAC, it is essential to recognize the effects of cold in order to prevent deep or prolonged anesthesia. MAC is increased by IV administration of amphetamine, a drug that releases catecholamines. In a clinical situation, an aggravated and aroused mean animal may have high levels of endogenous catecholamines, which would require a higher maintenance concentration initially. As catecholamine levels decrease, however, MAC would return to expected levels. Opioids, tranquilizers and other depressants reduce MAC and the interaction between anesthetics appear to be additive. This is a useful concept in understanding the benefits of balanced anesthesia.

Individual sensitivities vary not only within species but between anesthetics as well. MAC is a guide that is very helpful but it is not absolute. In any given population of animals, MAC may be higher or lower than published values (Barter et al 2004). From a clinical standpoint, some patients will require higher levels of anesthesia, others may be lower.

In addition to evaluating factors that influence anesthetic requirements, MAC is quite useful in comparing effects of various inhalation anesthetics using equipotent concentrations and multiples of MAC. For example, the effects of halothane and isoflurane on respiration can be compared at 1.0, 1.5, and 2.0 MAC to provide information on the comparative effects of both agents. MAC is useful in redefining "signs" of anesthetic depth; each anesthetic has its own criteria, precluding the use of a ubiquitous standard. In addition, the use of MAC to test theories of narcosis has provided some interesting correlations (Eger, 1974).

Metabolism of Inhalation Anesthetics

Inhalation anesthetics were in use many years before any thought was given to their biological instability. It was assumed that these drugs were inert, that is, they exited via the lungs just as they entered and were not metabolized. Biotransformation was demonstrated in laboratory animals, suggesting that inhalation anesthetics may be converted by the liver to CO_2 and other metabolites (Van Dyke and Chenoweth, 1965). Those initial studies spawned a new era of research to determine not only the extent of biotransformation but also what effect metabolites may have on the patients receiving the anesthetics as well as on personnel breathing trace concentrations. Studies have shown that halothane or methoxyflurane may be metabolized by as much as 50% whereas, less than 0.2% of isoflurane is changed.

The liver is the principal site of anesthetic metabolism. Eger defined metabolism as the fraction of anesthetic transformed as it traverses the liver (Eger, 1974). This would imply that metabolism is a function of hepatic accessibility. Anesthetics taken up in nonsplanchnic tissues would not pass through the liver and thus would not be subjected to metabolism.

Numerous studies have shown that drugs such as phenobarbital that cause enzyme induction will increase the fraction of anesthetic metabolism; anesthetics themselves may induce the enzymes that cause their destruction. Anesthetists excreted more metabolic products following exposure to halothane than nonanesthetists exposed to the same challenge (Eger, 1974).

Anesthetic partial pressure also appears to affect the rate of metabolism. In one study, the concentration of halothane entering and leaving the liver was measured in swine and the fraction removed calculated (Figure 3-34) (Sawyer et al. 1971). It was determined that at or near

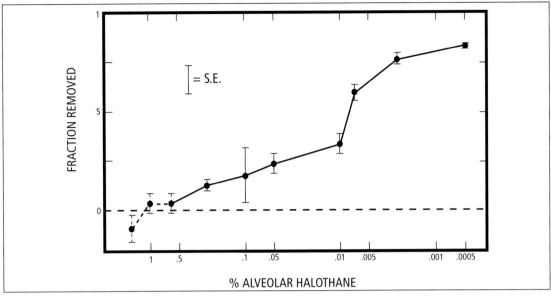

Figure 3-34 Comparison of the fraction of halothane removed by liver with calculated alveolar concentration. Dotted line indicates that values were not significantly different from zero (P > 0.05). (From Sawyer et al 1971).
Reprinted with permission. Sawyer, D C, The Practice of Small Animal Anesthesia, W.B. Saunders, 1982

anesthetic partial pressures, no detectable metabolism was evident. However, at low concentrations–similar to those breathed by anesthetists and operating room personnel–nearly complete metabolism occurred. This was most likely an effect of enzyme saturation and may apply to other anesthetics. It is reasonable to assume that the more soluble an anesthetic, the greater the metabolism, especially at subanesthetic concentrations. Halsey and colleagues measured hepatic extraction only at very low alveolar concentrations and demonstrated significant metabolism of halothane and methoxyflurane (Halsey et al. 1971). Metabolism of enflurane was small and no metabolism was detected for nitrous oxide, cyclopropane or isoflurane.

What are the implications of metabolism, first, to the patient and, second, to people exposed to trace concentrations discharged into room air? There have been reports of postsurgical jaundice and hepatitis in humans and animals, associated with halothane, methoxyflurane, fluroxene, and enflurane. The risk factor is very small and difficult to assess in veterinary anesthesia because a complete central record system is not available. From 1970 to 1997 at the Michigan State University Veterinary Teaching Hospital, two hepatitis cases in dogs, one from halothane and one from methoxyflurane, could be judged as possibly being due to anesthetic exposure (author personal observation). In man, the possibility of a rare occurrence of halothane-induced hepatic necrosis is difficult to determine and the incidence of nonfatal, nonicteric hepatic disease is unknown. The theory that postanesthetic hepatic necrosis might represent sensitivity or allergic response has not been substantiated. However, this appears to be the case because fever, eosinophilia, jaundice and occasionally skin rash usually follow a previous exposure. In small animal practice, the incidence of hepatic necrosis appears to be so low that sequential exposures of veterinary patients to the same inhalant need not be a concern. However, it would seem prudent to consider an alternative anesthetic in highly allergic veterinary patients. If such a syndrome as halogenated hydro-carbon-induced hepatic necrosis exists, it is most likely due to an unusual combination of circumstances, including abnormal enzymatic responses that may result in unusual metabolites (Bruce, 1979).

Methoxyflurane is metabolized by the liver to free fluoride and oxalate; both are nephrotoxic (Brunson et al. 1979). It is considered a nephrotoxin because this process is dose-related and could be reproduced in both man and animals with dogs being less susceptible (Messick et al., 1972). Although MOF is no longer available in the US, it is still available in some countries and should be used with caution in patients with renal disease.

Characteristics of Inhalation Anesthetics
Ventilation and Anesthesia

Ventilation is the process that provides for uptake of O_2 and elimination of CO_2. The lung is structured primarily for efficient transfer of gases between alveoli and blood in the pulmonary capillaries. In addition, the lung also has nonrespiratory metabolic and other functions, such as removing inhaled substances through ciliary activity and serving as a blood reservoir.

Ventilation refers to movement of air or anesthetic gases through passages and subdivisions of conducting airways into terminal respiratory units. The amount of inspired gases that reach the site for gas exchange i.e., alveoli (Figure 3-35) is determined by the distensibility of lung tissue and other factors that govern movement of air through conducting pathways (trachea, bronchi, and bronchioles).

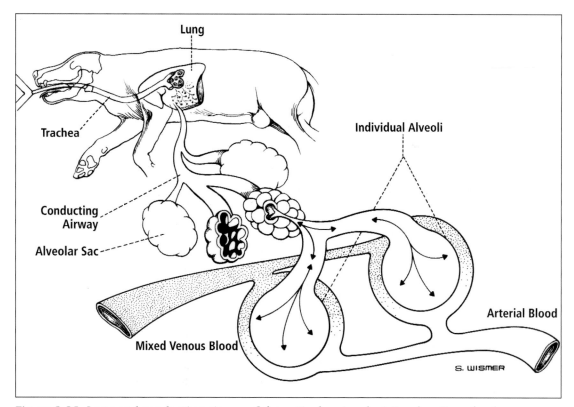

Figure 3-35 Lung and conducting airways. Schematic drawing depicting location of pulmonary alveoli in relationship to conducting airways and pulmonary capillary blood.
Reprinted with permission. Sawyer, D C, The Practice of Small Animal Anesthesia, W.B. Saunders, 1982

Muscular effort, or force from manual or mechanical ventilation, is required to cause inhaled gases to flow through the system. Since most inhalation anesthetics depress spontaneous ventilation, voluntary muscular effort by patients to increase ventilation is usually not possible during anesthesia.

The volume of gas passing in or out of the lungs with a single breath is referred to as the tidal volume (Figure 3-36) (Comroe et al., 1962).The number of breaths per minute (BPM) is called the rate of breathing. The product of these two is the minute ventilation (Ve) or minute volume (V_t x BPM = Ve). In Figure 3-37, total lung capacity (TLC), vital capacity (VC), inspiratory capacity (IC), functional residual capacity (FRC), inspiratory reserve volume (IRV), tidal volume (V_t), expiratory reserve volume (ERV) and residual volume (RV) are represented. During anesthesia, V_t (7 to 10 ml/kg) is crudely estimated by observing movement of the reservoir bag or chest area. When a deeper breath is provided by manual or mechanical ventilation, it encroaches upon some portion of the inspiratory capacity, which is approximated at six times V_t (Figure 3-36).

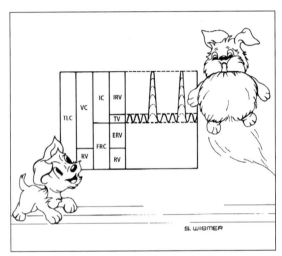

Figure 3-36 This figure illustrates relationships between various lung volumes. Of clinical importance are tidal volumes (TV) and inspiratory capacity (IC). Usually during either manually or mechanically controlled breathing, normal TV (i.e., volume that would be achieved during spontaneous breathing) is exceeded two to three times. However, should IC (estimated to be six times TV) be reached, overinflation of the lung in a closed chest will occur, as represented by the floating character. TLC = total lung capacity; VC = vital capacity; RV = reserve volume; FRC = functional residual capacity; IRV = inspiratory reserve volume; ERV = expiratory reserve volume; RV = reserve volume.
Reprinted with permission. Sawyer, D C, The Practice of Small Animal Anesthesia, W.B. Saunders, 1982

The term used to describe elastic properties of the lung is compliance, which is defined as a volume change produced by a unit pressure change. The elastic response that occurs with manual compression of the reservoir bag can be detected by the hand and one develops a feel for this elasticity or compliance. In the presence of respiratory disease, the lung may feel hard or stiff, thus compliance is low; that is, a high pressure must be used for any given change in volume.

Dead space refers to anatomical conduits occupied by residual air. Gas exchange occurs only in the alveoli; therefore, gas contained in the nose, mouth, trachea, larynx, pharynx and bronchi is defined as dead space gas. Increased dead space may occur because of a malfunctioning anesthetic circuit (e.g., faulty unidirectional valve in a circle rebreathing system) and by poorly perfused but ventilated alveoli. A decrease in anatomical dead space is achieved by tracheal intubation, which eliminates the large volume in the nose and mouth and part of the trachea. Excessive mechanical dead space will occur if the endotracheal tube extends proximally beyond the incisor teeth. The ideal length limits of the endotrachreal tube are the incisor teeth and the thoracic inlet.

Gas exchange occurs across the alveolar membrane and pulmonary capillary membrane by the process of diffusion. The more molecules of gas in the alveoli, the more rapidly diffusion will occur. The higher the partial pressure of gas in the alveoli, the higher the partial pressure will be in blood. In addition to inhaled gases, water vapor will always be present since each breath will be saturated with water vapor as it passes through the trachea and bronchi. Partial pressure of water ranges between 47 and 52mm Hg at 37 to 38.5°C.

In air, partial pressure of oxygen is about 160mm Hg at sea level. When it reaches the alveoli, PO_2 will drop in alveolar blood to 100mm Hg and in arterial blood to 95mm Hg. The PO_2 of venous blood returning from body tissues will be approximately 45mm Hg. Higher oxygen tensions are used during anesthesia to compensate for atelectasis and other induced ventilation-perfusion disorders. Therefore, during anesthesia, normal arterial PO_2 should be between 120 and 500mm Hg, depending on inspired oxygen tension and the degree of ventilation/perfusion mismatch. Significant control of respiration by circulatory oxygen is activated only during conditions of hypoxemia.

CO_2 is continuously produced by metabolism and eliminated by the lung. Normally, CO_2 pressure gradient is opposite to that of oxygen since the partial pressure of CO_2 is higher in venous blood than in alveoli. Respiratory control centers maintain arterial PCO_2 between 38 and 42mm Hg in the dog and 28 to 32mm Hg in the cat. Anesthetics depress the stimulatory response to elevations of CO_2 and this effect is dose related.

Anesthetics have a profound and sometimes unpredictable effect on ventilation. They affect not only the normal mechanisms of gas exchange but also patterns of breathing. Apnea, breath-holding and irregular breathing are common during induction especially at presurgical levels. In most cases, rhythmic breathing accompanies the onset of surgical anesthesia but one can expect a decrease in tidal volume and a variable effect on rate of breathing. Tachypnea may occur as a response to hypercapnia induced by anesthetics. Panting in anesthetized patients is most often observed in small canine breeds, especially terrier and toy groups, and may occasionally be seen in cats. Etiology of panting during anesthesia is not well understood but it is most likely not a response to physiological maintenance of core temperature. With tachypnea or panting, tidal volume may actually be reduced thus decreasing alveolar ventilation and resulting in respiratory acidosis. Also during surgical anesthesia, respiratory depression with decreased tidal volume and/or decreased rate of breathing may cause CO_2 in arterial blood ($PaCO_2$) to rise. Because of the influence of anesthetics on respiratory centers in brain, normal responses cannot compensate for hypercapnia. The anesthetized animal may appear to be ventilating adequately but in fact the $PaCO_2$ could be 50 to 60mm Hg or more instead of 40 to 45mm Hg. Intervention for this development is possible through controlled breathing by either manual or mechanical means. As a general rule, normal V_t of 10ml/kg should be doubled and rate should be controlled to between 8 and 12 breaths per minute. The effectiveness of controlled breathing is determined on the basis of presence or absence of spontaneous breathing. If ventilation is properly controlled, spontaneous efforts will not be evident. Adjustments in rate and depth are made accordingly to control gas exchange effectively. Assisted ventilation may be used to treat atelectasis but it is not effective in treating the problem, i.e., hypercapnia. With assisted ventilation, the patient initiates the breath and the tidal volume is delivered by the ventilator or anesthetist.

Mechanical Ventilators for Small Animal Patients
The only way to effectively maintain ventilation at normal levels during anesthesia is to control breathing. Does spontaneous breathing severely compromise every patient during anesthesia with isoflurane or sevoflurane? Probably not, especially in young healthy patients during surgical stimulation. However, for obese patients and those at risk because of disease, injury, or age, controlling ventilation to maintain $PaCO_2$ at or near normal levels may be very advantageous for a successful outcome. Tables are sometimes provided with each ventilator but the only method of monitoring effectiveness of controlled breathing is with capnography. Without knowing values of end tidal CO_2, it is very difficult to know which adjustments to make or not make to the ventilator. With or without a capnograph, it is best to start the procedure by setting the rate at 12 BPM. Then with the flow control set at minimum, increase the setting with each breath until chest excursions are a little above normal. Tidal volume should be about 10ml/kg with inspiratory pressure 10-15cm H_2O. The rate can then be adjusted up or down depending on specific patient needs and circumstances.

During anesthesia, the ventilator replaces the reservoir bag in a breathing system. It is usually connected at the bag mount with a corrugated hose. On some units, the ventilator may be connected directly to the breathing system. When the ventilator is in the controlled breathing mode, the APL valve of the breathing circuit must be closed. There is a relief valve built into the ventilator that automatically closes during inspiration and opens once the bellows fill toward the end of expiration and allows excess gas to be vented from the system.

The bellows thus becomes the reservoir bag but is out of touch from the anesthetist. Driving gas from the ventilator collapses the bellows in a similar manner that hand compression would collapse the reservoir bag. For inspiration, driving gas is delivered into the space between the bellows and chamber housing. The resulting pressure causes the bellows to compress and deliver gas to the breathing system and patient. During expiration, the bellows refills as breathing system gases flow from the patient and flow meters. Driving gas is vented to the room separately and once the bellows completely fill, excess gases from the breathing system are vented through the exhaust into the scavenging system.

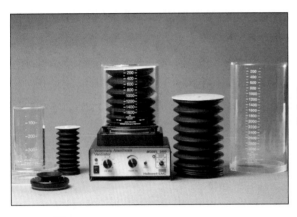

Figure 3-37 Hallowell Small Animal Ventilator with different size bellows.
Courtesy of Hallowell EMC, Pittsfield, MA.

Ventilators are pneumatically powered usually by oxygen. Controls regulate flow, volume, inspiratory time, expiration and pause and pressure of the driving gas. Depending on manufacturer, controls may be pneumatic, fluidic, or electronic. Most older ventilators use fluidic technology that uses moving streams of gas through channels cut into a block of solid material to perform sensing, logic, amplification and control functions. These circuits are modular, easy to maintain and are very compact. Newer ventilators may incorporate electronic controls and alarms that require a power supply in addition to a compressed gas source. For example, the ventilator by Hallowell EMC is an electronically controlled, pneumatic, time cycled ventilator with pressure limiting alarms (Figure 3-37). A small animal ventilator from Surgivet is shown in (Figure 3-38).

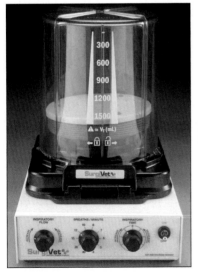

Figure 3-38 Surgivet Small Animal Ventilator.
Courtesy of SurgiVet, Inc. Waukesha, WI

Pressure-Limiting Valve

To prevent excess pressure being delivered by a volume cycled ventilator, the pressure-limiting valve is used to vent excess driving gas from the system. This may be preset by the manufacturer and can be as high as 80cm H_2O. If controls are present on the ventilator, they may be set by the operator between 10 and 60cm H_2O. For patients with high resistance airways, high inspiratory pressure may be needed but it is unlikely that inspiratory pressure beyond 60cm would be needed. With adjustable controls, one must avoid operator error by leaving the maximum pressure limit too high in patients with normal lungs especially after the ventilator has been used on a patient with high airway resistance or low compliance.

Bellows and Assembly

The accordion-like bag inside the plastic housing or chamber is called the bellows. There are two types depending on whether they are attached at the top or bottom of the unit. Ascending or standing bellows are in the upright position at the end of expiration and descending bellows are in a hanging or inverted position.

With standing bellows, the bag is compressed downward during inspiration. During expiration, the bellows expand upward. Tidal volume is regulated by adjusting inspiratory time and flow. For hanging bellows attached at the top of the chamber, there is usually a weight at the bottom of the bellows that assists in re-expansion. Tidal volume is controlled by limiting excursion of the bellows during filling.

What is the difference between these two designs? Starting with no fresh gas inflow from the anesthesia machine, a standing bellows is collapsed. It only expands when gas flows into the unit from flow meters or flush valve. There is full expansion at the end of expiration if there are no leaks in the breathing system. That is, the bellows returns to the same position at the top of the chamber during each cycle being filled with fresh and rebreathed gases. If there is a leak or disconnection in the system, the bellows will not refill to the same degree at the end of expiration and will not return to its previous position indicated by the scale on the chamber wall. If the leak is small, increasing flow meter setting may match the leak. Usually, this cannot keep up with the leak because positive pressure delivered to the circuit by the ventilator expresses a large quantity of gas through the break in the system. This assumes that flow meters are set properly and there is no obstruction to the spill valve outlet or scavenging system. Ventilators with standing bellows always have some level of positive end expiratory pressure in the range of 2-3cm H_2O. This is similar to airway pressure at the end of expiration maintained by the APL valve during spontaneous breathing on a circle system. There is no possibility of generating a negative airway pressure.

With a hanging bellows, weight in the bellows pulls it to the bottom of the chamber so it looks expanded even with no fresh gas provided from the anesthesia machine. A leak in the system will not be as remarkable because the bellows will still be hanging at the end of expiration. During the inspiratory phase, gas is discharged through the leak resulting in a reduced V_t delivered and air is sucked back into the system as the bellows makes its downward movement during expiration. The entrained air dilutes the O_2 and anesthetic concentrations. Airway pressure with a hanging bellows may be negative until the bellows have been refilled at end of expiration. The danger is risk of collapsed alveoli.

Exhaust Valve

This valve is interposed between the compressed driving gas and bellows housing. It automatically closes during inspiration and opens during expiration to allow driving gas inside the chamber to be discharged into the room. That port may be identified as "Exhaust" on the back of the ventilator. This outlet should never be blocked. On some units, the port may be on the inside of the ventilator housing and can only be heard, not seen.

Relief Valve

The relief valve, also called spill valve, overflow valve or pop-off valve functions in a manner similar to the APL valve of the breathing system. The APL valve must be closed for a mechanical ventilator to deliver gases to the patient so the relief valve is the only place for excess gases to be vented from the system. It is located inside the system at the bellows attachment. This valve automatically closes during inspiration and remains closed until the bellows returns to its fully expanded status. Once that occurs, the valve opens to discharge excess gas from the system. The port on the back of the ventilator should marked with "Exhaust" with either a 19 or 30mm opening to accommodate connection to the waste gas scavenging system. The minimum opening pressure for the relief valve is 2-3cm H_2O which allows the bellows to remain filled at end of expiration and pause.

Ventilator Hose

Tubing that connects the breathing system to the ventilator must have a standard 22-mm female-cuff that is the same as breathing circuit and the reservoir bag connection.

Controls

Depending on design, controls include Tidal Volume, Minute Volume, Frequency (Respiratory Rate), I:E Ratio, Inspiratory Flow Rate and Maximum Pressure Limit or Safety-Pressure Relief Valve. If the unit has Tidal Volume and Frequency controls, Minute Volume would be determined indirectly. With Minute Volume and Frequency controls, Tidal Volume becomes an indirect setting. On some ventilators, the I:E ratio is fixed and cannot be adjusted. On other units, this ratio is automatically determined from other settings. Inspiratory flow rate may be set directly on some ventilators while it is derived indirectly on others by controlling minute volume and the I:E ratio. The concept is to allow sufficient time for gases to be delivered during inspiration and enough time for gases to exit the lung. Typically, 1 to 1.5 seconds is provided for inspiration and 3-4.5 seconds for expiration. This would be an I:E ratio of 1:3 and frequency of 12-15 breaths per minute. For slower respiratory rates, expiratory time including pause will be longer with an I:E ratio of 1:4 or 1:5.

Ventilators for Specific Applications

There are units available for anesthesia and controlled ventilation specifically designed for animals under 7kg. The Anesthesia Work-Station* (AWS) has been used for short and long term anesthetic procedures on animals from the size of rats to cats (Figure 3-39). It incorporates a time-cycled volume ventilator with an adjustable pressure safety limit. The AWS has been shown to be effective for induction, stabilization, and maintenance of anesthesia, as well as providing precise respiratory control. There is also a dual mode ventilator that delivers standard intermittent positive pressure ventilation (IPPV) or high frequency oscillatory ventilation (HFOV) (Figure 3-40). The entire breathing system has a volume of less than 1cc. There are four variables to control: Oxygen flow, Frequency, Amplitude (Tidal Volume) and Mean Airway Pressure. In IPPV mode the frequency selectable ranges from 75 to 240 breaths per minute (BPM). The deliverable tidal volume is a maximum of 10 ml. However, this does not limit the usefulness of this unit since switching it to HFOV mode changes the frequency range to 750-2400 "breaths" or more accurately, cycles per minute. The "Tidal Volume" during HFOV is generally an order of magnitude less than it would be during IPPV and is used to set up an oscillation of the molecules of gas from the breathing system down to the alveoli. This unit can be directly connected to any type of scavenging system; direct vacuum, an active or a passive system.

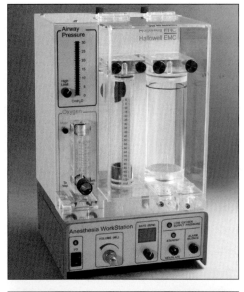

Figure 3-39 Hallowell Anesthesia Work Station.
Courtesy of Hallowell EMC, Pittsfield, MA.

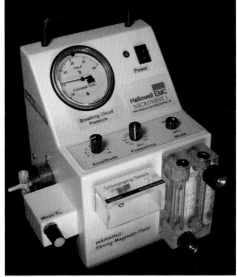

Figure 3-40 Hallowell "MicroVent 1" Ventilator for very small patients.
Courtesy of Hallowell EMC, Pittsfield, MA.

Agents
Gas
Nitrous Oxide

Nitrous oxide was first prepared by Joseph Priestley over 200 years ago but Humphrey Davy is credited for describing its "anesthetic" properties in 1799. Another 50 years passed before its analgesic effects were demonstrated by Horace Wells. A fellow dentist extracted one of Wells' teeth while Gardner Quincy Colton administered the gas. Its label "laughing gas" was coined during this time as ether frolics and laughing gas parties were popular. Since the late 1800's, use of N_2O in human anesthesia evolved through the 1960's and 1970's, especially with halothane, to the point that more techniques of general anesthesia were based on the use of N_2O than on the use of any other agent. Usual concentrations ranged between 50 and 80%, with the latter used only for brief periods during induction. These concentrations are not adequate for anesthesia of healthy patients because the MAC value for the human is 101% (Eger, 1974).

The popularity of N_2O in veterinary anesthesia also grew during the '70's when halothane became the predominant inhalation anesthetic. It was used at teaching institutions which influenced its use in practice by clinicians who learned to appreciate its advantages. Although its MAC value in the dog is 188%, 66% N_2O reduced halothane MAC by 22 ± 8.4% (De Young and Sawyer, 1980). Lack of potency is obviated by continuous or intermittent IV injection of opioids or use of inhalation anesthetics. This, combined with injection of a neuromuscular blocking agent for muscle relaxation, can be a very valuable adjunct especially in high-risk patients. Anesthesia produced with volatile liquid anesthetics is achieved with lower concentrations when N_2O is used as an adjunct compared to either agent used alone. Spontaneous breathing is enhanced by N_2O; alveolar ventilation appears to be improved by its sympathomimetic properties. This is not to imply that N_2O must be given whenever volatile liquids are used. However, such a combination may provide a more satisfactory induction and a better intraoperative and postanesthetic course. Excessive depth of anesthesia may be avoided and the circulatory and respiratory depression of the more potent agents is lessened to some extent by the mild sympathetic-stimulating properties of N_2O, thus providing a valuable adjunct to general anesthesia.

For patients in profound shock, debilitated or in a high-risk category, N_2O may be used in 50 to 66% concentrations and opioids such as morphine, oxymorphone, hydromorphone or fentanyl may be given to supplement analgesia as needed. Very low concentrations of inhalation agents may be used as an alternative for sick animals requiring anesthesia and surgery. The susceptibility of these patients to depressant drugs is much greater and deep anesthesia may be avoided with the more potent anesthetics if nitrous oxide is used as well. This is not to say that N_2O does not exert any adverse actions. When it is given alone, a mild direct depression to myocardial contractility has been shown, but the magnitude of change is much less than with other inhalants (Krahwinkel et al. 1975).

N_2O must not be used in the presence of pneumothorax or in any situation in which air is trapped in a body cavity. The high partial pressures of N_2O in blood coupled with its low solubility cause it to diffuse rapidly into air-containing body cavities (Eger and Saidman 1965b). This can also happen with methane in a bowel lumen (Steffey et al. 1979). The relative increase in volume results from the inability of another gas to diffuse out of the cavity and into blood at the same rate as the influx of N_2O because of the lower blood solubility of nitrogen or methane. The net result is distension of the bowel or, in the case of pneumothorax, an increase in intrathoracic pressure and a decrease in lung volume. The pressure-volume relationship compromises both ventilation and circulation and death occurs if the problem is not recognized. Therefore, in situations of bowel obstruction, air or nitrogen-containing gas is trapped and use of nitrous oxide must be avoided. Procedures such as pneumocystography using air or CO_2 may produce venous gas emboli. N_2O dissolved in blood will enlarge emboli should they occur and possibly cause death (Steffey et al. 1980).

N_2O should not be used in patients with respiratory dysfunction. In these patients, inspired oxygen tension must be high in order to avoid hypoxemia. This would include patients with significant space-occupying lesions in the thorax, diaphragmatic hernia, pulmonary disease, alveolar-to-arterial diffusion abnormalities, and pulmonary edema. One must properly assess the surgical patient in order to avoid potential difficulties.

During the first few minutes of induction with nitrous oxide, a higher concentration may be used because the PaO_2 increases above the inspired pressure owing to the second gas effect (Epstein et al., 1964; Stoelting and Eger 1969). Thus, in the healthy patient, 80% N_2O may be used to accelerate induction. At termination of anesthesia with N_2O, the patient must not be allowed to breathe room air abruptly. Because of the relative difference in solubility between nitrogen and N_2O, a large volume of N_2O diffuses from blood into the alveoli faster than the uptake of nitrogen from air into blood. This lowers the alveolar PO_2, causing hypoxemia (diffusion hypoxia) (Roesch and Stoelting 1972). This situation can be avoided by administering 100% oxygen a few minutes before tracheal extubation or by mask should the patient be inadvertently extubated while breathing N_2O. The same process will occur during mask induction with N_2O if a patient is allowed to breathe room air for more than 45 seconds during the process of a difficult intubation. Treatment of diffusion hypoxia is a simple process and therefore one need not panic at the signs of cyanosis. Under these conditions, the patient is given oxygen for a short time until the problem is resolved.

Concentration Effect and Second Gas Effect

These two factors influence the rate of induction of inhalation agents (Epstein et al. 1964; Stoelting and Eger, 1969). In addition to the mechanical aspects of ventilation, there is another effect on ventilation during induction and recovery. Uptake of anesthetics by blood in high concentration during induction tends to reduce volume of gas in alveoli. Before the next breath, gas moves into the alveoli from the bronchioles which has the effect of augmenting the volume of gas introduced to alveoli. During recovery, anesthetics move from blood to alveoli, thus increasing the volume of alveolar gas and effectively causing more gas to be expelled from the alveoli during exhalation. This is the concentration effect, which denotes that the higher the inspired concentration, the more rapid the relative rise in alveolar concentration. The higher the anesthetic concentration inspired, the greater the uptake and the greater the influence on alveolar ventilation. The increase in ventilation brought on by the anesthetic promotes an increase in alveolar concentration. A concentrating action also contributes to the concentration effect since higher inspired partial pressures tend to concentrate the anesthetic and blunt the effect of uptake. Thus, the concentration effect results in a more rapid induction of anesthesia and also aids in anesthesia recovery. This process occurs with diethyl ether and nitrous oxide, which are delivered in significantly large volumes. However, more potent gases such as halothane, isoflurane and sevoflurane are used in such low concentrations that the influence on second gas uptake is minimal. This was confirmed by a study in dogs in which N_2O did not improve rate or quality of mask induction with sevoflurane or isoflurane (Mutoh et al. 2001c).

The second gas effect occurs when two anesthetics are given together. Uptake of a large volume of the first gas in the mixture, e.g., N_2O, augments the inspired volume as does the concentration effect, thus increasing delivery of the second gas, e.g., halothane, to the alveoli. In addition, uptake of the first gas, N_2O, has a concentrating effect on the second gas which results in a more rapid alveolar rate of rise of the second gas than if it were used alone. Thus, one of the benefits of N_2O is a more rapid induction with certain inhalation anesthetics. Not only is anesthesia induction faster but the oxygen partial pressure will be higher since oxygen would also be considered a second gas. Significantly, the concentration effect and the second gas effect have their biggest impact during the first 5 to 10 minutes of induction.

Volatile Liquids
Diethyl Ether

Modern anesthesia had its birth in March 1842, when C.W. Long of Georgia first gave ether for a minor surgical procedure. Four years later, W.T.G. Morton, a Boston dentist, demonstrated its use for analgesia and anesthesia at the Massachusetts General Hospital on one famous October day. George Dadd, who turned from human to veterinary practice, regularly used ether for general anesthesia in the early 1850's.

Diethyl ether (C_2H_5-O-C_2H_5) is an excellent anesthetic and may still be used on very limited bases in veterinary practice. However, it is not available in the US. Cardiac output and arterial pressure usually remain normal but heart rate is increased. Diethyl ether does not sensitize the myocardium to catecholamine–induced dysrhythmias. Spontaneous respiration remains adequate because depression of ventilation is offset by increased activity of the sympathetic nervous system. It provides good analgesia and muscle relaxation but its flammability and explosive properties are its main disadvantages. Its high solubility in blood ($\lambda = 12.1$), high vapor pressure (450mm Hg at 20°C), and high MAC value ($3 \pm 0.5\%$) all combine to indicate the need for large amounts of the agent. Diethyl ether causes irritation to the tracheal mucosa and excess salivation that can lead to respiratory congestion. It has been commonly delivered by open drop technique although in-the-circle drawover wick vaporizers are a useful means for delivery. Because of its flammability and irritating properties, its limited availability and the advantages of the newer more potent anesthetics, diethyl ether is seldom used any more in small animal practice. It must be stored in sealed metal containers coated with copper or another metal that prevents light oxidation. Diethyl ether should never be kept in non-explosive-proof refrigerators or around any potential source of sparks or flames. The bodies of small animals euthanatized with diethyl ether should never be stored where a spark might ignite its vapors.

Halothane

Halothane is credited with revolutionizing the anesthesia specialty and brought with it a more scientific approach to understanding action and influences of inhalation anesthetics. Synthesized and developed by Suckling between 1951 and 1956, halothane has a molecular structure ($CF_3CHBrCl$) that features chemical stability, nonflammability and good potency. The fluoride group is inert and also provides stability and nonflammability. This agent gained popularity for human anesthesia beginning in 1959 and in the early to mid 1960s veterinarians slowly began to introduce it into practices. Halothane steadily increased in usage through the 70's and 80's until it was replaced as the most popular inhalation anesthetic in veterinary practice by isoflurane. It provides a rapid and smooth induction. Surgical anesthesia is easily maintained, vital functions remain stable yet anesthetic depth can be quickly adjusted. Because of halothane's relatively low solubility in blood ($\lambda = 2.5$), mask or chamber induction of small patients is easily accomplished. Emergence from anesthesia is smooth and animals will rest quietly during recovery providing analgesics have been used for pain relief. With relatively rapid return of protective reflexes and consciousness, most patients become ambulatory within 15 minutes.

Because of its high vapor pressure (243 mm Hg at 20°C) and high potency (MAC = 0.90 ± 0.12 per cent) halothane must be delivered from a calibrated or precision vaporizer. During clinical anesthesia, equilibration with VRG tissues may be achieved with 1.5-2.5% halothane. Once surgical anesthesia is reached in the healthy patient, vaporizer setting should be maintained between 1.0 and 1.5% until surgery begins. MAC will range between 0.8 and 1.1% and will be $22.2 \pm 8.4\%$ lower when combined with 66% N_2O (De Young and Sawyer, 1980). In general, vaporizer settings can be reduced by 0.5% when halothane is used with 66% N_2O because of the reduction in MAC and augmentation of alveolar ventilation caused by nitrous oxide.

Halothane decreases arterial blood pressure and myocardial contractile force but has little or no effect on heart rate except at deep levels. Peripheral vascular resistance (PVR) is reduced as a result of partial alpha blockade. There is no predominant action to account for the circulatory depressant effects of halothane. The combination of central autonomic inhibition, ganglionic blockade and suppression of the peripheral response to norepinephrine effectively robs sympathetic mechanisms of their compensatory action and peripheral vasodilation (Merin et al. 1976). Because of a reduction in perfusion pressure, muscle blood flow is reduced leading to the mild metabolic acidosis usually seen with halothane. Splanchnic and renal blood flow is also reduced but cerebral circulation increases because of vasodilation. This increased brain blood flow will raise cerebrospinal fluid (CSF) pressure that can lead to high normal or elevated CSF pressure. Halothane also increases blood flow to the uterus at surgical anesthesia levels as demonstrated in women, which may lead to increased bleeding during cesarean section; thus one must take steps to prevent or control a possible bleeding crisis.

Halothane sensitizes the myocardium to catecholamines, so indiscriminate injection of epinephrine is unwise. Severe ventricular dysrhythmias, tachycardia, and ventricular fibrillation may result. If local infiltration of 1:100,000 epinephrine (1μg/kg) is needed to control bleeding during halothane anesthesia, ventilation must be supported to prevent respiratory acidosis and hypoxemia, since an hypoxic and acidotic myocardium is much more susceptible to epinephrine-induced dysrhythmias.

Respiratory depression is usually evident at all anesthetic concentrations. However, when halothane is used with N_2O, arterial PCO_2 may be at or below normal levels. Halothane causes bronchodilation in the dog, which increases dead space. Typical with all anesthetics, it is common to need additional inflation of the cuff on the endotracheal tube after 15 minutes or more of anesthesia with halothane because of tracheal relaxation.

With the availability of isoflurane and sevoflurane, both of which have less respiratory and cardiac depressant effects, and the high metabolic profile of halothane, very few small animal practices use this anesthetic any more in the US. However, it is still widely used in countries outside America.

Methoxyflurane

Methoxyflurane ($CHCL_2$-CF2-O-CH_3) was introduced into human anesthesia by Artusia in 1959 and by 1963 it had gained popularity for use in veterinary patients. With the promotion of the anesthetic as well as equipment for delivery, use of inhalation anesthesia began to rise in prominence to replace long-acting barbiturates in clinical veterinary anesthesia.

Use of methoxyflurane in clinical veterinary practice continued through the 70's and 80's in the U.S. However, its use declined through the 1990's with the increasing popularity of halothane and isoflurane until it was withdrawn by the manufacturer from the U.S. market in 1999. It might be used to a limited extent from existing supplies in the US and is still available in a few European countries.

Enflurane

Enflurane ($CFHCL$-CF_2-O-CHF_2) was synthesized by Dr. Ross Terrell in 1963 along with its isomer isoflurane. It differed significantly from halothane and methoxyflurane in its greater biological stability. Organ injury was minimal or nonexistent and its relatively low solubility in blood made rapid changes in alveolar concentration possible along with rapid recovery. From 1972 until the early 1980's, it was the most widely used potent inhaled anesthetic for use in human patients. Its limitations especially that of causing seizure–like movement at deep levels of anesthesia, precluded its application for general anesthesia in dogs. This was found to occur in humans only in situations of hypocarbia induced by hyperventilation. Anesthesia with enflurane alone in the dog is accompanied in a high percentage of patients by signs of motor hyperactivity such as muscle twitching and movement of the head, body and extremities. These signs are more pronounced at deeper levels of enflurane anesthesia and are accompanied by the appearance of EEG seizure patterns.

Enflurane has a B/G coefficient of 2.0 and MAC of 1.7%. It is a stable nonflammable liquid, slightly less volatile than halothane (P_{vap} = 175 at 20°C). Enflurane produces rapid induction and maintenance when used with IV induction or tranquilizer premedication and rapid recovery. Cardiac rhythm tends to be stable and there is only mild sensitization of the heart to epinephrine. It increases salivary secretions and is a slight bronchoconstrictor. It is usually used with N_2O and provides good muscle relaxation. The cardiovascular system is stable and does not sensitize the heart to catecholamines. There are no reports of hepatic or renal damage from this anesthetic. Enflurane has a pungent odor that sometimes leads to breath-holding during mask induction. It causes profound respiratory depression so controlled ventilation is usually required. An average of 2.5-10% is metabolized to inorganic fluoride.

Clinical trials for use in veterinary anesthesia were conducted in late 1979 early 1980. Because of the muscle movement that occurred in the dog and poor results with trials in cats, enflurane never made any inroads for use in veterinary patients. Attempts were made to gain CVM FDA approval in the US for dogs but trials were aborted because of the induced hyperactivity during anesthesia. This anesthetic is used by a small percentage of veterinarians and has good application as long as sedatives or tranquilizers are used preanesthesia.

Isoflurane

Isoflurane (CF_3-CHCl-O-CHF_2), synthesized in 1965 also by Dr. Terrell, is an isomer of enflurane. Initial problems in purifying isoflurane delayed its development and not until its approval for use in human patients by the FDA in 1979 did it start to receive serious attention for use in veterinary patients. The physical properties of isoflurane approach those sought in an ideal anesthetic. It is nonflammable at all anesthetic concentrations. It is stable without the need of a preservative and resists breakdown by sunlight or strong alkalis. Isoflurane's solubility with a B/G coeffiecient of 1.5 is lower than that of enflurane and halothane (Table 3-3). From the early 1980's, isoflurane became the most widely used potent inhaled anesthetic in humans in the US and Canada. In 1986, it was approved by CVM FDA in the US for use in horses and in May, 1987, the NADA requesting approval for its use as an inhaled anesthetic in the dog was submitted. Approval was granted in June 1989 and it became generic when it no longer was covered by an US patent in January 1993. It is sold under many different labels in the US and Canada. It is also available throughout Europe, the United Kingdom and many other countries in the world.

Isoflurane is a fluorinated, chlorinated ethyl-methyl ether with a molecular weight of 184.5, specific gravity @ 25°C of 1.50 and boiling point of 48.5. At 20°C, vapor pressure of isoflurane is 238mmHg. In comparison, the Pvap for halothane is 243. Thus, a vaporizer calibrated for halothane but properly cleaned, filled with isoflurane and correctly operated will produce slightly higher concentrations of isoflurane than that indicated on the vaporizer dial for halothane (Steffey et al. 1982; Steffey et al.1983). This does not suggest that this is a proper procedure in clinical practice as delivery of isoflurane in halothane-specific vaporizers is not a recommendation provided by pharmaceutical companies or vaporizer manufacturers.

Relatively low solubility of isoflurane in blood and tissues permit rapid induction and recovery. Isoflurane has an ethereal odor and is somewhat pungent. Breath-holding may occur when this agent is delivered by mask. It is stable in soda lime and does not react with metal. A major difference between isoflurane and halothane or methoxyflurane is the almost complete biological stability of isoflurane. This has important implications for anesthetic metabolism and hepatic or renal toxicity.

MAC is 1.28% in dogs and 1.63% for the cat which means that maintenance levels will be slightly higher in cats compared to dogs (Steffey 1977). Isoflurane MAC does not change significantly with time. That is, anesthetic requirements do not increase or decrease during an anesthetic procedure. Surgical anesthesia is usually achieved between 1.2 and 1.5 MAC, thus one can expect to maintain anesthesia using vaporizer concentrations of 2.0 to 2.5% in a semi-open or semi-closed system. These concentrations will be lower in patients receiving tranquilizers, opioid analgesics, alpha$_2$ agonists or in aged animals.

Isoflurane depresses respiration in a dose-related fashion. It increases arterial PCO_2 and depresses the ventilatory response to increased CO_2 slightly more than halothane. The depressant effects of isoflurane can be offset by decreasing concentration of anesthetic, by assisting ventilation or by providing surgical stimulation. Isoflurane relaxes bronchial smooth muscle and is useful in patients with obstructive pulmonary disease. Clinical experiences indicate that respiratory depression may be evident shortly following induction and during surgical preparation when the patient is not being surgically stimulated. However, in healthy adult dogs, significant changes in arterial PCO_2 are not commonly seen in surgically stimulated patients breathing spontaneously.

In healthy P1 or P2 patients, surgical levels of isoflurane minimally depress myocardial function, cardiac output and tissue perfusion. It provides a larger margin of safety than halothane. Isoflurane has the highest cardiac anesthetic index (CAI) of the modern potent inhaled anesthetics. This index is obtained by dividing the concentration of anesthetic in the myocardium at cardiac failure by the concentration in the heart at 1 MAC. The CAI for isoflurane is 5.7 compared with methoxyflurane at 3.7 and halothane at 3.0 (Wolfson et al. 1978). Heart rate tends to increase especially during light levels of anesthesia. For example, heart rate for halothane in the dog is 90 to 120 BPM. In contrast, the rate during isoflurane anesthesia might be expected to be 120 to 140 BPM. Heart rate and rhythm are stable and isoflurane does not sensitize the heart to the effects of epinephrine. Isoflurane decreases TPR which lessens the work of the heart. The mild degree of arterial hypotension may be compensated by decreasing anesthetic concentration or by providing surgical stimulation even with the use of preemptive analgesia. The combination of peripheral vasodilation in the presence of near normal cardiac output is a desirable characteristic in maintaining or improving tissue perfusion.

Isoflurane produces muscular relaxation sufficient for virtually all surgical procedures. It also enhances the action of muscle relaxants. This includes not only the neuromuscular blocking agents but also the minor tranquilizers, diazepam or midazolam. Isoflurane does not produce convulsive activity. Cerebral spinal fluid flow or pressure does not increase during isoflurane anesthesia and autoregulation is retained at surgical anesthetic levels. About 20% of halothane undergoes metabolic degradation but only 0.17% of isoflurane is changed. The limited metabolism of isoflurane may be related to its physical stability and to its rapid elimination during recovery from anesthesia.

Isoflurane does not appear to produce liver injury even when given for prolonged periods or under conditions in which other anesthetics induce liver injury. No significant renal depression or injury follows isoflurane anesthesia. Margin of safety in older patients is lower usually because of the high probability of degenerative heart disease. Geriatrics have less ability to compensate for drug induced insults which means that it is essential to use anesthetics and techniques that produce minimal changes in organ function. Anesthetic requirements are lower in aged animals. Isoflurane is especially beneficial in patients with pre-existing conditions that may induce ventricular dysrhythmias such as myocardial trauma. Ventilatory support in high-risk patients is advisable regardless of the anesthetic procedure selected and this would also apply when isoflurane is used. Based on experiences with all of the potent inhaled anesthetics, isoflurane is an excellent anesthetic in most all respects. Its effects during surgical levels of anesthesia, or lack of them on the cardiovascular or respiratory system, make it a good choice in small animal patients at risk. It is the most widely used inhaled anesthetic in the US and has gained in popularity throughout the world.

Sevoflurane
Sevoflurane is a 1,1,1,3,3,3-hexafluroro-2-(fluoromethoxy) propane (CH_2F-O-$CH(CF_3)_2$ nonexplosive volatile liquid anesthetic with a blood-gas partition coefficient of 0.7 (Table 3-7). This is half that of isoflurane (1.5) and almost 4 times less than that of halothane (2.5). Comparative physical properties of sevoflurane along with other inhalation agents are listed in Table 3-3. The low solubility of sevoflurane offers certain advantages: more rapid induction, quicker change in anesthetic levels and faster recovery (Steffey 1992, Clarke 1999).

Sevoflurane was synthesized by investigators at Baxter-Travenol Laboratories in 1969. It was first reported as a potential inhalation anesthetic in 1971 and results of test studies in dogs and rats suggested that sevoflurane was somewhat unique and worthy of further study (Wallin et al. 1975). In dogs, anesthetic concentrations did not produce spontaneous cardiac arrhythmias and did not sensitize the heart to epinephrine. Subacute studies in dogs and rats, using closed-circle absorption with soda lime, revealed no toxicologically significant changes in animals anesthetized 2 hours daily for 2 weeks (Sawyer unpublished data). Follow-up studies were conducted in human volunteers with findings that were very favorable as well (Holaday 1983). Baxter-Travenol decided not to pursue further investigations and contracted with Maruishi Pharmaceutical Company in Osaka, Japan for final development. The Maruishi company was granted approval for clinical use of sevoflurane in humans from the Japanese Ministry of Health and Welfare in January 1990. Prior to that, Anaquest contracted with Baxter-Travenol in 1985 to develop sevoflurane for use in humans in the US but a year later elected not to continue and returned the rights of this drug to Baxter-Travenol. Maruishi then became interested in developing the anesthetic in the US along with their efforts to gain approval in Japan. However, they initiated a licensing agreement with Abbott Laboratories for completion of the clinical plan to cover global registrations as well as the US. An NDA was submitted to the US FDA August 1994 with approval granted July 1995. Numerous studies were conducted in dogs and in November 1999, Abbott Laboratories received CVM FDA approval for sevoflurane use as an anesthetic in this species.

The lower solubility of sevoflurane compared to that of isoflurane gives the advantage to sevoflurane for mask inductions for providing rapid changes in anesthetic levels which is advantageous for patients at risk. One must be capable of using this high performance anesthetic as inductions will be faster and levels of anesthesia will change more quickly in both directions–lighter and deeper. Minimum Anesthetic Concentration (MAC) values for dogs and other species is listed in Table 3-8. This would indicate that surgical levels of sevoflurane would be higher than other commonly used anesthetics in dogs. In comparison with isoflurane and halothane, dogs woke up quietly from sevoflurane and without any excitation and were able to stand on an average of 10 minutes earlier than after isoflurane and 85 minutes earlier than after halothane anesthesia (Tacke et al. 1998). On the basis of numerous studies and clinical use, sevoflurane is a suitable volatile liquid anesthetic for induction, maintenance and recovery of dogs and appears to have some advantages over other inhalation anesthetics.

With the approval of sevoflurane in the US, Japan and other countries, a great deal of information is available in the human and veterinary literature. As a result, this anesthetic is well characterized for its pharmacodynamic and pharmacokinetic properties. The mechanism of action of sevoflurane includes depression of excitatory transmission of glutamate in the CNS and potentiation of the effects of the inhibitory neurotransmitter GABA.

Induced hypocapnia is often used in neurosurgical procedures to decrease size of brain tissue. In concentrations up to 2.5 MAC, sevoflurane caused neither EEG nor gross motor evidence of seizure activity in dogs that were rendered hypocapnic, exposed to intense auditory stimuli, or both (Scheller et al. 1990). Cerebral metabolic activity is decreased at high MAC values but was not changed at lower levels of anesthesia. There is a profound effect on intracranial pressure (ICP) at deep levels of anesthesia. Sevoflurane was shown to dilate large and small cerebral pial vessels in dogs via activation of ATP-sensitive K+ channel activation (Iida et al. 1998). The effect on ICP is somewhat abolished by induced hypocapnia.

Sevoflurane has characteristics of low pungency and low airway irritability. Studies in unpremedicated human patients demonstrated that on a grading scale from most to least airway irritability, agents were graded as desflurane > isoflurane > sevoflurane (TerRiet et al. 2000). In a comparative study of respiratory reflexes at 1.2 and 2.4 MAC multiples in spontaneous breathing dogs, nasal administration of sevoflurane induced milder reflex inhibition of breathing than that of isoflurane or halothane (Mutoh et al. 2001a). In another study comparing mask induction with sevoflurane and isoflurane in dogs, both produced a smooth onset (Mutoh 2001b). Sevoflurane induced less reflex inhibition of breathing compared to isoflurane. Administration of a 2:1 mixture of N_2O to O_2 with isoflurane or sevoflurane did not improve the rate or quality of mask induction in dogs (Mutoh et al. 2001c) but did provide rapid induction in cats (Tzannes et al. 2000). These characteristics have been associated with faster and smoother induction and rapid emergence at least in dogs and cats. That was not the case when isoflurane and sevoflurane were used for mask induction in rabbits. Both anesthetics induced periods of apnea, significant reduction in heart rate and aversive behavior suggesting that this technique should be avoided in this species (Flecknell et al. 1999).

Effects of sevoflurane on laryngeal drive receptor activity are less than isoflurane and halothane which would support a more stable breathing pattern with sevoflurane (Mutoh et al. 1999). These characteristics have been associated with faster and smoother induction and rapid emergence in dogs. Increasing concentrations of sevoflurane in dogs impairs diaphragm function at 2 MAC anesthesia compared to lighter levels. This is thought to be through its inhibitory effect on neuromuscular transmission (Ide et al. 1991 & 1992).

In groups of 6 dogs each, respiratory effects were determined at 1, 1.5 and 2 MAC sevoflurane during spontaneous ventilation (Mutoh et al. 1997). Respiratory rate decreased significantly at 2 MAC from that at 1 MAC levels. Tidal volume and dead space-to-tidal volume were unchanged at either levels resulting in significantly decreased expired and alveolar ventilation at 2 MAC but not at 1.0 or 1.5 MAC sevoflurane. $PaCO_2$ increased and arterial PH decreased with deeper levels of anesthesia. They determined that at 1.0 MAC (light level) and 1.5 MAC (moderate level); sevoflurane can be used safely in the spontaneously breathing dog. Polis et al (2001a) confirmed these findings and more specifically indicated that mode of breathing could be spontaneous, controlled or at a PEEP of 5cm H_2O.

To assess the anesthetic index (AI) of sevoflurane with that of isoflurane, 8 dogs were mask induced with each anesthetic (Galloway et al. 2004). Anesthetic index is calculated as apneic concentration divided by MAC. The apneic concentration was determined during spontaneous breathing by increasing anesthetic concentration until dogs stopped breathing. The AI was significantly higher for sevoflurane compared to isoflurane. These effects support the respiratory depressant effects of sevoflurane especially at deep levels but appear to be minimal at light to moderate levels of surgical anesthesia. Sevoflurane is less irritating to respiratory reflexes which provide an advantage in using this anesthetic for mask induction in dogs.

Regarding the effects of sevoflurane on the cardiovascular system, many studies have been conducted comparing these changes to those induced by halothane, isoflurane, enflurane or desflurane. The latter two drugs are not approved in the USA for use in dogs so comparisons to halothane and isoflurane are more meaningful. From the references, sevoflurane causes a drop in peripheral resistance, mean arterial pressure and cardiac output. Cardiac index is either depressed less than that with isoflurane or doesn't change due to the rise in heart rate with sevoflurane. The arrhythmogenicity of sevoflurane is lower than isoflurane or halothane.

In dogs, the effects on the cardiovascular system appear to be similar to that of isoflurane as are effects on the respiratory system (Steffey 1992; Clark 1999). In dog studies, sevoflurane either reduced systemic resistance or maintained it. Some investigations in animals have shown that sevoflurane does not produce tachycardia. Sevoflurane was found to induce marked cardiovascular depression at 2 MAC compared to those found at 1.5 MAC during either spontaneous or controlled ventilation (Polis et al. 2001b). This suggested that sevoflurane could be used safely in healthy dogs better at 1.5 MAC compared to 2.0 MAC. Heart rate was found to increase with sevoflurane in a study comparing sevoflurane and isoflurane in chronically instrumented dogs (Bernard et al. 1990). Otherwise, effects on cardiac function and coronary blood flow were almost identical to those induced by isoflurane. Inhalation anesthetics increase heart rate *in vivo* in both animals and humans (Picker et al. 2001). Differences in the degree of increase between agents were shown to be related to differences in their vagolytic action. At equianesthetic concentrations in dogs, the greatest increase was 40 BPM for desflurane and least for halothane (8 BPM). At 2 MAC, sevoflurane increased heart rate an average of 21 BPM compared to that with isoflurane being 8 BPM. Thus, during inhalation anesthesia heart rate depends primarily on cardiac vagal activity but it is not known why some anesthetics inhibit the autonomic nervous system more than others with sevoflurane being intermediate with the agents studied. Kazama and Ikeda (1988a) compared cardiovascular effects of sevoflurane with that of halothane and isoflurane. With increasing MAC levels (1.0-3.0), heart rate did not change significantly for any of the 3 anesthetics and mean values were essentially the same as recorded by Picker et al. (2001). As anesthetic concentrations increased, cardiac index and dp/dt max decreased significantly for halothane, isoflurane and sevoflurane. Although arterial pressure of sevoflurane was significantly lower than that of isoflurane, cardiac index of sevoflurane was sustained and systemic vascular resistance did not change with increased sevoflurane levels. Central venous pressure and pulmonary artery pressure did not change. Coronary sinus blood flows at 1 and 2 MAC sevoflurane were significantly higher than those of halothane (Merin et al. 1991). These findings are consistent with studies reported in the dog that cardiac functions are sustained better through all levels of sevoflurane anesthesia than with those induced by halothane (Bruckner et al. 1979).

Effects of 2.5% and 5.0% end tidal sevoflurane on cardiovascular dynamics, coronary circulation and myocardial metabolism were determined in pentobarbital-pancuronium anesthetized dogs (Akazawa et al. 1988). Although they found that sevoflurane produced dose-dependent decreases in systolic arterial pressure, heart rate, cardiac index, left ventricular minute work index and systemic vascular resistance, left ventricular end-diastolic pressure remained unchanged. They concluded that sevoflurane causes rapid but easily controlled cardiovascular depression and does not appear to have unfavorable effects on coronary circulation and myocardial metabolism. Mutoh et al. (1997) compared cardiopulmonary effects of sevoflurane with halothane, enflurane, and isoflurane in 24 Beagle dogs. Although some of the effects of sevoflurane were greater than halothane and similar to those of isoflurane, cardiac index was unchanged because of the significant increase in heart rate. However, sevoflurane reduced heart rate, mean arterial pressure and left ventricular systolic pressure in a similar manner in dogs to that of isoflurane and desflurane (Hettrick et al. 1996). Myocardial contractility decreased along with left ventricular afterload. These findings support the concept that volatile anesthetics preserve optimal left ventricular-arterial coupling and efficiency at low anesthetic concentrations. As anesthetic levels increase, these alterations increase contributing to reductions of overall cardiac performance with these agents. Sevoflurane does not produce spontaneous cardiac arrhythmias and does not sensitize the heart to epinephrine (Wallin et al. 1975). Arrhythmogenicity of sevoflurane is even lower than isoflurane (Imamura and Ikeda 1987). Results of a study in dogs by Hirano (1995) suggested that sevoflurane is a less potent coronary arteriolar dilator than isoflurane and that neither anesthetic has any direct effect on the diameter of large coronary arteries. This would indicate that coronary "steal" is less likely to occur with sevoflurane. Effects on dose-related cardiovascular depression including heart rate; systolic, mean and diastolic blood pressure; and oxygen saturation were similar for both isoflurane and sevoflurane (Galloway et al. 2004).

Allogenic blood transfusion is an important therapeutic tool for a number of surgical conditions, especially those associated with trauma and major blood loss. Acute normovolemic hemodilution (ANH) consists of removal of a predetermined amount of blood and simultaneous infusion of plasma expanders such as crystalloids, colloids or both. This is a very useful technique to avoid blood transfusion in surgical patients. The changes in blood flow characteristics due to the decrease in blood viscosity, the consequent increase in cardiac output and heart rate and the increased oxygen extraction rate account for hemodynamic stability during the procedure. A factor in this equation is the depressant effects of inhalation anesthetics that could attenuate the hemodynamic response promoted by hemodilution thus impairing the increase in cardiac output and stroke volume necessary to maintain adequate oxygen transport. Fantoni et al. (2005) compared the effects of halothane, isoflurane and sevoflurane during ANH at 1 MAC in dogs. Cardiac index increased 157% in the sevoflurane group compared to that of isoflurane and halothane, 86% and 88% respectively. Results of this study demonstrated that 1 MAC halothane, isoflurane or sevoflurane did not impair the hemodynamic response to ANH in dogs and may be used for this procedure.

Sevoflurane does not have any significant effect on the hepatic circulation or function. Studies were performed in chronically instrumented dogs to investigate the effects of sevoflurane on liver function (Frink et al. 1992; Bernard et al 1992). Hepatic arterial blood flow was maintained at anesthetic levels up to 2 MAC. Portal vein flow was decreased at both 1.5 and 2.0 MAC. The same test concentration did not affect tissue oxygenation. Intrabiliary pressure was not changed at 1 MAC, but a significant reduction was evident at higher MAC levels. The only study available on the effects of inhalation anesthetics on liver enzymes was published by Topal et al. (2003). They used 21 clinically normal mongrel dogs with 7 dogs each anesthetized for 60 minutes with roughly 1.5 MAC halothane, isoflurane or sevoflurane. Dogs were recovered with venous blood samples taken preanesthesia; 24 hours, 48 hours, 7 days and 14 days postanesthesia. An elevated serum level of aminotransferase (AST) was found indicating anesthetic related hepatic toxicity. Liver cell damage was found after halothane anesthesia with levels exceeding 160 IU/L (normal = 10-88). Neither isoflurane or sevoflurane induced elevation of serum enzymes beyond normal limits and the highest with sevoflurane was found at 7 days postanesthesia; pretest, 19 ± 6; day 7, 38 ± 10.

Almeida et al (2004) anesthetized 2 groups of healthy dogs with 1.5 sevoflurane or desflurane for 105 minutes. They compared cardiovascular and intraocular pressure values preanesthesia, 45 minutes following induction and at 3-20 minute intervals before recovery. They found no clinically significant effects on IOP, MAP, HR, CI, or CVP.

The most important tissue groups during clinical anesthesia are vessel rich group (VRG), muscle group (MG) and vessel poor group (VPG). Time taken to reach 90% of maximal values ranged from 20-70 minutes in tissues including blood, liver, brain and muscle. With a blood/gas partition coefficient of 0.7 and low tissue blood coefficients, alveolar rate of rise is very rapid in the dog. Inspired (Fi) and alveolar-endtidal (Fa) concentrations of sevoflurane equilibrate rapidly (Kazama and Ikeda 1988a).

The metabolic stability of sevoflurane has never been an issue. It is estimated that metabolism is less than 2%.With its low blood and tissue solubility and biological stability, there has not been a need for metabolic studies since the early 1980's. Based on findings following 1 hour of sevoflurane in male human volunteers, very little biotransformation was found. Wallin et al. (1975) reported small increases in urinary excretion of inorganic fluoride in rats in the first 24 hours postanesthesia. Following exposure of 4% sevoflurane to dogs for 3 hours, sevoflurane was metabolized to inorganic fluoride and hexafluoroisopropanol with no induced renal effects (Martis et al. 1981). Plasma inorganic fluoride concentrations are increased after sevoflurane. However, no significant changes in renal function have been reported (Reichle and Conzen 2003).

Soda lime and barium hydroxide lime produce concentrations of a reaction product called Compound A that has been reported to cause renal and hepatic toxicity in rats (Altuntas et al. 2004; Sheffels et al. 2004; Stabernack et al. 2003). Carbon dioxide absorbents differ in their capacity to degrade sevoflurane to $CF_2 = C(CF_3)OCH_2F$, a fluoromethyl-2, 2-difluro-1-(trifluoromethyl) vinyl ether referred to as Compound A (Stabernack et al. 2000). Hepatotoxicity was not shown to be a factor with sevoflurane in rodents (Strum et al. 1987a) and long term anesthesia using rebreathing and non-rebreathing systems in cats did not produce toxic levels (Hikasa et al. 1988). The potential for production of toxic products may be increased when volatile anesthetics are used with dry standard absorbents (Strum & Eger 1994). Dehydration of baralime was shown to cause a 5 to10-fold increase in Compound A when sevoflurane was given in anesthetizing concentrations to swine (Steffey et al. 1997). This demonstrates the importance of frequent changes and use of fresh absorbents in a circle rebreathing system. Degradation of sevoflurane by soda lime is also temperature dependent and was shown to increase by a rate of 1.6% per hour per degree starting at 22°C (normal room temperature) reaching 57.4% per hour at 54°C (Strum et al. 1987b).

It appears that potassium hydroxide and sodium hydroxide contribute to this reaction as both baralime and soda lime include these chemicals. Because of the concerns about the possible toxic effects of Compound A, absorbents free of both NaOH and KOH were developed and shown not to generate Compound A in anesthetic systems with oxygen delivery of < 1L/min or > 2L/min in human patients (Bouche et al. 2002; Kharasch et al. 2001; Kobayashi et al. 2003; Struys et al.

2004; Versichelen et al. 2001). Renal tubular and hepatic effects of low-flow sevoflurane or isoflurane anesthesia with 1L/min in human patients were assessed using both conventional measures of hepatic and renal function and more sensitive biochemical markers of renal tubular cell necrosis. Moderate duration anesthesia during which compound A occurs appeared to be as safe as low-flow isoflurane anesthesia (Kharasch et al. 1997). Even after high loading with compound A during long-lasting low-flow sevoflurane anesthesia, no clinical or laboratory signs of renal impairment were observed in surgical human patients (Baum & Woehick 2003).

The only published studies in dogs were conducted to determine hepatic and renal function in beagles (Sun et al. 1997) and to determine concentrations of sevoflurane and Compound A in the anesthetic circuit when sevoflurane was delivered with an in-circuit vaporizer at oxygen flow rates of 250 and 500ml/min (Muir and Gadawski 1998). No significant changes were observed in liver or kidney function and no significant cardiorespiratory depression or clinically important concentrations of compound A found in dogs anesthetized with sevoflurane.

Concerns about Compound A have not been realized over years of clinical use. Halothane and isoflurane are also degraded by conventional CO_2 absorbents but the by-products have never been of any consequence. As a general rule, circle CO_2 absorption anesthetic systems designed for small animals have smaller absorbers than are used on human systems. In addition, veterinarians tend to use higher oxygen flow rates based on patient body weight ranging from 500ml/min to 2L/min. The higher end of this range is used for human patients. So these two factors would tend to minimize production and inhalation of Compound A with sevoflurane in dogs. It is also apparent that at clinical concentrations of sevoflurane over a timespan of more than a decade, toxicities have not been related to renal problems in animals and specifically in dogs. It is possible that levels of Compound A could be found with the use of sevoflurane in animals during close system anesthesia. However, the rate of breakdown with sevoflurane appears to be very small and no reports of toxicity from Compound A have been found in clinical veterinary anesthesia patients. With all the factors available, it appears that production of Compound A is not of great importance and has not affected the use of this anesthetic (Eger 2001).

Anesthetic requirements for volatile anesthetics are based on minimum alveolar concentration (MAC). Multiples of MAC are often compared with increasing numbers relating to deeper levels of anesthesia. Assessment in dogs indicated that MAC for sevoflurane was 2.36 ± 0.46%, a value of 1% higher (actual) than isoflurane and almost 3 times higher than halothane (Kazama & Ikeda 1988a). Surgical anesthesia would be considered as 1.5 MAC (about 3.5% sevoflurane). Lower blood/gas and tissue blood partition coefficients indicated that this anesthetic would offer faster inductions and recoveries than other volatile anesthetics (Strum & Eger 1987c; Yasuda et al. 1989). Absorption in breathing circuits and in CO_2 absorbents is lower than other agents as well (Table 3-9; Eger et al. 1998; Boller et al. 2005).

Compatibility with commonly used induction agents has been inconsequential and use of sedative/analgesic drugs has been shown to be advantageous (Mutoh et al. 2002; Mutoh et al. 2001b; Mutoh et al. 2001c; Mutoh et al. 1995a; Mutoh et al. 1995b; Ma et al. 1998a&b; Byron et al. 2003; Naganobu et al. 2004). Sevoflurane was shown to be an alternative to propofol anesthesia in female dogs undergoing urethral pressure profilometry (Byron et al. 2003). Clinical experiences with sevoflurane in dogs have been favorable offering some advantages over other volatile anesthetics (Hayashi et al. 1988; Mitsuhata et al. 1994; Haitjema and Cullen 2001).

There have been numerous clinical studies comparing sevoflurane and isoflurane in dogs. One such study compared isoflurane and sevoflurane for mask induction and recovery in adult dogs (Johnson et al. 1998). Results indicated that sevoflurane could be used as an inhalant for mask induction with smoother, quicker induction and comparable recovery to that of isoflurane. Experiences were reported on the use of sevoflurane in dogs undergoing mostly elective surgical procedures in a clinical setting in Australia (Haitjema 2001). They used 22 dogs of 12 different breeds and duration of anesthesia ranged from 34 to 112 minutes. The major advantages were rapid induction and recovery that were particularly advantageous for short procedures. Owing to sevoflurane's low blood-gas solubility coefficient, low pungency, less airway irritation and circulatory effects similar to those of isoflurane, it seems to be an ideal choice for inhalation induction. Rapid changes in anesthetic levels would also be an advantage when using sevoflurane in geriatric and high-risk patients. Titration of anesthesia is a critical component of this test so changing levels quickly can be accomplished with this inhalant.

A more rapid emergence may occur after anesthetic discontinuation of sevoflurane: 10 minutes faster than isoflurane and 85 minutes earlier than halothane (Taske et al. 1998). However, recovery times may not different as confirmed by studies comparing anesthetic effects of isoflurane and sevoflurane in dogs (Johnson et al. 1998; Gasthuys et al. 2001; Polis et al. 2001b). In addition, rapid recovery from surgical anesthesia in clinical settings is usually prevented by the use of sedatives and analgesics for pain control.

In a multisite study on clinical use of sevoflurane, comparable anesthesia was found with both isoflurane and halothane (Branson et al. 2001). They evaluated clinical safety and efficacy of sevoflurane as a volatile anesthetic in 196 dogs at 3 veterinary teaching hospitals. The average quality of induction, maintenance and recovery was good to excellent in all protocols. The 3 most common side effects during maintenance and recovery were arterial hypotension, tachypnea and apnea.

Exposure to volatile anesthetics will consistently trigger MH in susceptible animals and humans (Shulman et al 1981; Sawyer 2005). Comparative *in-vitro* studies indicated that although sevoflurane, isoflurane and halothane have similar effects on calcium sensitivity in skeletal muscle, sevoflurane induced smaller releases from sarcoplasmic reticulum (Kunst et al. 1999). The significance of this finding is not well understood. There have been a few suspected cases of sevoflurane induced MH in human adults, 3 cases in children but none have been reported in dogs (Gillmeister et al. 2004; Jonassen et al. 2004; Claussen et al. 1997; Kinouchi et al. 2001; Nishiyama et al. 2001). All of the human cases survived and no such reports were reported in the US.

Sevoflurane is a potent inhalation anesthetic. It is capable of producing a relatively rapid and smooth induction and may be used for maintenance of anesthesia with commonly used pre-anesthetic and injectable induction agents. Recommended levels for both induction and maintenance are supported by published reports. The most frequently reported adverse side-effects associated with sevoflurane anesthesia especially at deep levels are arterial hypotension, tachypnea, decreased cardiac output, decreased peripheral vascular resistance and respiratory depression. Cardiac index is preserved due to an increase in heart rate. Based on clinical reports, these conditions can be satisfactorily managed with appropriate monitoring and intervention during anesthesia which is actually more precise with sevoflurane than with isoflurane or halothane.

There are no data available regarding the safety of sevoflurane in pregnant and lactating bitches and dogs less than 3 months of age. Although the volatile agents tend to cause uterine relaxation, they are commonly used in low concentrations during cesarean section. In this regard, sevoflurane offers the advantage in patients admitted for emergency cesarean section with no intravenous access. Because of the lack of pungency and ease of administration for mask induction, less stress would be induced in the pregnant dog. There are no published reports for contraindications in the use of sevoflurane for cesarean section. When sevoflurane is used in geriatric and debilitated dogs, careful monitoring is advised during anesthesia.

There is a big difference between halothane and methoxyflurane. There is significant difference between halothane and isoflurane. Is the difference between isoflurane and sevoflurane of the same magnitude? The lower solubility of sevoflurane compared to that of isoflurane gives the advantage to sevoflurane for mask inductions for providing rapid changes in anesthetic levels for patients at risk. One must be capable of using this high performance anesthetic as inductions will be faster and levels of anesthesia will change more quickly in both directions–lighter and deeper. Another factor to consider is the ability of veterinary technicians to effectively and safely use two anesthetics that require different vaporizer settings with different pharmokinetics. It is obviously less complex with one agent compared to two.

Sevoflurane MAC is 2.4% in dogs which is 62% (0.9% actual) higher than isoflurane MAC. This means that delivered concentrations will be higher resulting in increased consumption of the anesthetic. Therefore, sevoflurane costs more and one uses more of it. Cost is relative and likely not to be a factor depending upon the type of practice, policies and clientele. Will the price of sevoflurane decrease in the future? Yes, because there will be competition for market share.

Are there circumstances where sevoflurane would be preferable over isoflurane? Yes, especially for mask inductions, rapid change in anesthetic levels and P3, P4, P5 patients. Is sevoflurane a better anesthetic and the preferred volatile liquid over isoflurane? That decision is up to the user but both anesthetics will be available for a long time. The point is that there is no such thing as safe anesthetics, just safe anesthetists. On the basis of numerous studies and clinical use, sevoflurane is an excellent volatile liquid anesthetic for induction, maintenance and recovery of dogs, cats and other animals and appears to have some advantages over other inhalation anesthetics.

Desflurane

Desflurane is a fluorinated methylisopropyl ether with a blood/gas partition coefficient of 0.42. It is exceptionally insoluble in blood and tissues; alveolar concentration reaches inspired concentration very quickly resulting in rapid induction of anesthesia (Yasuda et al. 1989). Its MAC value in beagle dogs was 7.2 ± 1% (Doorley et al. 1988). As a result, induction and maintenance concentrations will range from 6-11%. Because of the problems with volatility, it requires a specially designed vaporizer to contain, transfer and vaporize this anesthetic. The saturated vapor pressure at 20°C is 87% of one atmosphere (660mm Hg). This means that desflurane is nearly boiling at room temperature. The Tec 6 vaporizer is a gas/vapor blender, not the variable bypass type used for other volatile liquid anesthetics (Andrews 1993). It is a heated, thermostatically controlled, constant temperature, pressurized, electromechanically coupled dual circuit gas/vapor blender. It is not designed with a standard mount for veterinary anesthesia machines.

Desflurane stimulates the sympathetic system when inspired concentration is suddenly increased and causes a centrally mediated decrease in skeletal muscle tone. It causes a decrease in myocardial contractility but sympathetic tone is well preserved (Kersten et al. 1993). It does not sensitize the myocardium to circulating catecholamines but causes a dose dependent decrease in TPR leading to a decrease in arterial pressure. Heart rate may increase via an indirect autonomic effect. Desflurane is a respiratory depressant resulting in decreased tidal volume, although respiratory rate may increase. It is an irritant to the respiratory tract in concentrations greater than 6% meaning that it is unsuitable for use during gaseous induction. This anesthetic causes cerebral vasodilatation leading to increased cerebral blood flow. Hepatic blood flow is not decreased with desflurane and only 0.02% is metabolized, predominantly to trifluoroacetic acid. It is a trigger agent for malignant hyperthermia in the same manner as other inhalation anesthetics. Elimination is rapid due to its low solubility. Effects of desflurane are relatively similar to those of isoflurane and sevoflurane but it is considerably more expensive to use because of the high MAC values and specially designed vaporizer. As a result, this anesthetic will not find much application in clinical veterinary patients.

Reactivity, Stability, and Flammability

Anesthetics are soluble in the rubber and plastic breathing circuits of anesthetic systems (Lowe, 1971; Targ et al. 1989) (Table 3-9). Although solubility is less in plastic than in rubber, plastic circuits are usually not as resistant to deterioration and both will become useless with time. Absorption of anesthetics in the breathing components may be sufficient, especially with the more soluble agents, to affect a second patient given an anesthetic through the same circuit.

Table 3-9

Solubility of Anesthetics in Breathing Circuits

Agent	Rubber/ Gas @ 23°C	Polyvinylchloride Endotracheal tube	Polyethlene Circuit tube
Desflurane	10	35	16
Enflurane	74	120	2
Sevoflurane	23	68	31
Isoflurane	43	114	58
Halothane	199	233	128

Figures are rounded from referenced sources.
Targ AG, Yasuda N, Eger EI 2nd (1989). Solubility of I-653, sevoflurane, isoflurane, and halothane in plastics and rubber composing a conventional anesthetic circuit. *Anesth Analg* 69:218-225.
Steffey EP. Inhalation Anesthetics. In *Lumb & Jones' Veterinary Anesthesia, 3rd ed.* Williams & Wilkins, 1996.

All volatile liquids are excellent solvents and may corrode brass, solder and aluminum. Thymol, a nonvolatile preservative, is added to halothane but all of the other modern volatile liquid anesthetics are preservative-free. To minimize decomposition, all volatile liquids are stored in amber-tinted glass bottles for protection against light.

Nitrous oxide will support combustion but none of the modern agents are considered flammable in the anesthetic range. Because of its explosive nature, diethyl ether must never be stored in an area where a flame or spark may ignite the vapor. To prevent explosion, it must never be stored in a refrigerator that is not explosion-proof nor should animals that have been euthanized with the agent be refrigerated.

Part of the emphasis on development of new inhalation agents has been nonflammability. The fluorinated ethers (methoxyflurane, isoflurane, enflurane, sevoflurane, desflurane) and the fluorinated hydrocarbons (halothane) are all nonflammable in clinical concentrations at 20 to 25°C. Veterinary hospitals are generally not properly designed to permit the safe use of flammable agents but this is not a problem since no new flammable anesthetics will be developed.

References

Adriani J (1962). *The chemistry and physics of anesthesia.* Springfield, IL: Charles C Thomas.

American Society for Testing and Materials (1988). Specification for minimum performance and safety requirements for components and systems of anesthesia gas machines. (ASTM F-116-88). Philadelphia: ASTM.

Akazawa S, Shimizu R, Kasuda H, et al. (1988). Effects of sevoflurane on cardiovascular dynamics, coronary circulation and myocardial metabolism in dogs. *J Anesth* 2:227-241

Almeida DE, Rezende ML, Nunes N, Laus JL (2004). Evaluation of intraocular pressure in association with cardiovascular parameters in normocapnic dogs anesthetized with sevoflurane and desflurane. *Vet Ophthalmol* 7:265-269.

Altuntas TG, Park SB, Kharasch ED (2004). Sulfoxidation of cycteine and mercapturic acid conjugates of the sevoflurane degradation product fluoromethyl-2,2-difluoro-1-(trifluoromethyl)vinyl ether (compound A). *Chem Res Toxicol* 17:435-445.

American Society for Testing Materials (1989). Standard specification for minimum performance and safety requirements for anesthesia breathing systems (F1208-89). Philadelphia: ASTM.

Andrews JJ, Johnston RV Jr (1993). The new Tec6 desflurane vaporizer. *Anesth Analg* 76:1338-1341.

Ayre P (1937). Endotracheal anesthesia for babies with special reference to hare lip and cleft palate operations. *Anesth Analg* 16:330-332.

Bain JA, Spoerel WE (1972). A streamlined anaesthetic system. *Can Anaesth Soc J* 19:426-435.

Baraka A (1977). Functional classification of anaesthesia circuits. *Anaesth Inten Care* 5:172-178.

Barter LS, Ilkiw JE, Steffey EP et al. (2004). Animal dependence of inhaled anaesthetic requirements in cats. *Br J Anaesth* 92:275-277.

Baum JA, Woehick HJ (2003). Interaction of inhalational anaesthetics with CO2 absorbents. *Best Pract Res Clin Anaesthesiol* 17:63-76.

Baxter PJ, Garton K, Kharasch ED (1998). Mechanistic aspects of carbon monoxide formation from volatile anesthetics. *Anesthesiology* 89:929-941.

Bednarski RM, Muir WW III (1991). Closed system delivery of halothane and isoflurane with a vaporizer in the anesthetic circle. *Vet Surg* 20:353-356.

Bednarski RM, Gaynor JS, Muir WW III (1993). Vaporizer in circle for delivery of isoflurane in dogs. *J Am Vet Med Assn* 202:943-948.

Bernard J, Wouters PF, Doursout M, et al. (1990). Effects of sevoflurane and isoflurane on cardiac and coronary dynamics in chronically instrumented dogs. Anesthesiology 72:659-62.

Bernard JM, Doursout MF, Wouters P, et al. (1992). Effects of sevoflurane and isoflurane on hepatic circulation in the chronically instrumented dog. Anesthesiology 77:541-5.

Berry FA, Hughes-Davies DI (1972). Methods of increasing the humidity and temperature of the inspired gases in the infant circle system. *Anesthesiology* 37:456-462.

Best JL, McGrath CJ (1977). Trace anesthetic gases: an overview. *J Am Vet Med Assn* 171:1268-1269.

Boller M, Moens Y, Sabine BN et al. (2005). Closed system anaesthesia in dogs using liquid sevoflurane injection; evaluation of the square-root-of-time model and the influence of CO_2 absorbent. *Vet Anaesth Analg* 32:168-170.

Bouche MP, Versichelen LF, Struys MM, et al. (2002). No compound A formation with Superia during minimal-flow sevoflurane anesthesia: a comparison with Sofnolime. *Anesth and Analg* 95:1680-1685.

Bozkurt G, Memis D, Karabogaz G, et al. (2002). Genotoxicity of waste anaesthetic gases. *Anaesth Intensive Care* 30:597-602.

Branson KR, Quandt JE, Martinez EA et al. (2001). A multisite case report on the clinical use of sevoflurane in dogs. *J Am Anim Hosp Assn*. 37:420-432.

Bruce DL, Bach MJ, Arbit J (1974). Trace anesthetic effects on perceptual, cognitive, and motor skills. *Anesthesiology* 40:453-458.

BruceDL, Bach MJ (1976). Effects of trace anesthetic gases on behavioural performance of volunteers. *Br J Anaesth* 48:871-876.

Bruce DL (1979). Halothane and hepatitis: a direct relationship is unproven. *In* Eckenhoff, J.E. (ed.): *Controversy in Anesthesiology.* Philadelphia, W.B. Saunders Co.

Bruchner JB, Kielmann D, Hess W (1979). Sevoflurane: Effects on the circulation and myocardial oxygen consumption in comparison with halothane. *Proc Cent Europ Cong of Anes, Innsbruck, Aus*

Brunson DB, Stowe CM, McGrath CJ (1979). Serum and urine inorganic fluoride concentrations and urine oxalate concentrations following methoxyflurane anesthesia in the dog. *Am J Vet Res* 40:197-203.

Byron JK, March PA, DiBartola SP, et al. (2003). Comparison of the effect of propofol and sevoflurane on the urethral pressure profile in healthy female dogs. *Am J Vet Res* 64:1288-1292.

Clark KW (1999). Desflurane and sevoflurane. New volatile anesthetic agents. *Vet Clin North Am Sm Anim Pract* 29:793-810.

Collins VJ (1966). *Principles of Anesthesiology.* Philadelphia: Lea & Febiger.

Comroe JH, Forster RE II, Dubois AB, et al (1962). The lung volumes. In The Lung: *Clinical Physiology and Pulmonary Function Tests.* 2nd ed. Chicago, Year Book Medical Publishers, Inc.

Conway CM (1970). Anaesthetic circuits. In: Scurr C, Feldman S, eds. *Foundations of anaesthesia.* Philadelphia: FA Davis, p 37.

DeYoung DJ, Sawyer DC (1980). Anesthetic potency of nitrous oxide during halothane anesthesia in the dog. *J Am Ani Hosp Assn* 16:125-128.

Doorley BM, Waters SJ, Terrell RC, Robinson JL (1988). MAC of I-653 in beagle dogs and New Zealand white rabbits. *Anesthesiology* 69:89-91.

Dorsch JA and Dorsch SE (1994). The anesthesia machine. In *Understanding Anesthesia Equipment*, Dorsch and Dorsch eds, pp 95-97.

Dripps RD, Echenhoff JE, Vandam LD (1968). *Introduction To Anesthesia.* 3rd ed. Philadelphia: WB Saunders.

Ebert TJ, Frink EJ Jr, Kharasch ED (1998). Absence of biochemical evidence for renal and hepatic dysfunction after 8 hours of 1.25 minimum alveolar concentration sevoflurane anesthesia in volunteers. *Anesthesiology* 88:601-610.

Eger EI, Hylton RR, Irwin RH, Guadagni N (1963). Anesthetic flowmeter sequence—cause for hypoxia. *Anesthesiology* 24:396-397.

Eger EI II, Saidman LJ, Brandstater B (1965a) Minimum alveolar anesthetic concentration: A standard of anesthetic potency. *Anesthesiology* 26:756-762.

Eger EI II, Saidman LJ (1965b). Hazards of nitrous oxide anesthesia in bowel obstruction and pneumothorax. *Anesthesiology* 26:61-66.

Eger EI II, Ethans CT (1968) The effects of inflow, overflow, and valve placement on economy of the circle system. *Anesthesiology* 29:93-100.

Eger EI II (1974) *Anesthetic uptake and Action.* Baltimore. The Williams & Wilkins Co.

Eger EI II, Ionescu P, Gong D (1998). Circuit absorption of halothane, isoflurane, and sevoflurane. *Anesth Analg* 86:1070-1074.

Eger EI II (2001). Compound A: does it matter? *Can J Anesth* 48:427-430.

Evans AT (1998). Anesthesia case of the month. *J Am Vet Med Assn* 212:30-32.

Epstein RM, Rackow H, Salanitre E, Wolf GL (1964). Influence of the concentration effect on the uptake of anesthetic mixtures: the second gas effect. *Anesthesiology* 25:364-371.

Fantoni DT, Otsuki DA, Ambrosio AM, et al. (2005). A comparative evaluation of inhaled halothane, isoflurane, and sevoflurane during acute normovolemic hemodilution in dogs. *Anesth Analg* 100:1014-1019.

Ferstandig LL (1978). Trace concentrations of anesthetic gases: A critical review of their disease potential. *Anesth Analg* 57:328-345.

Ferstandig LL (1979). Trace concentrations of anesthetics are not proved health hazards. In Eckenhoff, J.E. (ed.): *Controversy in Anesthesiology.* Philadelphia, W.B. Saunders Co.

Flecknell PA, Roughan JV, Hedenqvist P (1999). Induction of anaesthesia with sevoflurane and isoflurane in the rabbit. *Lab Anim* 33:41-46.

Foregger R (1948). The regeneration of soda lime following absorption of carbon dioxide. *Anesthesiology* 9:15-20.

Frink EJ Jr, Morgan SE, Coetzee A, et al. (1992). The effects of sevoflurane, halothane, enflurane, and isoflurane on hepatic blood flow and oxygenation in chronically instrumented greyhound dogs. *Anesthesiology* 76:85-90.

Galloway DS, Ko JC, Reaugh HF, et al. (2004). Anesthetic indices of sevoflurane and isoflurane in unpremedicated dogs. *JAVMA* 225:700-704.

Gasthuys PI, Van Ham L, Laevens H (2001). Recovery times and evaluation of clinical hemodynamic parameters of sevoflurane, isoflurane and halothane anaesthesia in mongrel dogs. *J Vet Med, A Physiol Pathol Clin Med* 48:401-411.

Ghani GA (1984). Safety check for the Bain circuit. *Can Anaesth* Soc J 31:487-488.

Gillmeister I, Schummer C, Hommann M et al. (2004). Delayed onset of malignant hyperthermia crisis during a living donor liver transplantation caused by sevoflurane. *Anasthesiol Intensivemed Notfallmed Schmerzther* 39:153-156.

Haitjema H, Cullen LK (2001). Clinical experience with sevoflurane in dogs. *Aust Vet J* 79:339-341.

Hall J (1966). *Wright's veterinary anaesthesia.* 6th ed. London: Baltimore, Tindall & Cox.

Hall LW, Clark KW (1991). Apparatus for the administration of anaesthetics. In *Veterinary Anaesthesia, 9th Ed, Bailliere Tindall.* pp 163-164.

Halsey MJ, Sawyer DC, Eger EI II, et al. (1971). Hepatic metabolism of halothane, methoxyflurane, cyclopropane, ethrane, and forane in miniature swine. *Anesthesiology* 35:43-47.

Hamilton WK (1964). Nomenclature of inhalation anesthetic systems. *Anesthesiology* 25:3-5.

Harrison GR (2000). The contamination of volatile anaesthetics in an in-circle vaporizer with water during prolonged closed-circle anaesthesia. *Anaesthesia* 55:791-792.

Haskins SC, Sansome AL (1979). A timetable for exhaustion of nitrous oxide cylinders using cylinder pressure. *Vet Anesth* 6:6-9.

Haskins SC, Knapp RG (1982). Effect of low carrier gas flows (50% oxygen/50% nitrous oxide) on inspired oxygen tension in anesthetized dogs. *J Am Vet Med Assn* 180:735-738.

Hayashi Y, Sumikawa K, Tashiro C, et al. (1988). Arrhythmogenic threshold of epinephrine during sevoflurane, enflurane, and isoflurane anesthesia in dogs. *Anesthesiology* 69:145-147.

Heath PJ, Marks LF (1991). Modified occlusion tests for the Bain breathing circuit. *Anaesthesia* 46:213-216.

Hettrick DA, Pagel PS, Warltier DC (1996). Desflurane, sevoflurane, and isoflurane impair canine left ventricular-arterial coupling and mechanical efficiency. *Anesthesiology* 85:403-413.

Hikasa Y, Yamashita M, Takase K, Ogasawara S (1998). Prolonged sevoflurane, isoflurane and halothane anaesthesia in oxygen using rebreathing or non-rebreathing system in cats. *Zentralbl Veterinarmed A* (Japan) 45:559-575.

Hirano M, Fujigaki T, Shibata O, et al (1995). A comparison of coronary hemodynamics during isoflurane and sevoflurane in dogs. *Anesth Analg* 80:651-656.

Holaday DA, Smith FR (1981). Clinical characteristics and biotransformation of sevoflurane in healthy human volunteers. *Anesthesiology* 54:100-106.

Holaday DA (1983). Sevoflurane: an experimental anesthetic. *Contemp Anesth Pract* 7:45-59

Hughes JML (1998). Comparison of disposable circle and "to-and-fro" breathing systems during anaesthesia in dogs. *J Small Anim Pract* 39:416-420.

Humphrey D (1983). A new anaesthetic breathing system combining Mapleson A, D, and E principles: a simple apparatus for low flow universal use without carbon dioxide absorption. *Anaesthesia* 38:361-72.

Ide T, Kochi T, Isono S, Mizuguchi T (1991). Diaphragmatic function during sevoflurane anesthesia in dogs. *Can J Anaesth* 38:116-20.

Ide T, Kochi T, Isono, Mizuguchi T (1992). Effect of sevoflurane on diaphragmatic contractility in dogs. Anesth Analg 74:739-746.

Ide T, Sakurai Y, Aono M, Nishino T (1998). Minimum alveolar anesthetic concentrations for airway occlusion in cats: a new concept of minimum alveolar anesthetic concentration—airway occlusion response. *Anesth Analg* 86:191-197.

Iida H, Ohata H, Iida M, et al. (1998). Isoflurane and sevoflurane induce vasodilation of cerebral vessels via ATP-sensitive K+ channel activaition. *Anesthesiology* 89:954-960.

Imamura S, Ikeda K (1987). Comparison of epinephrine-induced arrhythmogenic effect of sevoflurane with isoflurane and halothane. *J Anesthesia* 1:62-68.

Johnson RA, Striler E, Sawyer DC, Brunson DB (1998). Comparison of isoflurane with sevoflurane for anesthesia induction and recovery in adult dogs. *JAVMA* 59:478-481.

Jonassen AA, Petersen AJ, Mohr S et al. (2004). Sevoflurane-induced malignant hyperthermia during cardiopulmonary bypass and moderate hypothermia. Acta Anaesthesiol Scand 48:1062-1065.

Kazama T, Ikeda K (1988a). Comparison of MAC and the rate of rise of alveolar concentration of sevoflurane with halothane and isoflurane in the dog. *Anesthesiology* 68:435-437.

Kazama T, Kazuyuki I (1988b). The Comparative Cardiovascular Effects of Sevoflurane with Halothane and Isoflurane. *J Anesth* 2:63-68.

Kennedy RR, Baker AB (2001). The effect of cardiac output changes on end-tidal volatile anaesthetic concentrations. *Anaesth Intensive Care* 29:535-538.

Kersten J, Pagel PS, Tessmer JP, et al. (1993). Dexmedetomidine alters the hemodynamic effects of desflurane and isoflurane in chronically instrumented dogs. *Anesthesiology* 79:1022-1032.

Kharasch ED, Frink EJ Jr, Zager R, et al. (1997). Assessment of low-flow sevoflurane and isoflurane effects on renal function using sensitive markers of tubular toxicity. *Anesthesiology* 86:1238-1253.

Kharasch ED, Frink EJ Jr, Artru A, et al. (2001). Long-duration low-flow sevoflurane and isoflurane effects on postoperative renal and hepatic function. *Anesth Analg* 93:1511-1520.

Kharasch ED, Subbarao GN, Stephens DA, et al. (2007). Influence of sevoflurane formulation water content on degradation to hydrogen fluoride in vaporizers. *Anesthesiology* 107:A1591.

Kinouchi K, Okawa M, Fukumitsu et al. (2001). Two pediatric cases of malignant hyperthermia caused by sevoflurane. *Masui* 50:1232-1235.

Kobayashi S, Bito H, Obata Y et al. (2003). Compound A concentration in the circle absorber system during low-flow sevoflurane anesthesia: comparison of Dragersorb Free, Amsorb, and Sodasorb II. *J Clin Anesth* 15:33-37.

Krahwinkel DJ, Sawyer DC, Eyster GE, Bender G (1975). Cardiopulmonary effects of fentanyl-droperidol, nitrous oxide, and atropine sulfate in dogs. *Am J Vet Res* 36:1211-1219.

Kunst G, Graf BM, Schreiner R et al. (1999). Differential effects of sevoflurane, isoflurane, and halothane on Ca2+ release from the sarcoplasmic reticulum of skeletal muscle. *Anesthesiology* 91:179-186.

Lack JA (1976). Pollution control by co-axial circuits. *Anaesthesia* 31:561-562.

Lamont LA, Greene SA, Grimm KA, Tranquilli WJ (2004). Relationship of bispectral index to minimum alveolar concentration multiples of sevoflurane in cats. *Am J Vet Res* 65:93-98.

Laredo FG, Cantalapiedra AG, Agut A, et al. (2000). Assessment of the Komesaroff machine for delivering sevoflurane to dogs (abstract). Proceedings of the Assn of Veterinary Anaesthetists, Madrid 1999. In *Veterinary Anaesthesia and Analgesia*. 27:60-61.

Laredo FG, Murciano J, Sanchez-Valverde MA, et al. (1997). Low flow closed anaesthesia: A review of 85 clinical cases. *Vet Anaesth and Analg* 24:29-32.

Laredo FG, Sanchez-Valverde MA, Cantalapiedra A, et al. (1998). Efficancy of the Komesaroff machine for delivering isoflurane to dogs. *Vet Rec* 143:437-440.

Lerche P, Muir WW III, Bednarski RM (2000a). Nonrebreathing anesthetic systems in small animal practice. *J Am Vet Med Assn* 217:493-497.

Lerche P, Muir WW III, Bednarski RM (2000b). Rebreathing anesthetic systems in small animal practice. *J Am Vet Med Assn* 217:485-492.

Lowe HJ, Titel JH, Hagler KJ (1971). Absorption of anesthetic by conductive rubber in breathing in breathing circuits. *Anesthesiology* 34:283-289.

Ma D, Sapsed-Byrne SM, Chakrabarti MK, Whitwam JG (1998a). Synergistic antinociceptive interaction between sevoflurane and intrathecal fentanyl in dogs. *Br J Anaesth* 80:800-806.

Ma D, Sapsed-Byrne SM, Chakrabarti MK, et al. (1998b). Synergism between sevoflurane and intravenous fentanyl on A delta and C somatosympathetic reflexes in dogs. *Anesth Analg* 87:211-216.

Martis L, Lynch S, Napoli MD, Woods EF (1981). Biotransformation of sevoflurane in dogs and rats. *Anesth Analg* 60:186-91.

Merin RG, Doursout MF, Chelly JE (1991). Effects of volatile anesthetics on the coronary circulation in chronically instrumented dogs. *Adv Exp Med Biol* 301:295-300.

Manley SV, McDonell WN (1980). Anesthetic pollution and disease. *J Am Vet Med Assn* 176:515-518.

Manley SV, McDonell WN (1979a). A new circuit for small animal anesthesia: the Bain coaxial circuit. *J Am Ani Hosp Assn* 15:61-65.

Manley SV, McDonell WN (1979b). Clinical evaluation of the Bain breathing circuit in small animal anesthesia. *J Am Ani Hosp Assn* 15:67-72.

Manning MM, Brunson DB (1994). Barotrauma in a cat. *J Am Vet Med Assn* 205:62-64.

McIntyre JWR (1986). Anaesthesia breathing circuits. *Can Anaesth Soc J* 33:98-105.

McMahon J (1951). Rebreathing as a basis for classification of anaesthesia circuits. *J Am Assoc Nurse Anesth* 19:133-158.

McMurphy RM, Hodgson DS, Cribb PH (1995). Modification of a nonrebreathing circuit adapter to prevent barotraumas in anesthetized patients. *Vet Surg* 24:352-355.

Merin RG, Kumazawa T, Luka NL (1976). Myocardial function and metabolism in the conscious dog and during halothane anesthesia. *Anesthesiology* 44:402-415.

Messick JM, Wilson DM, Theye RA (1972). Canine renal function and VO_2 during methoxyflurane anesthesia. *Anesth. Analg.* 51:933-941.

Middleton V, Poznak AV, Artusio JF, Smith SM (1965). Carbon monoxide accumulation in closed circle anesthesia systems. *Anesthesiology* 26:715-719.

Mitsuhata H, Saitoh J, Shimizu R, et al. (1994). Sevoflurane and isoflurane protect against bronchospasm in dogs. *Anesthesiology* 81:1230-1234.

Moyers J (1953). A nomenclature for methods of inhalation anesthesia. *Anesthesiology* 14:609-611.

Muir WW 3rd, Gadawski J (1998). Cardiorespiratory effects of low-flow and closed circuit inhalation anesthesia, using sevoflurane delivered with an in-circuit vaporizer and concentrations of compound A. *Am J Vet Res* 59:603-608.

Mutoh T, Nishimura, Kim HY, et al. (1995a). Rapid inhalation induction of anesthesia by halothane, enflurane, isoflurane and sevoflurane and their cardiopulmonary effects in dogs. *J Vet Med Sci* 57:1007-1013.

Mutoh T, Nishimura, Kim HY, et al. (1995b). Clinical application of rapid inhalation induction of anesthesia using isoflurane and sevoflurane with nitrous oxide in dogs. *J Vet Med Sci* 57:1121-1124.

Mutoh T, Nishimura R, Kim HY, et al. (1997). Cardiopulmonary effects of sevoflurane, compared with halothane, enflurane, and isoflurane, in dogs.

Mutoh T, Kanamaru A, Kojima K, et al. (1999). Effects of volatile anesthetics on the activity of laryngeal "drive" receptors in anesthetized dogs. *J Vet Med Sci* 61:1033-1038.

Mutoh T, Kanamaru A, Tsubone H, et al. (2001a). Respiratory reflexes in response to upper-airway administration of sevoflurane and isoflurane in anesthetized, spontaneously breathing dogs. *Vet Surg* 30:87-96.

Mutoh T, Kojima K, Takao K, et al (2001b). Comparison of sevoflurane with isoflurane for rapid mask induction in midazolam and butorphanol-sedated dogs. *J Vet Med* 48:223-230.

Mutoh T, Nishimura R, Sasaki N (2001c). Effects of nitrous oxide on mask induction of anesthesia with sevoflurane or isoflurane in dogs. *Am J Vet Res* 62:1727-1733.

Mutoh T, Nishimura R, Sasaki N (2002). Effects of medetomidine-midazolam, midazolam-butorphanol, or acepromazine-butorphanol as premedicants for mask induction of anesthesia with sevoflurane in dogs. *Am J Vet Res* 63:1022-1028.

Naganobu K, Maeda N, Miyamoto T, Hagio M, et al. (2004). Cardiorespiratory effects of epidural administration of morphine and fentanyl in dogs anesthetized with sevoflurane. *JAVMA* 224:67-70.

Nishiyama K, Kitahara A, Natsume H et al. (2001). Malignant hyperthermia in a patient with Graves' disease during subtotal thyroidectomy. *Endocr J* 48:227-232.

Occupational Exposure to Waste Anesthetic Gases and Vapors. No. 77-140. Washington, DC: Department of Health, Education, and Welfare (National Institute for Occupational Safety and Health), 1977.

Picker O, Scheeren TW, Arndt JO (2001). Inhalation anaesthetics increase heart rate by decreasing cardiac vagal activity in dogs. *Br J Anaesth* 87:748-754.

Polis I, Gasthuys F, Laevens H, et al. (2001a). The influence of ventilation mode (spontaneous ventilation, IPPV and PEEP) on cardiopulmonary parameters in sevoflurane anaesthetized dogs. *J Vet Med* 48:619-630.

Polis I, Gasthuys F, Van-Ham L, Laevens H (2001b). Recovery times and evaluation of clinical hemodynamic parameters of sevoflurane, isoflurane and halothane anaesthesia in mongrel dogs. *J Vet Med* 48:401-411.

Pypendop BH, Ilkiw JE (2004). Hemodynamic effects of sevoflurane in cats. *Am J Vet Res* 65:20-25.

Rees GJ (1950). Anaesthesia in the newborn. *Br Med J* 2:1419-1422.

Reichle FM, Conzen PF (2003). Halogenated inhalational anaesthetics. *Best Pract Res Clin Anaesthesiol* 17:29-46.

Robinson DA, Lack JA (1985). The Lack parallel breathing system. *Anaesth* 40:1236-1237.

Roesch R, Stoelting R (1972). Duration of hypoxemia during nitrous oxide excretion. *Anesth. Analg.* 51:851-855.

Sawyer DC, Eger EI II, Bahlman SH, et al. (1971). Concentration dependence of hepatic halothane metabolism. *Anesthesiology* 34:230.

Sawyer DC, Lumb WV, Stone HL (1971). Cardiovascular effects of halothane, methoxyflurane, pentobarbital and thiamylal. *J Appl Physiol* 30:36-43.

Sawyer DC (1973). Effect of anesthetic agents on cardiovascular function and cardiac rhythm. *Vet Clin North Am* 3:25-31.

Sawyer DC (1976). A personnel hazard: operating room environmental pollution. *J Am Ani Hosp Assn* 12:214-217.

Sawyer DC, Evans AT (1979). Evaluation of the Bain breathing circuit in small animal anesthesia. *Inhalation Anesthesia Using Fluothane™.* Ayerst Laboratories, NY.

Sawyer, DC, Rech, RH, Durham, RA, Langham, MA, Striler, EL. Comparisons of Induction Techniques and Maintenance Systems for Isoflurane Anesthesia in Cats. *Vet Surg* 20(2): 161 (Abstract), 1991.

Sawyer DC, Rech RH, Adams T, et al. (1992). Analgesia and behavioral responses of dogs given oxymorphone-acepromazine and meperidine-acepromazine after methoxyflurane and halothane anesthesia. *Am J Vet Res* 53:1361-1368.

Sawyer DC (2005). Malignant Hyperthermia. *The Merck* Veterinary Manual, ninth ed: 832-834.

Scheller MS; Nakakimura K; Fleischer JE; et al. (1990). Cerebral effects of sevoflurane in the dog; comparison with Isoflurane and Enflurane. *Br J Anaesthesia* 65:388-392.

Sheffels P, Schroeder JL, Altuntas TG, et al. (2004). Role of cytochrome P450A in cysteine S-conjugates sulfoxidation and the nephrotoxicity of the sevoflurane degradation product fluoromethyl-2, 2-difluro-1-(trifluoromethyl) vinyl ether (compound A) in rats. *Chem Res Toxicol* 17:1177-1189.

Shanks CA, Sara CA (1974). Estimation of inspiratory limb humidity in the circle system. *Anesthesiology* 40:99-100.

Shih A, Wu W (1981). Potential hazard in using halothane-specific vaporizers for isoflurane and vice versa. *Anesthesiology* 55:A115.

Shulman M, Braverman B, Ivankovich AD et al. (1981). Sevoflurane triggers malignant hyperthermia in swine. *Anesthesiology* 54:259-260.

Stabernack CR, Brown R, Laster MJ, et al. (2000). Absorbents differ enormously in their capacity to produce compound A and carbon monoxide. *Anesth Analg* 90:1428-1435.

Stabernack CR, Eger EI 2nd, Warnken UH, et al. (2003). Sevoflurane degradation by carbon dioxide absorbents may produce more than one nephrotoxic compound in rats. *Can J Anaesth* 50:249-252.

Steffey EP, Howland D Jr (1977). Isoflurane potency in the dog and cat. *Am J Vet Res* 38:1833-1836.

Steffey EP, Johnson BH, Eger EI II, Howland D Jr (1979). Nitrous oxide: effect on accumulation rate and uptake of bowel gases. *Anesth Analg* 58:405-408.

Steffey EP, Johnson BH, Eger EI II (1980). Nitrous oxide intensifies the pulmonary arterial pressure response to venous injection of carbon dioxide in the dog. *Anesthesiology* 52:52-55.

Steffey EP, Woliner M, Howland D (1982). Evaluation of an isoflurane vaporizer: the Cyprane Fortec. *Anesth Analg* 61:457-464.

Steffey EP, Woliner MJ, Howland D (1983). Accuracy of isoflurane delivery by halothane-specific vaporizers. *Am J Vet Res* 44:1072-1078.

Steffey EP, Hodgson DS, Kupershoek C (1984). Monitoring oxygen concentrating device. *J Am Vet Med Assn* 184:626, 638.

Steffey EP (1992). Other new and potentially useful inhalational anesthetics. *Vet Clin North Am Small Anim Pract* 22:335-340.

Steffey EP, Laster MJ, Ionescu P, et al. (1997). Dehydration of Baralyme increases compound A resulting from sevoflurane degradation in a standard anesthetic circuit used to anesthetize swine. *Anesth Analg* 85:1382-1386.

Stoelting RK, Eger EI II (1969). An additional explanation for the second gas effect: a concentrating effect. *Anesthesiology* 30:273-277.

Strum DP, Eger EI II, Johnson BH, et al. (1987a). Toxicity of sevoflurane in rats. *Anesth Analg* 66:769-773.

Strum DP, Johnson BH, Eger EI II, (1987b). Stability of sevoflurane in soda lime. *Anesthesiology* 67:779-781.

Strum DP, Eger EI 2nd (1987c). Partition coefficients for sevoflurane in human, blood, saline, and olive oil. *Anesth Analg* 66:654-656.

Strum DP, Eger EI 2nd (1994). The degradation, absorption, and solubility of volatile anesthetics in soda lime depend on water content. *Anesth Analg* 78:340-348.

Struys MM, Bouche MP, Rolly G, et al. (2004). Production of compound A and carbon monoxide in circle systems: an in vitro comparison of two carbon dioxide absorbents. *Anaesthesia* 59:584-589.

Sun L, Suzuki Y, Takata M, et al. (1997). Repeated low-flow sevoflurane anesthesia: effects on hepatic and renal function in beagles. Masui 46:351-357.

Taske S, Xiong S, Schimke E (1998). Sevoflurane (SEVOrane) as an inhalation anesthetic in dogs in comparison with halothane and isoflurane. *Tierarzti Prax Ausg K Klien Heim* 26:369-377.

Targ AG et al (1989). Solubility of I-653, sevoflurane, isoflurane, and halothane in plastics and rubber composing a conventional anesthetic circuit. Anesth Analg 69:218-225.

TerRiet MF, DeSouza GJ, Jacobs JS, et al. (2000). Which is most pungent: isoflurane, sevoflurane or desflurane? *Br J Anaesth* 85:305-307.

Topal A, Gul N, Hcol Y, Gorgul OS (2003). Hepatic effects of halothane, isoflurane or sevoflurane anaesthesia in dogs. *J Vet Med, A Physiol Pathol Clin Med* 50:530-533.

Tzannes S, Govendir M, Zaki S, et al. (2000). The use of sevoflurane in a 2:1 mixture of nitrous oxide and oxygen for rapid mask induction of anaesthesia in the cat. *J Feline Med Surg* 2:83-90.

U.S. Dept. of Health, Education and Welfare: Waste Anesthetic Gases and Vapors–Criteria Document. Washington D.C., Nat Inst. Of Occupational Safety and Health, March, 1977.

Van Dyke RA, Chenoweth MB (1965). Metabolism of volatile anesthetics. *Anesthesiology* 26:348-355.

Verichelen LF, Bouche MP, Rolly G, et al. (2001). Only carbon dioxide absorbents free of both NaOH and KOH do not generate compound A during in vitro closed-system sevoflurane: evaluation of five absorbents. *Anesthesiology* 95:750-755.

Wagner AE, Bednarski RM (1992). Use of low-flow and closed-system anesthesia. *J Am Vet Med Assn* 200:1005-1010.

Wallin RF, Regan BM, Napoli MD, Stern IJ (1975). Sevoflurane: a new inhalational anesthetic agent. *Anesth Analg* 54:758-766.

Waters RM (1936). Carbon dioxide absorption from anaesthetic atmospheres. In *Proceedings.* Royal Soc Medicine, pp 11-22.

Waterman AE (1986). Clinical evaluation of the Lack coaxial breathing circuit in small animal anaesthesia. *J Sm Ani Prac* 27:591-598.

Whitcher C, Hart R (1976). Occupational exposure to the inhalation anesthetics in the veterinary operating room (abstract). Submitted for criteria document on waste anesthetics. (See U.S. Dept. of Health, Education and Welfare, 1977)

Wingfield WE, Ruby DL, Buchan RM, Gunter BJ (1981). Waste anesthetic gas exposures to veterinarians and animal technicians. *J Am Vet Med Assn* 178:399-402.

Wissing H, Kuhn I, Warnken U, Dudziak R (2001). Carbon monoxide production from desflurane, enflurane, halothane, isoflurane, and sevoflurane with dry soda lime. *Anesthesiology* 95:1205-1212.

Wolfson B, Hetrick WD, Lake CL, Siker ES (1978). Anesthetic indices–further data. *Anesthesiology* 48:187-190.

Yasuda N, Targ AG, Eger EI II (1989). Solubility of I-653, sevoflurane, isoflurane, and halothane in human tissues. *Anesth Analg* 69:370-373.

Chapter 4
The Anesthetic Period: Maintenance

The Anesthetic Record

The record is an essential part of any anesthetic procedure and is of undeniable value to the patient, surgeon, and anesthetist. If blood pressure, pulse rate, respiration, ECG and other variables have been monitored, they should be recorded to better allow assessment of the patient's condition on a moment-to-moment basis. A good anesthetic record is also helpful if a patient must be anesthetized again and it is the only means of recording events occurring from the pre-anesthetic period through recovery. For medicolegal reasons, it is wise to keep accurate records because a written review of established events is far better than an account reconstructed from memory. A thorough record is an invaluable asset in any legal situation. In clinical practice, anesthetic records can be used to better assess procedures and techniques, to establish a good system of disciplined monitoring by technicians, and for educational benefits as well. The usefulness of anesthetic records has been evident at teaching hospitals and large veterinary centers for improved patient care, research, teaching, and the short time spent on making them pays great dividends.

Patient care should never be sacrificed for sake of the record. There are times when the patient demands the anesthetist's complete attention and it would be unwise to withdraw attention to maintain the record. However, one can recap events a short time later when a reasonably detailed account of the procedure can be made. Minimum content in the patient's record should be procedure, time interval, drugs given and dose, and variables monitored during anesthesia. If automated blood pressure has been used, a good rule of thumb is to record pre-incision pressures and pulse rate and the same at end of the procedure before recovery. Records should be kept in duplicate—one copy for the patient's record and the other for the clinic files and anesthesia log.

An automated anesthetic record is available with certain models of Multivariable Veterinary Monitors (Table 4-1). The monitor is connected with a serial cable directly to a computer (lap top) located in close proximity to the monitor. With specific patient information entered by the anesthetist as requested by the software, vital sign values recorded during the procedure are downloaded into the record. When the anesthetic procedure is completed, it can be entered into an electronic patient record and/or printed.

Records should also be kept for careful analysis of the circumstances related to death of every patient who has received an anesthetic. As a general rule, a death that occurs during the interval between induction and recovery is considered an anesthetic death. If anesthetic management in its broadest terms appears not to have contributed to the death, then other events may be given as the cause. It is best to be overcritical and not to dismiss anesthesia as the cause. Probably the most common cause of death during anesthesia is the lack of recognition of cardiac arrest. The most common cause of arrest is cardiovascular depression as a consequence of deeper anesthesia than is needed under the circumstances. Occasionally, an animal may expire during anesthesia and the cause cannot be attributed to anything other than the fact that the patient was anesthetized. This occurrence is relatively rare and may be in the range of one in 5,000 to 10,000 procedures.

Procedures Following Induction and Intubation

Following induction, using any of the drugs described in Chapter 2, the trachea is intubated and the tube connected to the appropriate anesthetic system. As a regular routine, the proper placement of the tube should be checked by palpation to verify that the end is positioned in the distal third of the trachea but not beyond the thoracic inlet. The carina is usually located between the 3rd and 4th intercostal spaces and keeping the end of the endotracheal tube in a position that can be gently palpated will avoid bronchial intubation. The tube should be secured in proper position with gauze or tape tied to the upper or lower jaw or behind the ears. Position of the tie will vary according to species, breed, and surgical procedure. In most dogs, the tie is made behind the canine teeth, whereas in some small canine breeds, brachycephalics, and felines and for procedures around the head such as the eye and mouth, the tie is made behind the head.

Table 4-1

ANESTHESIA REPORT

Patient Name:	Emily
Patient ID:	4322
Species:	Canine
Age	1 Yrs. 2 Months
Weight (kg):	20
Lead DVM:	Dr. Bob Trout
RVT:	Sally Roberts

Date: 03/08/07

Anesthesia start time: 1:40:00 PM
Anesthesia end time: 2:30:00 PM
Surgery start time: 1:50:00 PM
Surgery end time: 2:20:00 PM

Procedure:
OHE

Remarks:
Nice dog.

Pre Anesthetic Status:
Normal healthy patient

Pre Anesthesitic Agents:
BAG, 2ml, sub-cutaneous   (SC) at 1:15PM

Maintenance Agents:
IV Catheter, 20 ga; ET tube: 7.0; Induction: Ket Val 2ml IV at 1:40 PM; Isoflorene; Oxygen; Extubated at 2:30 PM

Carrier Gases:
Oxygen - 0.5 liters per minute (lpm)

Complications:
None noted.

Waveform   snapshot

Lead II

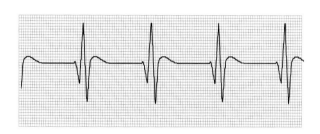

25 mm/sec

Tabular trends

TIME	NIBP S /	D	(M)	PPR	RR	mmHg ETCO2	SpO2%	P1 S /	D	(M)	P2 S /	D	(M)	T1
13:51	120	80	90	61										
13:52					60	16	38	98						
13:53					60	16	38	98						
13:53	120	80	90	61										
13:54					60	16	38	98						
13:55					60	16	38	98						
13:55	120	80	90	61										
13:56					60	16	38	98						
13:57					60	16	38	98						
13:57	120	80	90	61										
13:58					60	16	38	98						
13:59					60	16	38	98						
13:59	120	80	90	61										
14:00					60	16	38	98						
14:01					60	16	38	98						
14:01	120	80	90	61										

This is a simulated report that can be obtained when using certain anesthesia monitoring systems. With a laptop connected to the monitor, patient information is entered along with other data pertaining to the procedure. Once completed, final information is then added and a Waveform Snapshot automatically recorded with Tabular Trends of variables as listed. This Anesthesia Report can then be downloaded into the patient's electronic record and/or sent to a printer. Cardell monitoring systems courtesy of Sharn Veterinary, Tampa, FL.

The cuff of the endotracheal tube should be inflated as needed but care should be taken not to overinflate it and place undue stress on the tracheal endothelium. Compress the rebreathing bag until inspired pressure reaches 12 to 15cm H_2O or the lungs are one-half to two-thirds inflated. Simultaneously, inflate the cuff until the leak around the tube is barely detectable by palpation or auscultation. This procedure, when done properly, prevents injury to the trachea and protects the lungs from accidental overinflation because the space around the cuff acts as an escape vent for excessive pressure. Because of tracheal dilation produced by inhalation anesthetics, slight additional inflation should be made to prevent dilution of inspired anesthetic gases by room air breathed around the tube and to maintain better control of the airway. The cuff can become overinflated in the presence of nitrous oxide and therefore, it is a good practice to deflate and reinflate the cuff each hour of anesthesia (Stanley et al. 1974).

Procedures of induction and intubation should be done quickly and efficiently. Following intubation and cuff inflation, the esophageal stethoscope can be inserted in position for determination of heart and lung sounds (Figure 4-1). It is possible for the esophageal stethoscope to pass down the trachea so care should be taken to avoid this by inflating the cuff of the endotracheal tube first and not forcing the stethoscope when resistance is encountered. Palpation of the esophagus will assure proper location. This problem is most often seen in large dogs when a smaller tracheal tube is used (i.e., 8mm ID instead of a 10mm ID), when the cuff has not been inflated first or when the stethoscope has been inserted with unnecessary force.

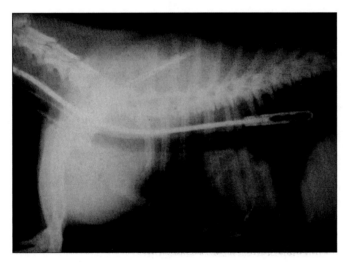

Figure 4-1 Thoracic radiograph showing esophageal stethoscope position positioned in an anesthetized dog to allow auscultation of heart and lung sounds.
Reprinted with permission. Sawyer, D C, The Practice of Small Animal Anesthesia, W.B. Saunders, 1982.

When the endotracheal tube is connected to the anesthetic system, care must be taken not to exceed recommended vaporizer settings. For patients weighing less than 5kg, it is prudent not to deliver excessive concentrations to avoid rapid uptake and profound cardiovascular depression. The level of inspired anesthetic will also vary depending on the patient's physical status, rate and depth of ventilation, type of anesthetic system, flow rate of fresh gases into the system, use of N_2O, and the adequacy of the intubated airway. In sick patients, vaporizer settings should be kept close to MAC levels and the patient should be closely assessed to avoid deep anesthesia. When a semi-open system such as the Bain circuit is used, vaporizer concentration must be decreased more quickly because dilution of inspired gas with expired gases in a semi-closed circle system does not occur in a semiopen system. When a circle system is used, total flow may be increased to accelerate induction in patients who are lightly anesthetized instead of moving the vaporizer setting above 1.5 MAC.

Frequent use of the flush valve in a circle system will serve to slow induction by inhalation agents. The valve may be used initially to wash out expired nitrogen in a circle system but because flushed oxygen bypasses the vaporizer, inspired anesthetic concentration will be diluted by oxygen delivered by the flush valve. If the reservoir bag does not fill as expected, total flow of O_2 should be increased until the problem (i.e., inadequate cuff inflation, leak in the system, improper endotracheal tube location and improper connection of the delivery tube) is identified. The flush valve should never be used in a semi-open system because the rapid inflow may overinflate the lung and thus damage alveoli. In addition, there is no reason to use the flush valve in these systems because as soon as the vaporizer is turned off, inflow of fresh gas is immediately delivered to the patient and is not delayed as it is by the large volume of the circle system.

It is very important to monitor depth of anesthesia during the induction process and to decrease vaporizer concentration in increments of 0.25 to 0.5% as the patient reaches desired level for maintenance. This will occur more quickly with a semi-open system and with small patients such as cats, puppies, and toy breeds. There should be a smooth transition from induction to mainte-nance as one must consider vaporizer settings, expected concentrations in the anesthetic system, inspired concentrations, alveolar concentration, and anesthetic levels in the brain. The relationship of MAC to the values needed for surgical anesthesia must always be considered with the objective of achieving surgical anesthesia at 1.2 to 1.5 MAC.

Unstable Physiology

Major goals for monitoring the anesthetized patient are to help assess anesthetic depth and detect trouble before severe consequences occur. There are a number of electronic devices available for monitoring anesthetized veterinary patients. Unfortunately, some of these systems do not accomplish the intended goal for early warning of impending problems. Observing patient responses to a painful stimulus (pinching a paw or tail), observing color of mucous membranes or presence of a blink reflex are used to help determine if a patient is too light or adequately anesthetized for a given procedure. Although palpation of pulse pressure in the tongue or limb can be helpful, one cannot use this as a means of estimating blood pressure. Detection of the pulse is good–not being able to palpate the pulse is not good. Observation of the ECG as discussed in this chapter is useful in detecting conduction abnormalities within the heart. Listening to heart and respiratory sounds through an esophageal stethoscope are commonly used to assess patient status during anesthesia. Audible monitors that amplify heart and respiratory sounds are unreliable in assessing hypotension and changes in heart rate are not consistent with low arterial blood pressure from either deep anesthesia or blood loss (Dyson 1997). The only way to effectively assess respiratory function is by capnography which measures end-expired carbon dioxide.

Perioperative Monitoring of the Anesthetized Patient

The primary instruments of monitoring are the veterinarinary technician's / anesthetist's senses of sight, hearing, and touch. Potent depressant drugs may alter physiologic reserves and in sick patients, may have profound consequences. Adjustments in therapy must be made because of alterations in physiologic function or surgical requirements.

Relaxation of the jaw is one of the best indicators of anesthetic depth. It should not be "sloppy loose," but rather a certain amount of muscular tone should still be present. A great deal of difference exists among breeds because of the size and strength of masseter muscles and adjust-ments must be made. For example, the jaw will feel "stiffer" in a Labrador retriever than in a Collie. Ideally, when the animal's jaw is opened widely with the anesthetist's finger on the top and bottom incisor teeth, slight tension should be present; if the animal tries to close its mouth, anesthesia should be deepened.

Rate and quality of pulse are assessed along with the rate and depth of ventilation. Heart and lung sounds are evaluated subjectively with the esophageal stethoscope (see Figure 4-1). Mucous membrane color, when pale or gray, is a good indicator of impending problems and may be used to warn of hypoxia, shock, metabolic acidosis, poor tissue perfusion, or cardiovascular depression.

The palpebral reflex disappears early with isoflurane and sevoflurane. The paw pinch reflex is a crude means of assessing whether the patient is sufficiently anesthetized prior to skin incision.

These simple observations for evaluating the patient's condition are sufficiently dependable and valuable that they should not be abandoned even when more sophisticated methods are employed. In the event of sudden power failure and loss of information from monitoring devices, the simple techniques described above are invaluable for maintaining safe anesthesia. Use of mechanical and electronic devices substantially enhances the breadth of patient monitoring during anesthesia and allow greater vigilance by both surgeon and anesthetist. In situations where minute-to-minute monitoring is not available, devices such as automated blood pressure monitors, pulse oximeters, ECG and audible monitors become even more essential.

All anesthetics depress cardiac and respiratory function in a dose related manner. Cardiac effects are primarily due to action of anesthetic agents on myocardial function and peripheral vasculature. The state of anesthesia can be looked upon as that interval between life and death. Because of the fragile interaction between disease, surgery, and physiology of the patient, interoperative monitoring is essential in being able to respond to complications before serious consequences occur.

Cardiac output would be the most accurate means of monitoring cardiac function but present technology does not provide practical means of effective measurement. However, by measuring blood pressure and pulse rate either by direct or indirect methods, valuable information can be obtained on a minute-to-minute basis to maintain good homeostasis. This also provides an effective means of monitoring anesthetic depth.

Monitoring adequacy of pulmonary function is also important. Rate of breathing, which is easy to measure, is an isolated measurement that provides very little information regarding the adequacy of ventilation. For example, 6 breaths per minute may be sufficient to maintain adequate levels of CO_2 and O_2 as long as each breath is large enough. In contrast, 20-30 BPM may be inadequate if tidal volumes are too small or dead space ventilation is too large. Therefore, monitoring CO_2 and/or O_2 will provide a much better assessment of ventilation during anesthesia.

The ECG is a direct measure of myocardial electrical activity which provides information regarding heart rate and rhythm. Although it offers no direct information regarding mechanical function of the heart, it provides information on intraoperative problems including dysrrhythmias, ischemic events and electrolyte imbalances that are important to assess during anesthesia. It does not provide information about the cardiac contractile state or hemodynamic status, which are useful in monitoring anesthetic depth. By monitoring the ECG, early detection and treatment of disturbances in cardiac rhythm can be made. The ECG should not be used as the sole means of monitoring cardiovascular function in the anesthetized patient.

Importance of the Veterinary Technician/anesthetist

Value of a technician trained in skills of monitoring anesthesia cannot be emphasized enough. From the perspective of achieving anesthesia safe as possible, the presence of a technician from beginning to end of the anesthetic procedure ranks as number one in importance. From that point, the order from best to least in value of monitoring anesthetic depth is non-invasive blood pressure (NIBP), capnography, pulse oximetry and ECG.

Circulation
Pulse Rate
Pulse in a superficial artery provides information on rate, rhythm and strength of the heart beat. Commonly, the femoral, metacarpal, metatarsal, coccygeal, cranial tibial, facial or lingual artery can be palpated with the last two sites very difficult to assess in very small patients. In general, if the systolic pressure is below 60mm Hg, femoral pulse may be difficult to palpate nor will the lingual artery be visible. Continuous auscultation of the chest not only provides information on

quality and amplitude of heart sounds but also provides information on the adequacy of the airway and the quality of ventilation. An esophageal stethoscope or external stethoscope bell taped in the appropriate position can be used for this purpose.

Heart rate or pulse rate, except at the extremes of light or deep anesthesia, is not a precise means of determining anesthetic depth. However, maintaining heart rate within acceptable limits is important. Usually, limits range from 70 to 160 BPM. Tachycardia is usually not treated pharmaco-logically. However, it is prudent to assess the cause, if possible, such as light anesthesia, inadequate pain management, hypotension, hypovolemia, anemia or response to anticholinergics. Lidocaine, 1mg/kg IV, may be used in the dog to protect the myocardium against potentially dangerous dysrhythmias, which may be associated with tachycardia. Lower doses must be used in cats.

Bradycardia, which can be a greater problem, may be mediated by vagal stimulation or a side effect of alpha$_2$ agonists or potent opioids, e.g. fentanyl. Atropine, given IV at 0.01mg/kg, may be used to treat bradycardia. Occasionally in some animals, especially athletes that have resting normal heart rates below 70 BPM, bradycardia is not due to cholinergic stimulation or anesthetic depression, does not require treatment and will not respond very much to anticholinergics.

Arterial Pressure

Cardiac output is the product of volume ejected from the heart per beat (stroke volume) and the rate the heart beats per minute (heart rate). The resultant pulsatile pressure generated in the vascular system causes distention of arterial vessels that has a maximum value, systolic arterial pressure (SAP), and a minimum value, diastolic arterial pressure (DAP). Mean arterial pressure (MAP) is the average pressure during the cardiac cycle that occurs as blood is pushed through vessels. It is not the midpoint between SAP and DAP and takes into account changes in vascular resistance. Blood flow through vessels is the transport system for oxygen, nutrients and metabolic products and is closely dependent upon blood pressure. Tissue perfusion is maintained between arterial pressures of 60 to 150mm Hg. When MAP falls below 60mm Hg, blood flow to essential organs such as brain, heart, lungs, liver and kidneys may be too low to adequately perfuse these essential organs. Sustained SAP over 170mm Hg can result in severe consequences such as blindness, stroke, hemorrhage and death.

The palpation method is the most common means of indirect assessment of arterial pressure. The traditional use of a stethoscope over a major artery with an occluding cuff in the dog or cat limb for detection of Korotkoff sounds is limited or impossible because of anatomical differences among breeds and between species. The smallness of many veterinary patients also presents a problem.

Prevention of arterial hypotension is a major concern during anesthesia so early detection is of prime importance. Assessment of blood pressure is essential in emergency situations to evaluate patient status, to monitor the effectiveness of therapy during intensive care and as a means of determining the presence of internal hemorrhage. Monitoring blood pressure as part of the anesthesia protocol will improve morbidity and mortality for not only patients at risk but healthy animals as well. Measurement of arterial blood pressure during anesthesia may accomplished by direct or indirect means and accuracy at low pressures would be considered to be most important.

Direct

Direct measurement of arterial blood pressure and pulse rate can be more accurate than indirect methods if proper procedures of calibration and recordings are followed and this method provides a means of continuous beat-to-beat monitoring. However, these measures do not have good clinical application because it is technically difficult especially in small patients and is time consuming. This procedure requires introduction of a catheter into a peripheral artery either by surgical cutdown or percutaneous placement. In most circumstances, the animal should be anesthetized before catheter placement. For percutaneous placement during anesthesia, the dorsal pedal artery (also called the anterior tibial artery) or the lingual artery are best used in dogs and the femoral artery in cats. In large dogs, the coccygeal artery can be used. Catheters located in appendage arteries can be secured with tape but it is best to suture or glue them in place if they are to be maintained for several days postsurgery.

Procedures for percutaneous placement and cutdown in small animals have been described (Haskins 1987). The percutaneous technique is best accomplished in animals larger than 10kg but with practice and skill, it is possible to place catheters in animals of small size. The standard procedure for percutaneous placement is to remove hair over the site and prepare the area aseptically. Using sterile gloves, the artery is palpated with two fingers of one hand to identify the exact position of the artery. It is best to have the leg extended to straighten the vessel. A small stab incision is made through skin overlying the artery with a 20 gauge hypodermic needle without penetrating the vessel. This incision is made to minimize damage to the over-the-needle catheter material. The catheter is positioned with the bevel up in one hand while palpating the artery with the fingers of the other hand. The needle tip and artery are palpated through the skin and the catheter inserted into the artery, steeply at first just so that the tip of the needle penetrates the upper wall of the artery. When flashback blood is seen in the catheter, one has to make sure that both the needle and catheter are in the lumen without the needle penetrating the opposite wall. The presence of the needle and catheter within the lumen can be verified by the reflux of blood into the hub of the needle and by feel. Without moving the needle, the catheter is gently rotated over the needle to its full length into the artery. Once assured of proper placement, the needle is removed and replaced with a stopcock or injection cap on the catheter end. It is then flushed with heparinized saline. An aneroid manometer (Haskins 1987) may be used to monitor mean pressure (Figure 4-2) or if attached to a pressure transducer and recorder, systolic, diastolic and pulse rate can be recorded continuously. Some recorders will electronically calculate MAP. Attaching the catheter to either system is facilitated by connecting one or two sections of extension tubing filled with heparinized saline (Goodger & Dunlop 1972). The manometer or transducer must be positioned at the level of the right atrium and the catheter flushed periodically with heparinized saline.

Direct measurement of blood pressure is the gold standard against which indirect methods are often compared. However, it is not feasible to take direct measurements from the same sites used for cuff or probe placement of indirect systems. Direct and indirect methods are remarkably different. Direct values are taken with a fluid-filled system connected to a transducer and indirect data obtained with an ultrasonic sensor or air-filled oscillometric system. Direct methods can be associated with inaccuracies related to the dynamics of a fluid-filled catheter and arterial line, site of catheter placement, possible air bubbles in the system and frequency responses of the measurement system.

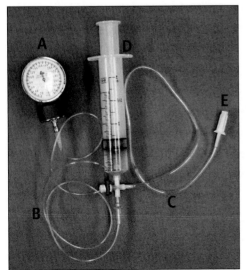

Figure 4-2 Equipment for monitoring direct mean arterial pressure. A, Aneroid manometer. B, 36-inch transmission set. C, Extension tubing and three-way stopcock. D, Heparinized saline in syringe used to fill tubing and catheter before connection to manometer. E, Connection to arterial catheter.
(Photo courtesy of Dr. David B. Brunson, University of Wisconsin.) Practice of Small Animal Anesthesia, WB Saunders, 1982.

Indirect

NIBP monitoring using Doppler or oscillometric technology offers a simple and effective means of repeatedly and harmlessly estimating arterial blood pressure in young, old, large, small, healthy, sick or high-risk patients. Application of automated NIBP monitoring is not technically difficult but does require a certain skill level and experience to achieve desired results. It has been an effective means of monitoring blood pressure for more than 20 years. It should be part of the routine physical examination with baseline data recorded as part of the medical record. Should medical problems occur in the future, comparisons can be easily made. In addition to monitoring anesthetized patients, it can be used to diagnose essential and secondary arterial hypertension, to monitor effects of drug and diet therapy for cardiac problems, and other diseases.

Doppler Technique

The Doppler flow detector is an electronic instrument that transmits a high-frequency signal toward the artery from a small crystal placed on the overlying skin. Sites of measurement include palmar aspect of the forelimb or hindlimb (metacarpal or metatarsal artery), anterior surface of the hind limb just below the hock (dorsal pedal artery) or tail (coccygeal artery). Hair over the site area must be clipped before the sensor is applied and an aqueous gel must be applied to the probe to ensure proper signal conduction. The detector consists of two piezoelectric crystals. One sends an ultrasonic beam to the arterial site. The other crystal receives reflected waves from underlying tissue and moving red blood cells (rbc's). If there is nothing moving under the sensor, frequency of the reflected waves will be the same as the emitted waves. When the reflected waves detect motion of rbc's in the vessel, there is a change in frequency made audible by the monitor, referred to as the Doppler-shift. The sound that occurs is caused by the difference between emitted and reflected sound waves. This sound is not pure and is described as a variable hissing or swishing noise that is proportional to the velocity of moving blood. Optimal probe position is based on the loudest blood flow signal. The probe must be fixed to the tail or limb site usually with adhesive tape and must be an air-free coupling between it and the skin. Because the sound beam is very narrow, one has to be sure that there is no loose skin that will cause the probe to shift off the site. A cuff with a width to limb circumference ratio of 0.4-0.6 is placed proximal to the probe with a snug fit. It must not be so tight that it obstructs venous blood flow. An aneroid manometer is connected to the cuff. Determination of blood pressure requires an operator to inflate the cuff placed above the Doppler probe. This effectively occludes the artery thus stopping wall motion and the audible signal of blood flow. The cuff is slowly deflated in 2- to 5mm Hg increments until clear flow sounds are audible. The manometer reading observed at the first brisk sound is recorded as SAP. If the cuff is deflated too rapidly, the first few sounds may be missed and the recorded pressure will be falsely low. Measurement of DAP, which relies on subjective judgment of sudden muffling of the Doppler signal toward the end of cuff pressure deflation, is much more difficult to determine. Without this component, MAP cannot be calculated. Pulse rate must be counted and hand recorded along with the blood pressure. This process should be repeated three to five times to ensure an accurate reading (Acierno and Labato 2004).

In a study evaluating the Doppler method of measuring SAP in cats, it was determined that a clinically useful calibration adjustment for indirect measurement to direct would be to add 14 mm Hg to the Doppler SAP value (Grandy et al. 1992). Also, this method was shown to underestimate SAP measurements in cats and that the Doppler appeared to be a better predictor of MAP compared to SAP (Caulkett et al. 1998). Direct to indirect comparisons would be helpful in learning how to use the Doppler system if one is to be dependent on this process for monitoring anesthetized patients, especially at low pressures where sounds will be of lower intensity. In addition, it is to be expected that accuracy between technicians will be different. Not every operator's hearing will be the same which results in further variation of values. Keeping the sensor in position can be a problem during anesthesia especially when the patient is moved.

Because the Doppler system is not automated, this is a major disadvantage unless the anesthetist can be dedicated to making regular measurements especially for patients at risk. When the technician is attending to other needs at times of patient instability, time may not be available to make repeated measurements as frequently as needed. However, by committing a skilled technician to this monitoring procedure, experience and attention to detail, it is possible to obtain clinically useful SAP measurements during anesthesia. One of the values in using the Doppler is that the sounds of blood flowing past the sensor on a continuous basis can be useful in assessing patient status.

Oscillometry

Automated devices have evolved to become a standard of excellence in clinical practice (Leblanc & Sawyer 1993). From a survey conducted in 1999, only 7% of veterinarians used automated blood pressure monitors in their hospitals. The "gold-standard" for automated NIBP monitors has been the Dinamap™ (Mitchell 1993). The Dinamap™ 1846sx and subsequently the Dinamap™ Vital Signs Monitor 8100 were marketed for use in human patients. Because of improved oscillometric technology in these monitors, published reports provided comparative information regarding accuracy, precision and cuff placement in veterinary patients (Nakada et al. 1990; Sawyer et al. 1991; Vincent et al. 1993; Bodey et al. 1994; Bodey et al. 1996; Hansen et al. 1997; Grosenbaugh & Muir 1998a; Dart & Dunlop 2000). In 1992, the Critikon Company developed the first oscillometric NIBP monitor for clinical veterinary patients. This monitor was manufactured for commercial distribution until 1997 at which time Critikon decided not to continue production of the unit. Final stocks of Dinamap 8300's were sold in 1999. Since that time, a number of different manufacturers have made the availability of non-invasive automated veterinary blood pressure monitors a common product for veterinary hospitals.

Technology

Oscillometry is the basis of operation for monitors that use microprocessor technology to detect oscillations produced by vascular pulsation in a peripheral artery. A compression cuff is placed around an appropriate location on an extremity and is automatically inflated to occlude the underlying artery. Each time the heart beats, oscillations occur within the artery which is transmitted to the cuff creating oscillations in pressurized air within the cuff. Signals are transmitted through the pressure hose to a transducer located within the monitor. A microprocessor analyzes oscillations and displays values of SAP, MAP, DAP and PR (Figure 4-3).

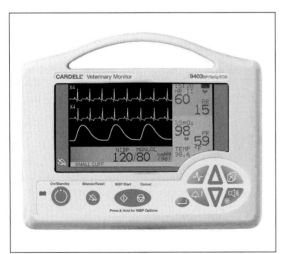

Figure 4-3 Cardell 9403 Veterinary Blood Pressure monitor. This model includes ECG, Pulse Oximetry and NIBP.
Courtesy of Sharn Veterinary, Tampa, FL.

Following cuff inflation sufficient to occlude blood flow in the artery, the monitor automatically begins the sequential deflation process. As the cuff is deflated, pulsations in the cuff are detected to be relatively constant. Amplitude of oscillations change as the cuff is deflated and greater flow is re-established beyond the cuff. As cuff pressure is stepped down, the monitor measures pattern and magnitude of pressure oscillations. The point of maximum amplitude is considered to be MAP. Based on the shape of the bell curve, SAP and DAP are determined. The process of this calculation for the different brands of monitors is proprietary by different manufacturers. A determination sequence begins when the START or STAT button is depressed or when time has expired in the cycle mode. Measurement cycles can be set at 1, 2, 3, 4, 5, 10, 15, 30, 60, and 90-minute intervals. One and three minute cycles are most commonly selected during anesthesia depending upon patient condition and circumstances. The first determination sequence initially inflates the cuff to a pressure of 150mm Hg. The monitor deflates the cuff one step each time it detects two pulsations of relatively equal amplitude. Time between deflation steps depends on the frequency of these matched pulses (PR). If the monitor does not detect a pulse within 1-2 seconds, it deflates to the next step. The process of finding two matched pulses at each step rejects artifacts caused by cuff movement at the measurement site and greatly enhances the accuracy of the monitor. If during the first determination, the monitor finds that inflation pressure did not occlude the artery, it will interrupt the stepped deflation process. The cuff will be pumped 30mm Hg above the initial pressure to 180mm Hg and the stepped deflation will start again. This process will repeat if necessary until the artery is occluded. At each step, the microprocessor stores cuff pressure, the matched pulse amplitude, and time between successive pulses. The monitor then deflates the cuff completely, analyzes stored data, updates the front panel displays, and sounds a short tone. This process takes place over a 20 to 30 second period. Data are stored in memory that can be accessed for the previous 80-100 measurements.

Alarm limits for high and low pressures are incorporated in the monitor. Monitors such as the Cardell™ have a wide range of pulse rates of 20 to 300 beats per minute (BPM) within which measurements can be made. Another feature is that the sensitivity appears to be excellent with the Cardell™ which is an advantage especially in patients less than 5kg.

Blood Pressure Cuffs
A complete array of cuff sizes is available for oscillometric monitors to facilitate measurements in animals of almost any size (Figure 4-4). Cuffs are disposable but with proper care, they can be used many times before a leak develops, the self-adherent attachment becomes clogged with hair and debris or attachment tubing separates from the cuff. Cuffs from different manufacturers are not interchangeable. The air bladder is usually incorporated in the entire cuff so that it is not necessary for them to be marked for placement over the artery. It is essential that a variety of size cuffs are provided with monitors ranging in size from small cuffs #1 to #5 (Figure 4-4) to one medium and one large tail cuff (not shown). Selection of appropriate size is very important as cuffs too narrow or too wide will produce inaccurate values.

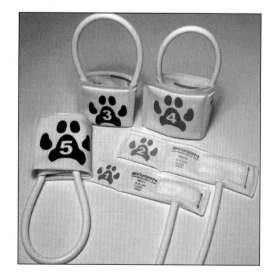

Figure 4-4 Blood pressure cuffs for Cardell oscillometric monitors. Five sizes (cuff width) are shown: #1 = 2.0cm; #2 = 2.5cm; #3 = 3.5cm; #4 = 4.0cm; #5 = 5.0cm.
Courtesy of Sharn Veterinary, Tampa, FL.

Cuff Placement

Cuffs should be wrapped snugly around the appendage so that the bladder is over the selected site (Figure 4-5). A cuff properly placed on an appendage site will not move during the measurement cycle, between inflations or when manipulated by the operator. If wrapped too tightly, the cuff will not function properly and can restrict blood flow when not inflated. The optimal cuff size is based on the cuff width to limb circumference (CW/LC) ratio. Studies in dogs have confirmed an optimal range of 0.4-0.6 (Valtonen & Eriksson 1970; Sawyer et al. 1991). It is relatively easy to avoid placing a cuff that is too small for the site since the self-adherent component (Velcro-like material) will not be sufficient to hold it in place when inflated. Selecting the next size larger will usually be sufficient. Tape should not be used to secure the cuff as it may suppress the signal and cause inaccurate measurements. Body weight cannot be used as a guide for cuff size since limb anatomy will be different for different body conformations. Removal of matted hair just over the measurement site is recommended; otherwise it is not necessary to clip the area. Proper care of cuffs is important to prevent damage between uses. Cuffs should not be placed loosely in a box or drawer as they usually end up in a tangle. This makes it difficult to find the intended size and cuffs are easily damaged as they are rapidly sorted to find a given size. One way to take care of this problem is to place a self-adherent strip in a convenient location where the monitor is used and attach the most commonly used cuff sizes to the strip.

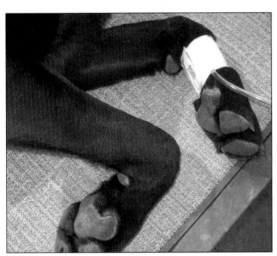

Figure 4-5 Cuff placement on forelimb around the metacarpus. Cuff should wrap around the appendage with a snug fit. That is, not so loose that the cuff can be rotated or so tight that the air bladder will restrict venous return.
Courtesy of Sadie, companion of Bob and Alice Schell, Tucson, AZ and Sitka, AK.

Sites of Measurement

Studies conducted on anesthetized animals have predominately used peripheral sites on the forelimb and hindlimb (Sawyer et al. 1991; Sawyer et al 1994; Bodey et al. 1994; Bodey et al. 1996; Kallet et al. 97; Grosenbaugh & Muir 1998b; Dart & Dunlop 2000; Sawyer et al. 2004). Precision based on coefficients of variation was better in conscious dogs when cuffs were placed around the base of the tail but proximal hindlimb cuffs gave the most accurate results in anesthetized dogs (Bodey 1994). Results from studies with the Dinamap 8300 demonstrated that the best site for cuff placement in dogs was over the anterior tibial artery (dorsal pedal) which is located just below the hock (Sawyer 1994). Two other acceptable sites were just proximal to the carpal pad or tarsal pad. In a subsequent study, the metacarpal site was shown to be most consistent with direct measurements (Sawyer et al 2004). As a result, any of the 3 sites, metacarpus, metatarsus, or dorsal pedal, can be used during surgery. Putting the cuff around the metacarpus is usually most convenient since it is usually most accessible should problems occur with the cuff. When securing patients to the surgery table by placing ties on appendages, the tie must be placed distal to the cuff site to avoid creating problems with measurements by occluding blood flow.

As indicated, the tail may be preferable in conscious dogs as it can be more conveniently used with animals in standing or sitting positions. Care must be taken to assure that the cuff site is located at the same approximate level of the heart. There are important considerations for not using the tail site for cuff placement during anesthesia. In addition to some dog and cat breeds not having a tail site available for cuff placement, Dunlop et al. (2000) suggested that blood pressure measurements might be compromised during conditions of low cardiac output. Normal blood pressures, e.g., SAP 80-140mm Hg, are usually associated with good tissue perfusion. Blood flow to the tail during intervals of hypotension and poor perfusion, such as might occur during deep anesthesia, blood loss or shock may be lower than in other body appendages. Consequently, adequate readings of NIBP would be better taken from the metacarpal or metatarsal area during anesthesia. The best site during anesthesia in cats is to place the cuff around the forelimb between the elbow and carpus (median artery). In small cats and dogs, the cuff should be placed above the elbow (brachial artery).

Measuring Blood Pressure in Cats

Studies have been published regarding use of oscillometric blood pressure monitors in cats (Bins et al. 1995; Branson et al. 1998). Results from some unpublished work comparing the Cardell to direct pressure measurements demonstrated excellent correlation with normal systolic and mean pressures in anesthetized cats based on 45 measurements from 3 sites, metacarpus, median, and tail (Sawyer et al. 2001). Caulkett et al. (1998) concluded from a study in eight anesthetized cats weighing 3.5 ± 0.8kg that the Dinamap 8300 provided the most accurate prediction of SAP compared to optical plethysmography and Doppler methods. Bodey and Sansom published an extensive study in 1998 using the Dinamap 1846sx (human model) with the tail as site of measurement in 203 conscious cats. They found blood pressure to rise with age, as SAP, DAP, MAP and pulse pressure were significantly higher in animals aged 11 years or older than in cats under 11 years old. One of the key findings of this study was that once the cuff was applied, cats were allowed to assume a comfortable position in a basket or padded cage. Most assumed sternal recumbency thus minimizing influence of cuff position and the heart. They recorded six or more readings from each cat and felt it was imperative that adequate time, e.g., 15 to 60 minutes, be taken to obtain repeatable readings.

Oscillometric monitors can be used effectively for blood pressure measurements in cats (Figure 4-6). From comparative studies with the Cardell monitor, very useful values can be obtained even with SAP below 70mm Hg and above 150mm Hg (Pedersen et al. 2002).

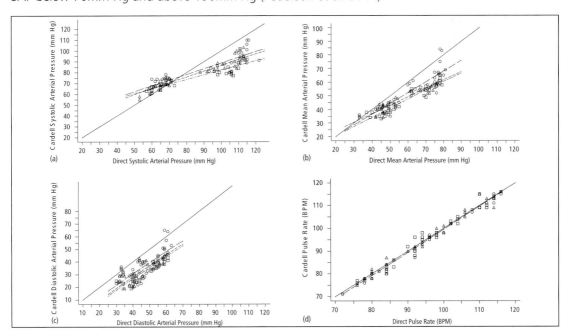

Figure 4-6 Four scatter plots of Cardell pressures versus direct pressures for low and normal measures. (Sawyer et AL 2004)
Reprinted with permission, Elsiever.

The anesthetic protocol can influence outcome of blood pressure readings as cats have an exquisite control of their peripheral vascular system. Most cats weigh less than 5kg and their peripheral arteries are smaller than in dogs of comparable size. If preemptive analgesia is not practiced, that is, administering analgesic drugs before surgery, release of endogenous substances will cause enough vasoconstriction to obviate pressure measurements even though good pressures would be recorded prior to skin incision or deep pain stimulation. NIBP measurements can be obtained in cats trained to lie quietly on a table, lap or chair and in anesthetized cats; there is plenty of evidence that this technology can be used in these animals. It is a greater challenge compared to dogs especially in conscious cats. When attempts at getting pressures in cats becomes difficult, most of the time it is not the fault of the monitor. Profound vasoconstriction is most likely the problem.

Causes for Inaccurate Measurements
Improper selection of size and placement of cuffs can contribute to spurious measurements. Cardiac arrhythmia may cause measurements to vary from one cycle to the next. Oscillometric devices are designed to select readings from steady pulses at each level in the measurement cycle and do not compensate for large deviations in pressure. Severe or sustained irregular heart rhythm (arrhythmia) will cause erratic or unattainable blood pressure readings. Certain injectable anesthetics and sedative drugs can cause arrhythmias that can interfere with blood pressure measurements. Movement at the site of measurement that include shivering may result in blood pressure and pulse rate values that are nonsense or unobtainable.

These monitors cannot distinguish vessel oscillations from other movement at the site. This can occur during light anesthesia, during recovery, or in conscious patients. A good signal can most often be obtained during anesthesia, when there is no movement of the patient either sponta-neously or by the surgeon, no muscle spasticity or movement of the limb site and no disturbance of the tubing between the cuff and monitor. It is important that there are no other sources of vibration in contact with the tubing such as suction pumps, fans, other analyzers or generators. The cuff should be at the approximate level of the heart. This is usually not a problem with patients in a prone position during anesthesia and surgery.

Small patients, especially those less than 2kg, offer a challenge for making blood pressure measurements. Selecting a site on an appendage closer to the trunk should be considered rather than sites like the tail, metacarpus or metatarsus. Placing the cuff between the hock and stifle, over the median artery between the carpus and elbow or above the elbow over the brachial artery may yield better results. Automated veterinary NIBP monitors are designed to make blood pressure measurements with pulse rates between 20 and 300 BPM. Rates outside of these limits would be unusual but if present, will yield inaccurate values or prevent measurements from being obtained.

Data
Results from NIBP studies using the following monitors demonstrate a tendency to underestimate direct blood pressure values: Dinamap 8300, Dinamap 8100, Dinamap 1846 sx, SDI VetBP 6000 and Cardell 9300 (Tabaru et al. 1990; Sawyer et al. 1991; Sawyer et al.1994; Bodey et al. 1994; Bodey et al. 1996; Grosenbaugh & Muir 1998a; Stepien & Rapoport 1999; Pedersen et al. 2002; Sawyer et al. 2004). In studies with the Cardell monitor, values at low pressures were not different from those measured directly but measurements within the normal or high range underestimated direct pressures by 18-23mm Hg (see Figure 4-6) (Sawyer et al. 2004). This is an important factor that further supports the value of automated NIBP during anesthesia. At high pressures, underesti-mation is not a problem and can be configured into determining the clinical welfare of the patient.

Summary
Blood pressure monitoring is invaluable for anesthetized patients and for following therapeutic responses in cardiac patients or those receiving critical or emergency care. This will allow the veterinarian to avoid prolonged intervals of hypotension and this is essential for maintenance of

adequate cerebral, coronary and splanchnic organ blood flows (Haskins 1996). Whether one uses SAP values of 80 or MAP of 60 as low alert thresholds during anesthesia, values can be followed not only for early warning but also to establish an upward trend of improved pressures as corrective measures are instituted. Most anesthetized patients should have indirect SAP values in the range of 80 to 120mm Hg. If indirect SAP is above l50mm Hg, arterial hypertension is evident (Mitchel 1993). Assessment must be made to evaluate other signs for light anesthesia, sympathetic responses from deep pain or other complications. In conscious patients, high pressures may be associated with disease, anxiety, fear, pain or other influences that must be determined. There is no question that automated indirect monitoring of arterial blood pressure in companion animals is in the best interest of veterinarians, clients and their pets. It should be a standard of practice not only during anesthesia but also as a diagnostic and therapeutic tool for better patient care.

Electrocardiography

ECG changes often occur in patients during anesthesia. Understanding what the ECG is revealing is valuable in managing patients compromised with the various drugs used to produce anesthesia/analgesia. Even though ECG findings may not indicate life threatening heart problems, they will often help the clinician make adjustments in the anesthetic protocol to allow the anesthetic episode to proceed safely and smoothly. ECG information may be absolutely crucial to patient survival in older patients and patients with heart damage or disease. There are times when underlying heart problems are not detected until the patient is anesthetized. These may be problems produced by anesthetic agents or drugs may have caused a pre-existing heart condition to become manifest. In any case, knowing what is happening with the patient's ECG will provide the best opportunity to effectively deal with a problem should it arise. If no abnormality is identified, there is comfort in knowing the electrical activity of the heart is functioning normally.

Value of ECG

The most valuable information provided by ECG is heart rate and rhythm. The ECG is not the first alert of impending problems related to anesthetic depth. Some would even say that there is little value provided by the ECG during anesthesia in normal healthy P1 and P2 patients, especially when NIBP and pulse oximetry are routinely used (Dodman 1992; Robertson 1992). The better the anesthetist understands information provided by the ECG as a measure of physiological events, the better they are be able to know when to alert the clinician that an adverse event is occurring. ECG monitors are readily available and designed specifically for use in veterinary patients. Some have multivariable capabilities combining NIBP, pulse oximetry, ECG and others (see Figure 4-3). Computerized analytical systems are also available in veterinary medicine (Figure 4-7). If an unknown arrhythmia appears on the monitor, the computer can be asked to render an analysis. The computer will never replace the clinician but because of this swift response, patient safety is greatly enhanced.

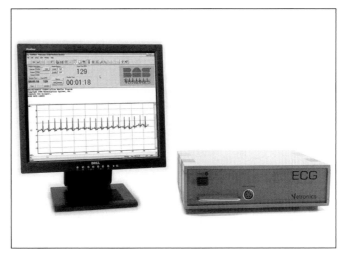

Figure 4-7 Vetronics systems monitor with computer. Screen demonstrates record that can be downloaded to patient record and printed.
Courtesy of Vetronics, W. Lafayette, IN

Lead Placement and Recording the ECG

Positioning Anesthetized Patients

For ECG monitoring during anesthesia, it is most important to position patients on the table for the procedure, not for the ECG. If standard lead placement is not possible, leads should be attached to the torso where they will be least subject to movement. It is preferable to view an upright QRS complex for monitoring ECG. A heart base to apex lead arrangement is best if the negative lead is placed at the base (point of right shoulder at thoracic inlet) and the positive lead at the apex (low on caudal left thorax). Standard right forelimb lead is negative and standard left hind leg is positive in lead two; so if these leads are properly placed and the machine is set to Lead II, an upright complex should be the result.

Positioning Conscious Patients

Standard position for recording diagnostic ECG in dogs is right lateral recumbency. Diagnostic tracings can be obtained in cats in either right lateral or sternal position. Limbs should be perpendicular to the spine and parallel with their opposite member. In awake cats and dogs, it is best to have the patient held by a technician or assistant. One lead should be applied first to determine comfort level and adjustment made as needed. Then the other clips can be placed in position. It is important that the patient be kept still which during anesthesia should not be a problem unless movement is caused by the surgeon. A moving conscious patient will allow clips to saw into skin tissue leading to discomfort and change in position of electrodes.

Lead Attachment

Leads should be attached just below the elbow on the front leg and just above the stifle on the hind leg. The following lead sequence should be applied for a 3 lead system: Right Foreleg *(RA-white)*; Left Foreleg *(LA-black)*; Left Hind Leg *(LL-red)*. For a 5 lead system, four limb leads can be applied *(RA, LA, RL, and LL)* with the exploring lead used for diagnostic purposes as needed. Otherwise, the exploring lead may be left unplugged.

Lead Contact

Sites where leads are attached to the body must be properly prepared to optimize contact. Dogs and cats have enough electrolyte material on their skin and hair so that merely moistening lead sites with 70% isopropyl alcohol is appropriate. This will usually be sufficient for ECG recording/monitoring for a short time, 30 to 60 minutes, depending upon the relative humidity. For monitoring during longer periods, an electrode paste should be used. It is best to first wet the hair at the lead attachment site with alcohol; then place paste on the moistened hair and skin. It is important that the paste be in direct contact with skin. For patients with dense undercoat, rub paste with fingers to assure that it has made contact with skin. Alligator clips are supplied with monitors and they must open wide enough to firmly but gently grasp the skin.

Acquiring an ECG signal

With electrodes placed on the body surface, the ECG measures tiny electrical signals generated by the heart. With these electrodes placed at standard anatomical locations on the body, information can be obtained about the size and shape of the heart as well as rate and rhythm. For purposes of monitoring heart rate and rhythm during anesthesia, electrodes may be placed almost anywhere on the body. Because most veterinarians learn to interpret lead II of the standard 6 or 7 lead veterinary electrocardiograms, this is the lead most often used for monitoring during anesthesia. Lead II is a bipolar lead with the positive electrode on the left rear leg and the negative electrode on the right fore limb. Most veterinarians prefer to look at an upright QRS complex and this approach produces an upright tracing in normal small animal patients. When it is not possible to use appendages for electrode placement, the negative electrode can be placed on the right anterior portion of the body and the positive electrode on the caudal left portion of the body. This will produce an upright QRS in patients with normal hearts.

When problems arise in obtaining a stable ECG signal, it is usually due to poor electrode contact with skin or movement of the electrode during the procedure for which the patient is anesthetized. Therefore, if limb movement is anticipated, as often occurs during an orthopedic procedure, electrodes should be placed at sites on the body that will not need to be moved.

Electrode site preparation is important to obtain a good ECG signal. If the procedure will be long, it will be necessary to clip the hair and place alcohol and electrode gel on the skin where the electrode will be attached. If hair is left at the electrode site, air will circulate between skin and electrode and will dry out the contact medium causing the electrode to lose electrical contact. If the procedure will be short or clipping the hair is undesirable, moistening the hair with alcohol followed with electrode gel at each electrode site will usually be sufficient. This procedure is especially useful in obtaining a good ECG signal in cats.

ECG Basics

Electrical signals generated within the heart trigger heart muscles to contract and move blood throughout the body. These electrical signals have little bearing on how forcefully blood is moved out of the heart. Therefore, information on the quality of blood flow and tissue perfusion must be garnered by other means.

There is a condition, known as electromechanical disassociation (EMD), where a textbook picture of an ECG may be seen on monitoring equipment and yet no mechanical events follow. The ECG pattern will have changed from the tracing seen at the beginning of the procedure and tissue perfusion and blood pressure will have changed as well. With careful monitoring, remedial action is often possible before this devastating situation is reached. This is a rare condition and patients usually die when EMD occurs. This condition has been seen during anesthesia especially in critical (P5) patients.

The ECG (Figure 4-8) begins with the firing of the sinoatrial (SA) node located high in the right atrium. There are specialized cells in the node that have the property of slow diastolic depolarization. These cells contain cellular elements to spontaneously release a burst of electrical activity. This action potential travels through three pathways made up of specialized cells that carry the electrical impulse to the atrioventricular (AV) node. The signal also spreads cell to cell through atrial muscle leading to depolarization and contraction. The impulse also travels to the left atrium through Bachman's bundle at the top of the atria and through muscle. This electrical activity produces the P wave on the electrocardiogram.

The AV node is capped with a thin layer of specialized cells called junctional tissue that cause the electrical impulse to slow down as it passes through. This results in a delay which permits atrial contraction to occur before the ventricles are signaled to contract, thus allowing the atrial contraction to top off filling of the ventricles before much stronger ventricular muscles contract. This "topping off" is very important even though atrial contraction accounts for only 30% of ventricular filling. It sets the final length on the ventricular myofibrils which determine force of contraction produced by the next heart beat. This is known as the Frank-Starling mechanism and is very important in normal cardiac function.

After the depolarization signal passes through junctional tissue on the top of the AV node, it speeds up as it passes through AV nodal tissue and travels over bundles of specialized cells that carry signals to the right and left ventricles. On the left side of the septum, bundles split again into anterior and posterior fascicles. The signal travels very rapidly through specialized conduction pathways but much slower when traveling through ventricular muscle. Cells in these specialized conduction pathways also have the property of slow diastolic depolarization. The rate at which slow diastolic depolarization occurs is most rapid in the SA node and becomes progressively slower as they travel farther down the conduction system. This is a very important redundant pacemaker system with the cells firing most rapidly serving as the pacemaker thus setting heart rate. Should a higher and therefore, faster pacemaker fail, a lower, but slower pacemaker will take over. Atrial and ventricular muscle cells do not have the ability to spontaneously depolarize. These seemingly disparate facts are important in understanding changes in rate and rhythm that can arise during anesthesia.

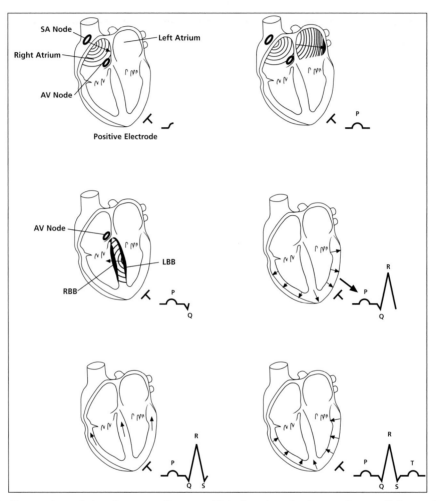

Figure 4-8 Generation of the electrocardiogram. This drawing depicts various cellular action potentials generated by groups of cells within the heart and how their activity is represented in the electrocardiogram recorded at the surface of the body. Sequence of electrical conduction and cardiac chamber activation as it relates to the ECG.
Reprinted with permission. Tilley LP and Burtnick NL, Electrocardiography for the Small Animal Practitioner. Made Easy Series, Teton New Media, 1999.

Heart Rate

Rate of the heart beat is influenced by several intrinsic and extrinsic mechanisms. An intrinsic mechanism causing the heart rate to speed up is an increasing venous return producing additional stretching of the right atrium. The heart rate will speed up to accommodate the increased blood flow and to prevent venous congestion. This mechanism is called the *Bainbridge Reflex*. An intrinsic mechanism tending to slow heart rate occurs with increased levels of physical fitness. This results in an increase in overall blood volume that leads to increased stroke volume; the so called "athletes heart." A slower heart rate occurs to maintain the same cardiac output as compared to when the individual was less physically fit. The autonomic nervous system has profound influences on the heart rate. Humeral influences also affect heart rate. Cholinergic and adrenergic effects slow and speed up the heart, respectively, when these mechanisms are actively engaged. The opposite effect will occur when each is blocked. Vagal influences tend to slow heart rate and the output of the adrenal gland and cardiac accelerator center in the medulla tend to increase heart rate. Therefore, drugs used during anesthesia that block or enhance these mechanisms can have a profound influence on heart rate. The absence of extrinsic mechanisms influences heart rate. Intrinsic heart rate in the awake dog is 140 bpm and 200 bpm in the cat. Effects on heart rate mitigated via the vagas nerve are mechanisms that must be dealt with most often during anesthesia.

Tachycardia

In dogs, heart rate above 160 pm is by definition tachycardia (Figure 4-9). If the rhythm is arising from the SA node as it normally does, it is called sinus tachycardia and represents normal body reaction to the need for increased blood flow. The fastest way the body has to increase cardiac output is to increase heart rate. The cat has a similar response but the sinus rate must be above 240 beats per minute before it is by definition, sinus tachycardia. When the "fight or flight" mechanism is invoked, the first stages result in a rapid increase in heart rate.

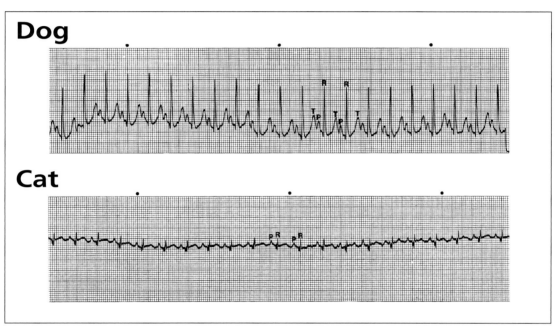

Figure 4-9 Sinus Tachycardia. A fast heart rate associated with regular sinus rhythm. Acceleration of the sinoatrial node beyond its normal discharge rate: > 160 bpm in dogs (180 in toy breeds, 220 in puppies, and 140 in giant breeds) and > 240 in cats. Rhythm is regular possibly with a slight variation in R-R interval. Light anesthesia and inadequate pain management may be associated with this condition.
Reprinted with permission. Tilley LP and Burtnick NL, Electrocardiography for the Small Animal Practitioner. Made Easy Series, Teton New Media, 1999.

Bradycardia

For dogs, a sinus rate below 60 bpm is by definition bradycardia (Figure 4-10). It is well known that in normal sleeping dogs, heart rate often drops below 30 bpm. So it is important to know the condition of the patient when a heart rate determination is made. Dogs under general anesthesia are technically sleeping but because they will be under the influence of particular drugs, the effect of that agent on heart rate must be understood to properly steer a course for that patient through that anesthetic episode. Cats with a faster heart rate will be considered bradycardic at a rate below 120 per minute. However, laid back, awake cats will often have a heart rate below 100.

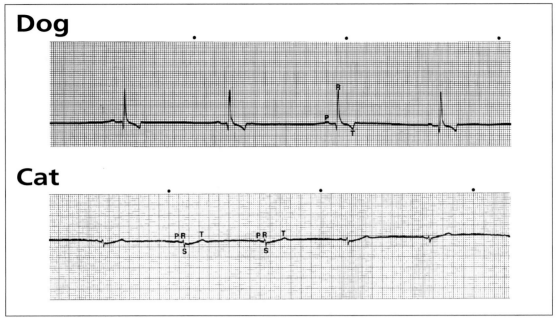

Figure 4-10 Sinus Bradycardia. This is a regular sinus rhythm with heart rate below normal discharge rates. Heart rates below 70 bpm may be normal during anesthesia for large breed dogs and athletes. In cats, it is often associated with a serious underlying disorder, which warrants attention and treatment. All criteria of NSR are met with the exception or a slow heart rate. Rhythm is regular with a slight variation in R-R interval and P-R interval is constant. Treatment is seldom required as long as blood pressure values are within acceptable limits.
Reprinted with permission. Tilley LP and Burtnick NL, Electrocardiography for the Small Animal Practitioner. Made Easy Series, Teton New Media, 1999.

Rhythm

The electrocardiogram is the gold standard for heart rhythm. The most important distinction that an observer of the ECG must unfailingly make is whether the rhythm seen is arising from above the ventricles or below the AV node. A supraventricular arrhythmia may be troublesome but is seldom life threatening. A rhythm that is originating from one of the ventricles, depending on frequency, is just one step from ventricular fibrillation and circulatory arrest.

To properly assess heart rhythm appearing on a monitor during anesthesia, the answers to two very simple and reciprocal questions are crucial: "Is there a P wave for every QRS? Is there a QRS for every P wave?" If the answers are in the affirmative and everything else appears normal, the heart is probably functioning normally. If there is a P wave triggering each QRS and QRS complexes appear normal, the rhythm is supraventricular. If there isn't a P wave triggering the QRS and the QRS complexes are not in the expected configuration, rhythm is ventricular. Accurately answering these two questions provides a clear path to take action or to be comfortable knowing the rhythm is normal.

Normal heart rhythm is a sinus rhythm manifested by the expected P, QRS, and T waves of a normal ECG (Figure 4-11). The SA node is the dominant pacemaker and initiates each heart beat. Depolarizing impulses are conducted as described above and mechanical events follow in proper sequence. In the dog, prominent vagal tone produces a cyclical slowing and speeding of the sinus rate known as sinus arrhythmia (Figure. 4-12). This is normal for the dog. Cats seldom have this arrhythmia.

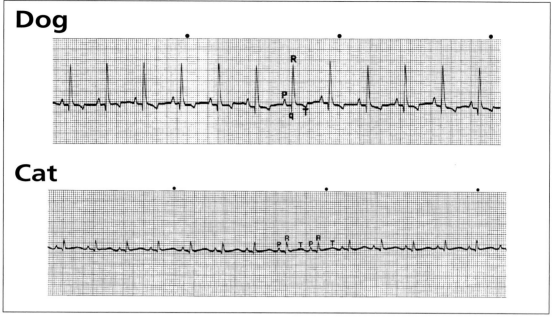

Figure 4-11 Normal sinus rhythm (NSR) in the dog and cat. Sinus rhythm is the normal mechanism for initiating cardiac systole. The normal cardiac impulse originates in the sinoatrial node and spreads to the atria, the atrioventricular node, and ventricles. The rhythm is regular at 70-160 bpm in dogs and 120-240 bpm in cats. A rapid heart rate often makes it difficult to determine where the signal is arising. It is crucial to know if a rhythm is supraventricular or ventricular. There is less than 10% variation in the R-R intervals in dogs. In cats, the difference between the largest and smallest R-R intervals is less than 0.10 sec. P waves are positive in lead II. P-QRS complexes are normal with a constant P-R interval. QRS complexes may be wide and bizarre if an intraventricular conduction defect is present.
Reprinted with permission. Tilley LP and Burtnick NL, Electrocardiography for the Small Animal Practitioner. Made Easy Series, Teton New Media, 1999.

Ventricular Prematurity

A heart beat that is initiated from a ventricle is potentially very dangerous for the patient. When a classical ventricular complex occurs, the QRS is bizarre in shape meaning it does not look like a normal QRS; it is wider than normal QRS complexes, has a T wave that is opposite in polarity to it's QRS complex and is followed by a compensatory pause. If the ventricular complex is occurring early, close on the heels of the previous normal QRS complex, it is called a *premature ventricular complex* or *PVC* (Figure 4-13). If this same appearing QRS complex is occurring late, perhaps after a one or more second delay following the previous normal QRS, it is called an escape beat. Both are arising from the ventricle and may look identical but have very different meanings for the health of the patient.

Because PVCs can signal conditions that can be ranked from benign to lethal, three rules have been established to generally guide the clinician in dealing with them. Intervention may be considered. 1) if PVCs are occurring singly at a rate greater than 20 per minute; 2) PVCs are appearing in runs of *three or more* (Figure. 4-14); 3) the *shape/configuration* of each of these PVCs are different (Figure. 4-15). A single PVC intermixed with normal complexes is seen in patients with normal hearts. If the PVCs are occurring interspersed with normal heart complexes and less than 20 per minute, they will usually not progress to troublesome ventricular arrhythmias. But, if the PVCs are occurring singly and more often than 20 per minute, the potential for progression to a life threatening arrhythmia is real. If PVCs occur in runs of three or more, this by definition is *ventricular tachycardia* (Figure. 4-14) and can easily progress to longer runs of rapid ventricular beats or to *ventricular fibrillation* (Figure. 4-16). In the former, blood flow is severely compromised affecting the

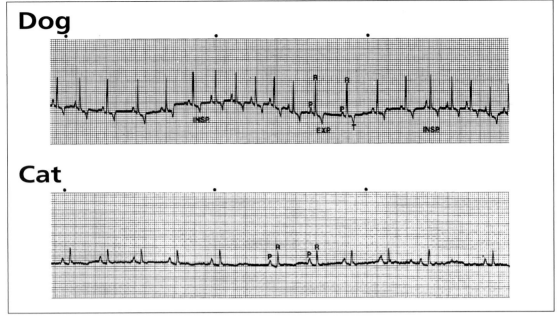

Figure 4-12 Sinus arrhythmia (SA) is a common rhythm seen in normal dogs associated with respiration when conscious. It is can be enhanced by drugs used during anesthesia or SA may not be seen in anesthetized dogs. Cats seldom have this rhythm. It is represented by alternating periods of slower and more rapid heart rates usually related to respiration, heart rate increasing with inspiration (insp) and decreasing with expiration (exp). All Criteria of NSR are met, except that variation of R-R intervals is greater than 10%. P wave, QRS complexes and P-R intervals are normal. A wandering pacemaker (P waves varying in configuration), a variant of SA, is often present. Reprinted with permission. Tilley LP and Burtnick NL, Electrocardiography for the Small Animal Practitioner. Made Easy Series, Teton New Media, 1999.

coronary circulation of the heart itself and in the latter, circulation ceases. If PVCs occur frequently and configuration of the QRS complexes is variable, this suggests that they are arising from more than one site in the ventricles. If more than one area in the ventricle is producing ectopic beats in this fashion, the ventricle has wide spread damage or disease. If any of these three conditions occur, an action plan must be taken immediately to deal with these potentially serious situations (Table 4-2).

One plan might be to carefully watch the rhythm with antiarrhythmic drugs drawn up ready to administer on a moment's notice should the patient's arrhythmia progress in severity. Another plan would be to treat the arrhythmia immediately. The cause of any arrhythmia must be given some consideration. Some of the causes to immediately look for are as follows: inadequate ventilation to the point the myocardium is hypoxic; blood volume is too low to allow proper myocardial perfusion; or something is occurring during surgery that is preventing adequate venous return. If a precipitating cause of an arrhythmia can be identified and eliminated, it may not be necessary to administer an antiarrhythmic drug.

Atrial Prematurity
A heart beat that is arising from above the ventricles is less likely to progress to a life threatening situation. Beats can be initiated in atria, junctional tissue on top of the AV node, or from the AV node. If these are occurring early, they are called atrial premature complexes (APCs) (Figure 4-17), *junctional premature beats* or *AV nodal premature beats* (Figure 4-18). The QRS that follows is usually of the same configuration as the normally conducted sinus nodal impulses for that patient but if the prematurity is early enough, QRS may be slightly altered because repolarization is not quite complete. If these beats are occurring late, they are part of the fail safe mechanism to be sure

Dog

Cat

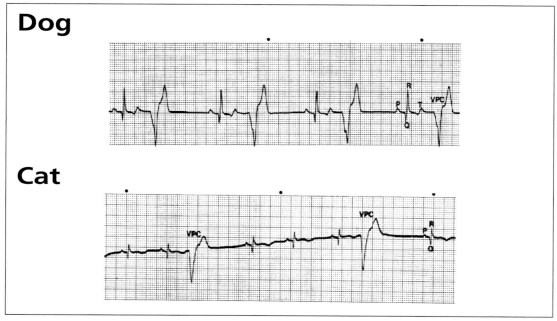

Figure 4-13 Premature Ventricular Complexes (PVCs) are synonymous with Ventricular Premature Complexes (VPCs). PVCs are cardiac impulses initiated within the ventricles instead of the sinus node. Mechanisms include increased automaticity and reentry. PVCS have direct effects on the cardiovascular system with secondary effects on other systems because of poor perfusion. QRS complexes are typically wide and bizarre. P waves are dissociated from QRS complexes and a PVC is usually followed by a compensatory pause. During anesthesia, incidence of PVCs of up to12 per minute are relatively common. However, great concern should be given when PVCs occur during anesthesia at more than 20 per minute and a plan must be established to treat the underlying problem. Cardiovascular monitoring must be continued while attempting to discover if the cause can be identified and eliminated. Reprinted with permission. Tilley LP and Burtnick NL, Electrocardiography for the Small Animal Practitioner. Made Easy Series, Teton New Media, 1999.

pacing activity within the heart is initiating a beat in as timely a fashion as possible. Many drugs used to create anesthesia/analgesia can alter normal pacemaker function and these fail-safe mechanisms may then temporarily appear.

Tachycardia

Tachycardia can be a problem even if it is from the SA node. Heart rates above 170 in the dog and above 250 in the cat can be detrimental to cardiac output. The higher the heart rate is above these numbers, the lower the cardiac output will be, because time for filling is progressively being reduced. Also, fast heart rates do not allow the heart to rest. Myocardial perfusion occurs mostly during diastole and is markedly diminished with high heart rates. Causes of these very fast rates must be determined and when identified, dealt with appropriately. Pain would be the most common cause and administration of proper analgesics will result in a slower heart rate. If sinus tachycardia persists, specific drug therapy may be necessary to lower the heart rate to a safer level.

Bradycardia

Bradycardia is common with certain anesthetic/analgesic agents. Some preanesthetic drugs may produce *bradyarrhythmias.* Anticholinergics used preanesthesia can produce bradyarrhythmias in patients if given in low doses. Some clinicians will administer a low dose of atropine anticipating they will avoid the cardioacceleration effects of the drug. This often works fine but a rare patient may become bradycardic even to the point of inducing a second degree AV block with this approach. Administration of an additional dose of atropine in that rare patient will return the patient to a rapid sinus rhythm (see Table 4-2).

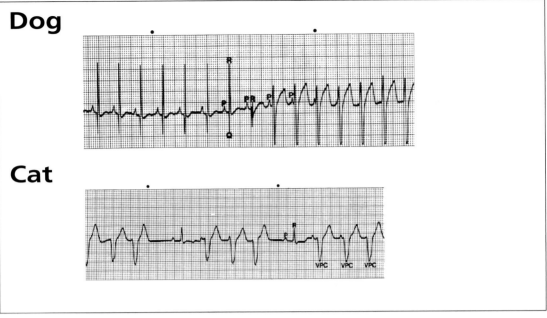

Figure 4-14 Ventricular Tachycardia. Runs of three or more PVCs (also called VPCs) are prone to progress to more serious arrhythmias that will compromise blood flow. V-Tach results from stimulation of an ectopic ventricular focus. Ventricular tachycardia may be intermittent (paroxysmal) or sustained. This is a potentially life threatening arrhythmia, usually signifying an important problem during anesthesia, myocardial disease or metabolic derangement. As a result, actions should be taken to suppress them. Direct effects are on the cardiovascular system, with secondary effects on other systems because of poor tissue perfusion. Ventricular rate is > 150 bpm with a regular rhythm. Ventricular tachycardia between 60-100 bpm is termed idioventricular rhythm. QRS complexes are wide and bizarre. Ventricular fusion and capture complexes occur commonly with ventricular tachycardia. There is no relationship between the QRS complexes and P waves. P waves may precede, be hidden within, or follow the QRS complexes.
Reprinted with permission. Tilley LP and Burtnick NL, Electrocardiography for the Small Animal Practitioner. Made Easy Series, Teton New Media, 1999.

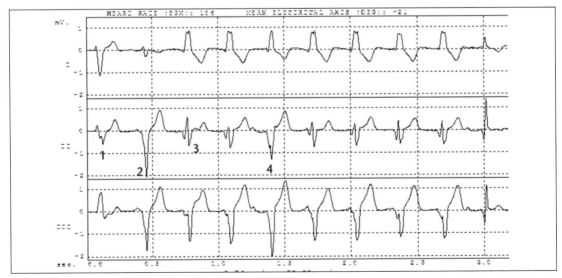

Figure 4-15 Multifocal PVCs that take on various shapes indicate they are arising from different ectopic areas in the ventricles (1,2,3,4). Multifocal PVCs indicate that damage and or disease is widespread through the ventricles. This arrhythmia is very serious and if not controlled quickly, progression to ventricular fibrillation can occur.
Courtesy of Vetronics, INC., West Lafayette, IN

215

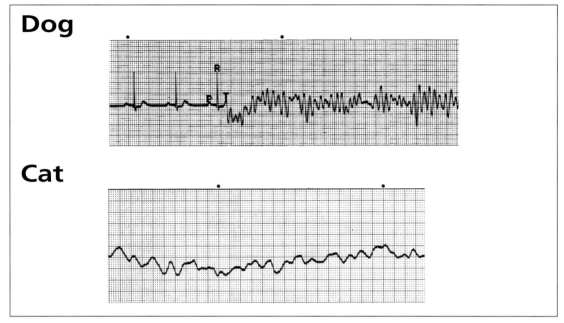

Figure 4-16 Ventricular fibrillation occurs when ventricular myocardial cells depolarize in a chaotic and uncoordinated manner. Blood pressure plummets within seconds and no pulse can be recorded or palpated. Cardiac output approaches zero, making this a life-threatening and generally terminal rhythm. It is associated with rapid, chaotic, irregular rhythm with bizarre waves or oscillations. No QRS complexes or P waves are observed. Oscillations may be large (coarse fibrillation) or small (fine fibrillation).
Reprinted with permission. Tilley LP and Burtnick NL, Electrocardiography for the Small Animal Practitioner. Made Easy Series, Teton New Media, 1999.

Heart Block

Heart blocks occur in two major categories. 1) *Atrioventricular block* (AV Block) where the pacemaker impulse is generated normally in the SA node but cannot get through the AV node or is delayed in reaching the ventricles. AV block is broken down into three categories: *First degree AV block* (Figure 4-19) is a prolongation of the PR interval. Impulses from the SA node get through but are delayed in reaching the ventricles. *Second degree AV block* is an intermittent blockage of some of the signals from the SA node so that there are more P waves than QRS complexes. This can range from an occasional impulse not getting through to multiple P waves before one gets through to the ventricles. *Third degree AV block* (Figure. 4-20) is a complete blockage at the AV area and no impulses can get through. The atria and ventricles are beating independently. In all of these cases, the overall heart rate is usually slow to very slow. 2) The second form of heart block is a *Bundle Branch Block*. The impulse arising normally reaches the conduction system in the ventricles but one of the bundles that branch to the ventricles is blocked. This is manifested as a *Right Bundle Branch Block*, (Figure. 4-21). The left bundle splits into an anterior fascicle and posterior fascicle. The left main bundle may be blocked (Figure 4-22) or there may be a block in either fascicle, e.g. a *Left Anterior Fascicular Block* (Figure 4-23). *Left Posterior Fascicular Block* is very rare.

AV heart block can be caused by anesthetic/analgesic agents and drugs commonly used to treat chronic heart disease. When AV blocks occur by these means, they are often atropine responsive. Right bundle branch block is a benign arrhythmia that has no influence on cardiac function and requires no treatment. The problem with right bundle branch block is that it looks similar to ventricular tachycardia and clinicians will often jump to this conclusion and administer antiarrhythmic drugs that have no positive effect and do not alter rhythm. The procedure might even be aborted unnecessarily. The patient would very likely have suffered no ill effects had anesthesia been continued.

Table 4-2

Antiarrhythmic Therapy

DRUG	D = Dog dose C = Cat dose
SINUS BRADYCARDIA	
Atropine Sulfate	D 0.01-0.04mg/kg IV IM C same
Propantheline Bromide	D small: 7.5mg, TID PO medium: 15mg, TID PO large: 30mg, TID PO C 7.5mg/kg PO TID-QID
Isoproterenol	D 0.04-0.09mcg/kg/min IV C same
Glycopyrrolate	D 0.005-0.01mg/kg IV IM C same
SUPRAVENTRICULAR TACHYCARDIA	
Esmolol	D 0.1-0.5mg/kg, IV Maintenance 0.05-0.2mg/kg/min IV C none
Propranolol	D 0.2-1mg/kg, TID PO 0.05-0.06mg/kg over 5-10 minutes C 2.5-5mg PO BID-TID 0.02-0.06mg/kg IV over 5-10 minutes
Diltiazem	D 0.5-1.5mg/kg PO TID titrate to effect C 0.5-2.5mg/kg PO BID-TID
VENTRICULAR TACHYCARDIA	
Lidocaine	D 2-8mg/kg slowly IV Maintenance 20-100mcg/kg/min IV C 0.25-0.75mg/kg IV over 5 minutes
Mexiletine	D 5-8mg/kg PO BID-TID C none
Procainamide	D 8-20mg/kg PO TID-QID 2mg/kg IV over 3-5 minutes to total dose of 20mg/kg CRI 20-50mcg/kg/min IV C 3-8mg/kg PO TID-QID

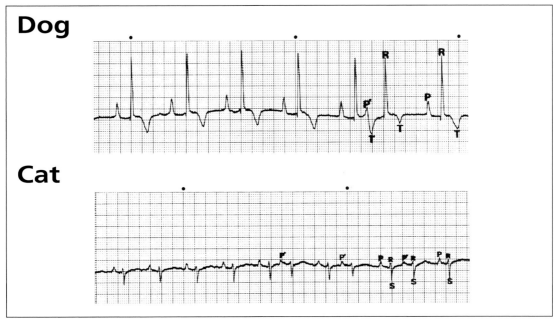

Figure 4-17 Atrial premature complexes (APCs) are common and usually are of no consequence. They are caused by supraventricular impulses originating from an ectopic atrial site (other than the SA node). However, if frequent, they will cause the heart to contract early thus compromising filling. Blood will be pumped by the ventricles so the danger of life threatening problems is relatively low. Heart rate us usually normal, rhythm is irregular due to the premature ectopic P wave that disrupts normal P wave rhythm. APCs are easy to miss because they look just like normally conducted beats except that the P wave unexpectedly touch the T wave of the previous beat. Anesthetists monitoring patients should be wary of this rhythm and be alert to the possibility of progressing to a serious ventricular rhythm.
Reprinted with permission. Tilley LP and Burtnick NL, Electrocardiography for the Small Animal Practitioner. Made Easy Series, Teton New Media, 1999.

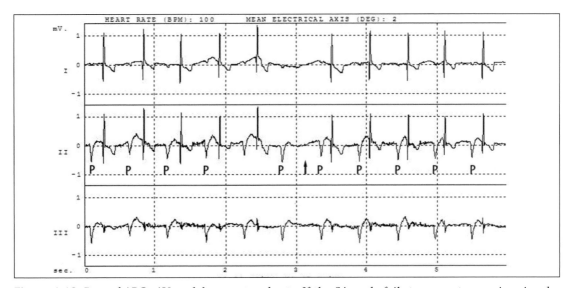

Figure 4-18 Run of APCs AV nodal premature beats. If the SA node fails to generate a pacing signal, the fail safe system will become active. The AV node which has a slower intrinsic pacing rate will become dominant and begin serving as the primary pacemaker. This usually causes no problems for the patient but the clinician should be concerned as to why the SA node is failing to function.
Courtesy of Vetronics, INC., West Lafayette, IN

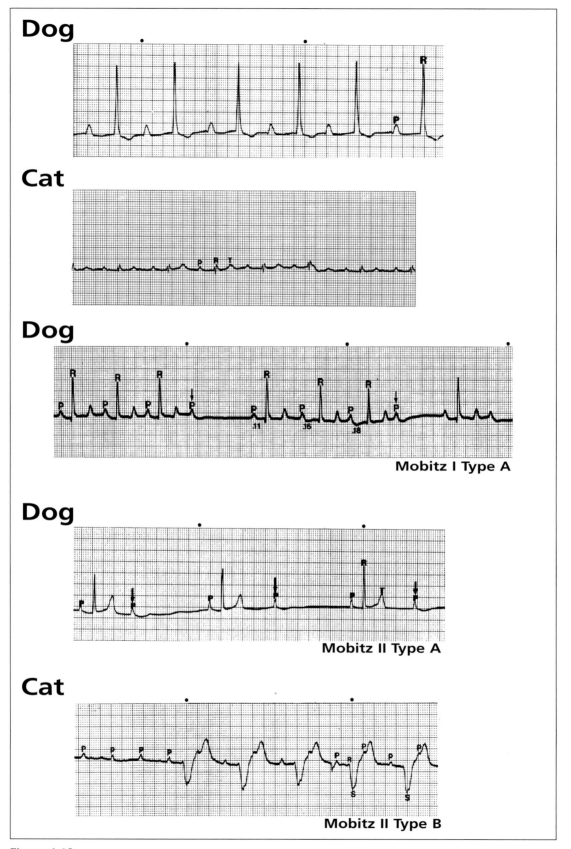

Figure 4-19

Figure 4-19 First-degree and Second-degree atrioventricular (AV) block. Sinoatrial heart blocks occur between the atria and ventricles. The least troublesome form of AV block is first degree AV block which is a delay in conduction of a supraventricular impulse through the AV junction and bundle of His. This rarely causes problems as it is only a prolongation of the PR interval. Second degree AV block is a condition where some impulses from the atria do not make it through to the ventricles. It is characterized by an intermittent failure or disturbance of AV conduction. One or more P waves are not followed by QRS-T complexes. Second degree AV block is classified into two types: Mobitz type I (Wenkebach) and Bobitz type II. Mobitz type I. Mobitz type II is more serious than type I because frequency and severity of the block is unpredictable.

Reprinted with permission. Tilley LP and Burtnick NL, Electrocardiography for the Small Animal Practitioner. Made Easy Series, Teton New Media, 1999.

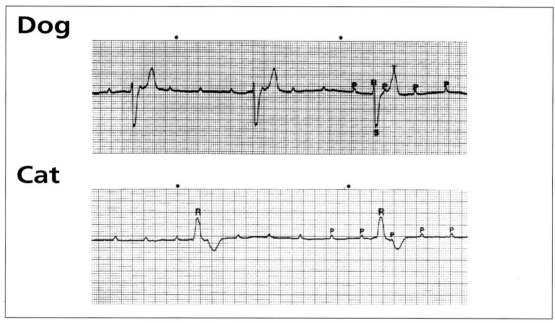

Figure 4-20 Third degree or complete AV block is a condition where none of the signals from the atria get through to the ventricles. There is no conduction between the atria and ventricles as P waves have no constant relationship with QRS complexes. The atrial rate (P-P interval) is normal but the idioventricular escape rhythm is slow. The P-P and R-R intervals are relatively constant except for sinus arrhythmia. Patients can survive with this arrthymia but they cannot increase their heart rate to accommodate increased demand for blood flow. This can obviously be a problem during anesthesia. Causes include aortic stenosis, isolated congenital defects, cardiomyopathy, endocarditis, myocarditis, myocardial infarction, and hyperkalemia. Treatment is with a temporary or permanent pacemaker.

Reprinted with permission. Tilley LP and Burtnick NL, Electrocardiography for the Small Animal Practitioner. Made Easy Series, Teton New Media, 1999.

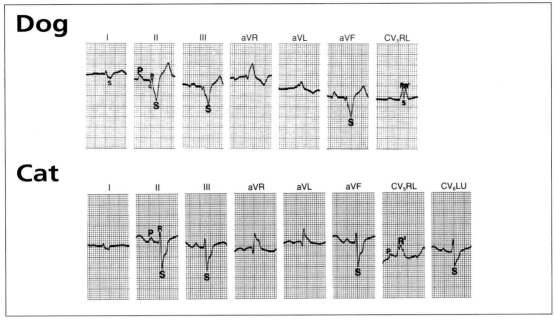

Figure 4-21 Right Bundle Branch Block (RBBB) is a benign but important arrhythmia because it takes on the appearance of ventricular tachycardia. Notice that each ventricular complex is preceded by a P wave. The pacing impulse is conducted normally until it reaches the right bundle. It is blocked and the right ventricle is depolarized by the signal traveling through the heart muscle from the left side of the ventricular septum. This causes the electrical depolarization to be late producing this bizarre complex. Treatment is not needed and the patient is in no difficulty as result of this arrhythmia. It should be of interest to the clinician regarding etiology of the blocked right bundle.
Reprinted with permission. Tilley LP and Burtnick NL, Electrocardiography for the Small Animal Practitioner. Made Easy Series, Teton New Media, 1999.

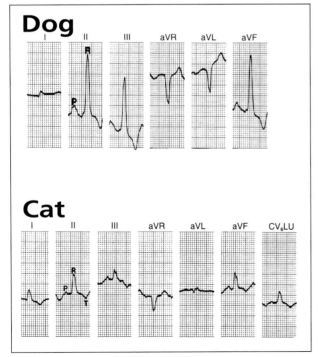

Figure 4-22 Left Bundle Branch Block (LBBB). Conduction delay or block of both the left posterior and left anterior fascicles of the left bundle. A supraventricular impulse activates the right ventricle first through the right bundle branch. The left ventricle is then activated late, causing the QRS to become wide and bizarre. The QRS is prolonged, positive in leads I, II, III, and AVF and the block can be intermittent or constant. LBBB is uncommon in dogs and cants and does not cause hemodynamic abnormalities.
Reprinted with permission. Tilley LP and Burtnick NL, Electrocardiography for the Small Animal Practitioner. Made Easy Series, Teton New Media, 1999.

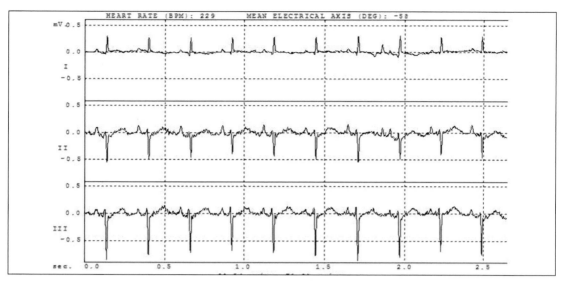

Figure 4-23 Left Anterior Fascicular Block is a common arrhythmia in cats with hypertrophic cardiomyopathy,. There is a severe left axis deviation (-60 degrees) with a qR pattern in Leads I and a rS pattern in Leads II, and III. Terminal QRS forces are slightly wide, suggesting partial right bundle branch block.
Courtesy of Vetronics, INC., West Lafayette, IN

Left bundle branch block often indicates very severe myocardial damage, with cardiomyopathy being the most common. Left bundle branch block will be diagnosed on the pre-anesthetic ECG and the patient should have a complete cardiac work-up before any drug is given. Left anterior fasicular block is quite common in cats with hypertrophic cardiomyopathy. Because the left ventricular chamber size and compliance may be severely restricted, risk status for anesthesia will be higher.

Summary
ECG monitoring during anesthesia provides important information on the patient's cardiac status. If nothing adverse is found, it is comforting to know that good patient management has prevented an adverse effect on the electrical activity of the heart.

Central Venous Pressure
Adequacy of circulating blood volume relative to cardiac compliance can be evaluated by measuring central venous pressure (CVP), which normally ranges from 3 to 8cm H_2O. Central venous pressure is measured at the level of the right atrium, usually with a catheter inserted via a jugular vein to the vena cava. If taken from a peripheral vein, venous pressure may be 8 to 12cm H_2O. An estimate of CVP can be made just by observing the hair over the jugular vein as it moves to the heart beat. In general, if arterial pressure, urine output and venous pressure are all low, either circulating blood volume is inadequate or venous capacitance is excessive. Low arterial pressure and oliguria combined with an elevated venous pressure (above 15cm H_2O) are suggestive of myocardial depression and the use of inotropic drugs may be indicated.

Venous pressure, either central or peripheral, may be used to assess changes in blood volume that may be caused by blood or water loss. Measurement may be made with a conventional manometer or by using the administration set and IV bottle already in place for fluid therapy and preferably connected to IV extension tubing. Disconnect the drip chamber from the bottle and allow the fluid to move down the tubing until it is even with or above the level of the heart. Mark the zero reference (level of the right atrium) on the tube and measure the fluid level with a centimeter ruler to obtain the venous pressure. Reinsert the drip chamber into the fluid bottle and either lower the bottle until blood forces the air back into the bottle or disconnect the line from the catheter to evacuate the air and reconnect it.

During rapid infusion of blood or crystalloid fluid, venous pressure often rises transiently above normal but usually falls with equilibration of fluid in the body compartments. If this does not occur, other causes must be determined and fluid administration must be modified.

Ventilation

Observation of the thorax and abdomen with the chest closed or the lungs with the chest open helps one assess adequacy of pulmonary ventilation. Auscultation of breath sounds through an esophageal stethoscope will provide information pertaining to both lung and airway problems.

Frequency, Tidal Volume, and Minute Ventilation

Rate of breathing is easily counted and with spontaneous breathing, tidal volume should be regular during maintenance anesthesia. It may be irregular and rapid during the light phase of anesthesia and at maintenance levels in times of deep pain, such as during manipulation of the ovarian pedicle or stimulation of the periosteum. Respiratory rate is usually maintained between 8 and 20 BPM although tachypnea or panting may occasionally be encountered. The combination of tachypnea, reduced tidal volume and increased physiological dead space serves to reduce alveolar ventilation. In these circumstances, controlled ventilation should be provided to maintain adequate alveolar ventilation. One of the best clues to depressed ventilation is the inability to maintain adequate levels of inhalation anesthesia with expected vaporizer settings. For example, for a patient in which 2% isoflurane is expected to be sufficient, but that requires above 3%; and assuming that there are no leaks in the system and the endotracheal cuff is properly inflated, depressed ventilation may be the cause.

Not all anesthetized patients have depressed ventilation but it is an expected consequence of general anesthesia. In patients anesthetized with isoflurane and sevoflurane at normal values during surgery, $PaCO_2$ is commonly maintained between 35 and 45mm Hg with spontaneous breathing. Of course, an excellent means of monitoring the adequacy of ventilation is to measure expired and/or arterial $PaCO_2$. Spirometry may be used to measure tidal volume. Because condensation of exhaled water vapor interferes with function of mechanical spirometers, intermittent rather than continuous use of spirometry is advisable.

Minute ventilation is the product of tidal volume (V_T) and frequency (f), and by subtracting estimated dead space (V_D) one can obtain an estimate of alveolar ventilation: $V_A = (V_T - V_p) \times f$. Estimated V_T is 10ml/kg and estimated V_D is 5ml/kg of body weight during spontaneous breathing (Severinghaus and Stupfel 1958). The whistle device placed on the inspiratory or expiratory side of the circle system breathing circuit, which is used to provide an indication of frequency, is not recommended because it increases the resistance to breathing.

Without analytical methods of measuring carbon dioxide and oxygen during anesthesia, one must rely on subjective clinical observations. Rate of breathing is useful from the standpoint of identifying abnormally slow (bradypnea) or rapid (tachypnea) breathing or absence of breathing (apnea). In addition, the character of the breathing effort is very important and provides information regarding anesthetic depth. Breathing should be regular and smooth both at the beginning and end of the breath. Exaggerated breathing determined either by the presence of large tidal volumes or rapid rate may be suggestive of light anesthesia. In contrast, slow, regular and shallow breathing may suggest CNS depression and deep anesthesia.

Auscultation

Monitoring heart and respiratory sounds is helpful in identifying abnormalities. As a general rule, breathing efforts that are difficult to hear even with an esophageal stethoscope are probably associated with respiratory depression and deep anesthesia. Abnormal breaths associated with snoring, wheezing, bubbling or muffled sounds should be investigated immediately to localize the problem.

Mucous Membrane Color

Cyanosis is usually associated with inadequate oxygenation but also may be indicative of poor tissue perfusion. If cyanosis occurs during anesthesia, it is a bad sign indicative of impending death. The patient should be checked immediately and controlled breathing instituted immediately. In addition, the anesthetic system must be examined to determine adequacy of oxygen supply and whether there is a problem with the endotracheal tube. Cyanosis may also be a sign of inadequate blood flow during shock, deep anesthesia, or cardiac arrest. This can be confirmed by the lack of heart sounds, weak or absent pulse, fixed and dilated pupils, etc. Immediate action is then required.

Oxygen

Adequacy of oxygenation of arterial blood can be estimated by looking for cyanosis. Conditions such as hypothermia, hypotension and pigmentation as well as the intensity and color of incident light all interfere with the use of cyanosis as a reliable sign of arterial oxygenation. Cyanosis can usually be seen when the PaO_2 is below 60mm Hg, but assessment of specific levels is difficult. Color of the oral mucous membranes, ocular sclera and blood in the surgical field is a more dependable indicator of oxygenation and tissue perfusion.

Measurement of PaO_2 is the most readily acceptable method for accurate assessment of oxygenation. Recent improvements in noninvasive PaO_2 monitoring using fiberoptic light transmission and computer analysis compensate for factors such as skin pigmentation and tissue thickness. Cost of these devices is high and precludes their routine use; perhaps they will become economically feasible in the near future.

The anesthetist must understand that color of the mucous membrane is not a reliable indicator of the adequacy of ventilation. If the membranes look pink, oxygenation may be adequate but the $PaCO_2$ is not necessarily optimal. However, when cyanosis is detected, both ventilation and tissue perfusion must be evaluated promptly.

Pulse Oximetry

Arterial PO_2 is a measure of the oxygenating efficiency of the lungs. In addition, the percent hemoglobin saturation (SaO_2) and the oxygen content can be measured to assess oxygenation of blood. Prior to 1972, visual inspection of mucous membrane color was the only noninvasive method used to assess a patient's arterial oxygen concentration (Butinar et al. 1991). Pulse oximetry has improved accuracy of this assessment and has become the standard of monitoring human patients along with blood pressure and ECG. It might be the only monitor used in patients undergoing procedures that only require conscious sedation. Pulse oximetry can be incorporated into multivariable monitors (see Figure 4-3) or may be stand alone units (Figure 4-24).

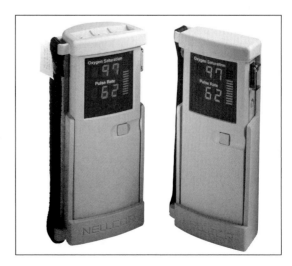

Figure 4-24 Nelcor Model N20 Pulse oximeters. Oxygen saturation is indicated at the top, pulse rate at the bottom. The indicator on the right side of the screen rises and falls with each pulse. On some monitors, the wave form is shown across the screen.
Courtesy of Nellcor, Pleasanton, CA.

Determination of SaO_2 by pulse oximetry is possible because oxyhemoglobin and reduced hemoglobin (desaturated) absorb light differently. Therefore each time a pulse of arterial blood passes under the light-emitting probe, the amount of light exposed to a photodetector on the opposite of the vascular bed will vary based upon the relative amount of oxyhemoglobin.

Values of arterial oxygen hemoglobin saturation greater than 90% are acceptable. However, hypoxia rapidly develops as this percentage drops below 90% and an alarm on the monitor will be activated when oxygen saturation is detected below 90%. Severe hypoxia (SaO_2 less than 85%) for short periods (less than 5 min) may result in cell death. The probe of the oximeter must be attached to any pulsating arterial bed. The tongue is the most useful site but the tail, toe web or ear pinna may also be used. Thick skin in some areas and dark pigmentation may alter accuracy of measurements. Most pulse oximeters provide an accurate assessment of pulse rate up to 250 BPM.

Pulse oximeters provide information on both pulse rate and SaO_2. More sophisticated monitoring devices provide a small screen illustrating the wave form of the pulse and will even indicate when a weak pulse is detected. In general, the 90-80-70 to 60-50-40 rule may be used to estimate PaO_2: O_2 saturation of 90% estimates a PaO_2 of 60, 80% estimates 50mm Hg, and 70% estimates 40mm Hg. Low oxygen levels must be corrected immediately which might be due to hypoventilation, hypercarbia, inadequate oxygen supply, problems with pulmonary function or reduced cardiac output.

Carbon Dioxide

A capnograph can be used to estimate alveolar and arterial levels of carbon dioxide (Moens & Verstraeten 1982). With the capnograph, hypoventilation (increased CO_2) or hyperventilation (decreased CO_2) can be assessed. The problem of obtaining a representative sample during shallow breathing must be taken into consideration but this is an excellent means of monitoring adequacy of ventilation in the anesthetized patient. Most veterinary capnographs use a side stream port inserted between the ET tube and breathing circuit. Sampling rate will be 50-150ml/min and gases from the exit port of the capnograph need to be captured and expelled in the anesthetic machine scavenging system.

CO_2 is the primary controller of breathing in medullary centers of the brain. Normal $PaCO_2$ is 36 (range 34-38) mmHg in the dog and 30 (range 29-31) mmHg in cats. $PaCO_2$ is measured with a blood gas analyzer from an arterial sample of blood and is discussed later in this chapter. Monitoring CO_2 levels in expired breaths using capnography can provide an estimate of $PaCO_2$ during anesthesia. Capnographs are readily available and may be used to monitor both rate of breathing and adequacy of respiration on a breath by breath basis (Butinar et al. 1991) (Figure 4-25). Shape of the tracing is important with baseline being essentially zero. A rising baseline reflects rebreathing of CO_2. The highest number is obtained at the end of the breath and is referred to as end-tidal (ET) CO_2. During anesthesia, ET CO_2 should be below 50mmHg in dogs and 40mm Hg in cats. Adjustments can be made by changing depth of anesthesia to improve efficiency of spontaneous breathing or controlling ventilation.

Methods most often used to assess respiratory function were discussed in the previous section. However, the best measure of effective pulmonary ventilation is CO_2 and with this variable, the anesthetist can evaluate status of inspired CO_2, (which should be below 0.3%) whether sponta-neous breathing is adequate, whether controlled ventilation has been provided appropriately and information about circulation as well. Capnography is of definite value in anesthesia for patients at risk.

Body Temperature

Thermal regulation is depressed by most anesthetics and therefore body temperature will fall during anesthesia. This tendency is further compounded by clipping, surgical prepping with cold

Figure 4-25 This multivariable monitor screen includes tracing for ECG at top, Respiratory Rate (RR) in the middle and capnograph at the bottom of the screen. Et CO_2 is listed as 38 mm Hg; Respiratory Rate (RR)15; NIBP Systolic/Diastolic (Mean Pressure) mm Hg. In the right vertical column, Heart Rate (HR Lead II is 120 BPM, RR is 15 breaths per min, %SpO_2 98; Pulse Rate (PR) 119 and Rectal Temp is 100.9°F. This screen photo is from a Cardell Veterinary Monitor, Model 9405.
Courtesy of Sharn Veterinary, Tampa, FL.

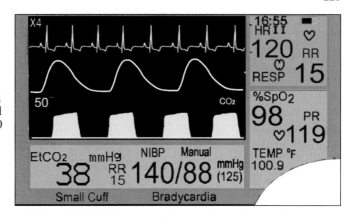

fluids including alcohol which induces evaporative loss of body temperature, administration of room temperature IV fluids, opening the chest or abdomen and placing patients on a large, cold surface such as an unpadded steel table. Cats and small dogs, that have a large surface-area-to-body-mass ratio, are particularly subject to hypothermia during anesthesia and this can occur in less than 30 minutes. Although less common, hyperthermia can occur in patients placed on overheated water blankets or insulated thermally by surgical drapes and in some arctic breeds that appear to conserve heat rather than to lose it. Occasionally cats may become hyperthermic after hydromorphone administration.

The routine use of a water blanket with thermostatically controlled heater and pump will prevent the drop of body temperature below 35°C (98°F) for most patients. Temperature of the pump should be maintained between 90 and 105°F as indicated on the pump dial. The highest temperature setting is best for animals larger than 5kg but the thermostat should be set at 37.5°C (100°F) for smaller patients in order to avoid hyperthermia.

Monitoring body temperature is especially useful for long procedures. It can be conveniently measured with a battery-powered electronic telethermometer and a thermistor placed in the esophagus at the level of the heart to obtain the best estimate of core temperature. Electronic digital thermometers for monitoring rectal temperature are available and temperature can be included as a component of multivariable monitoring systems. Although less convenient (but also less expensive), a mercury laboratory thermometer can be used to record rectal temperature. However, temperature in the rectum will fall more slowly and depending on the time course, will not provide a good estimate of core temperature. Clinical thermometers are not suitable because they do not register a continuous decrease in temperature.

It is best to avoid profound hypothermia during anesthesia, as it would prolong recovery. Hypothermia decreases MAC and increases the solubility of inhalation anesthetics. Therefore, if the anesthetist provides the same anesthetic concentrations during hypothermia as in normothermia, deep and prolonged anesthesia will be the consequence. Anesthetics depress the normal body mechanism in the CNS that maintain normal temperature. As a result, hypothermia is an expected consequence and is time related. With procedures lasting more than one hour, body temperatures between normal and 35°C are common and usually are not problematic. However, temperatures below 35°C will result in reduced anesthetic requirements and influence recovery from anesthesia. Oxygen should be provided during rewarming when shivering is present, to avoid hypoxemia.

Miscellaneous
Pressure in the anesthesia circuit is easily monitored with an aneroid manometer, available on most anesthetic machines. This is useful in helping the anesthetist ensure that the pressure applied to the patient's lung is within safe limits. Airway pressure produced when the lungs are inflated with a fixed volume is a rough measure of pulmonary compliance. Decreased compliance is a

signal of pulmonary edema, hydrothorax, or pneumothorax. This decreased compliance can also be "felt" by manually compressing the rebreathing bag.

Urinary Output

Catheterization of the urinary bladder provides the opportunity to monitor urine output. This is especially valuable in high risk patients undergoing major surgery and in patients recovering from anesthesia. Oliguria can result from reduced circulating blood volume, antidiuretic effects of anesthetics, stress of surgery or acute renal failure. Infusion of fluids should be made to maintain urine output at greater than 0.3ml/kg/hr.

Monitoring urinary output during anesthesia is indicated in patients with compromised renal function and is especially useful in long surgical procedures even in normal patients. Placement of a urinary catheter can be done while the anesthetized patient is being prepared for surgery (Haskins 1987). Once secured in place, the catheter is connected to a closed-system urine collection bag. The goal will be to maintain intraoperative urinary output at 1 to 2ml\kg\hr.

Anesthetic Depth

The recognizable phases of anesthesia were clearly described by Guedel as four stages: I, amnesia and analgesia; II, delirium; III, surgical anesthesia; and IV, premortem (Guedel 1971). For more accurate estimation of depth, stage III was arbitrarily divided into four planes. For the human patient anesthetized with ether, Guedel described respiratory changes, pupillary alterations, eye movements and swallowing and vomiting responses. Gillespie added reflex responses: laryngeal and pharyngeal reactivity, lacrimation and respiratory response to surgical incision (Gillespie 1943). This system applied only to the unpremedicated human patient allowed to breathe spontaneously during ether anesthesia, a situation that does not exist in modern practice. Anesthetists today use a more logical though less well-defined system than Guedel's, but one that is more appropriate. Anesthetics alter the patient's reaction to various stimuli. It is important to evaluate the stimulus and response in terms of the differences among animals, breeds and species, a problem unique to the veterinary anesthetist (Table 4-3).

Stimulus-response Assessment

Because of the routine use of premedicants and various IV induction techniques, classical stages of sedation, analgesia and delirium are usually not seen. Even during inhalation induction, Guedel's stages I and II are not easily separated and may be regarded as a single level, that of presurgical anesthesia. Signs indicative of change from presurgical to surgical anesthesia are loss of palpebral reflex, onset of muscle relaxation and onset of rhythmic breathing. If these have not occurred, the patient is still at the presurgical level and stimulation must be avoided. When they are present, degree of surgical anesthesia can then be evaluated.

Presurgical anesthesia, surgical anesthesia and anesthetic overdose define the magnitude of anesthetic depression. Surgical anesthesia may be subjectively divided into three planes: too light, adequate, and too deep (Table 4-3). The anesthetist must evaluate the intensity of nervous system stimulation, observe physiologic responses and then interpret the interaction of patient, stimulus, and anesthetic to deduce the level of surgical anesthesia. The difficulty of learning anesthetic assessment is brought into perspective when one compares the signs produced by isoflurane with those produced by ketamine in the cat. With isoflurane, muscle relaxation is present and palpebral responses are absent, whereas the opposite is the case with ketamine.

Stimulus

The intensity of pain stimulation is quite variable. High-intensity pain results from skin and joint capsule incision, periosteal stimulation, fracture manipulation, visceral or peritoneal traction, diaphragmatic stimulation, manipulation of the cornea and excessive distension of the urinary bladder. During surgical anesthesia at a level that previously seemed adequate, the patient may

Table 4-3

Evaluations of Response to Painful Stimulation During Anesthesia

Level of Anesthesia	Sensory Response	Motor Response	Reflexes		
			Circulatory	*Respiratory*	*Gastrointestinal*
Too light	Breathholding Deep breathing Stiff chest Phonation Laryngospasm Tachycardia Rise or fall in BP Movement with stimulus Coughing	Fine or gross movement Abdominal tightness	Bradycardia and hypotension or Tachycardia and hypertension Arrhythmias	Spasm: laryngeal bronchiolar Salivation Dysrhythmic breathing	Retching Vomiting Swallowing
Adequate	Minimal response	Quiet surgical field to painful stimuli followed by accommodation	Absence of troublesome CV, respiratory, and GI reflexes Relaxation of skeletal muscles		
Too deep	No response	Flaccid muscles Inability to re-establish normal breathing at the end of anesthesia	Bradycardia Tachycardia Hypotension	Arrest (in the absence of hypocarbia)	Intestinal atony Postoperative ileus

(Modified from Dripps, R. D., Eckenhoff, J. E., and Vandam, L. D.: Introduction to Anesthesia. 5th ed. Philadelphia, W. B. Saunders Co., 1977.)

show signs of light anesthesia such as tachycardia, tachypnea and even movement whenever one or more of these events occur. In anticipation, the anesthetist may increase the anesthetic concentration briefly, fully aware of the further depression of cardiopulmonary function and then return the concentration to the previous level when appropriate. Weak stimulation results from toe pinch, wound debridement, mild distension of the bladder and manipulation of fascia or muscle without traction. No appreciable change in maintenance levels should occur with muscle or connective tissue dissection or bowel resection and suturing. Inflammation of the tissue will usually increase intensity of the stimulus, and careful handling of tissue may decrease intensity. Younger animals may show increased intensity, whereas older animals and animals with a fair, poor or critical physical status may have a decreased response. For this reason, the high-risk patient is more difficult to monitor.

If the anesthetist is to maintain the appropriate level of anesthesia, surgical activity must be considered along with the patients' responses. Too often clinicians maintain anesthesia unnecessarily deep to prevent any type of movement instead of providing only the level appropriate for the type of surgery being performed.

Response
Evaluation of responses from painful stimulation during anesthesia is difficult for the beginner but with experience one finds the combination of signs to be a useful guide to anesthetic depth. The three components of evaluation are classified as sensory, motor and reflex functions. Intensity of these responses are separated into three levels: high = light anesthesia, adequate = acceptable anesthesia, and low = too deep anesthesia. These responses are collated in Table 4-3. A comparison of strength of the surgical stimulus and observation of intensity of response is what the good anesthetist learns and practices in order to deliver the appropriate anesthetic level. When the high-risk patient cannot tolerate deeper anesthesia, a balanced approach with use of a neuromuscular blocker may be needed to provide the degree of muscle relaxation needed.

Also, as uptake of inhaled anesthesia continues and approaches equilibration in body tissues, inspired concentrations should be gradually reduced to avoid deeper anesthesia than necessary. Surgical anesthesia usually appears to be deeper than it really is and one may need to lighten inspired concentrations to check the level. This is one of the great values of using NIBP to monitor anesthetic depth. As a general rule, induction should be carried a little deeper than seems necessary for incision to avoid difficulties of inadequate anesthesia. Then a middle course should be taken between light and unnecessarily deep anesthesia.

Levels of Anesthesia
Too Light
One of the most aggravating and typical problems using potent low solublity inhalation anesthetics, e.g., sevoflurane or isoflurane, is the situation when a patient responds to surgical stimulus or appears to wake up prematurely. This usually follows induction when the patient seems to be adequately anesthetized. The obvious problems should be eliminated first. Anesthetic equipment should be checked for leaks (preferably preanesthesia), the vaporizer examined for liquid level and all connections should be intact. The position of the endotracheal tube must be verified for proper placement and to determine that the distal end is not beyond the thoracic inlet and possibly in one main bronchus. One can feel for the tip by gently lifting the trachea and the trachea will bend where the end of the tube is positioned. A 50% shunt because of improper tube position will result in inadequate levels of anesthesia and is most evident with the less soluble anesthetics. If the tube is too short, the end of the ET tube may be in the trachea but the cuff may be located in the oral pharynx. Thus air is allowed to enter the trachea around the ET tube and dilute the inhaled gases.

Most often, the problem of patients being too light is related to the oxygen flow rate being too low. The common complaint in this regard is that there seems to be a problem with relatively big dogs compared to small dogs: small ones stay anesthetized, big ones wake up. The answer to this problem is to use a higher flow during induction to adequately deliver anesthetics to the alveoli. For example, guidelines listed above suggest providing 500ml/min oxygen for animals up to 25kg during maintenance but for induction, that flow rate should be doubled, e.g., 1000ml/min.

If surgery has already started and the patient responds, it may be necessary to administer a supplemental analgesic drug to return the animal to an adequate level of anesthesia while the source of the problem is resolved. Lack of preemptive analgesia may also be the problem.

Adequate

A quiet surgical field, good tissue oxygenation, acceptable NIBP and other measured variables and no ECG abnormalities, all equate to a good level of anesthesia and analgesia. If everything has been done correctly and essential monitoring systems are in place, all is well (Table 4-3).

Too Deep

One of the most obvious reasons for a patient being too deeply anesthetized is relative overdose. Inappropriate administration of inhalation agents or failure to monitor the patient adequately can result in deep anesthesia. Treatment of excessive inhalation anesthesia is accomplished by flushing the anesthetic unit (circle system), decreasing the vaporizer setting and ventilating the patient to lighten the level of anesthesia.

Overdose with an injectable agent is many times not easily resolved. Antagonists are not available for some injectable anesthetics, but deep sedation with an opioid can be reversed with naloxone. Geriatric, pediatric and sick patients have lower anesthetic requirements. Therefore, if doses of anesthetic drugs are given to these animals in the same way they are to normal healthy patients, excessive anesthesia may be the consequence. Obesity will also create a situation of excessive anesthetic depth. Doses of injectable drugs are calculated based on body weight but because fat does not play a role in the uptake and distribution of anesthetic drugs during clinical anesthesia, a relative overdose will likely be given. For example, a Beagle that weighs 25kg, but should weigh only 15kg, can possibly receive 60 to 100mg in excess of the calculated dose.

In very small patients or in patients undergoing longer procedures, a profound decrease in body temperature is a common sequel. Below 35°C, hypothermia decreases anesthetic requirements and also increases the solubility of inhalation agents thus allowing tissues including the brain to absorb more anesthetic. All of this contributes to excessive anesthesia in patients that are cold. Pregnant animals near term also have decreased anesthetic requirements as do animals with hyponatremia, shock, acute anemia, and those under the influence of other CNS depressants.

Fluid Therapy

IV administration of drugs, electrolyte solutions and blood is an integral part of anesthetic management. In the anesthetized patient, routine monitoring of variables such as blood pressure, pulse rate, venous pressure and ECG are all used to estimate adequacy or inadequacy of circulating intravascular volume. It is important to understand how this fluid compartment interacts with fluid compartments of the body and how they are influenced by what we do or do not do.

Body Fluid Compartments

There are two major compartments of total body water: intracellular and extracellular. Subdivisions of extracellular fluid (ECF) are the intravascular and interstitial compartments and all areas are in equilibrium. ECF volume accounts for about 20% of normal body weight or about 33% of total body water. Approximately 20% of ECF is intravascular (plasma volume) while the balance is interstitial fluid.

Several homeostatic mechanisms are used by the body to maintain proper balance between the size of the intravascular space and plasma volume. Mobilization of protein and the vasoactivity of the capacitance vessels are two primary mechanisms. Changes in ECF are reflected by proportional changes in both interstitial volume and plasma volume of the intravascular space. Therefore, maintenance of normal ECF volume is essential in maintaining adequate blood volume.

Water freely moves between these compartments, whereas size of molecules such as plasma proteins limits their movement. Certain electrolytes do not cross cell membranes with the result that water diffuses across the membranes to maintain osmotic equilibrium.

Concepts of Tonicity and ECF

For an understanding of the relationship of tonicity to solutes and solvents in the body, definitions of osmolarity and osmolality are presented in Table 4-4. The major extracellular cation is sodium. Two other osmotically active substances are urea and glucose. Therefore, in patients with uremia or severe hyperglycemia, these molecules will add to the total osmolality. Urea crosses cell membranes and does not cause acute shifts in water between the extracellular and intracellular compartments. However, sodium, glucose and mannitol do not readily cross cell membranes and can cause a loss of intracellular fluid (ICF). In clinical situations, such as fever or exposure of thoracic or abdominal viscera, water is lost without solute. Without fluid replacement, a hyperosmolar or hypertonic state exists. Hyperosmolarity exists if serum osmolality exceeds 340mOsm/L or serum sodium is greater than 160mEq/L. In contrast, hypo-osmolarity exists if serum osmolality is less than 240mOsm/L or serum sodium is less than 110mEq/L.

Table 4-4

Concepts of Osmolarity and Osmolality

1 Mol. Wt. (1 mole) = 6.06×10^{23} molecules (Avogadro's number)

1 Osmole = 1 mole/L of solution

1 Milliosmole (mOsm) = 1/1000 osmole/L

Osmolarity = osmoles/L of solution

Osmolality = osmoles/1000g solvent

Osmolality = osmolarity (in dilute solutions)

Osmolality of extracellular fluid = 280 to 305 mOsm/L

Hyperosmolarity = osmolality > 340mOsm/L or serum Na > 160mEq/L

Hypo-osmolarity = osmolality < 240mOsm/L or serum Na < 110mEq/L

When tonicity rises in the normal conscious patient, sensors in the posterior hypothalamus induce increased water intake by means of thirst and more antidiuretic hormone (ADH) is released from the posterior pituitary to increase water resorption from the renal tubules. This occurs at the expense of increasing ECF volume. The volume maintenance system then returns ECF volume toward normal. Through a complex mechanism of a decrease in renin release by the kidney and in angiotensin II and aldosterone, less sodium is retained from the proximal renal tubules. This lowers ECF tonicity, causing shifts of intracellular water and decreases in thirst and ADH in order to return ECF toward normal.

These homeostatic mechanisms may be upset by a number of factors especially those related to anesthesia and surgery: (1) restriction of water and electrolyte intake; (2) fluid and electrolyte deficits or excesses as a consequence of disease or injury; (3) iatrogenically produced deficits or excesses; and (4) inappropriate ADH secretion induced by anesthetics, stress, pain, blood loss and positive pressure ventilation.

Fluid Therapy for Elective Surgery

Use of isotonic fluids in the anesthetized patient undergoing surgery or diagnostic procedures helps maintain hydration necessary for adequate tissue perfusion and renal function and for prevention of severe hypotension. Because most animals have food and perhaps water withheld preoperatively, a certain amount of water and solute is lost. Water is lost primarily via kidneys, lungs, skin, mouth and gastrointestinal tract. In addition to these presurgical losses, anesthetized patients lose fluid as a result of blood loss, humidification of inspired gases, tissue edema and tissue trauma. Hypovolemia may also occur owing to vascular dilatation induced by drugs.

Use of Lactated Ringer's solution (LRS) is preferable for maintenance fluid therapy as there appears to be little advantage in using more complex solutions except in special circumstances. In patients who have not eaten for a period of days or in small patients susceptible to hypoglycemia, use of 5% dextrose is indicated. This will create a hypertonic solution and so the total volume given should not be excessive. The recommended rate of administration is 10ml/kg per hour of anesthesia for normal maintenance. The average "adult" drip set delivers 15 drops per ml while pediatric sets deliver 60 drops per ml. It is best to check with the manufacturer's specifications provided with the packaging. The rate may be increased as needed to meet losses due to a variety of causes. In situations in which blood loss is anticipated, drip rate may be started at 15 to 20ml/kg/hr to increase plasma volume ahead of time. Automated IV infusion systems are very much indicated for fluid administration during anesthesia and surgery.

For most circumstances, an IV catheter should be placed before anesthesia induction to provide an easy route for injection of anesthetics and for administration of emergency drugs should the need arise. In hard-to-handle patients for which preanesthesia catheter placement is not feasible, the catheter should be placed as soon as possible following induction.

For healthy patients undergoing short minor procedures, the decision not to use fluids may be indicated. However, this should be the exception, as even in a healthy patient the normal homeostatic mechanism will be disturbed by general anesthesia. High-risk and geriatric patients who require higher fluid intake for compensated renal disease and patients undergoing extensive surgery must certainly receive fluid therapy.

Caution must be exercised in patients with heart failure or pulmonary edema. For the heart patient, 5% dextrose in water is indicated under conditions of sodium restriction and the rate of administration may be decreased to prevent water intoxication. Fluid therapy must also be restricted in patients undergoing correction of patent ductus arteriosus. Because of the vascular shunt from the congenital anomaly, fluid overload may occur when the ductus is ligated. Therefore, a diuretic is indicated presurgically and only enough fluid should be given to provide a convenient means for drug administration, i.e., to keep the catheter open (TKO).

Use of Balanced Electrolyte Solutions for Replacement of Blood Loss

The recommendation of 10ml/kg/hr is based on meeting probable losses of water during anesthesia and surgery. In patients requiring intravascular volume replacement for hemorrhage of less than 20% of blood volume, replacement can be maintained with saline or isotonic electrolyte solution at the rate of two to three times the estimated blood loss. Blood volume in the dog is estimated at 90ml per kg of body weight. Blood volume in the cat is slightly less.

When blood loss exceeds 20% of the blood volume, whole blood replacement is indicated. Rate of administration depends on whether losses are continuing and on the status of intravascular volume as indicated by central venous and arterial pressures. As a general rule, blood replacement should be given at the rate of 1 to 3ml/kg/hr. If ACD anticoagulant solution has been used and crystalloid solutions are given concurrently through the same catheter, fluids containing calcium should be avoided.

Rapid Method of Monitoring (estimating) Blood Loss During Surgery

When excessive bleeding occurs, an assessment should be made to approximate the extent of blood loss. Gauze sponges should be inspected and their blood content estimated by weighing or observation. Since 1ml of blood weighs approximately 1gm, dry weight of the sponge is subtracted from the gross weight to obtain the net loss. By observing an opened sponge one can roughly estimate how much blood it contains. A 3-inch-square gauze sponge fully soaked may contain 7ml of blood and a 4-inch-square sponge 10ml of blood. To best determine the appearance, place 3, 5, 7, and 10ml of blood on sponges, wait a few minutes, open them completely and observe their appearance. In addition, volume of blood in a suction bottle can be subtracted from the volume of irrigating solutions and added to the volume estimated to be present on the drapes. Replacement of blood volume with crystalloid solutions such as Lactated Ringer's is on a 3:1 ratio. That is, for each ml of blood lost, replacement is made with 3ml of balanced electrolyte.

Blood Gases and Acid-Base Relationships

Veterinarians have long appreciated the advantages that acid-base measurement could bring but considered the technology too expensive and unreliable. This has changed with recent developments in blood gas analyzers that have led to increased automation, miniaturization and incorporation of sophisticated microchip programming. These changes have made machines not only considerably less expensive but easier and more reliable to use. Today there are hand-held analyzers being mass marketed that cost around $5000 with a per sample cost of $5-10. There are kits for these analyzers that can test up to 10 variables (pH, blood gases, electrolytes and some chemistry components). Studies comparing these analyzers against the standard bench-top workhorses have shown them to be very comparable. This increased use of point of service blood gas analysis represents a break-through in veterinary practice as clinicians will no longer have to wait for test results from external laboratories but rather can get immediate feed-back on therapeutic interventions and increased understanding of the disease process they are working to master. This on-site information is revolutionizing care of surgical and critically ill patients in both large and small animals. A photograph of a commercially available hand-held blood gas analyser and a close-up of its data screen are shown in Figure 4-26 and Figure 4-27.

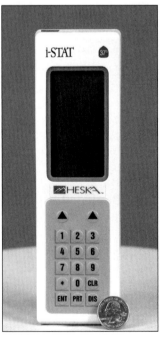

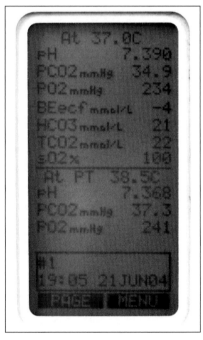

Figure 4-26 Photograph of the iSTAT® hand-held blood gas analyzer. Size is referenced to a quarter.

Figure 4-27 Close-up photograph of the screen of an iSTAT® blood gas analyzer. Data are shown at the apparatus' operating temperature of 37°C and corrected to body temperature. The cartridge used in this analysis only included blood gas variables.

Importance of Blood Gas Analysis

Hydrogen ion homeostasis is very important for proper functioning of biological systems. The hydrogen ion or proton (H^+) is the smallest ion and binds avidly to protein, increasing the net positive charge. This can change protein conformation and function so that vital enzymes throughout the body function aberrantly affecting such operations as oxygen carriage, nervous tissue conduction, myocardial contraction and hepatorenal metabolism. The effect of shifts in hydrogen ion concentration is magnified through the relationship with the CO_2 / HCO_3 buffer system. Changes in H^+ result in complementary shifts in CO_2 which can diffuse readily across lipid protein barriers such as cell walls and the blood-brain-barrier.

Fluids that bathe cells of the body have to be maintained in a delicate balance for cellular function to be normal. The major components of that internal milieu are the gases CO_2 and O_2, cationic and anionic electrolytes, protein and the hydrogen ion. The body works at keeping these components constant within very narrow margins so that the bodys' cells work optimally. This section looks specifically at the CO_2 and H^+ balance which is linked through dissolution of CO_2 in water to the formation of carbonic acid:

$$CO_2 + H_2O \rightleftharpoons H_2CO_3 \qquad (1)$$

The carbonic acid further dissociates to the bicarbonate and hydrogen ions

$$H_2CO_3 \rightleftharpoons HCO_3^- + H^+ \qquad (2)$$

These reactions form a unique open-ended biological buffer system where CO_2 can be either vented or retained in the system in support of tight control of hydrogen ion concentration (pH). Kidneys are also involved in this buffer system (CO_2 / HCO_3) because of their role in excretion of constantly produced hydrogen ion and retention of bicarbonate:

$$CO_2 + H_2O \rightleftharpoons H_2CO_3 \rightleftharpoons HCO_3^- + H^+ \qquad (3)$$

Hydrogen ion concentration is represented as its negative log, or pH (Table 4-5). Relationship between pH and a buffer such as HCO_3^- is expressed in terms of the Henderson-Hasselbalch Equation:

$$pH = pKa + \log \frac{BASE}{ACID} \qquad (4)$$

Usually a buffering system is optimal when the base:acid ratio approaches unity. Because the log of that value (one) is zero, pH and pKa (negative log of the acid dissociation constant for a particular buffer system) are equal. Although pKa of the CO_2 / HCO_3^- buffer system is 6.1 and well below the biological pH range, the buffer system still remains highly effective because of retention or removal of CO_2 (the acid component of the ratio). In the CO_2 / HCO_3^- buffer system, the base is represented by the bicarbonate ion concentration and the acid represented by concentration of carbon dioxide dissolved in plasma. For arterial blood, pH is normally about 7.4 and CO_2 tension is 40mm Hg; HCO_3^- concentration is 24mEq/L and the pKa 6.1. The concentration of dissolved CO_2 is calculated by multiplying the tension [40mm Hg] by the solubility coefficient [0.3]. The Henderson-Hesselbach equation then looks like:

$$pH = 6.1 + \log [24/(40 \times 0.3)]$$
$$= 6.1 + \log [2]$$
$$= 6.1 + 1.3$$
$$= 7.4$$

A commonly asked question is: why does the body so carefully maintain arterial blood pH at 7.4? The first point in the answer lies in deceptive nature of considering H^+ concentration in terms of pH. The true magnitude of change is more easily appreciated by remembering that pH is a log function of H^+ concentration and that a fall in pH from 7.4 to 7.3 represents an increase from 40mmol/l to 50mmol/l, a 25% increase (see Table 4-5). The biological basis for tight pH control lies in the changes in protein conformation that are brought about by changes in proton (H^+) binding as discussed above.

Table 4-5 Data and Graphical Display of the Relationship of [H⁺] and pH

	pH	[H⁺] nanomoles
acidic	7.00	100
	7.10	79
	7.20	63
	7.30	50
normal	7.35	45
	7.40	40
	7.45	35
alkalemia	7.50	32
	7.60	25
	7.70	20
	8.00	10

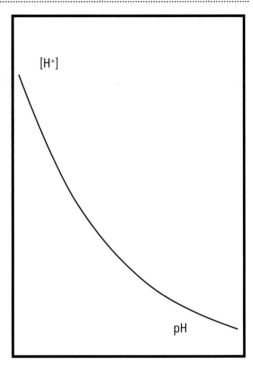

The body's initial response to acidemia is through the CO_2 / HCO_3^- buffer system to increase ventilation to lower CO_2 tension and allow pH to normalize. If acidemia continues or hyperventilation cannot normalize pH, kidneys start working to retain HCO_3^- (and conversely, excrete H^+). This latter mechanism is slowly activated and does not have appreciable effect for several hours. Both of these maneuvers increase the base/acid ratio in the Henderson-Hasselbalch equation. In acute and simple disturbances, extent of these shifts are predictable and must be allowed for when interpreting acid base data. The CO_2 / HCO_3^- buffer system is stressed here but there are other buffers that play a significant role in acid-base homeostasis (hemoglobin, phosphates and plasma & cellular proteins). However, the CO_2 / HCO_3^- buffer system, in addition to being an open system, is the easiest to measure and follow and the most rapid to respond. The compensatory activity of the four simple derangements are set out in Table 4-6.

Table 4-6 Primary Acid Base Pathology and Their Associated Compensatory Mechanisms

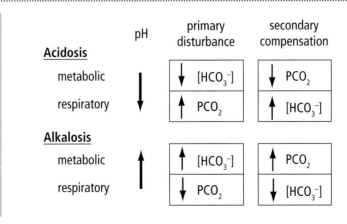

Analysis Methods

The oft stated data axiom of "garbage in, garbage out" holds also for blood gas analysis. The sampling and care of the sample is the biggest source of error in blood gas analysis. Except in some of the new hand-held units, the sample must be anticoagulated. In practice, anticoagulation is done by pre-heparinizing the sampling syringe. The common strength of heparin used is 1000 units/ml so most 1-3ml samples only need a couple of beads of heparin to prevent clotting. A problem commonly seen in small samples is that the syringe's hub (about 0.1ml) is filled with heparin and this dilutes the sample. Because heparin has a fairly neutral pH and gas tensions equal to those of the atmosphere, the main effect is to lower PCO_2 and shift PO_2 towards that of air (> 2mm Hg and 150mm Hg, respectively). The use of sodium heparin can introduce errors in electrolyte measurements (increased sodium and decreased calcium ion concentrations) if these are measured with the same sample. This error is lessened by use of minimal amounts of heparin but lithium heparin can be used if accuracy of electrolyte data is important. The second important requirement of sampling is that it must be done anaerobically with no addition of air or use of significant negative pressure. This means blood is drawn slowly into the syringe, preferably over at least one whole respiratory cycle with introduction of air bubbles being avoided. There are arterial blood gas sampling syringes made specifically for this purpose that are pre-heparinized and fill automatically under the influence of arterial blood pressure. The size of the sample will depend on the equipment but is minimally about 0.5ml. Samples of 2ml or more are less affected by sampling techniques because errors tend to be constant and the larger volume lessens effect of the error. In very small animals, such a sample is impractical and in those cases heparinized capillary tubes may have to be used.

A third sampling error exists when sampling is done from an indwelling arterial or venous line and insufficient discard volume results in inclusion of catheter dead space material in the sample. This occurs more often when the animal is small and clinical staff are anxious to minimize blood loss. This error can be avoided by using strict aseptic sampling techniques to allow return of the removed dead space and then flushing the line. Occasionally, inexperienced individuals will collect blood for blood gas analysis using Vacutainer tubes. Values from these samples are so distorted by the sampling method that they are of no use and have to be discarded.

Choice of which blood vessels to use for sampling is limited only by the operator's experience and the animal's positioning and/or cooperation. The femoral artery is considered the easiest but skilled personnel can usually get samples from the distal limb arteries in dogs. Animals that are anesthetized are obviously easier to sample and in all but very small patients, the lingual artery can be used. In some circumstances, an arterial catheter may already in place for blood pressure monitoring. Some words of caution about sampling by percutaneous arterial puncture or lingual artery: use a small gauge needle (certainly no larger that a 23ga and preferably smaller) and to minimize the chances of a hematoma, maintain mild digital pressure on the site for at least 3 minutes by the clock. If venous samples are taken, it is best to use as big a vein as possible (for example jugular vein) as the sample will be less affected by local pathology. Regardless of site, if numbing of the skin is required to minimize pain from sampling, EMLA cream may be used but it will require a 10-20 minute period (20-30 is more realistic)for the local anesthetics to work.

Once a sample is obtained, the operator should immediately turn the syringe upward, sharply tap the barrel to move any bubbles toward the neck of the syringe and then eject any air and blood from the dead space. Only then can the syringe be inverted or rolled to mix the heparin with the blood sample. If the sample is immediately put into the analyzer, there is no need to cap the syringe. If the measurement is delayed, commercially available caps or crimped needles can be used. It is strongly advised not to put stoppers onto bare needles after sampling to avoid accidental needle sticks to the operator. Although infection risks with animal blood-borne pathogens may be considered less than when handling human blood, they are still present. When there is a delay between sampling and measurement, the sample should be placed into an ice slush to chill it as quickly as possible. This will stop loss of oxygen from the sample by continued white cell metabolism. Although plastic syringes are almost universally used today for blood gas sampling, they are associated with a small oxygen loss because of diffusion. However this is not considered significant in the clinical setting.

Blood gas analyzers usually work at 37°C (human body temperature). Some will correct variables to manually-inputted body temperatures. In general, corrections for warmer body temperature will increase gas tensions while lowering pH (see data shown in Figure 4-28). This is usually clinically insignificant, except when an animal is very hypothermic. Oxygen is held in blood instead of passing to tissues and ventilatory drive is suppressed by lowered $PaCO_2$ and hypothermia *per se.*

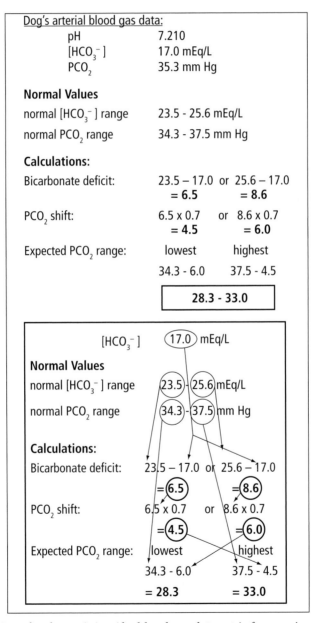

Figure 4-28 Calculations for determining if a blood gas data set is from a simple acid-base derangement or of multiple origins. See Making Diagnosis section in text for details.

The actual mechanics of equipment maintenance is routine, provided the manufacturer's instructions are followed. Regardless of equipment used, it is essential to have a good quality control program in place. Ampules of quality control (QC) standards are available and can be used to independently check the machine's accuracy and reliability. In human hospitals, quality control samples are run several times in every shift but this is not economical in veterinary practice. Instead, most practices run QC samples every day or every second day. Maintaining a log of the machine's behavior in these QC tests can provide trends that can warn of service needs or impeding electrode failure.

Analysis Results

Blood gas analyzers perform just three measurements–PO_2, PCO_2 and pH. Values are express in mm Hg or kPa for gas tension and units for pH. The kilopascal (kPa) unit used in Europe is equal to approximately 7.5mm Hg. All other data, including HCO_3^- concentrations, are calculated by the analyzer's programming. There are a number of acid-base terms and variables or indices provided by most blood gas analyzers and these are explained in Table 4-7. Normal acid-base values for dogs and cats are shown in Table 4-8 where mean values are given along with the 95% confidence intervals to provide some idea of the variability of these data within the population of normal animals. Note that there are no values for venous PO_2 because it is considered that samples taken from peripheral veins do not yield interpretable values. True central venous oxygen tension (PvO_2) as measured in the pulmonary artery, is usually in the range 44-46mm Hg and is used to evaluate total body oxygenation. Ranges for normal blood gas values demonstrate that clinicians must use some degree of tolerance when deciding whether particular sets of data are within normal limits and when interpreting an acid-base disorder as simple or mixed in origin.

In Table 4-8, it should be noted that venous blood gives a good estimation of arterial pH and PCO_2 by being about 0.05 pH units and 3-7mm Hg lower and higher, respectively, than arterial pH and PCO_2 values.

One problem that vexes clinicians can be when, after some difficulty, a blood sample is finally obtained only to find that results are ambiguous as to whether the sample is really arterial or venous. To clarify if the low oxygen tension is really arterial, confirmatory information can be gained by checking mucous membrane color, checking other indirect blood gas parameters such as pulse oximetry and end-tidal CO_2 or obtaining a confirmed venous sample for comparison. If all else fails, one can resort to the axiom that an artery is easier to hit than an unoccluded vein.

Interpretation of Blood Gas Data

The first step in making sense of blood gas data is to examine the patient and its history. This is important not only in appreciating the acid-base data, but in providing a clinician with a sense of priorities and underlying problems. To take an extreme example, there is no clinical advantage gained in puzzling over a set of blood gas data if the animal's mucous membranes are blue and the pulse is barely palpable. History and physical examination become even more important in complex derangements as described below. Interpreting blood gas results requires knowledge of normal values, how changes in one parameter affect the others, and hopefully some history to guide whether any changes are of acute or more chronic nature.

Steps in Making a Diagnosis

Evaluate

In evaluating an animal's acid-base status one looks first at the pH to decide if the pH has changed and, if so, in what direction:

7.35-7.45	normal
≤ 7.35	acidemia
≥ 7.45	alkalemia

Table 4-7

Blood Gas Terminology and Indices

ACID

substance that can donate hydrogen ions

$$[HCl \leftrightarrow H^+ + Cl^-]$$

BASE

substance that can accept hydrogen ions

$$[NH_3 + H^+ \leftrightarrow NH_4^+]$$

pH

hydrogen ion concentration expressed as a negative log.

As pH falls, hydrogen ion increases (the math of a negative logarithm which logs the reciprocal of the original unit). Normal pH of arterial blood is 7.4 which is a hydrogen concentration of 40nEq/liter. A rise in pH to 7.5 would mean a decrease in hydrogen ion concentration to 30nmole/liter while a fall in pH to 7.2 would mean an increase in hydrogen ion concentration to 80 nmole/liter. The pH of neutrality in traditional chemist terms is 7.0–by definition, lower pHs are acidic and conversely higher pHs are alkalotic.

pKa

Potential of an acid to release a proton or H^+ is defined as the ratio of the product of the dissociated ions to the undissociated parent acid and is termed Ka, or as its negative log10, pKa.

$$HA \leftrightarrow H^+ + A^-$$
$$\text{where } Ka = [H^+] [A^-] / HA$$

For most acids of biologic importance, Ka is in the range 10^{-1} to 10^{-7} (i.e. pKa of 1 to 7). As a corollary, when pH equals pKa, the buffer system is in equilibrium and concentrations of the acid and base are equal.

BUFFER

Compound that is capable of accepting or donating a proton or H^+. An example is how a weak acid and its anion (base) resist a change in pH when a strong acid or base is added to the system. Weak acids and bases are compounds whose potential for releasing / removing hydrogen ions in a solution depends on the pH of the solution.

HENDERSON-HASSELBACH EQUATION

$$pH = pK + \log \frac{[base]}{[acid]}$$

ACIDEMIA

Excess of hydrogen ions in the <u>blood</u> (a pH less than 7.35). Conversely alkalemia refers to a deficit of hydrogen ions in the blood and a pH greater than 7.45

ACIDOSIS

Pathologic condition resulting in an imbalance in the body's acid-base equilibrium where there is an excess of acid compared to available base (i.e. either an accumulation of acid or a loss of base). The converse condition is alkalosis where there is an excess of base compared to acid

continued

Table 4-7 continued

PRESSURE / TENSION

Henry's Law states that when a gas is in equilibrium with a liquid, it will be dissolved in the fluid in proportion to its partial pressure in the gas phase. The constant of proportionality is the partition coefficient and is expressed as either Bunsen or Ostwald units. The terms partial pressure and tension are interchangeable and are usually expressed in terms of mm Hg (Europeans use kPa or kilo-Pascal which is equal to 7.6mm Hg). An important example is that for each mm Hg of CO_2 tension, there is 0.3ml of CO_2 dissolved per dl of blood. There is no simple relationship between oxygen tension (PO_2) and oxygen content in blood.

TOTAL CO_2

Total concentration of carbon dioxide in blood obtained from the sum of CO_2 held dissolved in plasma (measured as CO_2 tension in mm Hg) and bicarbonate (measured in milli-Equivalents/liter). The measurement is performed by adding strong acid to plasma releasing all of the CO_2. Blood gas machines really just calculate the parameter. Total CO_2 is mainly determined by the bicarbonate in the sample and so is usually taken to reflect that. To be interpreted accurately, knowledge of pH is needed to partition the acid/base ratio. A normal value is between 24-27mEq/L under standard sample handling.

STANDARD BICARBONATE

Actual measured (or calculated) bicarbonate concentration corrected for a pH of 7.4 and a PCO_2 of 40mm Hg. It is normally 24mEq/L so deviations from that indicate a metabolic shift

BASE EXCESS

Difference between the calculated standard bicarbonate level and the normal value of 24. It is an index of magnitude of the metabolic shift in the acid-base equilibrium. It may include some additional correction factors such as hemoglobin to increase its accuracy. Calculations can be done with nomograms, calculators or computer programs associated with most blood gas analyzers. The normal range is −4 to +2mEq/L in dogs. To add to our confusion negative base excesses are often referred to as base deficits! There are modifications available that correct for other buffers such as hemoglobin and plasma protein—an example is Whole-blood buffer base.

ANION GAP

Estimate of anions not accounted for by just considering chloride and bicarbonate ions (protein, sulfates, phosphates, lactate, ketones, and exogenous anions such as salicy late). It is usually calculated as the difference between the sum of the major cations ([Na^+] and [K^+]) and the sum of easily measured anions [Cl^-] and [HCO_3^-]. Depending on laboratories and calculation methods (some laboratories just use [Na^+] as the sole cation) the anion gap is normally between 12 and 25mEq/L. It is important that the calculation and laboratory methods be consistent to avoid mis-interpretation.

Table 4-8

Normal Mean Values and 95% Confidence Limits for Blood Gas Variables for Dogs and Cats

	PO_2		PCO_2		pH		HCO_3^-	
	mean	95% CI	mean	95% CI	mean	95% CI	mean	95% CI
DOG								
arterial	90.9	87-95	35.9	34-38	7.453	7.44-7.47	24.5	24-26
venous			37.4	34-41	7.397	7.35-7.44	22.5	21-24
CAT								
arterial	97.2	91-103	29.9	29-31	7.456	7.45-7.47	21.0	20-22
venous			37.5	36-39	7.391	7.38-7.40	22.4	21-24

In simple derangements, the relationship between CO_2, H_2CO_3 and HCO_3^- (Equations 1 & 2) follows a defined path so that, as CO_2 increases or decreases, there are parallel changes in its dissolution to form carbonic acid and then dissociate to H_2CO_3 and H^+. Likewise, changes in H^+ (pH) affect the production of H_2CO_3 with corresponding changes in (HCO_3^-), as it is used or produced in buffering changes in H^+. Table 4-9 shows average rates of change for acute blood gas shifts. A very important principle to remember is that until the primary cause is corrected, compensation is never complete. This means that when acidosis is present, pH is always on the low side of normal. This guides the clinician as to what derangement is present. In unusual cases, there may be two or more pathological processes occurring that have opposing effects on pH and it will appear to be normal. In those cases, the animal is often so obviously ill that acid-base changes are expected but electrolyte and hydration changes are the only sign of the existing pathology.

Table 4-9

Adaptive Coefficients Used to Predict Compensatory Changes in Acid-base Parameters

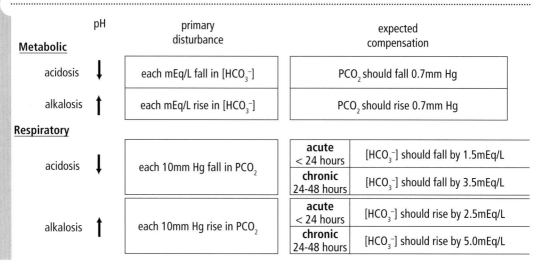

Compare

After deciding on the nature of the H+ derangement, the origin of that primary pH shift needs to be matched, by visual inspection, to the appropriate changed PCO_2 or HCO_3^- value:

Acidemia	pH ↓	↑PCO_2 > 45mm Hg	RESPIRATORY
	≤ 7.35	↓ HCO_3^- < 22mEq/l	METABOLIC
Alkalemia	pH↑	↓ PCO_2 < 35mm Hg	RESPIRATORY
	≥ 7.45	↑HCO_3^- > 26mEq/l	METABOLIC

Calculate

The third step is to calculate whether changes that have taken place can be explained as a simple derangement with normal compensation as in Table 4-8. This requires the clinician to use data in Tables 4-8 and 4-9 to calculate the compensation to be expected in a simple situation and to see if the compensation is appropriate or if some second factor is involved in the acid-base derangement. In Figure 4-28, these calculations are performed for the case of a dog with an initial diagnosis of metabolic acidosis [pH 7.21, bicarbonate concentration 17.0mEq/L, and a PCO_2 of 35.3mm Hg]. The expected compensation would be expected to lower the PCO_2 below the normal range. If the PCO_2 did not fall or was greater than the normal range, it would be presumptive that there is not a simple metabolic acidosis taking place. However, calculating the high and low PCO_2 compensatory points are necessary to eliminate another acid-base pathology factor being involved. This requires using the 95% confidence limits of both PCO_2 and HCO_3^- normal values. Multiplying the calculated high and low HCO_3^- shifts from normal by the metabolic compensatory coefficient of 0.7mEq/L yields the expected compensations of PCO_2. These calculations are shown in Fig 4-28 where the compensation ranges for PCO_2 were found to be 28.3 to 33.0mm Hg. The observed PCO_2 [35.3 mm Hg] is above this range and is therefore contributing to a co-existing respiratory acidosis (a situation often seen in animals with severe illness undergoing anesthesia and being allowed to breathe spontaneously). Conversely, if the PCO_2 had been below the predicted range, the diagnosis of concurrent respiratory alkalosis would have to be considered. Similar calculations are needed when the primary pathology appears to be respiratory in origin. In that case the chronicity of the condition has to be identified when calculating the compensatory ranges (Table 4-8). This difference between metabolic and respiratory compensatory predictions reflects the slowness of the renal compensatory mechanisms in respiratory acid base disorders.

Therapy

Unless the acid-base disorder is life threatening, consideration should be made to correcting the primary cause if possible rather than empirically correcting the acid-base derangement. For example, increase the inspired oxygen concentration (FIO_2) in hypoxia, use diuresis or dialysis in renal failure, analgesics for pain, reversal of opioid depression and so on. Quite often just rehydration starts the body's own correct processes in action and little other therapy is needed. Once the primary cause has been addressed, the derangement can be corrected empirically if it is deemed clinically necessary. In the case of metabolic disorders, this is usually when pH is below 7.2 or above 7.5 although these critical points vary between clinicians and depend upon the animal's physical condition. In all acid-base corrections, electrolytes must be carefully monitored and corrections made with all due caution.

Metabolic alkalosis, as often seen following protracted vomiting, can be treated with use of normal saline volume expansion which serves to both acidify and replace chloride. Serious metabolic acidosis requires addition of a base, typically sodium bicarbonate or one of the alkalinizing multielectrolyte solutions that contain acetate and/or gluconate (Normosol® and Multisol®). It should be pointed out that lactated Ringer's solution is not an alkalizing solution but in fact produces mild metabolic acidosis when infused in healthy animals. The use of sodium bicarbonate to correct metabolic acidosis is controversial. This is because of three main concerns:
(a) the sodium load associated with the drug and associated osmolarity (an 8.4% solution contains one mEq/ml of HCO_3^- and has an osmolarity of 2000mosm/l, nearly 7 times that of plasma.

(b) HCO_3^- is converted to carbon dioxide in neutralizing excess hydrogen ions. CO_2 is highly diffusible and can cross virtually all biological membranes. Until this newly created CO_2 is blown off, it can move into the CNS and cause a paradoxical acidosis.

(c) acute correction of severe and/or chronic acidosis can reveal uncorrected body depletion of potassium with secondary hypokalemia. This can be life-threatening if correction of acidosis occurs too rapidly. In addition to these concerns there are two further situations which dictate how sodium bicarbonate can be used:

- the animal must be at least eucapnic indicating an ability to excrete CO_2 produced in acid neutralization
- the animal must be able to handle the sodium load (i.e., not susceptible to cardiac fluid overload). In the operating room, anesthetists, who are skilled in acute fluid and electrolyte management and have the ability to increase ventilation to facilitate elimination of CO_2, will use HCO_3^- more readily to correct major metabolic acidotic situations before the animal is sent to recovery where it may well receive analgesics that possibly depress ventilation.

The amount of bicarbonate needed can be calculated by multiplying the base deficit by the fraction of the body in which it is distributed (extracellular fluid space or 30% of body weight) by the body weight in kilograms.

$$\text{Bicarbonate required} = \text{Base deficit} \times 1/3 \times \text{body weight} \qquad (4)$$

Usually only a half of this is ever needed as correction of acid base derangements is dynamic and partial changes often provoke the body into fluid and electrolyte shifts that complement the correction.

Respiratory acidosis and alkalosis in an anesthetized patient is usually quite easy to correct by increasing or decreasing minute ventilation through combinations of increasing ventilatory rate and tidal volume. These maneuvers need to be done with attention to monitoring cardiovascular function. In the conscious and un-intubated animal, the primary cause of the ventilatory disorder must be treated. The following sources are provided for further reading: Davenport (1974); DiBartola (2000); Halperin & Goldstein (1999); Rose & Post (2001).

References

Acierno MJ, Labato MA (2004). Hypertension in dogs and cats. *Compendium*. 26:336-346.

Bins SH, et al. (1995) Doppler ultrasonographic, oscillometric sphygmomanometric, and photoplethysmographic techniques for noninvasive blood pressure measurement in anesthetized cats. *J Vet Intern Med*. 9, 405-414.

Bodey AR, Young LE, Bartram DH, et al. (1994) A comparison of direct and indirect (oscillometric) measurements of arterial blood pressure in anaesthetised dogs, using tail and limb cuffs. *Res Vet Sci*. 57, 265-269.

Bodey AR, Michell AR, Bovee KC, et al. (1996) Comparison of direct and indirect (oscillometric) measurements of arterial blood pressure in conscious dogs. *Res in Vet Sci*. 61, 17-21.

Bodey AR and Sansom J (1998) Epidemiological study of blood pressure in domestic cats. *J Sm Ani Prac*. 39, 567-573.

Branson KR, Wagner-Mann CC, and Mann FA (1997) Evaluation of an oscillometric blood pressure monitor on anesthetized cats and the effect of cuff placement and fur on accuracy. *Vet Surg* 26, 347-353.

Butinar J, Petrun-Ulaga M, Cestnik V, et al. (1991).Pulse oximetry and capnometry-Methods of monitoring in veterinary anesthesia. *Proceedings, 4th International Congress of Veterinary Anaesthesia.* Utrecht, The Netherlands, August 25-30.

Caulkett NA, Cantwell SL, and Houston DM ((1998) A comparison of indirect blood pressure monitoring techniques in the anesthetized cat. *Vet Surg* 27, 370-377.

Dart CM, Dunlop CI (2000) Comparison of two indirect methods of blood pressure measurement with direct arterial blood pressure in anaesthetised greyhounds. *Proceedings of the 7th World Congress of Veterinary Anaesthesia, Berne, Switzerland,* pp 87-88.

Davenport HW (1974). *The ABC of Acid-Base Chemistry.* University of Chicago Press, Chicago; 6th edition.

DiBartola SP (2000). Introduction to acid-base disorders. In: DiBartola SP, ed. *Fluid therapy in small animal practice.* Philadelphia: W.B. Saunders Co, 2nd ed. pp 189-210.

Dodman NH (1992). The case against intraoperative ECG monitoring. Vet Clin of North Amer: Small Animal Practice. 22:440-443.

Dunlop CI, Dart CM, Quasem A, et al. (2000) Can peripheral blood flow measured either directly or indirectly estimate changes in cardiac output during anaesthesia in dogs? *Proceedings of the 7th World Congress of Veterinary Anaesthesia, Berne, Switzerland,* pp 89-90.

Dyson DH (1997) Assessment of 3 audible monitors during hypotension in anesthetized dogs. *Can Vet J.* 38, 564-566.

Edwards NJ (1990). Noninvasive Blood Pressure Monitoring and Treatment of Hypertension. *Academy of Vet Cardiology Proceedings.*

Gillespie NA (1943). The signs of anesthesia. *Anesth Analg* 22:275-282.

Goodger WJ (1972). Clinical management of intra-arterial catheters for blood pressure determinations and blood gas analysis. *JAAHA* 8:428-431.

Grandy JL and Dunlop CI (1992). Evaluation of the doppler ultrasonic method of measuring systolic arterial blood pressure in cats. AJVR 53:1166-69.

Grosenbaugh DA, Muir WA III (1998a) Accuracy of noninvasive oxyhemoglobin saturation, end-tidal carbon dioxide concentration, and blood pressure monitoring during experimentallly induced hypoxemia, hypotension, or hypertension in anesthetized dogs. *Am J Vet Res.* 59, 205-212.

Grosenbaugh DA, Muir WA III (1998b) Blood pressure monitoring. *Vet Med. January,* pp 48-59.

Guedel AE (1971). Inhalation Anesthesia. 2nd ed, NY. The Macmillan Co. pp 10-52.

Halperin ML and Goldstein MB (1999). Acid Base. In *Fluid, Electrolyte and Acid-Base Physiology–A problem-based approach.* Philadelphia:W.B. Saunders Co, 3rd ed. Pp. 4-224.

Hansen BD, Hardie EM, Carroll GS (1997) Physiological measurements after ovariohysterectomy in dogs: what's normal? *Appl Ani Behav Sci.* 51, 101-109.

Haskins SC (1987). Monitoring the anesthetized patient. *In Principles & Practice of Veterinary Anesthesia.* Edited by C.E. Short. Williams & Wilkins publisher.

Haskins SC (1992). Monitoring the anesthetized patient. *Vet Clin of North Amer: Sm Ani Prac* 22:425-431.

Haskins SC (1996) Monitoring the anesthetized patient. In Thurmon JC, Tranquilli WJ, Benson GJ, eds. Lumb and Jones' *Veterinary Anesthesia.* 3rd ed. Baltimore: Williams & Wilkins, pp 414-424.

Kallet AJ, Cowgill LD, Kass PH (1997) Comparison of blood pressure measurements obtained in dogs by use of indirect oscillometry in a veterinary clinic versus at home. *JAVMA* 210:651-654.

LeBlanc PH, Sawyer DC (1993). Electronic monitoring equipment. *Seminars in Veterinary Medicine and Surgery, Small Animal.* 8:119-126.

Mitchell AR (1993). Hypertension in companion animals. *Veterinary Annual.* Vol 33. Eds M E Raw and T J Parkinson. Oxford, Blackwell Scientific Publications. Pp 11-23.

Moens Y and Verstraeten W (1982). Capnographic monitoring in small animal anesthesia. *JAAHA* 18:659-678.

Nakada Y, Nishikibe M, Miyazawa H, et al. (1990). Basic Studies on Indirect Measurement of Blood pressure in Dogs. *Advances in Animal Cardiology.* No. 23:1-8 Tokyo, Japan.

Pedersen KM, Butler MA, Erbøll AK, Pedersen HD (2002). Evaluation of an oscillometric blood pressure monitor for use in anesthetized cats. *JAVMA* 221:646-650.

Riebold TW, Brunson DB, Lott RA, Evans AT (1980). Percutaneous arterial catheterization in the horse. *Equine Practice.* November: 1736-42.

Robertson S (1992). The case for routine intraoperative ECG monitoring. *Vet Clin of North Amer: Sm Ani Prac.* 22:437-440.

Rose BD and Post TW (2001). Clinical physiology of acid-base and electrolyte disorders, 4th ed. New York, McGraw-Hill Book Co.

Sawyer DC, Brown M, Striler EL, *et al.* (1991). Comparison of direct and indirect blood pressure measurement in anesthetized dogs. *Lab Ani Sci.* 41:134-138.

Sawyer DC, Striler EL, and Bohart G (1994) Indirect blood pressure measurements in dogs, cats, and horses: correlation with direct arterial pressures and site of measurement. *Proceedings of the 5th International Congress of Veterinary Anaesthesia,* Guelph, Ontario, p 209.

Sawyer DC, Guikema AH Siegel EM (2004). Evaluation of a new oscillometric blood pressure monitor in isoflurane-anesthetized dogs. *Vet Anaesth and Analg* 31:27-39.

Severinghaus JW and Stupfel M (1958). Alveolar dead space as an index of distribution of blood flow in pulmonary capillaries. *J Appl Physiol* 10:335-348.

Stanley T, Kawamura R, Graves C (1974). Effects of N_2O on volume and pressure of endotracheal cuffs. *Anesthesiology* 41:256-262.

Stipien RL, Rapoport GS (1999). Clinical comparison of three methods to measure blood pressure in nonsedated dogs. *J Am Vet Med Assn.* 215, 1623-28.

Tabaru H, et al (1990). Noninvasive measurement of systemic arterial pressure by Finapres in anesthetized dogs. *Japan J Vet Sci.* 52:427-430.

Valtonen MH and Eriksson LM (1970). The effect of cuff width on accuracy of indirect measurement of blood pressure in dogs. *Res Vet Sci.* 11:358-362.

Vincent IC, Michell AR, Leahy RA (1993). Non-invasive measurement of arterial blood pressure in dogs: a potential indicator for the identification of stress. *Res Vet Sci.* 54:195-201.

Chapter 5
The Anesthetic Period: Predictable Problems

Standard Surgical Anesthetic Procedures

In establishing a regimen for anesthesia in clinical practice, clinicians usually select a technique and procedure for normal healthy animals with which he or she has the most experience. This is a comfort zone that works. Protocols are modified as new procedures and drugs are presented, especially if an unfortunate outcome occurs. With the availability of various induction agents as listed in Chapter 2 that can be given IM or IV and inhalation techniques with isoflurane or sevoflurane, safer and better control of anesthetic depth, better predictability from patient to patient and smoother anesthesia recovery can be achieved. For normal, P1 and P2 patients, thiopental, propofol, ketamine/diazepam or ketamine/midazolam are often used to accomplish induction by injection to permit tracheal intubation with anesthesia maintained with an inhalation of preference.

The common anesthetic protocol recommended for the normal healthy dog undergoing elective surgery is: optional premedication with atropine or glycopyrrolate; light tranquilization with acepromazine (0.01 to 0.1mg/kg) for apprehensive patients or fear biters and 0.05 to 0.1mg/kg butorphanol or hydromorphone; induction with thiopental, propofol, or ketamine/benzodiazapine mixture; tracheal intubation; and maintenance with isoflurane or sevoflurane. The Bain circuit or preferred semiopen system is used for patients less than 7 kg but larger animals are maintained with a semiclosed circle CO_2 absorption system. An IV catheter is placed before induction and a balanced electrolyte drip started at a rate of 10ml/kg/hr. For cats, ketamine/benzodiazapine mixture is most commonly used followed by an inhalant. Regarding premedication, Table 5-1 provides information as to how drugs used for managing pain can influence actions of anesthetics.

With the wide selection of drugs and different conditions, Table 5-2 lists example protocols that may be used to guide clinicians in selecting appropriate combinations for different clinical situations. Appropriate substitutions are to be expected depending on personal preference, availability and geographical location.

Table 5-1 Optimizing Premedications: Synergism of Multimodal Analgesia

Premedication	Induction agent	Gaseous anesthetic
Mu-agonist Opioid	Lower end of dose range should be used because premedications provide sedation and analgesia.	Patients often will require much lower inhalant concentrations to maintain anesthesia when sedatives and analgesics are administered preemptively. This can range 0.5 to 2% depending on inhalant used.
• efficacious		
• relatively expensive depending on preferred drug		
• relatively safe	Selected Induction agent should be given slowly and to effect, as their need may be reduced as much as 50-70%	
• MOA: opioid receptors		
Alpha₂ Agonist		
• synergistic with opioids		
• at lower doses (Grimm et al. 2000)		
NSAID		
• sensitizes opioids to receptors		

Table 5-2

Example Protocols (These are only presented as guidelines for P1 and P2 patients. Modifications may be needed for patients at risk.)

Procedure	Anticipated Degree of Pain	Example Protocol A	Example Protocol B
Canine OHE and castration	Mild to moderate	**Premedication** Acepromazine#, 0.05-0.1mg/kg SC, IM + Buprenorphine*, 0.01-0.03 mg/kg SC, IM Or butorphanol, 0.1mg/kg SC, IM, ± Atropine, 0.01-0.04mg/kg SC, IM Or Glycopyrrolate, 0.005-0.01mg/kg SC, IM** **Intraoperative Analgesia** Incisional block: bupivacaine, 1.5mg/kg (with 1:200,000 epinephrine) **Postoperative Analgesia** Repeat dose of butorphanol at recovery. Dispense tramadol, 1-2mg/kg PO BID x 3 days; Deracoxib, 1-4mg/kg PO SID x 3 days starting 24 hrs after initial Deracoxib dose	**Premedication** Medetomidine, 0.005-0.020mg/kg IM + Morphine*, 0.5-1.0mg/kg IM Or Hydromorphone*, 0.2mg/kg IM ± Atropine, 0.01-0.04mg/kg SC, IM Or Glycopyrrolate, 0.005-0.01mg/kg SC, IM** **Postoperative Analgesia** Repeat dose of opioid 4-6 hrs following the initial dose, or sooner if needed. Deracoxib, 1-4mg/kg PO SID x 7 days starting 24 hrs after initial Deracoxib dose
Feline OHE	Moderate	**Premedication** Acepromazine#, 0.05-0.2mg/kg SC, IM + Hydromorphone*, 0.05-0.1mg/kg SC, IM; Or 0.1mg/kg butorphanol IM, SC ± Atropine, 0.01-0.04mg/kg SC, IM Or Glycopyrrolate, 0.005-0.01mg/kg SC, IM** **Intraoperative Analgesia** Incisional block: bupivacaine (with 1:200,000 epinephrine), 1.5mg/kg **Postoperative Analgesia** Repeat dose of opioid 4-6 hrs following the initial dose or at recovery with butorphanol. Dispense tramadol, 1-2mg/kg PO BID x 3 days	**Premedication** Medetomidine, 0.02mg/kg IM + Buprenorphine, 0.01-0.02mg/kg IM + Ketamine, 2-4mg/kg IM **Postoperative Analgesia** Repeat buprenorphine 6-8 hrs after initial dose. Buprenorphine, 0.01-0.02mg/kg buccal every 8-12 hrs for 2-4 days beginning 4-6 hrs after last IM dose

continued

Table 5-2 Continued

Procedure	Anticipated Degree of Pain	Example Protocol A	Example Protocol B
Feline castration	Mild to moderate	**Premedication** Acepromazine#, 0.05-0.2mg/kg SC, IM + Hydromorphone*, 0.05mg/kg SC, IM; Or 0.1mg/kg butorphanol IM, SC ± Atropine, 0.01-0.04mg/kg SC, IM Or Glycopyrrolate, 0.005-0.01mg/kg SC, IM**	Same as for OHE, but may omit the post-operative opioid.
Feline onychectomy	Moderate to severe	**Premedication** Acepromazine#, 0.05-0.2mg/kg SC, IM + Hydromorphone*, 0.05-0.1mg/kg SC, IM ± Atropine, 0.01-0.04mg/kg SC, IM Or Glycopyrrolate, 0.005-0.01mg/kg SC, IM** **Intraoperative Analgesia** Declaw block: bupivicaine, 1.5mg/kg maximum dose Or lidocaine 2.0mg/kg + bupivacaine 0.75mg/kg (without epinephrine) **Postoperative Analgesia** In hospital: hydromorphone*, 0.05mg/kg IM or SC, 4-6 hrs after initial dose and repeat as needed. At home: buprenorphine, 0.01-0.02mg/kg buccal every 8-12 hrs for 2-4 days beginning 4-6 hrs after last hydromorphone dose; Or tramadol, 1-2mg/kg PO x 5 da.	**Premedication** Apply 25µg/hr fentanyl patch 6-12 hrs before surgery OR at time of surgical prep (may cover half of the absorptive surface of the patch in cats < 5 kg) Medetomidine, 0.02mg/kg IM + Morphine*, 0.2-0.5mg/kg IM ± Atropine, 0.01-0.04mg/kg SC, IM Or Glycopyrrolate, 0.005-0.01mg/kg SC, IM** **Intraoperative Analgesia** Declaw block: bupivacaine , 1.5mg/kg maximum dose (without epinephrine) **Postoperative Analgesia** May need to repeat opioid dose 1-2 times to cover immediate postoperative pain or until fentanyl patch becomes effective. Remove fentanyl patch in 3-5 days.
Canine routine dentistry	Mild to moderate	**Premedication** Acepromazine#, 0.05-0.1mg/kg SC, IM + Buprenorphine*, 0.01-0.02mg/kg SC, IM; Or butorphanol, 0.1mg/kg IM, SC; ± Atropine, 0.01-0.04mg/kg SC, IM; Or Glycopyrrolate, 0.005-0.01mg/kg SC, IM**	**Premedication** Medetomidine, 0.005-0.010mg/kg IM + Morphine*, 0.5-1.0mg/kg IM Or Hydromorphone*, 0.2mg/kg IM ± Atropine, 0.01-0.04mg/kg SC, IM Or Glycopyrrolate, 0.005-0.01mg/kg SC, IM** + Deracoxib, 1-4mg/kg PO

continued

Table 5-2 Continued

Procedure	Anticipated Degree of Pain	Example Protocol A	Example Protocol B
Canine dentistry with extractions	Moderate to severe	**Premedication** Acepromazine#, 0.05-0.2mg/kg SC, IM + Buprenorphine*, 0.01-0.02mg/kg SC, IM ± Atropine, 0.01-0.04mg/kg SC, IM Or Glycopyrrolate, 0.005-0.01mg/kg SC, IM** + Deracoxib, 1-4mg/kg PO Infraorbital, mandibular, or other regional nerve blocks: bupivacaine, 1.5mg/kg maximum dose (± 1:200,000 epinephrine) **Postoperative Analgesia** Tramadol, 1-2mg/kg PO BID x 4-7 days + Deracoxib, 1-4mg/kg PO SID x 4-7 days starting 24 hrs after initial Deracoxib dose	**Postoperative Analgesia** ± Deracoxib, 1-4mg/kg PO SID x 7 days. Should be strongly considered with moderate to severe gingivitis. **Premedication** Medetomidine, 0.005-0.010mg/kg IM + Morphine*, 0.5-1.0mg/kg IM. Or Hydromorphone*, 0.2mg/kg IM ± Atropine, 0.01-0.04mg/kg SC, IM Or Glycopyrrolate, 0.005-0.01mg/kg SC, IM** + Deracoxib, 1-4mg/kg PO **Intraoperative Analgesia** Infraorbital, mandibular, or other regional nerve blocks. Bupivacaine, 1.5mg/kg maximum dose (± 1:200,000 epinephrine) **Postoperative Analgesia** Deracoxib, 1-4mg/kg PO SID x 7 days starting 24 hrs after initial Deracoxib dose
Feline routine dentistry	Mild to moderate	**Premedication** Acepromazine#, 0.05-0.2mg/kg SC, IM + Hydromorphone*, 0.05mg/kg SC, IM ± Atropine, 0.01-0.04mg/kg SC, IM Or Glycopyrrolate, 0.005-0.01mg/kg SC, IM** **Postoperative Analgesia** Tramadol, 1-2mg/kg PO BID x 4-7 da	**Postoperative Analgesia** ± Deracoxib, 1-4mg/kg PO SID x 7 days starting 24 hrs after initial Deracoxib dose. Should be strongly considered with moderate to severe gingivitis. **Premedication** Medetomidine, 0.02mg/kg IM + Buprenorphine*, 0.01-0.02mg/kg IM + Ketamine, 2-4mg/kg IM **Postoperative Analgesia** Repeat buprenorphine (IM or buccal) 6-8 hrs after initial dose or as needed if gingivitis is moderate to severe.

continued

Table 5-2 Continued

Procedure	Anticipated Degree of Pain	Example Protocol A	Example Protocol B
Feline dentistry with extractions	Moderate to severe	**Premedication** Acepromazine#, 0.05-0.1mg/kg SC, IM + Hydromorphone*, 0.05-0.1mg/kg SC, IM ± Atropine, 0.01-0.04mg/kg SC, IM Or Glycopyrrolate, 0.005-0.01mg/kg SC, IM** **Intraoperative Analgesia** Infraorbital, mandibular, or other regional nerve blocks: bupivacaine, 1.5mg/kg maximum dose (± 1:200,000 epinephrine) **Postoperative Analgesia** Tramadol, 1-2mg/kg PO BID x 4-7 da	**Premedication** Medetomidine, 0.02mg/kg IM + Buprenorphine*, 0.02mg/kg IM + Ketamine, 2-4mg/kg IM **Intraoperative Analgesia** Infraorbital, mandibular, or other regional nerve blocks. Bupivacaine, 1.5mg/kg maximum dose (±1:200,000 epinephrine) **Postoperative Analgesia** Repeat buprenorphine 6-8 hrs after initial dose. Buprenorphine, 0.01-0.02mg/kg buccal every 8-12 hrs for 2-4 days beginning 4-6 hrs after last IM dose
Canine laparotomy	Moderate to severe	**Premedication** Morphine*, 0.5-1.0mg/kg SC, IM; Or 0.1 mg/kg butorphanol; + Acepromazine#, 0.01-0.05mg/kg SC, IM ± Atropine, 0.01-0.04mg/kg SC, IM Or Glycopyrrolate, 0.005-0.01mg/kg SC, IM** **Intraoperative Analgesia** Incisional block: bupivacaine (with 1:200,000 epinephrine), 1.5mg/kg maximum dose Constant Rate Infusions: Morphine* (0.05 to 0.2mg/kg/hr) (Or other opioid CRI options). **Postoperative Analgesia** Oral morphine, 0.5-1.0mg/kg following discontinuation of CRI ± NSAID therapy for 7-10 days after discharge (if appropriate for gastrointestinal condition).	**Premedication** Hydromorphone*, 0.2mg/kg SC, IM + Fentanyl patch placed 12-24 hrs prior to surgery or at time of surgical prep. ± Atropine, 0.01-0.04mg/kg SC, IM Or Glycopyrrolate, 0.005-0.01mg/kg SC, IM** **Intraoperative Analgesia** ± Lidocaine CRI (0.025-0.050mg/kg/min) **Postoperative Analgesia** May need to repeat opioid dose 1-2 times to cover immediate postoperative pain or until fentanyl patch becomes effective Remove fentanyl patch in 3-5 days.

continued

Table 5-2 Continued

Procedure	Anticipated Degree of Pain	Example Protocol A	Example Protocol B
Feline laparotomy	Moderate to severe	**Premedication** Hydromorphone*, 0.05-0.1mg/kg SC, IM; Or 0.1mg/kg butorphanol IM, SC; ± Medetomidine, 0.02mg/kg IM ± Atropine, 0.01-0.04mg/kg SC, IM Or Glycopyrrolate, 0.005-0.01mg/kg SC, IM** **Intraoperative Analgesia** Incisional block: bupivacaine, 1.5mg/kg maximum dose Constant Rate Infusions: hydromorphone (0.03-0.05mg/kg/hr) (Or other CRI options). **Postoperative Analgesia** Buprenorphine, 0.01-0.02mg/kg buccal every 8-12 hrs for 2-4 days beginning 4-6 hrs after discontinuing CRI; Or Tramadol, 1-2 mg PO BID x 4-7da.	**Premedication** Morphine*, 0.25mg/kg SC, IM ± Acepromazine#, 0.05-0.1mg/kg SC, IM ± Atropine, 0.01-0.04mg/kg SC, IM Or Glycopyrrolate, 0.005-0.01mg/kg SC, IM** + Apply 25 µg/hr fentanyl patch 6-12 hrs prior to surgery or at time of surgical prep. **Postoperative Analgesia** May need to repeat opioid dose 1-2 times to cover immediate postoperative pain or until fentanyl patch becomes effective. Remove fentanyl patch within 3-5 days.
Canine cruciate repair or rear limb orthopedic procedure	Moderate to severe to excruciating	**Premedication** Acepromazine#, 0.05-0.1mg/kg SC, IM + Morphine*, 1.0mg/kg SC, IM; Or 0.1mg/kg butorphanol IM, SC; ± Atropine, 0.01-0.04mg/kg SC, IM Or Glycopyrrolate, 0.005-0.01mg/kg SC, IM** + Deracoxib, 1-4mg/kg PO **Intraoperative Analgesia** Epidural: 0.1mg/kg morphine or hydromorphone (not to exceed 7ml total volume) ± Bupivacaine, 1.0mg/kg Intra-articular: bupivacaine, 1.0 to 2.0mg/kg ± Morphine (1.0mg in 5ml saline)	**Premedication** Medetomidine, 0.005-0.010mg/kg IM + Hydromorphone*, 0.2mg/kg SC, IM ± Atropine, 0.01-0.04mg/kg SC, IM Or Glycopyrrolate, 0.005-0.01mg/kg SC, IM** + Deracoxib, 1-4mg/kg PO Appropriate size fentanyl patch applied 12-24 hrs preoperatively or at time of surgical prep. **Intraoperative Analgesia** Intra-articular: bupivacaine, 1.0-2.0mg/kg ± Morphine (1.0mg in 5ml saline) (for surgeries involving the joint)

continued

Table 5-2 Continued

Procedure	Anticipated Degree of Pain	Example Protocol A	Example Protocol B
		Postoperative Analgesia May need to repeat dose of morphine (oral or parenteral) every 4-6 hrs as needed after epidural analgesia is no longer effective. Deracoxib, 1-4mg/kg PO SID starting 24 hrs after surgery for 7 days.	**Postoperative Analgesia** Hydromorphone*, 0.2mg/kg IM, SC 4 hrs after initial dose. May repeat as needed until fentanyl patch is effective. Deracoxib, 1-4mg/kg PO SID starting 24 hrs after surgery for 7 days.
Canine forelimb orthopedic procedure	Moderate to severe to excruciating	**Premedication** Acepromazine#, 0.05-0.1mg/kg SC, IM + Morphine*, 1.0mg/kg SC, IM Or buprenorphine 0.01mg/kg SC, IM ± Atropine, 0.01-0.04mg/kg SC, IM Or Glycopyrrolate, 0.005-0.01mg/kg SC, IM** +Deracoxib, 1-4mg/kg PO	**Premedication** Medetomidine, 0.005-0.010mg/kg IM + Hydromorphone*, 0.2mg/kg SC, IM ± Atropine, 0.01-0.04mg/kg SC, IM Or Glycopyrrolate, 0.005-0.01mg/kg SC, IM** +Deracoxib, 1-4mg/kg PO Appropriate size fentanyl patch applied 12-24 hrs preoperatively or at time of surgical prep.
		Intraoperative Analgesia Brachial plexus block: bupivacaine, 1.0 to 2.0mg/kg (for procedures distal to the elbow) Consider ketamine CRI (0.5mg/kg IV followed by 10µg/kg/min during surgery and 2µg/kg/min for 24 hrs following surgery)	**Intraoperative Analgesia** Intra-articular: bupivacaine, 1.0-2.0mg/kg (for surgeries involving the joint)
		Postoperative Analgesia Morphine*, 1.0mg/kg SC, IM 2 hrs after initial dose and repeat as needed. Deracoxib, 1-4mg/kg PO SID starting 24 hrs after surgery for 7 days.	**Postoperative Analgesia** May need to repeat opioid dose 1-2 times to cover immediate postoperative pain or until fentanyl patch becomes effective. Remove fentanyl patch in 3-5 days. Or Tramadol 1-2mg/kg PO BID x 7 da; Deracoxib, 1-4mg/kg PO SID starting 24 hrs after surgery for 7 days.

continued

Table 5-2 Continued

Procedure	Anticipated Degree of Pain	Example Protocol A	Example Protocol B
Feline forelimb orthopedic procedure	Moderate to severe to excruciating	**Premedication** Acepromazine#, 0.05-0.1mg/kg SC, IM + Morphine*, 0.2mg/kg SC, IM Or Buprenorphine 0.01mg/kg SC, IM ± Atropine, 0.01-0.04mg/kg SC, IM Or Glycopyrrolate, 0.005-0.01mg/kg SC, IM** **Intraoperative Analgesia** Brachial plexus block: bupivicaine, 1.5mg/kg (for procedures distal to the elbow) **Postoperative Analgesia** Buprenorphine, 0.01-0.02mg/kg buccal every 8-12 hrs for 2-4 days beginning 4-6 hrs after initial dose of opioid. Alternative with Tramadol 1-2mg/kg PO BID 4 da depending upon procedure.	**Premedication** Medetomidine, 0.02mg/kg IM + Hydromorphone*, 0.05-0.1mg/kg IM ± Atropine, 0.01-0.04mg/kg SC, IM Or Glycopyrrolate, 0.005-0.01mg/kg SC, IM** + Apply 25µg/hr fentanyl patch 8-12 hrs prior to surgery or at time of surgical prep. **Intraoperative Analgesia** Consider ketamine CRI (0.5mg/kg IV followed by 10µg/kg/min during surgery and 2µg/kg/min for 24 hrs following surgery) **Postoperative Analgesia** May need to repeat opioid dose 1-2 times to cover immediate postoperative pain or until fentanyl patch becomes effective.
Feline rear limb orthopedic procedure	Moderate to severe to excruciating	**Premedication** Acepromazine#, 0.05-0.2mg/kg SC, IM + Morphine*, 0.25mg/kg SC, IM ± Atropine, 0.01-0.04mg/kg SC, IM Or Glycopyrrolate, 0.005-0.01mg/kg SC, IM** **Intraoperative Analgesia** Consider epidural morphine or hydromorphone, 0.1mg/kg **Postoperative Analgesia** Buprenorphine, 0.01-0.02mg/kg buccal every 8-12 hrs for 2-4 days beginning 4-6 hrs after initial dose of opioid. Or alternative with Tramadol, 1-2mg/kg PO BID 4 da depending upon procedure.	**Premedication** Medetomidine, 0.02mg/kg IM + Hydromorphone*, 0.05-0.1mg/kg IM ± Atropine, 0.01-0.04mg/kg SC, IM Or Glycopyrrolate, 0.005-0.01mg/kg SC, IM** + Apply 25µg/hr fentanyl patch placed 8-12 hrs prior to surgery or at time of surgical prep. **Intraoperative Analgesia** Ketamine CRI (0.5mg/kg IV followed by 10µg/kg/min during surgery and 2µg/kg/min for 24 hrs following surgery) **Postoperative Analgesia** May need to repeat opioid dose 1-2 times to cover immediate postoperative pain or until fentanyl patch becomes effective.

continued

Table 5-2 Continued

Procedure	Anticipated Degree of Pain	Example Protocol A	Example Protocol B
Canine pancreatitis	Moderate to severe to excruciating	**Premedication** Hydromorphone 0.1mg/kg + 0.1 mg/kg midazolam IM **Intraoperative Analgesia** Consider epidural morphine or hydromorphone, 0.1mg/kg Or Interpleural lidocaine, 1.5mg/kg followed by interpleural bupivacaine (No epinephrine), 1.5 mg/kg every 3-6 hrs Parenteral opioids **Postoperative Analgesia** Tramadol, 1-2mg/kg PO BID 7 da depending upon severity of condition.	**Premedication** Buprenorphine 0.01mg/kg SC, IM; Constant Rate Infusions: Lidocaine, 0.025-0.050mg/kg/min ± Morphine, 0.1mg/kg/hr And / or ketamine 0.5mg/kg IV loading dose followed by 2µg/kg/min + parenteral opioid Or fentanyl 2-5µg/kg/kg IV loading dose followed by 2-5µg/kg/hr Consider microdoses of medetomidine, 0.001-0.002mg/kg IM or IV
Canine osteoarthritis	Mild to severe	**Postoperative Analgesia** Weight management + controlled exercise Deracoxib, 1-2mg/kg SID PO + Tramadol 1-2mg/kg PO BID as needed.	**Postoperative Analgesia** Weight management + controlled exercise Deracoxib, 1-2mg/kg SID PO: + Tramadol, 1-5mg/kg PO BID PRN; ± Polysulfated glycosaminoglycan, 2mg/lb, IM twice weekly for 4 weeks If refractory to standard NSAID therapy or if progressed to severe stages, consider adding nontraditional pharmaceuticals (e.g., acetaminophen+codeine, amantadine, gabapentin) and/or alternative therapies (e.g., acupuncture, physical therapy).

*Consult other references for dosages of other drugs from the same class.

**Anticholinergics (eg, atropine and glycopyrrolate) have been listed as an option in a number of protocols. Use of anticholinergics should always be based on patient evaluation, anesthetic protocol and experiences of the veterinarian. These agents should fit into the protocol on an individual patient basis and should not necessarily be a routine component of every protocol. Further, the lower end of the atropine dose may not always be effective in alleviating bradycardia.

Maximum dosage of acepromazine in cats is 1 mg total dose and is 3mg total dose in dogs. Acepromazine dosages as low as 0.01mg/kg may be effective in dogs but higher dosages are generally required for adequate sedation in cats. *These lower dosages can only be achieved by diluting the drug with sterile water from the bottle at 10mg/ml to 1 or 2mg/ml.*

The FDA has not approved some of these drugs or the listed routes of administration for use as canine or feline analgesics; these constitute extra-label indications under the Animal Medicinal Drug Use Clarification Act (AMDUCA). It is the veterinarian's responsibility to comply with the rules and regulations required by this Act. Refer to the FDA/CVM website)www.fda.cvm.org) and the publication, "FDA and the Veterinarian" (http://www.fda.gov/cvm/index/fdavet/cov12.htm

Shock Patient and High Risk Anesthesia

Categories of risk are listed in Chapter 1. If the subject is sick enough to be in the poor or critical category, P4 or P5 respectively, the risk of anesthesia is high. The anesthetist must be very careful in establishing the anesthetic and pain management protocol and select drugs and techniques that do not significantly compromise organ function either during the procedure or following recovery. Just because the patient makes it through the procedure does not mean the job is done. Compromised organ function or failure may not materialize until a number of days post recovery.

In order to maintain tissue perfusion, MAP of at least 60mm Hg should be maintained and values less than that may create conditions conducive to organ failure. Use of automated NIBP to monitor arterial pressure levels is essential to prevent prolonged episodes of hypotension.

The goal is to control everything possible with the use of monitoring systems, administration of balanced electrolyte solutions and manual or mechanical ventilation. Without this capability, it may be best to refer the patient to facilities where not only a high level of anesthetic and pain management is practiced, but 24 hour care can be provided as well. The sections that follow provide information with details of managing patients at risk.

Balanced Anesthesia

Balanced anesthesia describes the use of different drugs in combination to target specific receptors, which will result in safe and effective anesthesia. Drugs that produce different components of anesthesia are used together, namely those agents providing unconsciousness, analgesia, muscle relaxation and attenuation of autonomic reflexes. Hence, by combining different agents, lower drug doses may be used, minimizing side effects produced by each agent. Balanced anesthesia may be achieved using drugs in combination with either inhalational or intravenous anesthetic agents. Opioids are often used to provide analgesia and may be administered pre-operatively or intra-operatively. Neuromuscular blocking agents may also be included in the drug protocol to provide muscle relaxation.

Neuromuscular Blockade

Agents providing muscle relaxation may be used during balanced anesthesia reducing requirements for inhalational agents, thus reducing cardiovascular depression resulting from deep anesthesia. Muscle relaxation facilitates surgical exposure and may be of particular benefit during thoracotomy and laparotomy. Risk of movement is minimized, making their use advantageous in intraocular surgery and in delicate surgeries such as spinal surgery. Some authorities still advocate their use for intubation of certain species although this is no longer commonly used in small animals. When using these agents, it is important to remember that all skeletal musculature is paralyzed and therefore intermittent positive pressure ventilation (IPPV) is mandatory. Also, depth of anesthesia should be closely monitored since these agents have no analgesic or sedative properties and some of the usual signs used to monitor anesthetic depth, such as eye position, are lost.

Before using these agents in clinical practice, a basic understanding of neuromuscular physiology is required.

Physiology of the Neuromuscular Junction

Myelinated motor nerve fibers carry impulses from the ventral horn of the spinal cord and branch to innervate multiple muscle cells (the motor unit) in order to cause muscle contraction. At the nerve terminals, the myelin sheath disappears and the nerve terminal lies in close proximity to the surface of muscle fibers in a specialized junction surrounded by the Schwann cell. This highly specialized junction is known as the neuromuscular junction (Figure 5-1).

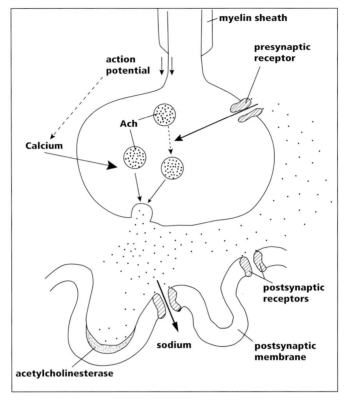

Figure 5-1 Neuromuscular junction

Acetylcholine is produced by the motor nerve cell body and transported down the axon to be stored in vesicles at the nerve terminals. Occasionally a single vesicle of acetylcholine is released into the synaptic cleft causing a miniature end-plate potential, however, this is not significant enough to cause depolarization of the muscle membrane. When an action potential reaches the terminal part of the nerve, an influx of calcium ions causes mobilization of acetylcholine vesicles. The vesicles release acetylcholine from the terminal end plate by exocytosis. Acetylcholine diffuses across the synaptic cleft and reversibly combines with the postsynaptic receptors on the muscle cell membrane, causing opening of ion channels increasing membrane permeability to Na^+, K^+ and Ca^{2+}. These single channel currents summate to form an end-plate potential, which, if large enough, will cause depolarization of the postsynaptic membrane and perijunctional membrane. The resulting action potential will propagate along the muscle membrane causing muscle contraction. The amount of acetylcholine released is far in excess of that required to cause depolarization. Acetylcholine also acts on presynaptic receptors causing movement of acetylcholine containing vesicles towards the motor endplate, preparing the terminal for further stimulation. The action of acetylcholine is rapidly terminated by acetylcholinesterase present at the junctional cleft. Some of the choline produced from hydrolysis is taken up at nerve terminals for resynthesis of acetylcholine.

Drugs that modify the action of acetylcholine at the postjunctional receptors are called neuromuscular blocking agents. These drugs are classed as either depolarizing or non-depolarizing agents depending on their effects at the motor endplate.

Depolarizing Neuromuscular Blocking Agents
As the name suggests, these agents produce depolarization of the motor endplate prior to onset of neuromuscular blockade. Drugs such as succinylcholine are structurally related to acetylcholine, initially producing similar effects by binding to the postsynaptic receptors, but being less rapidly removed from the motor endplate (Figure 5-2). Muscle fasciculations are commonly seen following administration of depolarizing neuromuscular blocking agents and can cause myalgia in

humans. Reversal agents used for non-depolarizing neuromuscular blockade will actually cause prolongation of blockade by depolarizing agents. If large doses or prolonged infusions are used then dual blockade may develop. Depolarizing neuromuscular blocking agents are now rarely used in small animal practice.

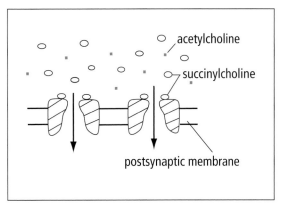

Figure 5-2 Motor endplate. Depolarizing neuromuscular blocking agents attach to the postsynaptic receptor and cause an initial depolarization of the membrane. This is followed by a period of inexcitability when the perijunctional tissue can no longer be depolarized. The succinylcholine molecules gradually dissociate and are metabolized by cholinesterases.

Non-depolarizing Neuromuscular Blocking Agents

Non-depolarizing neuromuscular blocking agents do not produce depolarization of the motor endplate and their effects on the neuromuscular junction are primarily due to competition with acetylcholine for receptor sites on the postsynaptic membrane (Figure 5-3). Hence, these drugs are commonly referred to as competitive neuromuscular blocking agents. By reversibly binding with post-synaptic receptors, depolarization by acetylcholine is gradually decreased as the number of available receptors is reduced. As the non-depolarizing agent is redistributed from the neuromuscular junction or if acetylcholine builds up at post-synaptic receptors to compete with the drug for receptor sites, normal neuromuscular function resumes. These drugs may also bind to pre-synaptic receptors causing a reduction in acetylcholine vesicle transport to the nerve terminal and a subsequent reduction in acetylcholine release. This may account for the phenomenon of "fade", that is seen when monitoring neuromuscular function.

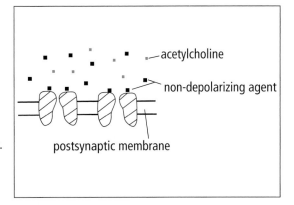

Figure 5-3 Postsynaptic membrane. Non-depolarizing neuromuscular blocking agents attach to the postsynaptic receptor but do not cause depolarization. Postjunctional stimulation is abolished until non-depolarizing agents dissociate and enough receptors are free to bind acetylcholine to allow significant sodium current.

Considerations for Use of Neuromuscular Blocking Agents

Since all skeletal muscles are paralyzed, equipment must be available for providing either manual or mechanical IPPV. Capnography is useful in determining whether ventilation is sufficient during blockade and adequacy of spontaneous ventilation should be determined prior to recovery from anesthesia.

Monitoring depth of anesthesia relies on changes in blood pressure since no respiratory changes can be seen and cranial nerve reflexes are abolished. If the patient is inadequately anesthetized during neuromuscular blockade, movement is possible. Subtle signs may be noticed such as twitching of the tongue and salivation. It is imperative to maintain an adequate plane of anesthesia during neuromuscular blockade and provide sufficient analgesia.

Any drugs or disease states that interfere with acetylcholine release, binding at receptor sites or receptor numbers will alter behavior of neuromuscular blocking agents. Some antibiotics may potentiate action of non-depolarizing neuromuscular blocking agents. Aminoglycosides, polymixins and lincosamides may potentiate neuromuscular blockade by a mixture of pre- or post-junctional effects. Inhalational anesthetic agents also potentiate neuromuscular blocking agents. Other drugs modify calcium flow into the nerve terminal by blocking calcium channels, such as verapamil, or by interfering with enzymes that control calcium flow such as theophylline. Use of organophosphates may cause reduction in plasma cholinesterases, therefore, duration of action may be prolonged for drugs metabolized by this route. Cholinesterase production may also be reduced in hepatic failure.

Extreme care should be taken when using neuromuscular blocking agents in the presence of neuromuscular disease, such as myasthenia gravis. Non-depolarizing neuromuscular blocking agents have been used in low doses since these patients are particularly sensitive to their effects. However, monitoring of neuromuscular blockade is essential if these drugs are employed. Effects of some agents may be modified by acid base derangements and alterations in temperature.

Neuromuscular blockade is often not monitored, although this is not ideal due to the unpredictable duration of action between patients. Residual blockade may be present in recovery, leading to poor ventilation, poor recoveries and hypoxemia once taken off 100% delivered oxygen and allowed to breathe room air. Therefore, it is helpful to monitor blockade using a peripheral nerve stimulator.

Monitoring Neuromuscular Blockade

Monitoring is useful to allow the assessment of blockade present. This is particularly helpful to assess duration of action of drugs used, requirements for top up doses and prediction of successful recovery or reversal of neuromuscular blockade. Monitoring neuromuscular blockade relies on supramaximal stimulation of a peripheral motor nerve, such as the peroneal, ulnar or facial nerve, and measurement of the evoked response of the corresponding skeletal muscle. Two electrodes are placed along or across the nerve. The peroneal nerve is located lateral to the stifle (Figure 5-4) while the ulnar nerve can be located on the medial aspect of the elbow. The facial nerve can be located as it crosses the zygomatic arch. Limb muscle twitches are eliminated before those of facial muscles allowing more sensitive assessment. Monitoring neuromuscular function can be achieved simply by visual assessment although feeling twitch strength is more sensitive. More accurate measurements can be made by electromyography (EMG) or mechanomyography. Several patterns of nerve stimulation may be employed but only the most useful in clinical practice will be described.

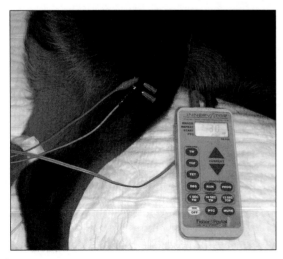

Figure 5-4 Nerve stimulator. A nerve stimulator attached across the peroneal nerve.

Train of Four Stimulation (TOF)

Four supramaximal stimuli at a frequency of 2Hz (2 stimuli per second) are applied to the nerve and the evoked response assessed. The ratio of amplitude of the fourth twitch is compared to that of the first and correlates well to the degree of neuromuscular blockade present when non-depolarizing neuromuscular blocking agents are used. A progressive decline in height of the four twitches is seen during partial non-depolarizing neuromuscular blockade, a phenomenon known as "fade" (Figure 5-5A). All four twitches are abolished with profound neuromuscular blockade. TOF ratio decreases when 70-75% of receptors are blocked.

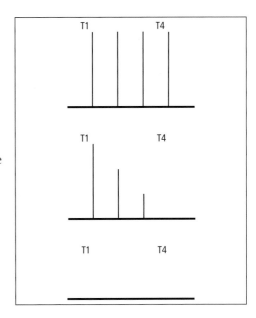

Figure 5-5A Train of four–fade. Response to train of four (TOF) stimulation in the presence of no non-depolarizing neuromuscular blockade at the top, in the presence of partial non-depolarizing blockade in the middle and with complete blockade at the bottom.

Tetanic Stimulation

With non-depolarizing neuromuscular blocking agents, fade can be seen during a supramaximal tetanic stimulation at 50Hz over 5 seconds (Figure 5-5B).

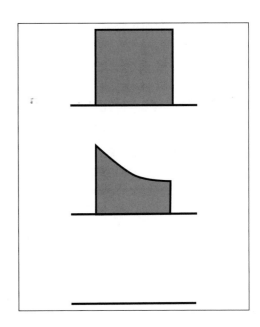

Figure 5-5B Tetanic stimulation–fade. Response to tetanic stimulation: top, no blockade; middle, partial blockade; bottom, complete blockade.

Post-tetanic Count

During deep non-depolarizing neuromuscular blockade when TOF has been completely abolished, post-tetanic count may be used to assess the expected duration of neuromuscular blockade. EMG techniques are required to detect twitches in response to single pulses following a tetanic stimulation. This effect is due to increased mobilization of acetylcholine following tetanic stimulation.

Double Burst Stimulation (DBS)

This form of stimulation consists of two sets of three 50Hz impulses generated 750ms apart, each resulting in a miniature tetanic response. During visual assessment of peripheral nerve stimulation, DBS is considered superior to TOF. Once the TOF appears to have fully returned, DBS will often still show some residual fade (Figure 5-5C). Once both twitches are considered to be equal in strength, it is generally considered that there is no clinically significant residual blockade present. Some non-depolarizing neuromuscular blocking agents are suitable for administration as a CRI. When monitoring blockade in patients receiving an infusion, it is useful to adjust the infusion rate to maintain presence of the first twitch of the TOF.

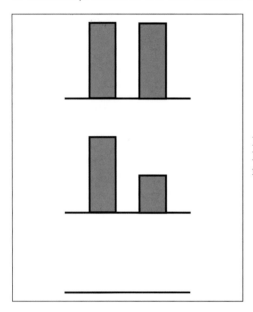

Figure 5-5C Double burst stimulation- residual fade. Response to double burst stimulation: top, no blockade; middle, partial blockade; bottom, complete blockade

Reversal of Neuromuscular Blockade

Depolarizing neuromuscular blockade cannot be reversed. Once non-depolarizing neuromuscular blockade is wearing off anticholinesterase drugs may be used to allow concentration of acetylcholine to increase and compete for available receptors. Neostigmine (0.04mg/kg IV) is most commonly used to antagonize non-depolarizing neuromuscular blocking agents. Administration of anticholinesterase agents may be associated with profound muscarinic effects such as bradycardia, salivation and intestinal hypermotility. Since these side effects may take several minutes to develop following neostigmine administration, heart rate should be closely monitored. Atropine (0.02 to 0.04mg/kg IV) may be given prior to its administration to minimize these effects and must be available whenever using this class of drug. Edrophonium is an anticholinesterase with a shorter duration of action and may be used at 100 to 250µg/kg but it is advisable to monitor neuromuscular blockade since repeated doses may be required. If neuromuscular blockade is monitored by a peripheral nerve stimulator, reversal should not be attempted until at least one twitch is detectable following TOF stimulation.

When neuromuscular blockade is monitored, it may not be necessary to antagonize actions of neuromuscular blocking agents. If TOF or DBS returns to full strength, there should be no clinically significant neuromuscular blocking agents present and reversal is not required once adequate ventilation has resumed. Return of full ventilatory function should always be assessed prior to discontinuation of the anesthetic and this can be done by measuring end-tidal CO_2 and by measuring tidal volume with a volumeter.

Agents
Depolarizing Neuromuscular Blocking Agents
Succinylcholine
Succinylcholine (0.1-0.5mg/kg) has a rapid onset of action with a relatively short duration (up to 10 min) except in dogs where the effect can last more than 20 minutes. This agent is hydrolyzed by plasma cholinesterases, produced by the liver. Dogs are paralyzed by small doses of succinyl-choline whereas cats are more resistant to these effects. Plasma cholinesterase levels differ between species so duration of action is species dependent. Muscle fasciculations are commonly seen and may result in muscle pain or discomfort post-procedure. It has been reported to precipi-tate malignant hyperthermia in susceptible patients and should be avoided in trauma or burn patients due the risk of hyperkalaemia following stimulation of extrajunctional receptors that develop in these cases.

Non-depolarizing Neuromuscular Blocking Agents
There are many non-depolarizing neuromuscular blocking agents available and the most widely used drugs in veterinary clinical practice include pancuronium, vecuronium, atracurium and mivacurium. In general, onset of action is dose-dependent with higher doses having a more rapid onset time.

Pancuronium
Pancuronium is bis-quaternary aminosteroid. It can cause an increase in heart rate, blood pressure and cardiac output due to its vagolytic actions. It relies heavily on renal elimination and blockade may be prolonged in renal failure. A dose of 0.06mg/kg has a duration of approximately 30 minutes in the dog.

Vecuronium
This is an analogue of pancuronium but has minimal cardiovascular side effects. Elimination is predominately via the biliary system and may be used in patients in renal failure. Vecuronium is unstable in solution and is presented as a dry powder to be reconstituted and used within 24 hours. The drug has a reliable duration of action in dogs and cats of approximately 20 to 30 minutes following a bolus of 0.06 to 0.1mg/kg. Vecuronium is not markedly cumulative and top-up doses of 20µg/kg may be administered to prolong blockade once the first twitch of the TOF has returned. IV infusions of vecuronium following bolus injection have been used in dogs to maintain first twitch of the TOF (Clutton 1992). The authors used a dose of 0.2mgkg/hour titrated to effect.

Atracurium
Atracurium is a bisquaternary isoquinolone. It is unique since its action is terminated by Hofmann elimination and metabolism by esterases. Hofmann elimination refers to the drug's spontaneous breakdown at physiological pH and temperature. The metabolite, laudanosine, has been associ-ated with seizures in the dog at extremely high concentrations but these levels are not encountered clinically. The elimination half-life of atracurium is not altered in renal or hepatic failure making it the neuromuscular blocking agent of choice in these patients. Rapid administra-tion of high doses of atracurium may result in histamine release and the drug should be administered over 75 seconds. Atracurium should be stored at 4 to 10°C.

Duration of action depends on the initial dose given. Blockade lasts approximately 15 minutes in the dog following 0.2mg/kg IV, while 0.4mg/kg will have duration of about 30 minutes. In cats, blockade lasts 30 minutes following 0.25mg/kg. Top up doses of 0.1 to 0.2mg/kg may be administered to prolong duration of blockade once the first twitch has returned. Atracurium has also been used as a CRI at approximately 0.5mg/kg/hour, following a loading dose of 0.5mg/kg (Jones & Brearley, 1987) with signs of spontaneous recovery seen 10 to 15 minutes after discontinuation of the infusion. However, dose should ideally be titrated to effect to maintain first twitch of TOF to allow lower total doses to be used and allow a more rapid recovery time.

Cis-atracurium
Cis-atracurium is an isomer of atracurium with five times its potency. There is minimal histamine release and is primarily metabolized by Hofman elimination relying less on plasma esterases. In the dog, a dose of 0.1mg/kg has a duration of action of 25 to 35 minutes and maintenance doses of 0.02 to 0.04mg/kg may be used.

Mivacurium
Mivacurium is a newer benzylisoquinolone with minimal cardiovascular effects, although histamine release may occur during rapid administration. Metabolism is primarily by hydrolysis by plasma cholinesterases. Its duration of action is prolonged in dogs but predictable in cats in the absence of hepatic dysfunction. Duration of action may also be prolonged in liver disease. A dose rate of 0.1mg/kg has been reported to have a rapid onset of action followed by 20 to 25 minutes to complete recovery in cats (Corletto et al. 2002).

Muscle Relaxation
As part of a balanced anesthetic protocol, local and regional anesthetic or analgesic techniques may be used. When employed correctly, this approach will reduce the anesthetic requirements for certain procedures and in some cases may enable procedures to be carried out in conscious patients. Local analgesia may prevent central sensitization making postoperative pain much easier to manage with systemic analgesic agents. When longer acting agents are employed, local techniques can provide postoperative pain relief as part of a multimodal approach to pain management.

Local Anesthesia
Local anesthetic drugs cause a reversible blockade of conduction along nerve fibers. Most local anesthetic drugs penetrate the nerve fiber in the lipophilic non-ionized form. Once inside the axon, drugs become ionized and block sodium channels preventing generation of action potentials. Local anesthetic agents exist as both ionized and non-ionized forms. The pH at which the concentrations of these two forms are equal is known as the dissociation constant (pK_a).

All nerve fibers are susceptible to blockade, however, those with small diameters tend to be more sensitive than those with larger diameters leading to differential blockade. The aim of local analgesia is to block impulse propagation along the sensory fibers, ideally with no effect on motor nerves. Different sensory modalities are affected to an unequal extent by local anesthetic drugs, with pain fibers being more sensitive to their effects than pressure sensory fibers and motor fibers. This may be a function of relative diameters of nerve fibers with smaller, unmyelinated C fibers that mediate nociception being more sensitive compared to larger, myelinated motor fibers. Uptake of local anesthetics and their binding to receptor sites may also be dependent on the frequency of discharge since the anesthetics will cause frequency dependent blockade in rapidly firing neurons. Anatomical distribution of different sensory fibers with a nerve bundle may explain why fast pain fibers are blocked before the C fibers. Agents, such as bupivacaine and ropivacaine, also cause differential blockade due to certain physicochemical properties. Due to the high lipid solubility of these agents, they diffuse across unmyelinated C fibers at low concentrations but do not diffuse across myelinated motor fibers due to high dissociation constants (pK_a values).

Potency of the local anesthetic drugs is related to their lipid solubility. Onset of action is partly determined by their pK_a values while extent of tissue protein binding governs duration of action. If a drug has a pK_a value close to physiologic pH, such as lidocaine, then a larger proportion of the drug is present in the lipophilic, non-ionized form and is available for diffusion across the axonal membrane leading to a rapid onset of action.

Agents
There are relatively few local anesthetic agents used for veterinary medicine and onset of action, lack of toxicity and duration of effect largely govern choice of local anesthetic drugs. Since some drugs at low concentrations cause vasodilation, this can cause increased systemic uptake therefore reducing duration of effect. Vasoconstricting agents such as epinephrine or felypressin are often included in preparations to allow a longer duration.

Procaine
Procaine is an amino ester with a fairly rapid onset of action of 10 to 15 minutes. Due to low protein binding and fast metabolism due to hydrolysis by circulating cholinesterases, the drug only possesses a short duration of action of 30 to 60 minutes. Low concentrations of the drug cause vasodilation so it is often formulated with a vasoconstricting agent.

Lidocaine
Lidocaine is a commonly used amino amide with a rapid onset of action of 10 to 15 minutes due to its low pKa value of 7.7. Lidocaine is 65% protein bound giving a duration of action of 60 to 120 minutes. When used in conjunction with epinephrine, duration of effect is increased. The drug is commonly employed for IV regional anesthetic (IVRA) techniques, local infiltration, peripheral nerve blocks and central nerve blocks (epidural and intrathecal).

Lidocaine has a low therapeutic index and the CNS effects of toxicity occur at lower plasma levels than the cardiovascular effects. IV doses of 22 ± 6.7mg/kg in dogs and 11.7 ± 4.6mg/kg in cats cause convulsions. In dogs, initial signs of CNS toxicity such as salivation and muscle fasciculations are seen at 36% of this dose. It is therefore recommended that doses of less than 12mg/kg are used in dogs while less than 6mg/kg are recommended for cats. If lidocaine is given IV to reduce isoflurane requirements for anesthesia in cats, greater cardiovascular depression will likely occur than with equipotent doses of isoflurane alone (Pypendop & Ilkiw, 2005). Therefore, lidocaine is not recommended for this purpose in cats.

Mepivacaine
Mepivacaine is an amino amide that is commonly used in equine practice for diagnostic nerve blocks. It has a pKa value of 7.6 affording a rapid onset of action of 5 to 10 minutes. There is 75% protein binding leading to a longer duration of effect as compared to lidocaine, with blockade lasting 90 to 180 minutes. It causes less tissue irritation and has a higher therapeutic index than lidocaine and is used for local infiltration and epidural blockade.

Bupivacaine
Bupivacaine is the most widely used local anesthetic drug in small animal anesthesia due to its prolonged duration of effect. It is an amino amide and has a relatively slow onset time of 10 to 30 minutes due to its high pK_a value of 8.1. It is highly protein bound (96%) and has a long duration of effect of 4 to 6 hours or up to 12 hours depending on site of administration. Low concentrations have a vasodilatory effect. Use of epinephrine may reduce systemic absorption but does not significantly affect duration of blockade. It is used for local infiltration techniques, peripheral nerve blockade and central nerve blockade.

Bupivacaine is bound to myocardial tissue to a greater extent than other agents and may also affect calcium and potassium channels, leading to significant cardiotoxicity at very high doses. In dogs, IV doses of 5 ± 2.2mg/kg can result in convulsions while the dose is lower in cats, 3.8 ± 1mg/kg. Maximum doses of 2mg/kg in cats and 4mg/kg in the dog are consequently recommended.

Levobupivacaine is the S(–) enantiomer of racemic bupivacaine and has less CNS and cardiovascular toxicity. When used via the epidural route, there is less prolonged motor blockade coupled with a longer duration of sensory blockade as compared to its parent compound.

Ropivacaine
Ropivacaine is an amino amide with an onset time of 5 to 10 minutes (pK$_a$ 8.1). Protein binding properties are similar to bupivacaine leading to a comparable duration of effect. Cardiotoxicity is approximately half that of bupivacaine. Ropivacaine causes vasoconstriction at low concentrations.

Adverse Effects of Local Anesthetic Drugs
Toxicity may be experienced if excessively high doses of local anesthetic drugs are administered. Peak plasma concentration is dependent on the dose, tissue vascularity and site of injection. The highest systemic absorption occurs following intercostal nerve block, followed by epidural administration, brachial plexus nerve blockade and then subcutaneous infiltration. If recommended dosing limits are adhered to and inadvertent IV injection avoided, side effects should not be encountered.

CNS effects are first seen as muscle twitching and sedation. Convulsions are seen with higher doses leading to coma and respiratory arrest. Supportive treatment includes anticonvulsants, such as diazepam or thiobarbiturates, and intermittent positive pressure ventilation. At higher toxic doses, local anesthetic agents affect the cardiovascular system. The drugs directly affect cardiac conduction as well as medullary centers resulting in hypotension, decreased myocardial contractility, bradycardia and bradyarrhythmias, QRS widening with ST distortion and eventually cardiac arrest. Bupivacaine is highly bound by myocardial protein leading to high localized concentrations and more potential for cardiotoxicity. Bupivacaine may also affect calcium and potassium channels as well as sodium channels resulting in enhanced cardiotoxicity. Local anesthetic agents may also cause local tissue and nerve damage.

Techniques
Topical Application
Local anesthetic agents may be applied topically to the larynx to better facilitate endotracheal intubation by blocking restrictive responses. Local anesthetics may also be applied to skin prior to venipuncture. A eutectic mixture of lidocaine and prilocaine (EMLA) is the most widely used formulation for this purpose and is applied under an occlusive dressing for at least 20 minutes. Intraoperative splash blocks can be employed and are used primarily following auricular surgery where such blockade may add to patient comfort. This is achieved by topical application of 1mg/kg of bupivacaine or ropivacaine using a sterile syringe onto the tissue layers during wound closure.

Local Infiltration
Local infiltration involves subcutaneous injections of local anesthetics to desensitize unmyelinated nerve endings and nociceptors. Local anesthetic drugs may be injected adjacent to the surgical wound to provide analgesia. Injection of bupivacaine near the wound site has been shown to be beneficial when combined with IP bupivacaine in dogs following ovariohysterectomy (Carpenter et al. 2004). In humans, postoperative opioid requirements are reduced following local infiltration of bupivacaine (Dierking et al. 1994). There is no significant increase in wound infection or postoperative morbidity with the use of surgical wound infiltration (Dahl et al. 1994). During procedures such as limb amputation, where many sensory nerve fibers are transected, nerves can either be bathed in local anesthetic prior to transection or local anesthetic drugs may be injected into the perineural tissue. Infiltration of tissues around distal extremities using local anesthetic may be used to produce a ring block. Vasoconstrictors should not be employed while performing a ring block due to risk of ischemic injury distal to the block.

Regional Analgesia

This involves injection of local anesthetic adjacent to major or minor nerve trunks to block sensory impulse transmission. In some instances, drugs can be introduced adjacent to nerves whereas with other blocks, such as the brachial plexus block, the drug is introduced in adjacent fascial planes and connective tissue. Use of nerve stimulators is commonly employed in human anesthesia to enable accurate identification of the nerve bundle by assessing motor function. This allows injection of agents immediately adjacent to the desired nerve trunk. Use of nerve stimulators in veterinary anesthesia is a relatively new concept but has allowed more accurate placement of brachial plexus blockade while enabling new local nerve blocks to be performed, such as paravertebral blocks.

Central nerve blocks may be performed using epidural or intrathecal injections of local anesthetics. Another method of regional anesthesia involves IV injection of local anesthetic distal to a tourniquet for surgery of distal limbs (IV Regional Anesthesia IVRA). Local anesthetic may also be instilled into body cavities such as intraarticular injection or interpleural administration.

Nerve Blocks of the Head

Blockade of branches of cranial nerves may be beneficial in dental procedures and surgery of the head, such as mandibulectomy or maxillectomy. The infraorbital nerve innervates the upper dental arcade, nose, soft and hard palates. Analgesia of structures cranial to the infraorbital foramen can be accomplished by injecting local anesthetic as the nerve exits the foramen. The needle may also be inserted into the foramen itself to block more proximal branches. The foramen is located dorsal to the rostral edge of the fourth upper premolar and is identified under a bony ridge lying under the levator nasolabialis muscle. The foramen may be approached either intraorally by elevating the lip or through the skin. A 22G 3/4-1 inch needle should be inserted under this bony rim until it "locks" into place indicating correct placement (Figures 5-6 A and B). A 0.5 to 1ml dose of bupivacaine may be injected following aspiration to ensure accidental penetration of a blood vessel has not occurred. The maxillary nerve can be blocked by introduction of the needle perpendicular to the skin ventral to the zygomatic arch where it joins the maxilla (Figures 5-7 A and B). A 3/4-1 inch needle should be inserted up to the needle hub in larger dogs and 1.5ml bupivacaie injected after negative aspiration.

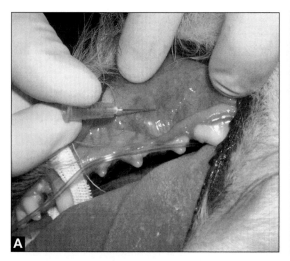
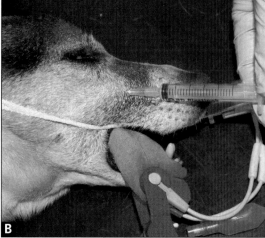

Figure 5-6A&B Needle placement for infraorbital nerve block. The foramen is approached either through oral mucosa (Fig A) or through the skin (Fig B) with the needle inserted under the bony rim so that it locks in place.

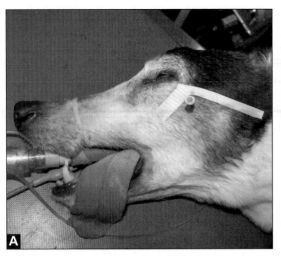 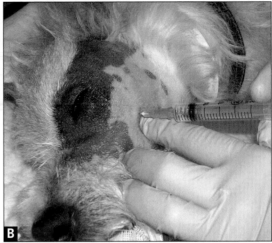

Figure 5-7A&B Maxillary nerve block. (Fig A) White tape has been placed over the maxilla and the zygomatic arch. The needle is inserted perpendicular to the skin, ventral to the angle created by these two landmarks. (Fig B) Injection of local anesthetic over the maxillary nerve.

The inferior alveolar nerve innervates the lower dental arcade and mandible. The nerve may be blocked as it exits the middle mental foramen ventral to the first and second premolars to provide analgesia of the lower incisors (Figure 5-8). The foramen can be easily palpated in dogs and the needle either inserted or else anesthetic solution injected over the foramen. For more extensive surgery, the nerve may be desensitized with 1.5ml bupivacaine injected on the ventromedial aspect of the ramus of the mandible, rostral to the angular process (Figure 5-9).

Blockade of the auriculotemporal nerve and great auricular nerve may be used in patients undergoing auricular surgery, such as total ear canal ablation and lateral bulla osteotomy (Buback et al. 1996). The former nerve can be blocked between the caudodorsal aspect of the masseter muscle and rostral aspect of the vertical ear canal. The great auricular nerve is located ventral to the wing of the atlas and caudal to the vertical ear canal. Bupivacaine is deposited in a line from the wing of the atlas to the caudal aspect of the vertical ear canal.

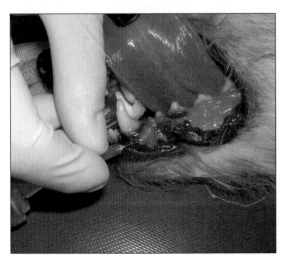

Figure 5-8 Inferior alveolar nerve, mental foramen. Needle placement for mental nerve block. The middle mental foramen can be palpated ventral to the first and second premolars.

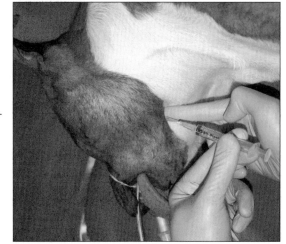

Figure 5-9 Inferior alveolar nerve, rostral placement. The needle is introduced ventromedially to the mandible, rostral to the angular process.

Brachial Plexus Block

Brachial plexus block may be performed blind to produce analgesia distal to the elbow. Recently the use of a nerve stimulator for locating specific nerves within the brachial plexus has allowed analgesia to be achieved distal to the shoulder joint. A spinal needle of approximately 10cm is inserted medial to the shoulder joint and directed toward the costochondral junction (Figures 5-10 A and B). The radial artery may be palpated as a marker in thinner dogs. When in position, the needle is aspirated to check that a blood vessel has not been penetrated. Bupivacaine (1mg/kg) is injected at this site. As the needle is withdrawn, an additional 1mg/kg of bupivacaine is injected. Depending on the accuracy of placement, blockade will develop within 15 to 30 minutes. It is difficult to accurately block the median, ulnar, musculocutaneous and radial nerves. Volume of anesthetic injected is important in the success of the blockade and 1ml/kg has been used along with bupivacaine concentrations above 0.25%. If a nerve stimulator is used, smaller volumes of anesthetic may be deposited adjacent to individual nerve bundles allowing a more rapid onset of blockade.

Use of a nerve stimulator to accurately locate various nerves and and then injecting bupivacaine provides long lasting analgesia distal to the shoulder (Futema et al. 2002). Onset of action is rapid with early loss of motor function followed by sensory blockade due to anatomical differences in fiber location.

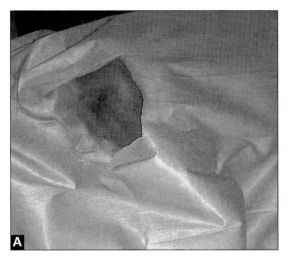
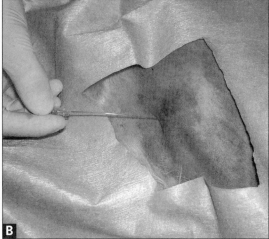

Figure 5-10A&B Brachial plexus block. The area over the costochondral junction if surgically prepared and draped (Fig A) and then a 7.5-10cm needle is introduced medial to the costochondral junction (Fig B). Often the radial artery may be palpated and used as a landmark for placement of the needle tip. Following drug administration, the needle is withdrawn and further local anesthetic placed.

Intercostal Nerve Block

Selective intercostal nerve blockade may be used to provide consistent analgesia following intercostal thoracotomy in dogs (Berg and Orton 1986; Pascoe and Dyson 1993) or to manage pain after rib fractures, while avoiding respiratory depression. Nerve blocks are commonly performed before closure of the chest since nerves can be more accurately located and there is reduced risk of severe hemorrhage from intercostal arteries and veins, which run alongside the nerves. Nerves lie caudal to the ribs and can be blocked by instilling local anesthetic dorsally walking the needle off the caudal border of each rib. The syringe should always be aspirated prior to injection. A dose of 0.25mg/kg bupivacaine should be instilled at each site in dogs. Three nerves cranial to the incision and three caudal should be blocked to ensure adequate blockade.

Paravertebral Nerve Blocks

Paravertebral nerve blocks are commonly used in large animal patients. However, they are being introduced into small animal anesthesia with use of nerve stimulators to provide segmental analgesia of the chest or abdominal wall.

Epidural Analgesia

The spinal cord is surrounded by pia mater and then the subarachnoid space, which contains CSF. This in turn is surrounded by the dura mater. The epidural space lies between dura and spinal canal and contains blood vessels, fat and lymphatics and the intervertebral foraminae connect to the paravertebral tissues. A needle or catheter can be introduced into the epidural space (Figure 5-11) to deliver analgesic drugs that diffuse across into the spinal cord via the dura mater, pia mater and CSF. The drug penetrates nerve roots at the level of the intervertebral foraminae where the dura is relatively thin and invaginated increasing the surface area available for diffusion. Either a spinal needle or Tuohy needle may be used to administer an epidural injection (Figure 5-12).

Epidural administration of local anesthetic agents can provide excellent analgesia and muscle relaxation for surgery of the abdomen and pelvic limbs and can be used as part of a balanced anesthetic technique. In high-risk patients, epidural anesthesia can moderate the need for general anesthesia, although the degree of cooperation or sedation required may outweigh the potential advantages. Epidural analgesia can provide pre-emptive and prolonged postoperative analgesia. Intraoperatively, epidural analgesia can decrease inhalation anesthetic requirements, resulting in improved hemodynamic function. Local anesthetic agents may be used alone or in conjunction with other agents such as opioids or alpha$_2$ adrenoceptor agonists. Motor blockade produced by local anesthetics during and after anesthetic recovery may not be desirable in some patients. More recently NMDA antagonists, e.g. ketamine, have been used for epidural administration. For analgesia cranial to the diaphragm, opioids alone have been shown to be effective at producing

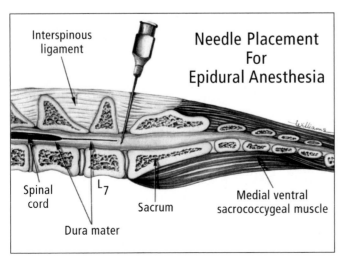

Figure 5-11 Diagram showing correct placement of an epidural needle at the lumbosacral junction.
Reprinted with permission. Sawyer, D C, The Practice of Small Animal Anesthesia, W.B. Saunders 1982

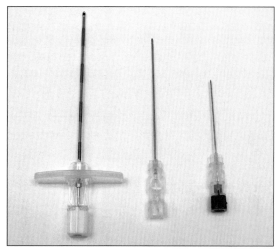

Figure 5-12 Spinal needles. A selection of spinal needles including a Tuohy needle on the left, which may be used for epidural injection or placement of an epidural catheter. Note that the Tuohy tip has the opening on the side compared to others with the beveled opening at the end.

prolonged analgesia (Popilskis et al. 1991). The use of local anesthetics and opioids (Valverde et al. 1989 & 1991) have been found to reduce MAC requirements of inhalational agents in small animal patients although cardiorespiratory effects vary according to agent used and extent of blockade. A combination of bupivacaine and morphine administered into the epidural space is recommended to provide prolonged post-operative analgesia in dogs (Hendrix et al. 1996; Troncy et al. 2002).

Epidural local anesthetics block conduction at the intradural spinal nerve roots, blocking nociceptive input from involved dermatomes to the spinal cord and therefore minimizing central sensitisation. There may also be some inhibition of spinal cord transmission and blockade at paravertebral sites. The quality and extent of analgesia is related to the volume and concentration of anesthetic. Higher doses of local anesthetic drugs will also cause motor blockade and muscle relaxation. Sympathetic blockade may be encountered leading to vasodilation and possible hypotension, which can be treated with IV fluids and vasopressor agents.

Epidural administration of opioids is commonly employed to provide analgesia via opioid receptors in the substantia gelatinosa. Dural transfer and diffusion into the spinal cord play an important role in onset times and analgesia, and these depend on molecular weight and structure as well as lipid solubility. Increased lipophilicity may also increase systemic uptake and therefore decrease duration of action. Duration of analgesia is longer than with systemic administration of certain agents and systemic side effects may also be lower.

Synergism between local anesthetic agents and opioids administered epidurally has been widely reported and may result from interaction with opioid receptors or decreased nociceptive input facilitating action of opioids. One retrospective study in dogs and cats found an apparently greater reduction in anesthetic requirements in patients receiving a mixture of bupivacaine and morphine epidurally as opposed to animals receiving morphine alone (Troncy et al. 2002). This would suggest that a combination of local anesthetic and opioid via this route may be beneficial. Lower doses of local anesthetic may also be employed resulting in less depression of motor function postoperatively.

Epidural alpha$_2$ agonists can provide significant analgesia via action at alpha$_2$ adrenoceptors in the spinal cord, inhibiting the release of neurotransmitters, norepinephrine and substance P. Systemic absorption leads to alterations in hemodynamic function and may limit their use in small animal patients. Alpha$_2$ agonists may be beneficial when used with opioids and local anesthetics epidurally. However, one study in dogs undergoing cranial cruciate repair demonstrated little benefit for postoperative analgesia of using medetomidine and morphine as compared to morphine alone (Pacharinsak et al. 2003).

Epidural injections are moderately easy to perform for the experienced practitioner and are associated with relatively few complications. If prolonged analgesia is required over a period of days, analgesic agents may be administered into the epidural space via an epidural catheter, either as intermittent bolus injections or constant rate infusions. Epidural catheters may be advanced cranially to provide specific segmental analgesia for certain procedures. Both techniques of administration are used extensively in small animal patients.

Technique of Epidural Injection

Epidural injections in both dogs and cats are usually placed at the lumbosacral junction. The spinal cord in adult dogs normally terminates at the level of the caudal lumbar vertebrae whereas it extends further back to mid-sacrum in cats. In young dogs, termination may also be beyond L7.

1. The patient is positioned in sternal or lateral recumbency with the hindlegs pulled forward (Figure 5-13A).
2. Hair over the lumbosacral junction is clipped and site prepared in an aseptic manner following positioning.
3. Wings of the ilium are palpated and an imaginary line drawn between them. This line should pass over the dorsal spinous process of L7 at the midline.
4. The lumbosacral space can be palpated as a depression just caudal to the dorsal spinous process of L7 (Figure 5-13B). Moving further caudally, the fused sacrum may be palpated in the midline.
5. The area is draped and surgical gloves worn. An epidural kit is prepared containing spinal needles, loss of resistance syringe and analgesic drugs (Figure 5-13C).
6. Some operators prefer to make a small stab incision through the skin for introducing the spinal needle.
7. Bevel of the spinal needle is directed rostrally and the needle inserted on the midline at the center of the palpated depression. The needle is inserted perpendicular to the skin. As it is advanced, different fascial planes may be appreciated. As the ligamentum flavum is penetrated, there is a sudden loss of resistance to advancement, which is often described as a distinct pop. This sensation may just be appreciated as a change in resistance depending on the type of spinal needle used (the "pop" is easier to feel when using a wider bore needle).
8. Once the ligament has been penetrated, the needle should not be advanced further, since blood vessels occupy the ventral part of the spinal canal making accidental penetration of a vessel more likely with further advancement.
9. If bone is encountered before reaching the ligamentum flavum, the needle is withdrawn to just below the skin and then redirected either cranially or caudally as determined by palpation of the lumbosacral depression.
10. The stylet is removed and needle hub checked for presence of either blood or CSF (Figure 5-13D). If CSF is encountered, the needle can be withdrawn slightly and rechecked for proper placement: otherwise a spinal injection can be made with half the calculated volume
11. If blood is encountered the needle may again be repositioned, however, it is often easier to withdraw the needle and start again with a new needle between L6-7.
12. Loss of resistance is then used to positively identify correct location of the needle. One half ml of air is injected using a glass syringe (a plastic syringe may be used although there is a little more resistance from the plunger). If a small amount of air can be injected without encountering resistance, correct placement is confirmed (Figure 5-13E). Following injection, the plunger should be watched to ensure it does not spring back which would suggest resistance. Following injection of air into the epidural space, air bubbles may persist for 24 hours. If too much air is introduced, bubbles created may lead to displacement of local anesthetic solution and cause "patchy" blockade. If nitrous oxide is subsequently used during inhalational anesthesia, bubbles may expand (Petty et al. 1996) exacerbating development of incomplete blockade. For this reason, injection of too much air should be avoided. If resistance is encountered, the needle should be repositioned and re-tested.
13. Drugs may then be injected slowly. Ideally the syringe should also contain a small air bubble (Figure 5-13F). As the plunger is depressed, the air bubble should not be compressed if correct placement in the epidural space has been achieved.

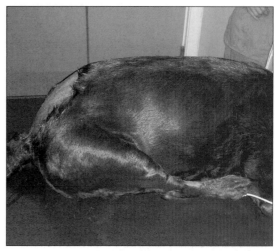

Figure 5-13A Positioning for epidural injection. Canine patient positioned in sternal recumbency with its legs pulled forward prior to epidural injection.

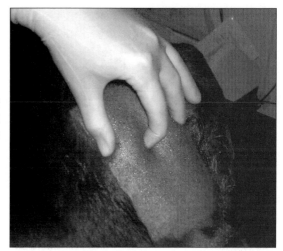

Figure 5-13B Palpation. Palpation of the wings of the ilium and the depression over the lumbosacral junction immediately caudal to the dorsal spinous process of L7 in the midline.

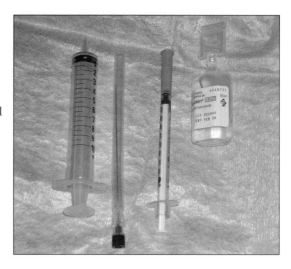

Figure 5-13C Equipment. Equipment for epidural injection including spinal needle, loss of resistance syringe and local anesthetic.

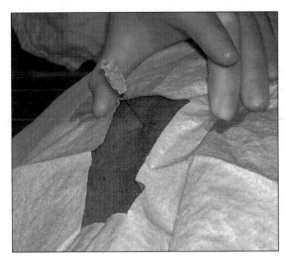

Figure 5-13D Needle insertion. After inserting the needle through the ligamentum flavum, the needle hub is checked for flow of CSF or blood

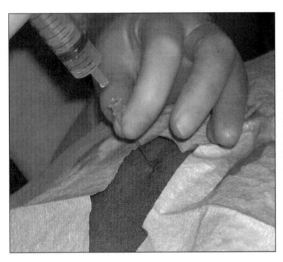

Figure 5-13E Air bubble to confirm placement. A small volume of air is injected using loss of resistance in syringe to check for correct placement. If the plunger bounces back following injection this demonstrates incorrect placement and the needle should be repositioned.

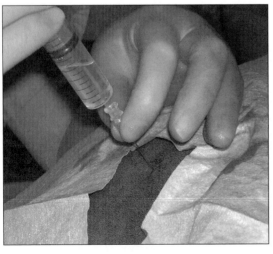

Figure 5-13F Air bubble compressed. Epidural drugs are administered slowly. A small air bubble has been retained in the syringe to detect presence of any resistance. If resistance is encountered, the air bubble will be compressed suggesting incorrect placement of the needle.

Placement of an Epidural Catheter

An epidural catheter may be placed at the lumbosacral junction. A Tuohy needle (Figure 5-14) is used to introduce the catheter into the epidural space. Needle placement is the same as that for epidural injection. However, the Tuohy needle needs to be introduced into the epidural canal at a shallower angle. Before placement of an epidural catheter, the procedure should be practiced on a cadaver to get a feeling for the degree of resistance encountered while feeding the catheter through the Tuohy needle (Figure 5-15).

Distance of insertion into the canal along with length of the needle should be estimated prior to placement so that the tip of the catheter can be positioned at the correct location. Once the needle has been placed and tested for correct placement, the catheter is fed through the needle into the epidural space. For hindlimb procedures, the catheter can be placed at the level of the caudal lumbar vertebrae. For abdominal procedures, the tip should lie at L 1-2 while for thoraco-tomies the tip may be placed more cranially at T 5-6. Verification of correct placement may be made by radiography or fluoroscopy. A positive response to administration of analgesic agents may also demonstrate correct positioning in the conscious patient.

A filter is connected to the catheter (Figure 5-16), which is then secured in place using a Chinese fingertrap suture along with butterfly tape and sutures. Since dislodgement of catheters is the most common complication of epidural catheter failure in dogs, it is important to ensure good stabilization at the outset. It is also wise to label the site with the words "epidural catheter" so that nursing personnel are aware to take extra care in this area.

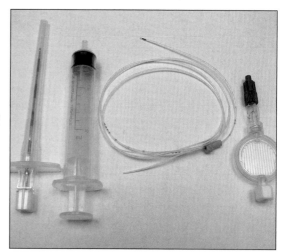

Figure 5-14 Tuohy needle, syringe, catheter and filter placement. Equipment used for placement of an epidural catheter. A Tuohy needle is used to introduce the catheter into the epidural space and then withdrawn. A filter is then attached to the catheter to enable clean injection of drugs.

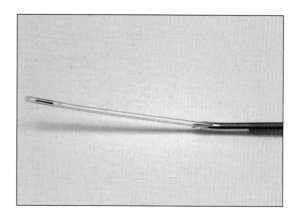

Figure 5-15 Epidural catheter being threaded through the tip of a Tuohy needle.

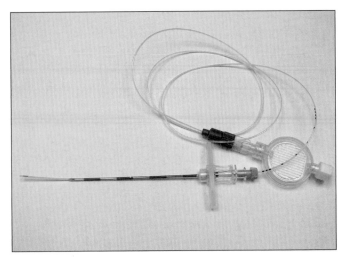

Figure 5-16 An epidural catheter with filter attached.

Drugs Administered into the Epidural Space

Local Anesthetics

Appropriate volume and concentration of local anesthetic remains controversial in the veterinary field. A 0.2ml/kg dose of either 2% lidocaine or 0.5% bupivacaine should provide adequate blockade up to the level of L1. A volume of 0.1ml/kg should be adequate for perineal surgery. Hendrix and colleagues (1996) calculated volume according to the distance from the occiput to the lumbosacral space with 1ml for every 10cm in distance administered. Many factors can interfere with cranial spread, including volume of injectate, concentration of anesthetic, rate of injection, direction of needle, size of epidural space and epidural fat (Klide and Soma 1968). Higher concentrations of local anesthetic are recommended for complete blockade; however, lower concentrations may be used to minimize motor blockade. Higher volumes of local anesthetic tend to increase duration of effect at more proximal dermatomes (Duke et al. 2000). Bupivacaine is more commonly used in veterinary patients due to its prolonged duration of action, which has been reported as up to 9 hours depending on the method of evaluation. Ropivacaine has been used recently with similar results to those found with bupivacaine (Feldman and Covino 1988; Duke et al. 2000). A recent study in dogs highlighted the fact that when administering local anesthetic agents via the epidural route, there is great inter-individual variation in onset, duration and cranial spread (Duke et al. 2000)

Opioids

Epidural use of opioids provides long lasting analgesia that is not associated with the systemic side effects commonly encountered with parenteral use, such as sedation. Use of opioids is not associated with motor blockade and there is no sympathetic blockade making it safe for procedures as far cranial as the forelimb. The technique may be used for thoracotomy or upper abdominal surgery where cranial spread of local anesthetic agents may be undesirable. Ideally, preservative free preparations should be used although preservative containing preparations of morphine have been used without significant complications.

Morphine has low lipid solubility and has a slow onset of action of up to an hour followed by a prolonged duration of effect, potentially as long as 24 hours (Valverde et al. 1989b). Due to its low lipid solubility, morphine may spread cranially and so injections made at the lumbosacral space can provide analgesia for procedures such as thoracotomy or forelimb amputation. In dogs, 0.1mg/kg morphine diluted in 0.13 to 0.26ml/kg sterile saline provided analgesia as far cranial as the forelimb (Valverde et al. 1989b). Oxymorphone, which has higher lipid solubility, has a more rapid onset time of 15 to 30 minutes with a duration of at least 8 hours when administered at a dose of 0.1mg/kg in dogs (Popilskis et al. 1991).

Alpha₂ Adrenoceptor Agonists

Alpha₂ agonists have been administered into the epidural space in dogs to provide profound long lasting analgesia. These drugs tend to have high systemic absorption and may be associated with sedation and hemodynamic effects (Vesal et al. 1996). Inclusion of medetomidine with epidural morphine in dogs offered only minor benefits in pain scoring postoperatively following cruciate surgery (Pacharinsak et al. 2003).

Contraindications to Epidural Injection

Epidural injection should not be performed if there is infection over the lumbosacral junction. The area should always be surgically prepared to preclude introduction of infection. The technique should be avoided if there is evidence of coagulopathy. Traumatic injury to the area or an obese patient may make identification of the lumbosacral space difficult but if the depression can be palpated, then an epidural technique may be beneficial.

Complications Associated with Epidural and Intrathecal Analgesia

Epidural local anesthetic administration may lead to hypotension due to sympathetic blockade. Aggressive treatment with intravenous crystalloids is usually successful although vasopressor agents may also be of benefit. Epidural administration of morphine has been associated with pruritis in dogs (Valverde et al. 1989, Troncy et al. 2002). Postoperative urinary retention may be seen following administration of morphine in the epidural space of dogs (Troncy et al. 2002; Herpinger 1998) and after intrathecal administration (Kohn-Boun et al. 2002). This is probably due to inhibition of the detrusor reflex (Drenger et al. 1986).

Prolonged regrowth of hair may be associated with clipping for lumbosacral epidural injection and it is best to advise owners prior to surgery that this may occur. Following epidural catheterization, there is a low complication rate with those being of only minor consequence in one study (Swalander et al. 2000). The most frequent problems encountered in 81 dogs were dislodgement of the epidural catheter or inflammation at the site of percutaneous entry.

Intrathecal or Spinal Anesthesia and Analgesia

Local anesthetics, opioids and alpha₂ agonists may also be administered into the subarachnoid space in small animals. It may be performed intentionally by introduction of the spinal needle cranial to the lumbosacral space in dogs. In cats or young dogs, it is common to encounter CSF when performing an epidural injection, and instead of repositioning the needle, drug dosages can be reduced and given intrathecally. Since intentional intrathecal injection is not commonly done in small animal practice, the technique shall not be described. Some authors have suggested that the dose of epidural drugs should be reduced by 50-75% for administration into the subarachnoid space although the same dose may be administered without adverse consequences.

Intraarticular

Intraarticular injection of local anesthetics may be employed following joint surgery, such as cruciate repair, once the joint capsule has been sealed. Local anesthetic agents such as bupivacaine 0.5mg/kg or lidocaine 1mg/kg may be injected into the joint, or an opioid such as intraarticular morphine may be used. Peripheral opioid receptors have been identified in synovial tissue following inflammation (Keates et al. 1999). Intraarticular bupivacaine or morphine provided better postoperative analgesia than intraarticular saline in dogs, with bupivacaine showing the greatest effect (Sammarco et al. 1996). In one study in dogs undergoing cranial cruciate repair, 0.1mg/kg morphine diluted in 1ml/10kg sterile saline provided effective, long lasting analgesia comparable with epidural morphine, although it did not eliminate requirement for supplemental analgesia (Day et al. 1995).

Interpleural Local Analgesia

Following thoracotomy, local anesthetic agents can be injected via a chest drain into the interpleural cavity (Figure 5-17). This technique is also suitable for cases of pleuritis, either via a thoracostomy tube or via a catheter secured in the pleural cavity. The local anesthetic diffuses across the pleura to induce intercostal nerve block with gravity dependent spread and no central effects. The regional analgesic technique offers potential advantages over systemic analgesics as it avoids central effects such as sedation or respiratory depression while allowing good ventilation and patient assessment. Interpleural bupivacaine (1.5mg/kg) did not produce any undesirable hemodynamic effects in healthy dogs (Kushner et al. 1995) and was found to produce similar analgesia to systemic morphine or selective intercostal nerve blockade following lateral thoracotomy in dogs (Thompson and Johnson 1991). Repeated administration is easy to perform. In a comparison with IV buprenorphine in clinical patients undergoing lateral thoracotomy, those receiving interpleural bupivacaine at 1.5mg/kg every four hours demonstrated superior respiratory function (Conzemius et al. 1994) and this has also been shown in comparison to patients receiving systemic morphine (Stobie et al. 1995; Thompson and Johnson 1991). Interpleural bupivacaine appeared to produce similar effects on pulmonary function as IM morphine in patients undergoing median sternotomy (Dhokarikar et al. 1996). Despite risk of blockade of the phrenic nerve, vagal nerve and recurrent laryngeal nerve, these do not appear to be of clinical relevance. Interpleural bupivacaine should not be used following pericardectomy due to the risk of cardiotoxicity.

Occasionally pain has been associated with injection of interpleural bupivacaine in conscious animals, although this is followed within minutes by analgesia. This may be minimized by using slow injection of a 0.25% solution. It is best to use a dose of 1 to 1.5mg/kg bupivacaine every 6 hours for the first 48 hours following surgery. Analgesia develops rapidly and evacuation of the chest drain can be recommenced 15 minutes after instillation of bupivacaine. Systemic opioids and NSAIDs should also be employed as part of a balanced analgesic protocol.

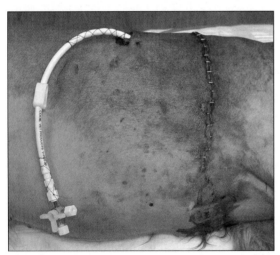

Figure 5-17 Local injection via pleural cavity. Interpleural bupivacaine can be injected via an indwelling thoracostomy tube for analgesia following thoracotomy.
Photograph courtesy of Prue Neath.

Intravenous Regional Anesthesia (IVRA)

Local anesthetic agents such as lidocaine may be administered IV via a limb vein distal to a tourniquet to allow surgery of the distal limb, such as toe amputation. The tourniquet pressure should be 100mmHg higher then that of SAP to minimize systemic absorption. This provides analgesia for distal limb surgery until shortly following tourniquet release. A double tourniquet may decrease tourniquet associated pain and discomfort. IVRA has been used in the dog at recommended dose rates of 0.5 to 5mg/kg of lidocaine (Kupper 1997; Skarda 1996). The technique has also been used experimentally in cats, with 3mg/kg lidocaine providing analgesia for up to 20 minutes following removal of the tourniquet (Kushner et al. 2002). Efficacy of blockade depends on effectiveness of tourniquet placement, pressure at which local anesthetic is injected and period of ischemia in the distal limb. Drugs such as bupivacaine, which are extensively protein bound, should not be used for this technique.

Use of Nerve Stimulators

Use of nerve stimulators in human anesthesia is commonplace. It allows accurate placement of smaller volumes of local anesthetic to be deposited close to nerve fibers leading to decreased onset time and more successful blockade. There is scarce literature regarding use of nerve stimulators in veterinary patients but clinical experience shows that it allows accurate location of mixed sensory and motor nerves in anesthetized or sedated veterinary patients. Needles used are insulated and connected to the nerve stimulator so that a current can be applied at the tip of the needle. If a current of less than 1mAmp is passed across a mixed nerve, there is selective stimulation of motor fibers causing muscle contraction. This allows the needle to be guided close to the nerve bundle.

A contact electrode is attached to skin and a stab incision is made through the skin to allow insertion of the stimulating needle. A stimulating current of 1mAmp is set as the needle is advanced. When muscle contractions become visible, current is decreased incrementally and the needle advanced or retracted until contractions are just visible at 0.2 to 0.3mAmp. This suggests correct placement of the needle tip adjacent to the nerve. Following aspiration, local anesthetic is injected causing muscle contractions to cease almost immediately. Current is then increased to 1mAmp to rule out accidental intravascular injection.

Catheters may also be placed using the same technique to allow prolonged administration of regional analgesia. Currently, technique for use of the nerve stimulator has only been reported in dogs for performing brachial plexus nerve blocks (Futema et al. 2002). At present, this technique is used for regional anesthesia of the head and further development of this technique should prove useful in veterinary patients (Figure 5-18).

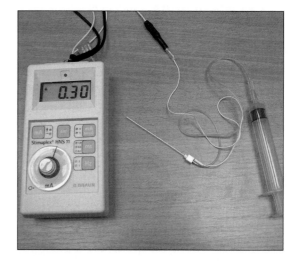

Figure 5-18 Nerve stimulator and needle

Modifications for Breeds

There are hundreds of different breeds of dogs and cats, each with its own unique challenges for the small animal practitioner. Breeders may provide information to owners and have them sign a contract indicating that a certain anesthetic drug or combination should not be used in a designated breed, even indicating that it might be fatal. The only breed that has specific contraindications with scientific support is the Greyhound. Thiobarbiturates are not metabolized in the same manner as in other dogs which may lead to longer recoveries. This does not mean that thiopental should never be used in this species but to recognize the possibility of an undesirable response if a member drug in this class is used. The specific problem is discussed in more detail later in this chapter and chapter 2.

No breed of dog or cat has been identified with scientific basis to have a specific contraindication for any injectable anesthetic, inhalation anesthetic or adjunctive drug used in association with anesthesia. This includes drugs such as tranquilizers, analgesics and muscle relaxants. This is not to say that there are not differences in dosages between breeds or species or even differences between individuals. For example, opioids are effective drugs in dogs and cats but effective doses in cats are usually less than in dogs.

When a client presents information to the veterinarian with concerns about a specific drug or combination of drugs even with reference from a breeder journal as often happens, how should the veterinarian respond? If the owner has signed an agreement with the breeder that "xyz" drug or combination must never be used in this breed, obviously the veterinarian is not a partner in that agreement. However, if the veterinarian is so informed but elects to use said drug and there is an undesirable outcome, then what? It is possible that the veterinarian would not be held liable from a legal standpoint but if the veterinarian's intent was not communicated to the owner, things could get a little difficult.

It would be essential that the veterinarian advise the owner of his or her intentions to use the drug alone or in combination with other drugs for the intended procedure. If there is an acceptable and equally effective alternative to the drug in question, the owner should be so informed. However, if the veterinarian feels said drug or combination is the most effective protocol for the intended procedure and that the veterinarian is not comfortable with any alternative, that information should be communicated to the owner. Most of the time, veterinarians have owners sign a release allowing them to use any and all drugs for the intended procedure including analgesics and anesthetics. Maintaining a good patient/client relationship with the veterinarian is in the best interest of all concerned so communicating clearly with the owner would be the best plan.

Cats, Kittens Small Dogs, and Puppies

One important objective in dealing with very small patients is to obtain exact weight. A baby scale or electronic scale may serve the purpose very well. Pharmaceutical companies rarely have information on dose responses in very young animals such as puppies and kittens. This applies to animals that may be only weeks old to a few months. Some drugs might be given by IM injection but identifying a vein for IV induction may be problematic. Sometimes establishing a venous access is best done after patient is induced with an inhalant. For this reason, inhalation anesthetics might be the best choice for induction and maintenance. For animals less than 8kg, mask or chamber induction may be the method of choice.

Mean cats and toy breeds that fit the category of "little alligators" are best induced in a chamber with isoflurane or sevoflurane. For those animals that may be more cooperative because of better attitude or under the influence of proper preanesthetic medication, a mask may be useful for induction.

One important issue for these small animals is being able to dose injectable drugs accurately. Using a "0" dead space syringe or TB syringe with a maximum volume of 1/3 to 1/2ml will be very helpful. However, preparing a dilute concentration will also aid in this process. As an example, it is very difficult or virtually impossible to provide an accurate dose of acepromazine (10mg/ml) with a standard small syringe unless the drug is diluted from 10mg/ml to 2 or even 1mg/ml. Dead space of a small syringe can contain 0.05 to 0.1ml. This means as much as 1mg of acepromazine can be in the dead space and if drawn into the syringe with a diluent such as sterile water, concentration will be greater than intended. Care in preparing the diluted drug is essential to avoid overdose.

Brachycephalic Breeds and Dogs with Problem Airways

Although most of these comments apply primarily to bulldogs, they should be considered appropriate to all brachycephalic or flat nosed breeds (Figure 5-19). The Chow Chow and Shar Pei are mentioned as having difficult airways as these dogs present unique difficulties that are focused around problems with their respiratory system. This applies not only to induction and intubation but maintenance and recovery as well. This information is provided by a seasoned small animal practitioner who has a special interest in the challenge of providing veterinary services to owners of English Bulldogs. Dr. Foster offered his insight in using inhalants for induction and maintenance for many years until propofol became available in the USA. Since some veterinarians may not have access to propofol, the use of inhalants is offered as an alternative protocol.

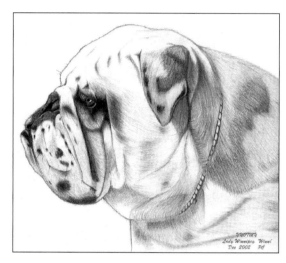

Figure 5-19 English Bulldog. Drawing of Ynotmy Lady Winnipet, an English Bulldog, by Paula Casey who lives in New Zealand.

Preanesthetic Considerations

A complete physical exam and blood work is recommended prior to any brachycephalic dog being anesthetized. Perform the same routine laboratory tests on these patients that one would do for any other case so it is best to follow the minimum diagnostic guidelines found in Chapter 1. However, with these special breeds, the anesthetist has to be aware that these dogs present a greater risk for anesthesia that is not just based on age, weight and disease. For any given risk category, increase by one level for these dogs.

When doing the physical exam, pay special attention to evaluate presence of stenotic nares. When the diagnosis is made, surgical correction will not only be of benefit to the patient but if mask induction is the selected method, one has to be sure the dog does not become obstructed with a mask over its nose without being unduly stressed. In this situation, an IV induction with propofol might be a better choice.

The preferred pre-anesthetic protocol is acepromazine/butorphanol. This may not be sufficient analgesic for severe pain, e.g. fracture. In all these special breeds, rarely if ever is atropine or glycopyrrolate used pre-anesthesia or during anesthesia because of its tendency to thicken mucous secretions, thereby making it very difficult for the dog to express secretions during recovery. Other analgesics may be used alternatively along with acepromazine even in animals over 10 years of age.

Generally, the pre-anesthetic is given IM or SC 20-40 minutes prior to induction. If need be, it can be given IV but one should also be aware that the effect will dissipate much faster. Usually, it is only necessary to repeat the opioid during recovery. Prior to induction, it is best to place an IV catheter and deliver a balanced electrolyte during the procedure. In all C-sections, especially in the English Bulldog, these animals do much better if fluids are running during surgery and there is much less chance that the patient will develop episodes of arterial hypotension or shock due to manipulation of the abdominal organs.

Anesthesia Induction

The preferred induction method for flat nosed breeds and those with known or potential airway problems is with propofol. Prior to the availability of propofol, induction with an inhalant by mask was used almost exclusively. Dogs are prepared in the manner discussed earlier, but then induced with sufficient amount of propofol to allow intubation. As discussed later in this chapter, it is used exclusively for all Caesarian section inductions and anesthesia is maintained with isoflurane or sevoflurane.

Most colleagues are skeptical when they hear that mask induction can be used on most Chow Chows and bulldogs. The smaller brachycephalic breeds less than 7kg can be induced in an induction chamber (see Chapter 2). When doing a mask induction in these breeds, it is best to muzzle them with gauze. This serves two purposes. The first concern is that it is more difficult for them to bite the anesthetist during mask induction. Second, since dogs also occasionally try to bite the mask during the excitement phase of induction, this helps prevent masks from being destroyed. They also seem more concerned about being muzzled than having the mask over their nose.

For the dog with stenotic nares, it is best not to muzzle as they do quite well if the mask is removed a couple of times during induction so they can mouth breath as needed. Then gently place the mask over the nose again. Propofol is a preferred method but pre-oxygenation is strongly advised.

For mask induction of the English Bulldog and Chow Chow, it is helpful to cut a larger hole in the gasket so that the mask will better conform to the face (Figure 5-20). Opthalmic ointment should be used to prevent corneal drying. The Boxer is one breed that usually does not require mask induction but does well with IV propofol. The exception to this for Boxers would be the very old dog in which case mask induction may be preferred.

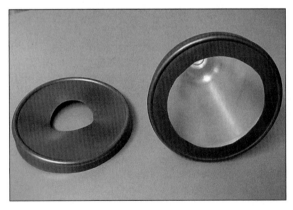

Figure 5-20 Face Mask Gasket. Gasket is cut larger for English Bulldog and other flat nose breeds. Normal gasket opening is on left.

When performing mask induction, use a gentle half-nelson hold on the animal at the onset. The left arm is placed over the top of the dog's neck with the left hand going under the throat to grasp the wrist of the right hand holding the mask in position. This half-nelson grip serves to secure the dog without putting pressure on the trachea. By holding the animal close to the chest with the left arm, the anesthetist has fairly good control of the average dog. Most dogs that are sedated properly will not struggle very much with just gentle handling. It is helpful to have another assistant at the rear of the dog if needed and a third at the front of the dog to hold the front legs if the dog struggles too much.

Another important point is that for most Chow Chows, it very advantageous to have the owner present during induction to hold the front feet. Most owners understand why these dogs need special attention. Try as much as possible to schedule all procedures on this breed so that they can be done first on the surgery schedule with the owner present during induction. There are many Chow Chows that behave entirely differently in a cage with the owner absent than they do otherwise. There may be some risk of liability if the dog unexpectedly bites the owner while in an excitement phase during induction.

When the dog is on the prep table and properly prepared for mask induction, it is time to begin. From this point, one should follow the mask induction instructions in the text to the letter. Allow the animal to just have oxygen flow through the mask on the nose first and then gradually increase the percentage of anesthetic from the vaporizer (see Gradual Mask Induction, Chapter 2.)

With the Chow Chow and English Bulldog, the preferred anesthetic is isoflurane for the majority of the procedures. The major advantage of the isoflurane of course is quicker induction time and the much quicker recovery time. *The author did not have any experience with sevoflurane at the time of this writing but this anesthetic would provide even more efficient inductions and recovery.* For soft palate resections, tonsillectomies and laryngeal sacculectomies, recovery will be quick with isoflurane (or *sevoflurane*) when removing the endotracheal tube for observation and then reinserting it, halothane is much preferred. An alternative for this procedure would be to include an opioid to facilitate this process.

Tracheal Intubation

English Bulldogs, almost without exception, have very narrow or hypoplastic tracheas and proper selection of endotracheal tubes is very important. An adult of this breed is usually intubated with a 6.0 to 7.5mm ID tracheal tube. It is best not to force too large a tube as this will irritate the trachea and create problems during recovery. One must be very careful not to over-inflate the cuff for the same reason.

Once the dog has reached a sufficient level of anesthesia to permit opening the mouth, the mask can be removed. The vaporizer is turned off while the endotracheal tube is inserted and following intubation, the vaporizer setting is returned to the desired position. With the dog in sternal recumbency, the assistant should grasp both upper lips with their hands and lift them up so that the mouth opens and the glottis can be visualized. By grasping the (very large) tongue with gauze, one can intubate most dogs. These dogs often have excessive soft tissue in the pharyngeal area so use of a long bladed laryngoscope is very helpful if not essential. This is especially the case if there is difficulty placing the tube in Chow Chows with dark mouths. Also, it is good to have lidocaine available should the dog develop laryngospasm.

Maintenance of Anesthesia

During induction of the English Bulldog, one has to be aware that they not only have hypoplastic tracheas, but their tidal volume and lung capacity is about 1/3 to 1/2 that of other breeds. This has not been documented in comparative studies, just offered as an observation from personal experience. The problem during maintenance with this breed also involves breathing. For some reason, most owners believe that a good bulldog is a fat bulldog. This usually means that spontaneous ventilation will be compromised because of decreased chest wall compliance. As a result, manual or mechanical IPPV should be used throughout the procedure.

Patient monitoring is discussed in Chapter 4. Because elective procedures in these dogs are an increased risk than in other breeds, they should be monitored more closely during anesthesia. The presence of a veterinary technician at all times and having complete monitoring equipment will pay large dividends.

Recovery

When the procedure is completed, the inhalant is turned off and the animal is allowed to breathe oxygen while still intubated until signs of recovery begin. Even when the Bulldog is taken to the recovery area, it should be kept on oxygen before extubation. Having a technician stay with the animal during the recovery process is absolutely essential for a successful outcome. Because of the unique anatomy of the English bulldog, Chow Chow and other brachycephalic breeds, it should be a rule in any practice that a skilled technician stay with the animal until it is standing. The endotracheal tube connected to an oxygen source should be left in place as long as possible. Should the airway become obstructed, 2 to 3 minutes will be available to correct the problem before severe hypoxia occurs. If allowed to breathe room air, cyanosis will occur in less than 1 minute. These animals especially seem to tolerate the tube even when almost completely recovered from anesthesia. Always place the animal in sternal recumbency for recovery as this seems to be the least stressful position for them. Bulldogs seem to prefer this position a good share of the time anyway. Once they start to object to the tube and making chewing efforts, the tube should be removed.

Once the trachea is extubated, the head must be extended in line with the neck and the tongue pulled out as much as possible to maintain the airway. If the neck is allowed to flex, the airway will usually become obstructed. It is also essential that the technician feel free to call for help if needed. Excessive stridor or respiratory effort often responds well to extension of the tongue and these breeds tolerate this well.

Recovery is when bulldogs are most likely to vomit foamy phlegm and one must be ready to clear this from the back of the throat if necessary. It is good to have some large gauze sponges on long shaft forceps available so the technician can remove phlegm early during recovery without causing too much stress to the patient.

A good protocol with these animals is to use any type of lemon concentrate to squirt in the back of the throat. This probably results in increased salivation to loosen phlegm and makes it easier for them to cough it up. A squirt bottle works well for this purpose. This should only be done when the dog is completely recovered. This is an old bulldogger's trick obtained from several breeders.

Once the patients are up on their feet and breathing normally, animals can be left unattended but still under observation. However, one must be aware that unless they are in a relatively cool and calm area, these dogs can become hyperexcitable and can develop hyperthermia even if at normal room temperature. Be especially careful with all black Chow Chows. They overheat most easily of any breed during recovery. By observing these patients closely for any signs of hyperexcitability, they can be treated with 0.02-0.05mg/kg IV acepromazine if needed.

Anticipate the unexpected and be sure technicians are trained in maneuvers to prevent and resuscitate an obstructed airway. Special attention to flat nose breeds, Chow Chow and Shar Pei is necessary to assure a successful outcome.

Sight Hounds

It is apparent that Greyhounds have prolonged recovery from thiopental and propofol. Mean recovery times from recumbency to standing were 3 to 4 times longer for Greyhounds anesthetized with thiopental or thiamylal than for mixed-breed dogs, with recovery times for some Greyhounds lasting more than 8 hours (Robinson et al 1986). Studies in Greyhounds demonstrated that thiopental was metabolized differently and the metabolic products were pharmacologically active leading to longer recoveries compared to other breeds (Sams et al 1985; Robinson et al 1986). Prolonged recoveries have also been attributed to a lower ratio of body fat to muscle resulting in a slower rate of redistribution from muscle to fat. Hematological differences such as a higher packed cell volume and lower serum protein and impaired biotransformation of drugs by the liver contribute to problems of anesthetic management of these dogs (Court 1999a; Court et al, 1999b). In addition, studies in Greyhound dogs demonstrated that recovery times were 55 to 72% longer following anesthesia with propofol than non-greyhounds (Robertson et al 1992). Pharmacokinetic studies confirmed that metabolic clearance of the drug is slower in Greyhounds (Court et al 1999b) probably due to a difference in propofol biotransformation by a specific hepatic cytochrome P-450 isoenzyme (CYP).

Although Greyhound dogs have been the only "sight hound" used in these studies, veterinary anesthesiologists consider the abnormal metabolic profile in Greyhounds to apply to all sight hounds in this group. This includes but is not limited to Afghan Hound, Irish Wolfhound, Italian Greyhound, Russian Wolfhound, Scottish Deerhound, Saluki, Borzoi and Whippet. Thus the recommendation to avoid thiobarbiturates applies to all sighthound breeds unless proven otherwise. This does not mean that these drugs should never be used in these breeds as long as the consequences are recognized. For long surgical procedures, extended recovery might not even be noticeable. However, for a short examination or anesthesia for radiography, it might be prudent to avoid both drugs if quick recovery is planned. It is also possible to use either anesthetic in combination with other drugs and at lower dosages. Proper anesthetic management includes sedative premedication and appropriate use of preemptive analgesia. Propofol, a ketamine/diazepam combination or methohexital are advised as useful alternative IV protocols.

Modifications for Specific Procedures
Thoracic Surgery

Most patients scheduled for thoracotomy have compromised cardiovascular and/or respiratory systems. Thoracic anesthetic procedures are altered to accommodate the compromised physiological capabilities of these systems. Valvular regurgitation or intracardiac shunting may increase time necessary for drugs to reach the brain and decreased cardiac output will delay induction. A patient with little or no cardiac reserve cannot compensate for normal induction or maintenance techniques. Cardiac dysrhythmias may also be potentiated by anesthetics and direct vagal stimulation may occur during thoracotomy. Patients with compromised cardiovascular function require a slow induction at lower anesthetic doses and concentrations. Cardiac depression, a side effect of most anesthetics, is dose-related. At lower doses, less depression occurs and the cardiovascular system has a longer time to adjust to the anesthetic insult. Adequate oxygenation is important for a depressed or irritable myocardium. Patients may have poor respiratory function owing to intra-alveolar, alveolar membrane, interstitial or intrapleural disease. Ventilation and exchange of oxygen and anesthetic gases may be severely hindered. Space occupying lesions outside the lungs, i.e., pneumothorax, diaphragmatic hernia, tumors or fluid decrease the functional capacity. Respiratory disease may necessitate IPPV immediately following induction. It is best to provide oxygenation prior to induction and to intubate the patient rapidly. Balanced techniques discussed in this chapter have great application for these patients. With the patient in lateral recumbency with the chest open, a massive pulmonary shunt develops as the "up lung" receives most of the ventilation and the "down lung" undergoes more perfusion. One can minimize the shunt by compressing the "up lung". This forces inspired air into the "down lung". Inflation pressure must also be increased after the thorax is opened as lung is exposed to atmospheric pressure. It is best to inflate lungs to 10 to 20cm H_2O during closed-chest procedures and to 20 to 30cm H_2O or higher with the chest opened. A tidal volume must be provided to expand lungs adequately as confirmed by observing excursions during thoracotomy.

It is best to keep inspiratory time between 1.0 and 1.5 seconds. Prolonged inspiratory time may collapse alveolar capillaries and impede venous return. Rate of ventilation should be 6 to 10 BPM. Ventilation must be sufficient to prevent spontaneous respiratory effort and capnography is very useful in these patients to keep expired CO_2 between 30 and 45mm Hg. For better control of anesthetic depth, either isoflurane and sevoflurane can be used and maintenance concentrations will be in general lower than during spontaneous ventilation.

For high-risk patients, a balanced technique using opioids, local anesthetics and neuromuscular blocking agents helps keep cardiovascular depression to a minimum. It is ideal for patients that are unable to tolerate cardiovascular depression from inhalation agents. Including an epidural opioid for these patients not only provides good pain management but allows lower concentrations of anesthetics to be used for maintenance. In critically ill patients, neuromuscular blocking agents have good application.

For successful thoracic anesthesia, one must be aware of the physiological alterations occurring with thoracic disease and during thoracotomy as well as the limitations of each anesthetic agent. Using good monitoring procedures including NIBP to avoid hypotension and ECG for identifying conduction defects are essential. After the thorax is closed and trapped air is evacuated, rate and depth of breathing should be decreased until spontaneous respiration resumes. PCO_2 will rise to normal levels and stimulate the respiratory center so that spontaneous breathing resumes. It is best not to disconnect the patient from the anesthesia machine until it is time to extubate. High oxygen tensions should be maintained and monitoring blood pressure and oxygen levels should continue until the animal is spontaneously breathing and responsive. Observe the patient closely in recovery and have oxygen readily available in case hypoxemia occurs. There must be a balance between having the patient's pain managed properly and not having respiration overly depressed. A painful patient will not breathe properly and overuse of central depressants will impede adequate ventilation. There is where local anesthetics and epidural opioids as described in this chapter can be very useful.

Abdominal Surgery

Abdominal disorders that require special consideration for anesthesia are bowel obstruction and the gastric dilation-volvulus complex. Nitrous oxide will increase the volume of trapped air and therefore must be avoided. One must also recognize that because water evaporates from exposed abdominal viscera at an increased rate, fluid administration of a balanced electrolyte solution must be increased to replace the loss. A rate of 20ml/kg/hr is recommended as a guide instead of 10ml/kg/hr. Visceral manipulation will often induce bradycardia and treatment with atropine may be indicated.

For pyometritis in the dog, balanced inhalation anesthesia or neuroleptanesthesia is preferred. For the cat, balance techniques with isoflurane or sevoflurane, muscle relaxants and use of local anesthetics may be the best choice. CRI ketamine with an opioid is a good technique to master for these cases.

Diagnostic Procedures
CSF Tap

Anesthetic techniques for diagnostic procedures are varied according to specific needs. Cerebrospinal fluid tap is being done with increasing frequency in veterinary medicine. Inhalation agents cause an increase in cerebral blood flow which in turn may cause falsely elevated cerebrospinal fluid pressure readings. Placing the patient in the cervical flexion position, the position required for CSF tap, can result in airway obstruction if the endotracheal tube is too short. Therefore, attention must be given to intubate correctly and avoid kinking of the tube. An armored ET tube can be used to prevent airway obstruction.

The trachea should be intubated to the thoracic inlet and the patient ventilated with oxygen. Verify that the airway is open after the neck is placed in flexed position and monitor heart and respiration closely. Be prepared to control ventilation if necessary, as apnea following the tap will sometimes interrupt spontaneous breathing. One must avoid hyperventilation because hypocarbia will decrease cerebral blood flow. Hemorrhage into the subarachnoid space from the spinal needle or protrusion of the brain stem through the foramen as a result of rapid reduction in cisternal pressure can result in a cardiopulmonary emergency, so the patient must be closely monitored.

Myelography

Myelography is a diagnostic procedure employing radiopaque media injected into the subarachnoid space. Although newer drugs used in this procedure minimize side effects, some may produce convulsions, respiratory and cardiovascular depression and other complications. An inhalation anesthetic technique is commonly used following standard premedication and the use of thiopental, a dissociative combination or propofol for induction. In high-risk patients requiring myelography, it may be advisable to avoid using a barbiturate for anesthesia induction and to choose an alternative technique. From in vitro studies, it was shown that sodium methiodal displaced protein-bound thiopental from brain homogenates, thus providing indirect evidence for a possible increase in the free (active) form of thiobarbiturate in the brain (Bonhaus et al. 1981). This provides partial evidence for some of the anesthetic complications encountered with myelography. IV fluids are administered to enhance excretion of contrast material and to provide a route for administration of emergency drugs. Fast-acting corticosteroids can be used IV to reduce irritation of the spinal cord. Heart and respiratory function must be monitored closely because apnea may occur without warning. It may be necessary to support ventilation and/or cardiac function. Light levels of general anesthesia should be continued for 1 hour postmyelogram to provide time to decrease concentration of contrast media from the brain. It is also best to keep the patient's head elevated. If seizures occur after extubation, they are controlled with 5 to 15mg (0.4mg/kg) diazepam or if severe with light doses of propofol given to effect.

Radiographic Imaging

CAT/CT scans and Magnetic Resonance Imaging (MRI) have unique requirements for anesthesia. Animals must be anesthetized for these procedures and monitoring must be from a distance. For CT imaging, the anesthetist must be shielded from radiation exposure but monitoring systems can be placed next to the patient so they can seen through windows in the screening wall.

For MRI, metal objects must be kept out of the area of the magnet. Therefore, either CRI anesthesia, e.g., propofol, a non-metallic anesthetic machine or a Bain circuit with a 13-15ft delivery hose must be used. MRI compatible laryngoscopes, IV poles and anesthetic machines are available. Monitoring patients from a distance poses a number of problems because most monitors are not MRI compatible. Monitoring NIBP and CO_2 is possible. A 15ft (457cm) hose is available for the Cardell NIBP monitor (Sharn Inc, Tampa) and the detected signal will be accurate. The normal tube length is 8ft (244cm). Capnography is also possible with a longer sample tube.

Modifications for Specific Conditions
Geriatric Patients

Age is an important factor in patient assessment because the margin of safety with patient responses to anesthetic drugs is wider in young patients than in old animals. Young adult and middle-aged companion animals will be expected to react in a more predictable manner than will neonatal, pediatric, senior, or geriatric patients. The newly born and nearly dead represent the widest extremes of the life experience. Very young and very old patients are in a changing physiological status, maturation for the young and degeneration for the old. Therefore, it would be expected that the margin of safety would be narrow for these patients and the degree of uncertainty the greatest (P3, P4 or P5 Risk Status–see Chapter 1). Increasing physiological age may not parallel increasing chronological age for all species and breeds. Transition from young adult to middle age to old age cannot be arbitrarily defined but life expectancy of species or breed in question must be taken into consideration. The last quarter of expected natural life span has been suggested as the geriatric phase of life for dogs and that is a reasonable estimate for cats as well (see Chapter 1). For example, a sporting dog such as Labrador retriever might have an average life expectancy of 10 to 12 years, thus their geriatric period might begin age 9. However, a large working dog, e.g., Great Dane, would start that period at about 6 years of age and be considered aged at 9. Cats are a little more difficult to classify, as there appears to be few if any feline breeds that have short life spans. Perhaps cats over 14 years of age should be considered starting their geriatric period.

When considering age as part of the criteria for assessing preanesthetic risk for dogs and cats, it is helpful to compare age of animals to that of human years. In this regard, both age and size (body weight) are necessary to classify pets as adult, senior or geriatric. The neonatal period is the first 2 weeks of life. Companion animals are considered kittens and puppies (pediatric) until they are 3 months old. From 3 to 18 months of age, they would be referred to as young adults. Thereafter, they would be called middle aged adults until animals become seniors at age 6 for dogs over 50 pounds or 9 years for smaller dogs and cats. The geriatric period begins when animals reach 10 to 14 years, depending on body weight.

Risks of Anesthesia

There is a widely held doctrine that compared to younger patients, major surgery in geriatrics (even those free of concomitant disease) is associated with a markedly higher incidence of intraoperative and postoperative complications and/or death. When examining the role that patient's age itself plays as a risk factor for geriatric individuals undergoing anesthesia and surgery, distinction between physiologic age and chronologic age becomes important. Compared to younger patients, older patients may be at greater risk for perioperative morbidity and mortality as a result of anesthesia and surgery because of two separate factors: first, an increased prevalence of age-related, concomitant disease, and second, a decline in basic organ function (independent of disease) due to aging, per se. A prospective study in human patients of 193,103 anesthetics demonstrated that the rate of complications relates far more closely to the number of associated diseases with which the patient presented rather than to the patient's age. The greater incidence of morbidity and mortality in older patients most likely reflects the fact that old patients present more commonly with a greater number of associated preexistent diseases.

Basal Metabolism and Thermoregulation

Basal metabolic rate declines with age. Thus, all anesthetic agents may be metabolized and excreted more slowly. In addition, intraoperative hypothermia is more likely in geriatrics due at least in part to the decrease in metabolic rate with aging. Older patients show exaggerated intraoperative decreases in temperature compared to young patients, even during short and relatively minor surgical procedures. The lesser heat production of older patients due to a slower metabolic rate contributes to their more exaggerated intraoperative heat loss. In addition, healthy younger patients exposed to a cold environment reduce their heat loss to the environment by intense cutaneous vasoconstriction. The reduced autonomic peripheral vascular control of the geriatric makes this protective ability less efficient. During anesthesia, this lack of autonomic peripheral vasoconstriction may help to explain the greater change in body temperature in geriatrics when undergoing a surgical procedure in a cold operating room.

Several adverse effects can result from hypothermia in old patients. First is an increased incidence of shivering. The greater the severity of hypothermia in recovery, the greater the incidence of shivering that places increased demands on cardiac and pulmonary systems. To minimize adverse metabolic effects associated with anesthesia and surgery, it is good anesthetic practice to maintain all patients, especially geriatric patients, in a thermo-neutral environment during the entire perioperative period.

Pharmacokinetic and Pharmacodynamic Differences

Pharmacokinetic variables determine the relationship between the dose of a drug administered and concentration delivered to the site of action. Pharmacodynamic variables determine relationship between concentration of the drug at the site of action and intensity of effect produced. Physiologic changes occur during aging which impact on pharmacokinetic and pharmacodynamic responses of elderly patients to administered drugs. For example, changes occur in plasma protein binding, percentage of body content that is lipid or lean, efficiency of metabolism and elimination of drugs and finally in a geriatric patient's sensitivity to administered drugs.

Protein Binding

All anesthetic agents are to some extent bound to plasma proteins. The portion of drug that is bound to protein is unable to cross membranes to produce the desired drug effect. On the other hand, the portion that remains free in plasma is able to cross membranes, including the blood brain barrier, and is responsible for drug effect. In old patients, protein binding of anesthetic drugs is less efficient resulting in an exaggerated pharmacologic effect. Four factors may explain reduced binding to serum protein in geriatrics. First with aging, the circulating level of serum protein, especially albumin, decreases in quantity reducing available protein binding sites for a variety of anesthetic drugs. Second, qualitative changes may occur in circulating protein, which reduces the binding effectiveness of available protein. Third, co-administered drugs may interfere with the ability of anesthetic agents to bind to available serum protein binding sites. Fourth, certain disease states may inhibit plasma protein binding of anesthetic drugs. Thus, an exaggerated clinical effect may be expected from administered anesthetic agents that are highly protein bound, if delivered to an old patient with reduced protein-binding efficiency.

Change in Body Composition

Important age-related changes in body composition include loss of skeletal muscle (lean body mass) and an increase in percentage of body fat. Therefore, injection of anesthetic drugs will initially be dispersed in a contracted blood volume in the old patient producing higher than expected initial plasma drug concentration. The increase in percentage of body fat that occurs with age results in an increased availability of lipid storage sites and a greater reservoir for deposition of lipid soluble anesthetic drugs. The greater sequestration of anesthetic drugs in lipid storage tissues of old patients allows for a more gradual and protracted elution from these storage sites. This increases time required for drug elimination resulting in greater residual plasma concentrations that contribute to prolonged anesthetic effects.

Hepatic and Renal Function

Hepatic and renal function is also reduced with age. Age-related reduction in renal blood flow is accompanied by a gradual loss of functioning glomeruli. The combination of these changes produce a predictable decline in glomerular filtration rate that in old age is only 60% of that found in younger patients. These renal changes result in reduced ability of an older patient to excrete administered drugs and their metabolites. The combination of reduced hepatic and renal elimination and a more protracted elution of drug from lipid stores contribute to a more gradual fall in plasma drug concentration in geriatric patients.

Central Nervous System

Classically, it has been thought that physiologic function of most organs, including brain, undergoes a gradual decline during the aging process. Reduction in neuronal density that occurs with age is accompanied by a parallel reduction in cerebral blood flow and cerebral oxygen consumption. Regional cerebral blood flow remains tightly coupled to cerebral metabolic activity in healthy geriatrics just as it does in mature adults. Absence of a quantitative relationship between age-related brain atrophy (accompanied by reduced cerebral blood flow) and general level of mental function, however, suggests that at the time of maximum brain weight, there is considerable redundancy of neuronal function within each cortical, subcortical and spinal region. It is generally agreed that geriatric patients have a reduced requirement for anesthetic agents. This may not be distinguishable in any given patient, but is observed in cross-sectional studies comparing old to younger animals and is believed to be due, at least in part, to a reduction in pre-existent CNS activity.

A classic example of age-related reduced anesthetic requirement is reduction in anesthetic potency (MAC), in both animals and man (Eger 1974). The requirement for inhalation agents decreases linearly with age. The reduced anesthetic requirement for geriatric patients applies not only to inhalation anesthetics but also to local anesthetics, opioids, barbiturates, benzodiazipines and other anesthetic agents. Old patients achieve a comparable level of sedation at diazepam plasma concentrations significantly lower than that required in young adult humans. Similarly, the effective dose of acepromazine in dogs and cats is considerably lower in old animals compared to young patients. Opioids have a much more profound effect on geriatrics and induction doses of barbiturates required in old patients may be more than 30% lower than that required for mature adults. This greater sensitivity to the same dose of thiopental may also be due to a reduced initial volume of distribution in the geriatric resulting in a higher plasma concentration following the same administered dose.

Anesthetic Procedures

No single anesthetic technique has been shown to be superior for geriatric patients. In addition to the important cardiopulmonary complications associated with anesthesia and surgery, risk of postoperative deterioration of mental function in this patient group may be of equal or even greater importance in affecting their quality of life postoperatively. Selection of the anesthetic technique should be influenced by not only by patient's clinical condition and surgical requirements, but also by the veterinarian's and veterinary technicians/anesthetists skill and experience. In general, a fragile geriatric patient should be handled gently and the anesthetic regime maintained in as simple a fashion as possible. This implies that there are increased risks of anesthesia because of a variety of factors. Margin of safety in older patients is less usually because of the high probability of degenerative or valvular heart disease. Their ability to compensate for drug induced insults is less, which means that it is important to use anesthetics and techniques that produce minimal changes in organ function. The practice of using pre-emptive analgesia is essential in geriatrics as analgesics should always be given preoperatively. Depending on the circumstances, induction with isoflurane or sevoflurane can be accomplished by mask starting at low concentrations (0.5%) and gradually working up to levels sufficient for endotracheal intubation.

A local anesthetic along with a neuroleptic combination may be preferable to general anesthesia. However, oversedation of a geriatric may lead to hypoventilation, an unprotected airway, and possibility of protracted and prolonged CNS depression postoperatively. An opioid and benzodiazepine induction followed by isoflurane or sevoflurane and an opioid epidural is a good choice for major surgical procedures involving the thorax, abdomen and hind limbs.

Proper hydration and non-invasive monitoring of arterial blood pressure and/or CO_2 levels are paramount in avoiding hypotension associated with deep levels of anesthesia and in maintaining good organ function intraoperatively and postoperatively. Ventilatory support in a geriatric patient is advisable regardless of the anesthetic procedure selected. Good patient monitoring in the postoperative period is essential to assure a successful outcome.

Summary

Aging is a process that results in decreased capacity for adaptation and produces a gradual decrease in functional reserve of many organ systems. Aging itself is not a disease process but instead, serves as a reminder for development of many age-related disease states. A thorough understanding of physiological changes that occur with aging and altered pharmacokinetic and pharmacodynamic responses of old patients to a variety of anesthetic drugs will help in the design of an optimal protocol for each patient. Appropriate anesthetic management must, therefore, be based on a thorough medical evaluation preoperatively, with possible correction of any detected abnormality. Intensity of monitoring during and following anesthesia will likely be greater than that for younger animals but should be determined on an individual basis taking into consideration patient condition and proposed surgical procedure. Because geriatric patients are not only pharmacologically but also physically fragile, they require great care during positioning and moving. Arthritis is common in geriatric patients and positioning for surgery should be done as carefully as possible to avoid post-anesthetic soreness. Once the patient has recovered from anesthesia, rapid discharge to the home environment will pay great dividends. By giving geriatric patients the safest anesthetic experience possible, veterinarians can contribute to the increase in life span and directly enhance maintenance of full function as nearly as possible to the end of life.

Trauma Patients

The most important consideration for trauma patients is to improve their physical status before surgery. Except in injuries of a life-threatening nature, fracture repair procedures may be done up to 5 days following injury with no change in the chance of successful repair. Depending on the severity of the injury, a delay of 24 to 48 hours will greatly improve the patient's ability to tolerate the stress of surgery and anesthesia. Allowing time for return of fluid balance and recognition of complications will be greatly beneficial to a successful outcome. In general, the anesthetic protocol is more important than selection of the specific agent. Isoflurane or sevoflurane are preferred for greater control of depth, along with the use of preemptive analgesic drugs and pain management procedures intraoperatively. Balanced anesthetic procedures as discussed earlier in this chapter should be considered. If not managed properly, potent inhalant anesthetics can produce severe hypotension, low cardiac output, depressed ventilation and acidosis. In patients already under stress from trauma, deep anesthesia should be avoided.

In an emergency situation such as diaphragmatic hernia, acute fluid loss or hemorrhage, the quicker the decision for surgical intervention can be made, the better. Vigorous replacement of blood loss with balance electrolytes should be at a 3:1 ratio. If blood loss exceeds 20% administration of fresh whole blood is indicated. In P3, P4, and P5 patients, a balanced anesthesia technique is essential with great attention paid to avoiding deep anesthesia. Of course, nitrous oxide must not be used in patients with pneumothorax or any condition compromising respiration.

Drugs such as ketamine that stimulate the CNS should be avoided in patients with head trauma. If there is a history or indication of seizure activity, phenothiazine tranquilizers must also be avoided. The long-standing nature of this myth is not supported by any scientific evidence. Even so, it is better to make this statement until evidence to the contrary can be provided.

For all trauma patients, thoracic radiographs should be taken preanesthesia to rule out pneumothorax or other pathologic conditions of the lung. After a reasonable period of cage rest and treatment, a patient with a pneumothorax may be operated, but a few precautions should be taken. A delay of up to 5 days will provide time for repair of damaged lung tissue. When the patient is not distressed and is able to breathe adequately at a normal rate, without tachypnea, surgery can be performed. The patient should be allowed to breathe spontaneously during anesthesia as long as it is effective. However, if controlled breathing is needed, small tidal volumes should be used at inspired pressure below 12cm H_2O and at a rate of 12 to 15 breaths/min. High inflation pressures should be avoided to preclude reinjury of lung tissue. It is also best to monitor arterial blood pressure and oxygen saturation in trauma patients and to include display of the ECG to detect unsuspected myocardial conduction defects. Fractures involving the forelimbs usually also have concurrent chest trauma and are associated with the highest incidence of anesthetic complications. Pelvic fractures are a close second. Therefore, preanesthetic evaluation of arterial blood pressure and ECG is advisable, especially in patients with front-quarter trauma.

Pregnancy
Cesarean Section

Anesthesia for cesarean section requires special consideration. There are many successful techniques, perhaps as many different ones as there are veterinarians. Some general concepts regarding anesthesia for this procedure are offered. Animals are usually presented during off-duty hours and require more than one person for conduct of surgery and anesthesia. Choice of anesthetic will depend on (1) species, (2) temperament, (3) available assistants, (4) client's concern for the offspring, (5) economics, and (6) condition of the mother.

Consideration must be given to adverse effects of anesthetic agents on the fetus. Such agents must provide immobility and adequate analgesia for the mother. If labor has been prolonged, she may be in a higher risk category because of hypovolemia, hypoglycemia and/or toxemia. The anesthetic procedure must allow for rapid return to a conscious state postanesthesia. A distended uterus may decrease tidal volume owing to pressure on the diaphragm and there is the potential that aortocaval compression in dorsal recumbency may produce hypotension. Positioning for C-section has been a concern but studies by Probst et al. (1983 &1987) demonstrated that supine hypotension did not occur in halothane anesthetized large, full-term pregnant bitches. Dorsal recumbency was an acceptable position for cesarean sections and tilting the bitch 10 to 15 degrees toward right or left lateral recumbency or true lateral recumbency was not preferable to dorsal recumbency.

Drugs that depress the mother will also affect the fetus. The rate of placental transfer is directly related to the lipid solubility and concentration of the un-ionized form of the drug. It is best to keep anesthesia time to a minimum. Place an IV catheter, start fluids as soon as possible and be prepared for surgery before the anesthetic procedure begins. Administer an anticholinergic regardless of anesthesia technique used. Inhalation agents cross the placenta rapidly but the low solubility of isoflurane and sevoflurane keep fetuses from being overly depressed. However, using incision blocks with a local anesthetic will allow concentrations of inhalants to be lowered just before pups are removed. Epidural anesthesia is safe for the fetus but usually must be used in conjunction with other agents; it induces hypovolemia due to peripheral sympathetic blockage and may take more time to perform if the clinician is not familiar with the procedure.

An anesthetic technique that is very successful is essentially the same as for elective procedures. Atropine and butorphanol premed, placing the IV catheter for administration of balanced electrolyte and induction with propofol. Doses of injectable drugs should be given to effect considering the pregnant weight of the bitch or queen. Following tracheal intubation, maintain with isoflurane and infiltrate 0.5% bupivacaine in the incision site. Once the pups or kittens are extracted, anesthesia can be maintained with the inhalant. Pups or kittens are kept warm until the mother is able to accept them and they are able to nurse. Butorphanol can be used postoperatively and oral tramadol upon discharge. One must always be concerned with drugs that may transfer into milk and produce some degree of sedation in pubs or kittens.

Risk of Abortion Associated with Anesthesia

Anesthesia for the pregnant animal requiring surgery before term increases the risk of abortion. Surgical stress, hypotension, and tissue hypoxia may all contribute to this possibility. If anesthesia is needed for a nonelective procedure, considerations need to be made for the welfare of the mother first and of the offspring second. If possible, a balanced technique with an epidural block probably provides the least risk, but opioids or inhalation agents may also be used. In no situation can the clinician assure that the pregnant animal can be anesthetized without the risk of abortion postanesthesia and this should be clearly communicated to the owner.

Urethral Obstruction

In anesthetizing cats with urethral obstruction, the most effective and simple procedure is to use inhalation induction by chamber or mask with isoflurane or sevoflurane. If using the chamber, induction is accomplished and light anesthesia then maintained by mask to permit insertion and stabilization of a urethral catheter. Recovery will be quick and uneventful. Ketamine/diazepam or ketamine/midazolam may be administered for acute obstruction; however, it must be used with great caution or not at all in patients with chronic urethral obstruction and renal dysfunction. High plasma levels of K^+ are often found with urethral obstruction and can lead to severe consequences if not treated.

Liver Disease

Patients with elevated serum enzyme levels indicative of liver disease must be anesthetized with great care. It is best to avoid any agent that requires hepatic metabolism for clinical recovery. Many homeostatic functions of the liver are influenced by anesthetics through their effects on splanchnic blood flow and the role of the liver in biotransformation of anesthetic agents. Liver disease must be severe before biotransformation of drugs such as short-acting barbiturates, succinylcholine and opioids is affected. However, acute liver disease and extensive tissue replacement by primary or metastatic hepatic neoplasms is associated with a high anesthetic death rate.

Maximal possible improvement in liver function should be attempted preoperatively. Prothrombin and serum albumin should be at minimally acceptable levels, as should sodium bromosulfophthalein excretion and alkaline phosphatase. Unless otherwise contraindicated because of a previous history of postanesthetic hepatitis, isoflurane or sevoflurane are acceptable inhalants. If induction by inhalation is not feasible, such as in a patient that has elevated liver enzyme levels and depressed liver function but is still difficult to manage physically, chemical restraint may be required. An opioid combined with midazolam may be used to get the patient under control with additional doses of the narcotic given along with an inhalant by mask and then intubated. A balanced technique as appropriate for the situation may be used to continue the procedure.

Kidney Disease

Excretion of anesthetic drugs and their metabolites by the kidney and its role in acid-base regulation, fluid balance and metabolism are important considerations in anesthetic management of patients with kidney disease. Certainly in patients with minimal kidney function, drugs such as thiopental, ketamine and propofol should be avoided. Even succinylcholine must be used with great caution but there are neuromuscular blockers that can be used as described earlier in this chapter. Tonicity of blood will be increased by elevated urea levels and high potassium may precipitate ventricular asystole or fibrillation. Anesthetic drugs, hypoxia, hypercarbia and low cardiac output may exacerbate the elevation in K^+. Fluid administration is essential but volume must be carefully monitored and fluids low in, or devoid of, potassium should be used. The geriatric canine patient will commonly have some degree of interstitial nephritis and one must be careful not to precipitate a crisis by administering drugs that are potential nephrotoxins to sick patients.

Endocrine Disease

Each abnormality calls for a specific anesthetic approach. Diseases of the pituitary-adrenal axis may require correction of electrolyte balance, replacement therapy with steroids and use of nonsympathetic stimulating agents such as halogenated compounds. Atropine should not be used in the presence of thyrotoxicosis and drugs with sympathetic stimulating properties should be avoided to preclude the possibility of high thyroxine release. In order to keep insulin levels under control in patients with insuloma, atropine should not be given.

Heart Disease

The goals of any anesthetic procedure are (1) to avoid an increase in myocardial irritability, (2) to avoid significant ventricular dysrhythmias and (3) to prevent profound circulatory depression that might lead to hypotension, poor tissue perfusion of vital organs and possibly cardiac arrest. The patient with primary heart disease is more susceptible to myocardial depression; therefore balanced anesthetic techniques are advisable in order to preserve adequate cardiovascular function. The use of sodium-containing fluids must be avoided and fluid load must be carefully monitored. One must understand the circulatory effects of the anesthetics used in order to ensure adequate oxygenation, elimination of carbon dioxide and maintenance of a safe blood pressure levels. A modest decrease in arterial pressure will decrease afterload and stroke work, thereby decreasing myocardial oxygen consumption. On the other hand, drugs that increase heart rate and myocardial action also increase the work of the heart and oxygen demand. An appropriate balance must therefore be attained during anesthesia to avoid poor tissue perfusion and any conditions that would increase myocardial oxygen demand. This issue is dealt with earlier in this chapter but it is obvious why the high risk patient, e.g., P3, P4 or P5, provides such a challenge for anesthetic management.

Diabetes

Diabetic animals often require special metabolic management, may have other concurrent diseases and are higher anesthetic risks because of interactions between anesthetics and insulin. Insulin release is stimulated by beta-adrenergic agonists and inhibited by epinephrine and norepinephrine through their alpha-adrenergic actions. Stresses associated with anesthesia that increase circulating catecholamines cause glycogenolysis and inhibition of insulin release, conditions that elevate blood sugar. Non-insulin-dependent diabetics, Type 2, have the ability to meet part of their insulin requirement with endogenous insulin production but need a boost to improve uptake of glucose by tissues. These patients are not commonly seen in veterinary medicine. Insulin-dependent Type 1 diabetics produce little or no insulin relative to their demands and, therefore, need exogenous insulin. In an unstressed state and on a stable diet, such patients may have adequate balance, but during the perioperative period they require close observation. One must be aware of the insulin requirements and the lability of disease when considering anesthesia in a diabetic animal. Hypoglycemia must be avoided; if any compromise is to be made, it must be made on the side of a transient hyperglycemia.

A number of methods have been proposed for anesthetic management of the diabetic: giving no insulin on the day of anesthesia, giving half the daily insulin dose, using sliding scale coverage with regular insulin governed by blood glucose levels and continuous IV insulin. For simple procedures in the unstressed, marginally diabetic patient with adequate endogenous insulin production, no change in management is indicated. In other cases, half of the usual daily NPH insulin dose should be given the morning of surgery. IV dextrose should be given preinduction and continued until the patient has recovered from anesthesia. The rate of administration of 5% dextrose in lactated Ringer's solution or a similar balanced electrolyte is the same as with other anesthetized patients, i.e., 10ml/kg/hr. This would be a hypertonic solution so avoid excess volume that may cause cardiac compromise in a patient with underlying heart disease. Many diabetic animals are elderly and often have concomitant diseases. Early in the day is the best time for anesthesia of these animals. If the procedure is not to be done until the afternoon, a small amount of food should be given at least 4 hours preinduction or a dextrose drip started after the morning insulin-dose is given. Another technique is to add 0.5 unit of insulin per 100ml of 5% dextrose-containing fluid and to administer the solution at the normal rate, 10ml/kg/hr. During the anesthetic procedure, especially those lasting more than 60 minutes, periodic checks of urine and/or blood glucose levels are advisable. Signs of hypoglycemia, which must be avoided, are: depression, seizures, tachycardia, hypertension, and other signs of sympathetic hyperactivity. Another sign is delayed recovery so glucose measurement during recovery of these patients is essential.

Epilepsy

A few precautions need to be taken in anesthesia of the epileptic. Anesthetics, of course, will suppress seizures during the procedure, but phenothiazine tranquilizers, which may lower the seizure threshold, and any cerebral stimulant must be avoided. If epileptic condition is being controlled with a cerebral depressant, induction dose of short-acting anesthetics may be decreased. Depending on drugs used to control seizures, one must be aware that hepatic enzyme induction is a consequence to chronic phenobarbital therapy and that increased metabolism of inhalation anesthetics or other agents may lead to complications.

Obesity

The obese patient presents special problems in anesthesia, mostly regarding ventilation and potential overdose of injectable drugs. Because of increased weight of excess fat and because of the insignificant role of fat in the uptake and distribution of anesthetic agents, a relative overdose of injectable anesthetics will be unintentionally given unless an allowance is made and the dosage reduced. In the obese patient, increased chest wall mass leads to decreased chest wall compliance. This adds to the work of breathing and may be coupled with a decreased parenchymal compliance secondary to reduction in lung volume, premature airway closure and increased pulmonary blood volume. Because of increases in adipose tissue distributed to the chest wall and abdomen and therefore an increase in intra-abdominal pressure, the work of breathing is greater and lung volume is reduced. Depression of alveolar ventilation by anesthetics contributes to this problem; therefore controlled breathing should be instituted immediately following induction and should be continued throughout the procedure.

Airway problems may be encountered after induction and extubation. Thus, oxygenation before induction is indicated, and attention to adequate oxygenation during recovery must be paid. Use of pulse oximetry is essential to monitor adequate oxygen levels while the patient regains full recovery.

It appears that metabolism of volatile anesthetic agents in markedly obese patients differs quantitatively and qualitatively, particularly with halothane, from that in nonobese patients. That is not a problem when using isoflurane or sevoflurane. With prudent management of the anesthetic levels and awareness of the longer duration of action of retained anesthetics, recovery of the properly ventilated obese patient will be prompt. Normal breathing patterns must return quickly postanesthesia to allow patients to resume ambulating early after operation.

Anemia

On rare occasions, a patient with chronic anemia will require anesthesia. Such a patient may have a hematocrit 50 to 75% below normal. Anesthesia carries a certain degree of risk in the anemic patient not only because of the loss of blood cells but also because of the underlying disease causing the chronic problem. Certainly attempts should be made preanesthesia for blood cell replacement or blood substitutes. Blood volume is usually normal and oxygenation is usually adequate with the patient at rest. Anesthesia for an anemic patient is best induced with isoflurane or sevoflurane only. MAC for the patient with severe anemia will be lower, so anesthetic concentrations must be as low as possible. If a short-acting barbiturate or propofol is used, the induction dose must also be reduced because protein-binding sites are fewer, resulting in an increase in the active form of the drug available for action. This same circumstance occurs in animals with a low total protein. Experience with anemic patients has been remarkably good, although it is difficult to assess their status regarding tissue perfusion during the procedure because of their pale or blanched mucous membranes. The patient should be closely monitored, including NIBP, pulse oximetry, CO_2, and ECG with attention given to evidence of myocardial hypoxia indicated by S-T segment depression or ventricular dysrhythmias. It is important to keep cardiac output as close to normal as possible in order to maintain adequate tissue perfusion. Precluding other complications, recovery from anesthesia by the anemic patient is usually uneventful.

Malignant Hyperthermia

Malignant hyperthermia (MH) is a hypermetabolic syndrome involving skeletal muscle. It is characterized by hyperthermia, tachycardia, tachypnea, increased oxygen consumption, cyanosis, cardiac dysrhythmias, metabolic acidosis, respiratory acidosis, muscle rigidity, unstable arterial blood pressure and death. There also may be electrolyte abnormalities, myoglobinuria, creatine kinase elevation, impaired blood coagulation, renal failure and pulmonary edema (Sawyer 1981; Nelson 1991). Although MH was initially recognized as a fatal syndrome in humans, the term describing its occurrence in swine was subsequently called Porcine Stress Syndrome (PSS). MH has been estimated to occur in 1 out of 15,000 general anesthetic procedures in humans. The prevalence of susceptible human patients is estimated at between 1 in 200 and 1 in 5000 of the general population (Britt and Kalow 1970). MH is most prevalent in swine, but this syndrome has also been reported in dogs (especially Greyhounds), and cats (Short and Paddleford 73; de Jong et al. 1974; Bagshaw et al. 1978; Cohen 1978; Kirmayer et al. 1984; Bellah et al. 1989).

MH was first described as an inherited syndrome in 1960. Five years later, Dr. Beverly Britt, an anesthesiologist at Toronto General Hospital, described a suspected case of MH. During an operation on a 10-year-old girl, the surgeon complained of the patient's muscle rigidity, a symptom now recognized as a warning sign of MH (Katz 1980). Shortly after a second dose of succinylcholine had been administered, body temperature jumped to 45°C, arterial blood pressure decreased and resuscitative efforts were unsuccessful. The anesthesiologist later discovered that this girl was a member of a family with a long pedigree that had a number of unexplained anesthetic deaths. The family, founded by a pirate in the 1600's, had numerous marriages between relatives and parents produced large families with big children. Six years after the young girl's death, Dr. Britt traveled to northern Quebec to obtain blood samples, muscle biopsies and to trace the family history in more detail. She eventually confirmed that MH was likely responsible for the girl's death and cause of many unexpected family member deaths as well. This provided data to confirm the genetic nature of this disease.

Currently, the question regarding unexplained anesthetic deaths is part of the family history questionnaire filled out by patients and should be included on history forms for veterinary patients as well. In addition, anytime a suspected case of MH occurs, it is prudent for the veterinarian to notify owners of siblings and the breeder, if applicable. However, MH can occur sporadically without any pedigree history. Many times, MH will have occurred following a prior anesthetic procedure but because of subtle symptoms that might go unrecognized, the syndrome would not have been suspected or diagnosed (Leary et al. 1983).

Etiology

An autosomal recessive gene that has variable penetrance determines susceptibility to MH. The causative mutation has been localized to a C-to-T transition in the gene that controls the Ca^{2+} release channel (ryanodine receptor) of sarcoplasmic reticulum in skeletal muscle (MacLennan and Phillips 1992). Loss in regulation of muscle cell Ca^{++} is believed to be the primary etiologic event for induction of MH. It is consistently triggered in genetically susceptible animals by excitement, apprehension, exercise or environmental stress (O'Brien and Rand 1985; Dickinson and Sullivan 1994). This is particularly true in pigs but exercise–induced MH has also been reported in dogs suggesting the existence of canine stress syndrome (Rand and O'Brien 1985). Exposure to volatile anesthetics or depolarizing neuromuscular blocking agents will consistently trigger MH in susceptible subjects. In fact, the halothane test can be used as a screening method.

Subsequent to the initial challenge or stress, the hypersensitive ryanodine receptor floods the myoplasm of skeletal muscle with Ca^{2+}. Muscle contracture and hypermetabolism develop rapidly as a direct result of this uncontrolled and sustained increase in myoplasmic Ca^{2+}. ATP depletion in skeletal muscle occurs as energy requirements for contracture exceed supply. Increased aerobic and anaerobic metabolism results in excessive CO_2 and lactic acid production, while thermogenesis and peripheral vasoconstriction increase core body temperature (Strazis and Fox 1993). As the MH episode progresses, combination of increased temperature, acidosis and ATP depletion leads to rhabdomyolysis. Myoplasmic enzymes and electrolytes are released from cells and additional Ca^{2+} enters the myoplasm. Contracture and its subsequent energy requirements are further enhanced and eventually, due to temperature and pH changes, contracture proceeds independent of myoplasmic Ca^{2+} levels. Death occurs due to an increase in K^+, which causes cardiac dysrhythmia and arrest.

Clinical Findings

Rapidity with which clinical signs develop varies. Symptoms include muscle stiffness or fasciculations that progress to muscle rigor. Ventricular tachycardia develops early and continues until serum K^+ reach cardiotoxic levels. In unanesthetized animals, open-mouthed breathing, tachycardia and hyperventilation may progress to apnea. Blanching and erythema followed by blotchy cyanosis are seen in skin of light-pigmented animals. Core body temperature rapidly increases and can reach

45°C antemortem. In anesthetized animals, there will be rapid depletion of CO_2 absorbent and the breathing circuit canister possibly too hot to touch. Usually, hypothermia is an expected consequence during general anesthesia so detection of hyperthermia is a key symptom along with the presence of tachycardia and tachypnea. The disease is usually fatal. Rigor mortis develops within minutes and muscle temperature is significantly increased. Affected muscles from an animal that dies acutely from MH are pale, soft and appear exudative or wet.

Diagnosis

Diagnosis is based on development of clinical signs in an animal exposed to a volatile anesthetic and/or stressful event. The acute nature of the disease and its relationship to a stressor enables differentiation of MH from other fatal disorders. Numerous laboratory tests have been developed to aid in the identification of MH-susceptible animals, but none enables rapid diagnosis of MH in an acute situation. Most screening tests lack the sensitivity and specificity to identify MH-susceptible animals or carriers. The Caffeine Contracture Test involves in vitro exposure of extracted muscle tissue to caffeine and halothane. Muscle from MH susceptible subjects will contract when exposed to lower concentrations of caffeine and halothane, compared with normal muscle. This test has limited application in animals since special laboratory facilities are required and the test must be run within minutes after the specimen is obtained. A molecular genetic test is specific for the MH gene (Gallant et al. 1989). This DNA-based assay is performed on a small sample of anticoagulated blood to detect mutation in the ryanodine receptor gene and can identify homozygous MH-resistant and MH-susceptible animals as well as heterozygous carriers. It has been reported to more accurately predict both the homozygous and heterozygous forms of the MH gene than does the halothane challenge test (Rempel et al. 1993).

Treatment

Often, MH episodes are not treated primarily because they are not identified soon enough. During anesthesia, early detection is essential for a successful outcome. Exposure of the animal to the volatile anesthetic must be eliminated. Breathing tubes and CO_2 canister must be changed and dantrolene sodium should be given at 4-5mg/kg, IV (Bagshaw et al. 1981).

It is imperative that dantrolene be administered early in the course of the disease because muscle blood flow is significantly reduced as the disease progresses. Additional dosages of dantrolene may be given as needed. Dantrolene is expensive and unfortunately is not usually available in most veterinary practices. Supportive treatment includes fluid therapy and management of acidosis through ventilatory support and administration of sodium bicarbonate. Increases in core body temperature can be managed by surface cooling and/or chilled saline lavages. If an MH anesthetic event is detected in cold climates, moving an animal outside and to a snow bank may be a life-saving maneuver. Other supportive measures include oxygen enrichment of inspired gases and treatment of cardiac dysrhythmias.

If a documented MH survivor or a suspected susceptible animal requires anesthesia and surgery, 3- 5mg dantrolene/kg should be given PO 1 to 2 days preanesthesia. A tranquilizer-opioid combination can be given as preanesthetic medication and propofol used to induce anesthesia (Allen 1991). Acepromazine and droperidol inhibit development of MH and propofol has not been reported to trigger MH (Gallen 1991). Volatile anesthetic agents must be avoided as well as ketamine which may also may trigger an MH episode. The CO_2 absorber should be cleaned and new absorbent used along with a new breathing circuit and endotracheal tube. Amide local anesthetics are safe to use in MH susceptible patients. Finally, the procedure must be kept as short as possible. When MH occurs, it most often will happen when anesthetic procedures exceed one hour. All of these maneuvers are precautionary to reduce the possibility but may not prevent initiation of an MH crisis.

References

Allen G (1991). Propofol and malignant hyperthermia. *Anesth Analg* 73:358.

Bagshaw RJ, Cox RH, Rosenberg H (1981). Dantrolene treatment of malignant hyperthermia. *JAVMA* 178:1029.

Bagshaw RJ, Cox RH, Knight DH, Detweiler DK (1978). Malignant hyperthermia in a Greyhound. *JAVMA* 172:61-62.

Bellah JR, Robertson SA, Buergelt CD, McGavin (1989). Suspected malignant hyperthermia after halothane anesthesia in a cat. *Vet Surg* 18:483-488.

Berg BJ & Orton EC (1986). Pulmonary function in dogs after intercostal thoracotomy: Comparison of morphine, oxymorphone and selective intercostal nerve block. *Am J Vet Res* 47:471-474.

Bonhaus DW, Sawyer DC, and Hook JB (1981). Displacement of protein-bound thiopental by sodium methiodal (Skiodan) may contribute to anesthetic complications during canine myelography. *Amer J Vet Res* 42:1612-1614.

Britt BA, Kalow W (1970). Malignant hyperthermia: a statistical review. *Can Anaesth Soc J* 17:293-315.

Buback JL, Boothe HW, Carroll GL et al (1996). Comparison of three methods for relief of pain after ear canal ablation in dogs. *Vet Surg* 25:380-385.

Carpenter RE, Wilson DV, Thomas Evans A (2004). Evaluation of intraperitoneal and incisional lidocaine or bupivacaine for analgesia following ovariohysterectomy in the dog. *Vet Anaes Analg* 31:46-52.

Clutton RE (1992). Combined bolus and infusion of vecuronium in dogs. *J Vet Anaesth* 19:74-77.

Cohen CA (1978). Malignant hyperthermia in a greyhound. *JAVMA* 172:1254-1256.

Conzemius MG, Brockman DJ, King LG et al. (1994). Analgesia in dogs after intercostal thoracotomy: a clinical trial comparing intravenous buprenorphine and interpleural bupivacaine. *Vet Surg* 23:291-198.

Corletto F, Brearley JC (2002). Clinical use of mivacurium in the cat. *Proc of the Assoc of Vet Anaes.*

Court MH (1999a). Anesthesia of the sighthound. *Clin Tech Small Anim Pract* 14:38-43.

Court MH, Hay-Kraus BL, Hill DW, et al. (1999b). Propofol hydroxylation by dog liver microsomes: assay development and dog breed differences. *Drug Metab Dispos* 27:1293-1299.

Dahl JB, Moiniche S, Kehlet H (1994). Wound infiltration with local anesthetics for postoperative pain relief. *Acta Anaesthesiol Scand* 38:7-14.

Day TK, Pepper WT, Tobias TA et al. (1995). Comparison of intra-articular and epidural morphine for analgesia following stifle arthrotomy in dogs. *Vet Surg* 24:522-530.

Dickinson PJ, Sullivan M (1994). Exercise induced hyperthermia in a racing Greyhound. *Vet Rec* 135:508.

de Jong RH, Heavner JE, Amory DW (1974). Malignant hyperpyrexia in the cat. *Anesthesiology* 41:608-609.

Dhokarikar P, Caywood DD, Stobie D et al. (1996). Effects of intramuscular or interpleural administration of morphine and interpleural administration of bupivacaine on pulmonary function in dogs thaht have undergone median sternotomy. *Am J Vet Res* 57:375-380.

Dierking GW, Ostergaard E, Ostergaard HT et al. (1994). The effects of wound infiltration with bupivacaine versus saline on postoperative pain and opioid requirements after herniorrhaphy. *Acta Anesthesia Scand* 38:289-292.

Drenger B, Magura F, Evron S et al. (1986). The action of intrathecal morphine and methadone on the lower urinary tract in the dog. *J Urol* 135:852-855.

Duke T, Caulkett NA, Ball SD et al. (2000). Comparative analgesia and cardiopulmonary effects of bupivacaine and ropivacaine in the epidural space of the conscious dog. *Vet Anaes Analg* 27:13-21.

Eger EI II (1974) *Anesthetic uptake and Action.* Baltimore. The Williams & Wilkins Co.

Feldman HS, Covino BG (1988). Comparative motor-blocking effects of bupivacaine and ropivacaine, a new amino amide local anesthetic, in the rat and dog. *Anesth Analg* 67:1047-1052.

Futema F, Teach Fenton D, Costa Abler Jar JO et al. (2002). A new brachial plexus technique in dogs. *Vet Anaes Analg* 29:133-139.

Gallant EM, Mickelson JR, Roggow BD, et al. (1989). Halothane-sensitivity gene and muscle contractile properties in malignant hyperthermia. *Am J Physiol* 257:C781-786.

Gallen JS (1991). Propofol does not trigger malignant hyperthermia. *Anesth Analg* 72:406-416.

Hendrix PK, Raffe MR, Robinson EP et al. (1996). Epidural administration of bupivacaine, morphine, or their combination for postoperative analgesia in dogs. *JAVMA* 209:598-607.

Grimm KA, Tranquilli WJ, Thurmon JC, Benson GJ (2000). Duration of nonresponse to noxious stimulation after intramuscular administration of butorphanol, medetomidine, or a butorphanol-medetomidine combination during isoflurane administration in dogs. *Am J Vet Res* 61:42-47.

Herpinger LJ (1998). Postoperative urinary retention in a dog following morphine with bupivacaine epidural analgesia. *Can Vet J* 39:368-652.

Jones RS, Brearley JC (1987). Atracurium in the dog. *J Small Anim Prac* 28:197-201.

Katz D (1980). Malignant hyperthermia: a family history. *MDA News,* May: 6.

Kirmayer AH, Klide AM, Purvance JE (1984). Malignant hyperthermia in a dog: case report and review of the syndrome. *JAVMA* 185:978-982.

Keates HL, Cramond T, Smith MT (1999). Intraarticular and periarticular opioid binding in inflamed tissue in experimental canine arthritis. *Anesth Analg* 89:409-415.

Klide AM, Soma LR (1968). Epidural analgesia in the dog and cat. *JAVMA* 153:165-173.

Kona-Boun J, Pibarot P, Quesnel A (2003). Myoclonus and urinary retention following subarachnoid morphine injection in a dog. *Vet Anaes Analg* 30:257-264.

Kupper W (1977). Die intravenose regionalanasthesie (Bier) beim Hind. *Zbl Vet A* 24:287-297.

Kushner LI, Fan B, Shafer FS (2002). Intravenous regional anesthesia in isoflurane anesthetized cats: lidocaine concentrations and cardiovascular effects. *Vet Anaes Analg* 29:140-149.

Kushner LI, Trim CM, Madkusudhan S et al. (1995). Evaluation of the hemodynamic effects of interpleural bupivacaine in the dog. *Vet Surg* 24:180-187.

Leary SL, Anderson LC, Manning PJ (1983). Recurrent malignant hyperthermia in a Greyhound. *JAVMA* 182:521-522.

MacLennan DH, Phillips MS (1992). Malignant hyperthermia. *Science* 256:789-794.

Nelson TE (1991). Malignant hyperthermia in dogs. *JAVMA* 198:989-994.

O'Brien PJ, Rand JS (1985). Canine stress syndrome. *JAVMA* 186:432-433.

Pacharinsak C, Greene SA, Keegan RD et al. (2003). Postoperative analgesia in dogs receiving epidural morphine plus medetomidine. *J Vet Pharmacol Ther* 26:71-77.

Pascoe PJ, Dyson DH (1993). Analgesia after lateral thoracotomy in dogs. Epidural morphine versus intercostal bupivacaine. *Vet Surg* 22:141-147.

Petty R, Stevens R, Erickson S et al. (1996). Inhalation of nitrous oxide expands epidural air bubbles. *Reg Anesth* 21:144-148.

Popilskis S, Kohn D, Sanchez JA et al. (1991). Epidural versus intramuscular oxymorphone after thoracotomy in dogs. *Vet Surg* 20:462-467.

Probst CW, Webb AI (1983). Postural influence on systemic blood pressure, gas exchange, and acid/base status in the term-pregnant bitch during general anesthesia. *Am J Vet Res* 44:1963-1965.

Probst CW, Broadstone RV, Evans AT (1987). Postural influence on systemic blood pressure in large full-term pregnant bitches during general anesthesia. *Vet Surg* 16:471-473.

Pypendop BH, Iikiw JE (2005). Assessment of the hemodynamic effects of lidocaine administered IV in isoflurane-anesthetized cats. *Am J Vet Res* 66:661-668.

Rand JS, O'Brien PJ (1987). Exercise-induced malignant hyperthermia in an English springer spaniel. *JAVMA* 190:1013-1014.

Rempel WE, Lu M, el Kandelgy S, Kennedy CF, et al. (1993). Relative accuracy of the halothane challenge test and a molecular genetic test in detecting the gene for porcine stress syndrome. *J Anim Sci* 71:1395-1399.

Robertson SA, Johnston S, Beensterboer J (1992). Cardiopulmonary, anesthetic, and postanesthetic effects of intravenous infusions of propofol in greyhounds and non-greyhounds. *Am J Vet Res* 53:1027-1032.

Robinson EP, Sams RA, Muir WW (1986). Barbiturate anesthesia in greyhound and mixed-breed dogs: comparative cardiopulmonary effects, anesthetic effects, and recovery rates. *Am J Vet Res* 47:2105-2112.

Sams RA, Muir WW, Detra RL, et al. (1985). Comparative pharmacokinetics and anesthetic effects of methohexital, pentobarbital, thiamylal, and thiopental in greyhound dogs and non-greyhound, mixed breed dogs. *Am J Vet Res* 46:1677-1683.

Sammarco JL, Conzemius MG, Perkowski SZ et al. (1996). Postoperative analgesia for stifle surgery: a comparison of intraarticular bupivacaine, morphine or saline. *Vet Surg* 25:59-69.

Sawyer DC (1981). Malignant hyperthermia. *JAVMA* 179:341-344.

Short CE, Paddleford RR (1973). Malignant hyperthermia in the dog. *Anesthesiology* 39:462-463.

Skarda RT (1996). Local and regional anesthesia and analgesic techniques: dogs. In *Lumb and Jones' Veterinary Anesthesia,* 3rd edition. Thurmon JC, Tranquilli WJ, Benson JG (eds). Williams & Wilkins, Baltimore, USA. pp. 426-447.

Stobie D, Caywood DD, Rozanski EA et al. (1995). Evaluation of pulmonary function and analgesia in dogs after intercostal thoracotomy and use of morphine administered intramuscularly or interpleurally and bupivacaine administered interpleurally. *Am J Vet Res* 56:1098-1099.

Strazis KP, Fox AW (1993). Malignant hyperthermia: A review of published cases. *Anesth Analg* 77:297-304.

Swalander DB, Crowe DT Jr, Hittenmiller DH et al. (2000). Complications associated with the use of indwelling epidural catheters in dogs: 81 cases (1996-1999). *JAVMA* 216:368-370.

Thompson SE, Johnson JM (1991). Analgesia in dogs after intercostal thoracotomy: a comparison pf morphine, selective intercostal nerve block and interpleural regional analgesia with bupivacaine. *Vet Surg* 20:73-77.

Troncy E, Junot S, Keroack S et al. (2002). Results of preemptive epidural administration of morphine with or without bupivacaine in dogs and cats undergoing surgery: 265 cases (1997-1999). *JAVMA* 221:666-672.

Valverde A, Dyson DH, Cockshutt JR et al. (1991). Comparison of the hemodynamic effects of halothane alone and halothane combined with epidurally administered morphine for anesthesia in ventilated dogs. *Am J Vet Res* 52:505-509.

Valverde A, Dyson DH & McDonell WN (1989a). Epidural morphine reduces halothane MAC in the dog. *Can J Anaesth* 36:629-632.

Valverde A, Dyson DH, McDonell et al. (1989b) Use of epidural morphine in the dog for pain relief. *Vet Comp Ortho Trauma* 2:55-58.

Vesal N, Cribb PH, Frketic M (2003). Postoperative analgesic and cardiopulmonary effects in dogs of oxymorphone administered epidurally and intramuscularly, and medetomidine administered epidurally: a comparative clinical study. *Vet Surg* 25:361-369.

Chapter 6
The Anesthetic Period: Other Small Animals

Birds

Recent popularity of birds as pets and renewed interest in rehabilitation of raptors has lead to a demand for veterinarians who are willing to work on the medical problems of sick or injured birds. Because of the unique pulmonary physiology of the avian species, birds are more subject to respiratory compromise and respond more rapidly to inhalation anesthetics than mammals of similar size.

Anatomy

The avian lung is characterized as a cross-current flow of air to blood (Fedde 1980). In other words the avian lung functions as a one-way circuit. This is in contrast to mammals where the lungs are inflated, the breath is held for 1 to 3 seconds and the gases are exhaled. In birds, the complete respiratory cycle requires 2 inhalations and exhalations. On the first breath, inspired gases flow from the trachea into abdominal and caudal thoracic air sacs as well as through the parabonchial gas exchange surface of the lung (Figure 6-1A). Gases in the parabonchi are pushed into the cervical, clavicular and cranial thoracic air sacs. On expiration, gases from the abdominal and caudal thoracic air sacs flow through parabronchial lung providing a continual flow of fresh gases to gas exchange surfaces of the lung (Figure 6-1B). At the same time, gases in the cervical, clavicular and cranial air sacs are exhaled out the trachea (Fedde 1980). Thus gases entering the avian respiratory system on one breath are not exhaled until the following breath.

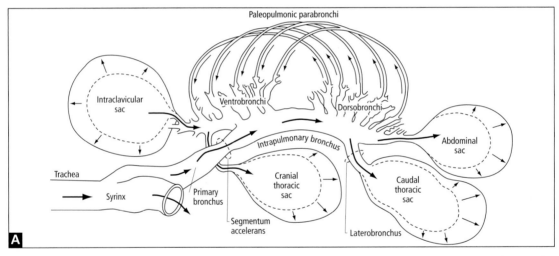

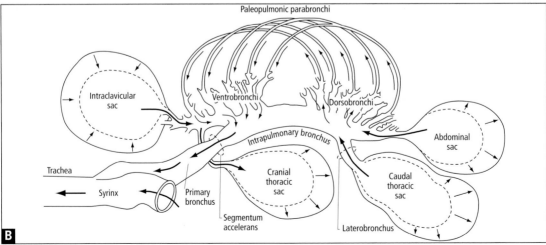

Figure 6-1A&B Anatomical illustration of respiration in birds: A = inspiration, B = expiration.

This unique pulmonary design provides a highly efficient ventilation system and has several profound effects on anesthetic management of birds. The avian lung is more efficient in delivering oxygen and removing CO_2 because there is a longer transit time of the inspired gases through gas exchange portion of the lung than in mammals and there is more time for oxygen uptake. The ratio of gas exchange surface to the lung volume, excluding the air sacs, is also larger facilitating gas exchange. Lastly, although the total volume of the avian lung is much larger than mammals on a per kilogram basis, the unidirectional flow of gas through the gas exchange parabonchi results in relatively continual fresh gas delivery to blood (Fedde 1980). In essence the avian lung has a very small functional residual capacity (FRC). The negative aspect of this setup is that during apnea birds become hypoxemic rapidly. Birds must breathe continually in order to maintain oxygenation of blood.

Anatomically, birds lack a complete muscular diaphragm separating the thorax and abdomen. Negative pressure is created in the thorax by active contraction of inspiratory muscles. The sternum moves ventrally in what has been called a bellows movement of the chest. Expiration is also an active process that lifts the sternum and forces air out of the thorax. Since anesthetic drugs decrease skeletal muscle function, respiration is significantly depressed at surgical levels of anesthesia.

Although intubation is usually easy to perform in birds because the larynx is located at the base of the tongue, visualization can be challenging in some species due to the size and shape of the bill. The trachea can also present important challenges for the anesthetist since there are significant species-related variations in length and shape of the trachea. Of most significance is that tracheal cartilages form complete rings in birds. For this reason some clinicians feel that it is better to use only non-cuffed endotracheal tubes since the trachea cannot expand as it does in mammals. Cuffed endotracheal tubes can be used to both protect the airway from aspiration and to enable positive pressure ventilation if care is taken to inflate the cuff only enough to enable ventilation to a pressure of 15cm H_2O.

Physical Restraint and Preanesthetic Preparation

Most birds can be physically restrained and examined without sedation or anesthesia. Knowledge of the species and skill in capture are required but most birds do not present a major threat to people. However, physical restraint can be extremely stressful to small non-predatory species and can potentially result in cardiac arrest. In these species, light levels of anesthesia are often recommended instead of physical handling.

Both physical and chemical restraint are contra-indicated when a bird is severely ill. Whenever possible, the bird should be stabilized prior to extensive physical restraint or anesthesia. Continued stress will result in death. Minimal handling should be used to treat with emergency therapy and stabilize the bird before further stress.

Frequently it is best to hospitalize the bird a day before surgery in order to allow recovery from stresses of transporting and preoperative evaluation. When possible, the bird should be kept in its own cage and on its normal diet. Do not withhold food prior to anesthesia as hypoglycemia and hepatic glycogen depletion can occur within 12 hours if fasted. This is especially true for small birds. Raptors (carnivores) have greater reserves and can be safely fasted 4-6 hours prior to anesthesia to avoid regurgitation.

A simple test to evaluate the bird's ability to handle stress is to determine the respiratory recovery time. First, observe the resting respiratory rate of the bird prior to handling. Second, measure the respiratory rate following a handling period of 2 minutes or longer. The respiratory rate should return to normal within 3-5 minutes. Birds that fail to return to base line have a reduced capacity to handle stress and are considered to have a higher risk of anesthetic complications.

If possible the PCV and TP should be assessed prior to general anesthesia. If the PCV is greater than 55%, the bird is likely dehydrated. Fluids should be administered and anesthesia delayed until rehydration has occurred. The general condition of the bird should be evaluated during the physical examination. Palpation of the pectoral muscles or legs will aid in the evaluation of the nutritional and health status of the bird. An accurate body weight should be obtained to facilitate drug dosage calculations and for estimation of the bird's blood volume. Blood loss can be a serious threat to survival in small birds and excellent hemostasis is essential. Table 6-1 provides normal values for selected avian species.

Table 6-1

Normal Ranges for Body Weight, PCV, and TP Values for Selected Birds

Avian Species		Typical Wt. Range	PCV(%)	TP(g/dl)
Psittacines	Parakeet (Budgie)	30-40gms.	37-53	0.5-6.0
Cockatiels		75-85gms.	45-57	2.2-5.0
Parrots		200-600gms.	43-55	3.0-5.0
Raptors	Red Tailed Hawk	1.3kgs.	34-44	3.3-4.5
	Great Horned Owl	1.8kgs.		
Cranes		4.0kgs.	41	3.1

Compiled from Fowler 1986.

Anesthetic Techniques
Inhalation Anesthesia

Inhalation anesthesia is the preferred method of chemical restraint and general anesthesia for most avian species. In general, birds are easily physically captured and restrained, enabling placement of an anesthetic mask over the face. Modern inhalation anesthetics have low blood:gas solubilities which are associated with rapid onset and adjustment of anesthetic depth. The high efficiency of the avian respiratory system further facilitates short induction times and minimal struggling. Equally important is the rapid recovery associated with inhalation anesthesia. Birds awaken quickly following isoflurane and sevoflurane minimizing risk of self trauma during recovery. On recovery, little to no residual sedation is expected so the bird is nearly fully functional within a short time after anesthesia is discontinued.

Although the elimination pathways and degree of biodegradation have not been studied in birds, it is reasonable to assume from clinical experience that almost all isoflurane and sevoflurane are exhaled rather than metabolized. This decreases concern of anesthetic induced toxicity to liver and kidneys. Additionally, if blood pressure and ventilation are maintained within or near normal values, post anesthetic hepatic and renal function should be unchanged.

Isoflurane

Isoflurane is a better choice for birds than halothane. Several studies have shown why the cardiovascular system is more stable than with halothane (Ludders et al. 1989; Ludders 1992; Ludders et al. 1990; Curro et al. 1994). Minimal anesthetic concentration for birds (MAC$_B$) is the effective alveolar dose for half of the animals tested (ED50) and this has been determined in several avian species representing different types of birds. These studies have confirmed that the MACB is similar to MAC in mammals (Ludders et al. 1988; Ludders et al. 1989; Ludders 1992; Ludders et al. 1990; Curro et al. 1994; Goelz et al. 1990). MACB of halothane was 0.85% and 1.05% in chickens and ducks and MAC for isoflurane was determined to be 1.32% in ducks, 1.35% in Sandhill cranes and 1.44% in cockatoo.

Inhalant anesthetics are known respiratory depressants and appear to cause apnea in birds at lower relative anesthetic depths than in mammals. When studied in ducks, apnea occurred at concentrations approximately 1.5 times the concentration to produce light anesthesia (Ludders et al. 1990; Curro et al. 1994). Since hypoventilation increases the difficulty of maintaining a stable anesthetic plane and presence of hypercarbia can have adverse effects on the cardiovascular system, ventilatory support should always be provided to anesthetized birds. Assisted ventilation should occur every 5 to 10 seconds, the peak inspiratory pressure should not exceed 20cm H_2O and tidal volume should be approximately 10ml/kg.

Inhalation anesthetics cause a dose-dependent decrease in MAP. For this reason blood pressure is one of the best indicators of changes in anesthetic depth. Abnormal cardiac rhythms have been observed during anesthesia of birds. Halothane has been associated with greater instability of cardiac function in birds and is the primary reason why isoflurane is considered the inhalation anesthetic of choice (Goelz et al. 1990; Abou-Madi 2001).

Sevoflurane
Sevoflurane is also a good choice for avian species. The principle advantages of sevoflurane are lower solubility and thus faster onset and recovery. In a comparative study in racing pigeons, induction and recovery times with sevoflurane were significantly shorter than with isoflurane (Kobel 1998). The greater speed will be of greatest advantage in large avian species such as ostriches and emus. Secondly, the less pungent odor of sevoflurane should theoretically improve ease of chamber or mask inductions although this has not been studied in avian species. The cardiovascular and respiratory effects of sevoflurane are similar to those of isoflurane and sevoflurane provides an acceptable alternative to isoflurane.

Semi-open or non-rebreathing systems should be used for delivery of inhalant anesthetics and oxygen in birds weighing less than 4kg. Circuits such as the Bain apparatus have the advantage of being light weight and thus have less likelihood of pulling on the endotracheal tube or mask. Fresh-gas flow rates should be in the 150-200ml/kg/min range.

Injectable Techniques
Injectable anesthetic techniques are available for avian species but should be reserved for situations where inhalation anesthesia is not feasible. Even in remote field situations, inhalation anesthesia can and should be used. The principle advantage of injectable techniques is that they don't require special equipment, they are inexpensive, readily available and simple to learn. The principle disadvantage of injectable anesthetic techniques is that elimination depends on hepatic and renal function. Drugs cannot be removed rapidly resulting in prolonged and/or rough recoveries compared to inhalation anesthesia.

Sites of injection for IM administration include the large muscles of the upper leg and pectoral flight muscles on each side of the sternum. The volume and concentration of anesthetic drugs should be kept as low as possible to avoid muscle damage in small birds. Drugs can be administered IV using jugular, brachial and saphenous veins.

Local Anesthetics
Local anesthetics are both safe and effective in avian species. They provide excellent analgesia and can be used for minor procedures in combination with gentle physical restraint in cooperative birds. Because of the small size of many pet birds, over dosage can be a serious risk with use of local anesthetics. Accurate body weight is essential and calculation of the maximal acceptable dosage must be performed. Lidocaine is commercially available as a 2% concentration. In order to safely use this drug, it should be diluted 1:10 with sterile water to make a 0.2% concentration. Dosage for birds should not exceed 8mg/kg.

Benzodiazepine Tranquilizers

Benzodiazepine tranquilizers have been used extensively for avian sedation and anesthesia. Unlike dogs and cats, sedation with these drugs is frequently effective in birds. In addition to producing a calming, quieting effect, benzodiazepines decrease anxiety and fear associated with handling and anesthesia induction. Furthermore, diazepam and midazolam are excellent muscle relaxants which facilitate anesthesia and surgery. When combined with butorphanol, benzodiazepines produce sedation, relaxation and analgesia for handling, anesthetic induction and surgery.

Recommended dosages for diazepam or midazolam are 0.1-0.2mg/kg IV and 0.2-0.5mg/kg IM, respectively. Midazolam is recommended in place of diazepam because midazolam lacks the solubilizing agent propylene glycol and this allows it to be absorbed well from muscle and have fewer cardiovascular depressant effects. Additionally, the water soluble formulation allows midazolam to be mixed with other drugs thereby decreasing the number of injections. Persistent sedative effects can be reversed by administration of flumazenil (0.05mg/kg). Half of the dose should be given IM or SC. The other half can be given IV.

Alpha$_2$ Agonists

Alpha$_2$ agonists have been used for sedation and as a part of injectable anesthesia techniques in many avian species. Like other animals, alpha$_2$ agonists have been associated with severe adverse effects, including respiratory depression and bradyarrhythmias. In general, alpha$_2$ agonists should be avoided in birds. Even though they can be antagonized with atipamezole, yohimbine or tolazoline, the marked cardiovascular depressive effects can be life threatening. When used at low dosages in conjunction with ketamine, alpha$_2$ agonists can be useful for chemical restraint of birds where inhalation or IV anesthetics cannot be used.

Opioids

Analgesic properties of opioids have been clearly demonstrated in studies of both awake and anesthetized birds (Paul-Murphy et al. 1999; Paul-Murphy & Ludders 2002). Studies in pigeons demonstrated that these birds have a higher number of kappa receptors than mu receptors (Mansour et al. 1988). This has correlated well with both clinical impressions and research studies that have demonstrated the efficacy of butorphanol. Although much additional research is needed to elucidate differences between avian species and effectiveness of clinically available opioid analgesics, use of butorphanol is currently recommended for perioperative analgesia in birds. Dosage of 1-3mg/kg has been shown to lower isoflurane requirements and to raise the pain response threshold in awake birds. Respiratory depression has not been significant when butorphanol has been used to treat pain.

Dissociative Agents

Dissociative anesthetics have a wide margin of safety in birds. When used alone, effects from ketamine are characterized by high muscle rigidity, inadequate analgesia and rough recoveries. For this reason, they should always be used in combination with a benzodiazepine tranquilizer. Ketamine can be administered IV, IM, orally and intraosseously (IO). Onset is rapid following IV or IO administration and dosage can be markedly reduced compared with the IM route. IV dosages are usually in the 4-8mg/kg range.

Effects of tiletamine / zolazepam (Telazol®) are similar to ketamine/midazolam but anesthesia is usually longer and recoveries have been reported to be associated with sustained struggling and wing-flapping. Onset is usually very rapid and smooth and for this reason the drug has been used in ratites for chemical capture.

Propofol

The addition of propofol for anesthesia in animals has given avian veterinarians another drug for induction and maintenance of anesthesia. Cardiovascular and respiratory effects of propofol are similar to those of ultrashort-acting barbiturates. However, unlike the barbiturates, propofol has a short duration of action due to rapid biodegradation by the liver and extra-hepatic enzymes. Thus propofol can be used for prolonged periods of time without resulting in rough or prolonged recoveries. In a study of propofol in pigeons, anesthesia was characterized as smooth and with good muscle relaxation (Fitzgerald & Cooper 1990). Propofol will produce profound respiratory depression and ventilatory support must be provided if apnea occurs. Slow administration and decreased dosage are advised when used with midazolam and butorphanol as premeds. Propofol must be administered via either the IV or IO routes and dosages in the 2-4mg/kg are recommended.

NSAIDs

The perioperative administration of NSAIDs to decrease pain associated with tissue injury is appropriate and these drugs will act synergistically with opioid analgesics, local anesthetics and general anesthetics. Marked avian species differences have been noted with NSAIDs and caution needs to be taken when using these drugs in a species for the first time. For example, half-lives of meloxicam and salicylic acid were 3 times longer in pigeons and chickens when compared to ostriches, ducks and turkeys (Baert & DeBacker 2003). In lame broiler chickens, carprofen was effective at improving speed of walking (1mg/kg SC) and lame birds self-selected oral carprofen indicating improved comfort (Danbury et al. 2000; McGeown et al. 1999). Studies in ducks indicated that flunixin and ketoprofen suppressed thromboxane levels for 4 hours and reduced the levels for approximately 12 hours. This study supports the premise that NSAIDs could provide an analgesic effect for several hours (Machin et al. 2001). As new clinical trials and research studies are published, NSAIDs will become a mainstay in avian analgesic adjunctive therapy.

Monitoring

Good anesthetic monitoring includes assessment of the patient's tissue perfusion, gas exchange by the lungs and the extent of CNS drug depression. This is often expressed as repeated evaluation of the cardiovascular, respiratory and nervous system. Since many variables can be used to assess these systems, the anesthetist should use a combination of monitoring approaches to ensure the bird is doing well during anesthesia.

As mentioned previously, it is essential for birds to breathe spontaneously during anesthesia. Thus observation and measurement of respiratory rate is fundamental to good monitoring. However, even without overt apnea, it should be assumed that the bird is likely in a hypoventilated condition. Anesthetic drugs depress muscle function and the respiratory center in brain. IPPV during anesthesia is the best insurance against elevated CO_2. Any interruption to breathing can be life threatening. It is critical to observe respiratory rate and depth due to the narrow interval between apnea and cardiac arrest. Side stream end tidal CO_2 monitors will underestimate the expired CO_2 in very small animals due to the entrainment of inspired gases by the analyzer. Normal respiratory rates for Psittacines are 50-80 bpm while larger birds such as raptors will have respiratory rates in the 10-15 BPM range.

Heart rate and rhythm should be monitored continuously during anesthesia. Doppler flow detectors provide an auditory signal that can provide an indication of strength, rhythm and rate of the pulse. The Doppler probe can be placed over the brachial or tarsal artery or it can be positioned in the thoracic inlet to pick up movement of the heart. The advantage of the Doppler flow detector over the ECG is that it monitors blood flow rather than electrical activity. The ECG will aid in the measurement of heart rate rhythmicity. Stainless steel suture passed through skin on the wings and legs can be used to ensure an atraumatic and consistent connection. The alligator clips from the ECG can then be attached to the suture. Small birds will have heart rates over 200 BPM.

Indications of depth of anesthesia in birds are similar to those in other animals. Muscle and pain reflexes are used to determine the degree of depression. Palpebral reflexes disappear at medium levels of surgical anesthesia (Arnall 1961). Like other species, corneal eye reflexes should be present. If absent, the anesthetic plane is too deep and appropriate steps should be taken to decrease depressive effects of anesthetic drugs. Muscle tone can be assessed by extending or flexing wings or feet. CNS awareness to pain is assessed by toe pinch (pedal reflex) or by feather plucking at the surgical site. Table 6-2 is provided to aid in assessment of anesthetic depth.

Table 6-2

Signs of Anesthesia in Birds

	Induction and Narcosis	Light	Medium	Deep
Signs:	Eyelids closing, wings starting to droop, head lowered	Eyelids relaxed, recumbent	Eyes open, relaxed and diminished reflexes	Eyes open, no reflexes
Voluntary Movements	Can be aroused and is sensitive to pain.	Absent	Absent	Absent
Respirations	Deep, rapid, regular without stimulation	Deep and rapid	Slow, deep and regular	Slow, regular and shallow
Corneal reflexes	Present	Present	Slow or intermittent	Absent
Palpebral	Present	Present	Absent	Absent
Pedal reflexes	Present	Present	Slow or intermittent	Absent
Cere reflexes	Present	Present	Absent	Absent

* Modified from Arnall 1961.

Fluids
Volume support in the form of fluids should be a part of the anesthetic regimen. Fluids can be administered orally, SC, IV or IO. The standard fluid administration rate during anesthesia is 10-15ml/kg/hr with daily maintenance fluids equaling 40-60ml/kg. Any crystalloid fluid is acceptable based on the bird's electrolyte and acid-base status. These would include 0.9% saline, 5% dextrose, LRS, 50% LRS + 50% 5% dextrose, 0.45% NaCl + 2.5% Dextrose. Dextrose 5% in water should not be administered via the SC route because of its hypertonicity. In any traumatic or disease situation, it is safe to assume 10% dehydration, which should be corrected prior to anesthesia or added to the standard fluid administration during anesthesia.

Hydration should be monitored during anesthesia if aggressive fluid therapy is administered. PCV and TP should be monitored hourly and body weight measured to determine success of fluid therapy. Blood glucose should be checked periodically but too frequent blood sampling can be detrimental to small birds. Even hourly sampling may be too frequent.

Recovery
Recovery is an extremely important part of successful anesthetic management in birds. Hypothermia due to open body cavities, removal of feathers, prolonged anesthesia and air conditioned operating rooms will produce severe drop in body temperature and prolong the bird's recovery. The use of circulating water pads and convective warm air heaters reduce the occurrence

and severity of hypothermia. During recovery, it is best to keep the bird in a warm environment and monitor core body temperature. Heating lamps directed onto the bird during surgery can sometimes reduce the loss of body heat but care must be taken to avoid burning skin. Surgeons can determine whether the heat from the light is too intense.

Trauma during recovery can occur if the bird is allowed to struggle prior to the return of full consciousness. Recovery cages should be padded to prevent injury and the bird can be recovered wrapped loosely in a towel. Another excellent method to reduce self-trauma during recovery is to place the bird inside a piece of notebook paper that has been taped into a tube shape. These methods will prevent wing flapping and struggling prior to the bird being able to coordinate its movements. Removal of perches should be done so that the bird cannot fall while not fully recovered.

Anesthetic Complications/Emergencies
The most common anesthetic complication is respiratory depression and/or arrest. This is usually managed by the use of manual or mechanical IPPV. Ventilation can be provided by squeezing the reservoir bag on the anesthetic apparatus or by use of an appropriate mechanical ventilator. Ventilatory support should be instituted if apnea occurs or if respiratory rate is below 6 BPM in birds greater than 4kg or less than 12 BPM in smaller birds. In addition to ventilatory support, check anesthetic and O_2 delivery equipment in advance to assure the apparatus is properly functioning, reevaluate bird and anesthetic drugs protocol and adjust the anesthetic plane as indicated.

In situations where cardiac depression or arrest is present, treatment is identical to that for mammals. Anticholinergics should be given in cases of bradycardia. The dose for atropine is 0.04mg/kg IV or IM. In cases of cardiac arrest, epinephrine is the catecholamine of choice at 0.01ml/kg IV or endotracheally. Dilution of epinephrine is 10:1 in sterile water. Because the small size of many pet birds, emergency drugs should be pre-calculated and drawn-up prior to starting anesthetic procedures to ensure rapid availability of appropriate dosage.

Guinea Pig, Hamster, Rat, Mouse, Gerbil
Patient Preparation
As with other species, it is important to carry out a clinical evaluation and obtain a case history in order to formulate an anesthetic plan. Obtaining a clear and relevant history may be difficult if the owner of the pet is a child so that undertaking a thorough clinical examination is particularly important. Remember that significant pathology may be present, without any obvious clinical signs of ill health, so that it is advisable to treat all small rodents as "high risk cases" and plan accordingly. If clinical signs are present, then it is particularly important to attempt to correct or at least stabilize any abnormalities, before anesthetizing the animal. Since many small rodents are fed ad lib, it may not be possible to assess whether food and water consumption are normal.

Common underlying disease conditions include chronic respiratory disease in rats and mice and chronic renal disease in older guinea pigs and rats. Note that the lifespan of these animals is relatively short, so it is possible to be dealing with a geriatric patient without being aware of this (Table 6-3). In older hamsters, amyloidosis may have produced renal and hepatic impairment, and arterial thrombosis may be present.

Non-specific signs of abnormality in all of these species include a ruffled fur coat or general signs of lack of grooming, soiling of the perineum and nasal or ocular discharge. In rats, secretions from the Harderian glands can accumulate around the eyes and nose and this is a non-specific sign of stress or ill-health. The discharge is black or brown but when wiped with a damp swab will appear red. Skin tone can be assessed as in other species but it may be difficult to detect signs of dehydration until this is pronounced. If dehydration is suspected, then it should be corrected pre-operatively by administration of fluids, using the same general approach as with cats and dogs. IV access is more difficult but fluid administered by the IP route is absorbed reasonably quickly. If more rapid administration is required, or prolonged therapy planned, then the IO route may be useful. Fluid requirements are relatively high in these small mammals and rates of approximately 100ml/kg/24h should be used.

It is helpful if the animal's normal activity and response to observation and examination can be assessed. This will be of value in assessing post-operative recovery particularly when attempting to evaluate post-operative pain. Guinea pigs often respond to observation by freezing (not moving) and may vocalize when handled. Other rodents tend to be active and inquisitive but may also be aggressive if unaccustomed to handling (see below). Heart rate and respiratory rate can be noted but these animals almost always show marked tachypnea and tachycardia (Table 6-3) in response to examination and handling. Any abnormal respiratory pattern or noise is often related to significant underlying respiratory disease. It is also critically important to weigh the animal as this is not only essential for accurate dosing with both anesthetic and other drugs but body weight is also useful in monitoring post-operative recovery. If a small mammal fails to eat or drink following recovery, it will lose approximately 10% of its bodyweight in 24 hours. Any weight loss should be minimized by good perioperative care and any fall in body weight should have been corrected within 2-3 days. There is often a fall in body weight following surgery in guinea pigs but this may be masked by gut stasis as a result of handling of the bowel during surgery or post-operative pain. If this occurs, the animal is at risk of developing serious complications, including enterotoxemia, and administration of gut-motility stimulants (e.g. cisapride, 0.5mg/kg by mouth bid) is advisable. Although it is common practice in many clinics to take pre-anaesthetic blood samples as a routine, practical difficulties limit this in small rodents. None of these species vomit, so it is unnecessary and undesirable to withhold food or water. Their high metabolic rate makes prolonged fasting hazardous and in the case of the guinea pig withdrawal of food may predispose to gut motility disturbances. Food and water may be removed 1-2 hours before induction of anesthesia to reduce the likelihood of food being present in the oropharynx.

Table 6-3 Average Life Span and Other Biological Data Relating to Rodents and Rabbits

Species	Average lifespan (years)	Adult body weight (gms)*	Heart rate BPM**	Respiratory rate BPM***
Gerbil	2	85-150	260-300	90
Guinea Pig	3.5	700-1200	150-250	50-140
Hamster	1.5	85-150	250-500	80-135
Mouse	1.5	25-40	350-600	80-200
Rabbit	8	2000-6000	135-325	40-60
Rat	2.5	250-500	250-350	70-115

* In general, males have a significantly higher body weight than females.
** Beats Per Min
*** Breaths Per Min

Restraint
Physical Restraint
Most pet rodents should be accustomed to handling, but they may be frightened or apprehensive because of the stress of transport to the veterinary clinic and by the presence of predators (dogs and cats) in the consulting area. Care should be taken to block potential escape routes before opening the cage or transport box. Sites for injection are listed in Table 6-4. Injections should be made by an assistant whenever possible as it is difficult to do this while providing firm but gentle restraint of the animal.

Table 6-4

Pre-anesthetic Agents and Their Effects in Rodents
(Analgesics are listed in Table 6-6)

Drug	Effects	Dose rates
Acepromazine	Sedates but does not immobilize small rodents.	Mouse, Hamster, Gerbil, 3-5mg/kg IP or SC Rat, Guinea Pig, 2.5mg/kg IP or SC
Atropine	Similar to other species.	40µ/kg SC or IM
Diazepam and midazolam	Both benzodiazepines have marked sedative effects, but this is not usually sufficient to provide complete immobility.	Mouse, Hamster, Gerbil, Guinea Pig, 5mg/kg IP, Rat 2.5mg/kg IP
Medetomidine	Both agents produce sedation and analgesia. Higher dose rates often immobiise the animal. Atipamezole can be used to reverse either agent (at 0.5-1.0mg/kg)	Hamster, Mouse, Rat, 30-100µ/kg SC or IP
Xylazine		Hamster, Mouse, Rat. 5mg/kg SC or IM

Hamster

Cup the animal in both hands (Figure 6-2) and carry out a general examination. To restrain the animal, immobilize it by covering it with one hand (Figure 6-3) and grasp the skin overlying the shoulders and back. A large area of skin should be included; otherwise the animal can turn and bite the handler. With the animal restrained in this way, an assistant can carry out IM, IP, or SC injections (Figure 6-4).

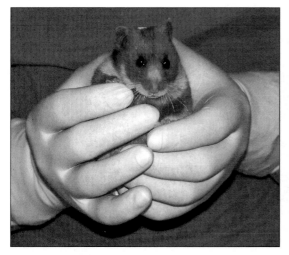

Figure 6-2 Restraining a hamster for initial examination.

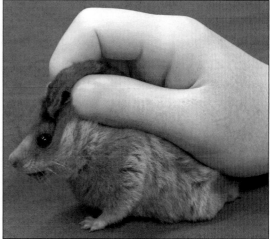

Figure 6-3 Immobilizing a hamster prior to firm restraint by grasping the scruff of the neck.

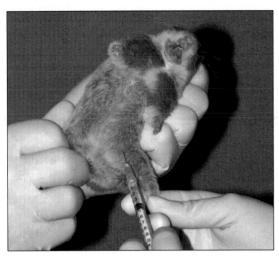

Figure 6-4 Restraint of a hamster for IP injection.

Gerbil

These rodents can be extremely active and restraint is further complicated by the fragility of the skin of the tail, which is easily damaged, resulting in de-gloving injuries. The animal should be immobilized by covering with the one hand and then grasped around the shoulders with the operator's thumb positioned below the animal's mandible.

Guinea Pig

Guinea pigs should be grasped around the shoulders and as they are lifted their hindquarters should be supported (Figure 6-5). This should be carried out as rapidly and smoothly as possible since animals that initially respond by "freezing" may subsequently become very active making them difficult to immobilize.

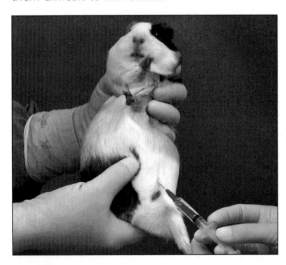

Figure 6-5 Holding a guinea pig while an assistant administers an IM injection.

Mouse

Pick up the mouse by the base of the tail and lift it onto a towel or other similar material. Most mice will grasp the material and try to pull away and they can then be further restrained by grasping the skin overlying the shoulders. The grip on the tail can then be transferred as shown in Figure 6-6 so that the animal can be restrained with one hand.

Rat

These animals should be picked up around the shoulders. The thumb is positioned under the mandible to prevent biting while supporting the rat's hindquarters as shown in Figure 6-7.

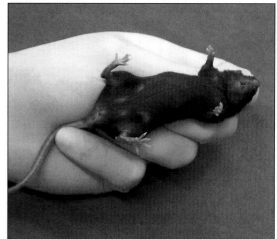

Figure 6-6 Restraint of a mouse

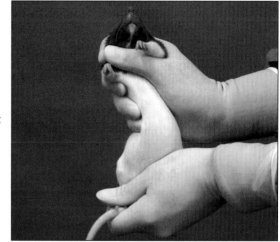

Figure 6-7 Restraint of a rat

Chemical Restraint

Preanesthetic agents are not often used in small mammals and injectable anesthetic regimens often consist of a "cocktail" of drugs administered as a single injection. However, sedatives can be used to provide restraint for non-painful procedures such as radiography. Pre-operative administration of opioids can be used to reduce anesthetic requirements as in other species. Also, atropine can be administered if necessary to reduce salivary and bronchial secretions and to prevent vagal responses to visceral and other surgical manipulations. Reducing bronchial secretions can be helpful in animals with chronic respiratory disease. Details of specific agents are given in Table 6-5. The agents produce similar side-effects to those seen in other species and have comparable contraindications.

Inhalation Anesthesia

All of the commonly used volatile anesthetic agents can be used to induce and maintain anesthesia in rodents. Isoflurane, halothane, sevoflurane and desflurane are well tolerated in most species. In guinea pigs, induction with isoflurane is often accompanied by signs of irritation such as ocular discharge. Although halothane is well tolerated, there have been reports of hepatic damage in this species. Sevoflurane in guinea pigs seems less suitable than in other rodents and its use is not recommended.

Although induction using a face mask is possible, it is usually more convenient to place the animal in an appropriate size chamber as described in Chapter 3. MAC values are broadly similar to those

Table 6-5

Anesthesia Dose Rates and Predicted Effects in Rodents

	Hamster	Gerbil	Guinea Pig	Mouse	Rat
Ketamine and medetomidine	100mg/kg + 0.25mg/kg IP	?	40mg/kg + 0.5mg/kg IP	75mg/kg + 1mg/kg IP	75mg/kg + 0.5mg/kg IP
Ketamine and Xylazine	200mg/kg + 10mg/kg IP	50mg/kg + 2mg/kg IP	40mg/kg + 5mg/kg IP	80mg/kg + 10mg/kg IP	75mg/kg + 10mg/kg IP
Tiletamine/ Zolezepam (Telazol)	50-80mg/kg IM	60mg/kg IM	40-60mg/kg IM	80-100mg/kg IM	20-40mg/kg IM
Ketamine and acepromazine	150mg/kg + 5mg/kg IP	75mg/kg + 3mg/kg IP	125mg/kg + 5mg/kg IP	100mg/kg + 5mg/kg IP	75mg/kg + 2.5mg/kg IP
Ketamine and diazepam (or midazaolam)	70mg/kg + 2mg/kg IP	50mg/kg + 5mg/kg IP	100mg/kg + 5mg/kg IP	100mg/kg + 5mg/kg IP	75mg/kg + 5mg/kg IP

of other species. Induction is rapid, usually being completed within 2-3 minutes depending upon the anesthetic agent used. At this point, either the animal can be removed from the chamber to allow a very rapid procedure to be carried out or it can be maintained with a face-mask, again at similar concentrations to those used in dogs and cats (eg 1.5-2% isoflurane). Recovery is rapid with animals regaining their righting reflex within 5-10 minutes after 30 minutes of anesthesia. Nitrous oxide is of limited value in these species as the MAC value is very high (e.g. > 200% in rats), so it is not generally used.

Suitable anesthetic induction chambers including small sizes for rodents can be purchased commercially or constructed from clear plastic containers. It is important that the anesthetic is delivered in a controlled and precise manner using a calibrated vaporizer. Attempting to use liquid anesthetic on a cotton wool pad or swab placed in the chamber is extremely hazardous since dangerously high concentrations of the agent are produced very rapidly.

Because of the ease of induction, control of anesthetic depth and rapid recovery, inhalation anesthetics are often considered the method of choice for small mammals. They can also be used very effectively as adjuncts to injectable anesthetic regimens. If full surgical anesthesia is not produced after use of an injectable combination, administration of low concentrations of a volatile agent is usually safer than administering additional doses of injectable agent(s).

Injectable Anesthesia

A range of different anesthetic agents can be used in small rodents. A suitable depth of anesthesia is produced but reliability and safety of different combinations varies considerably. This variability arises both because of the differing efficacy of anesthetics in different individuals and administration of anesthetics by IP, SC or IM injection rather than IV. When anesthetics are administered by the IV route, dose administered can be adjusted to suit individual animal responses. Although IP, SC and IM injections are easy to carry out, the animal receives a total estimated dose and it is not possible to take account of individual, breed and strain variations. This variation can be very large in rodents so that over or under dosing can be a significant problem. Two approaches can be adopted to manage this problem. Anesthetic mixtures with a wide safety margin that can be reversed wholly or partially with specific antagonists should be selected. In addition, since deepening anesthesia by administering additional anesthetic can be unpredictable, a balanced anesthetic approach by supplementing with a volatile anesthetic should be adopted. As an alternative to using inhalation anesthesia, additional analgesia can be provided by infiltration of the surgical site with local anesthetic. This is a safe technique provided the total dose of local anesthetic is calculated accurately. Although the toxic doses of local anesthetics are very similar in small rodents, dogs and cats, the very small size of rodents makes inadvertent overdose easy. It is safest to dilute the drug before use in order to better obtain accurate dosages.

Individual anesthetic agents and combinations of agents are listed in Table 6-5. Probably the most useful combination for routine use in small mammals is the combination of ketamine and medetomidine. This mixture of agents provides surgical anesthesia in gerbils, hamsters and rats. In mice, the effects are slightly more variable but a surgical plane of anesthesia is produced in most animals. In guinea pigs, the effect is even less uniform and some animals will be insufficiently deeply anesthetized to allow surgery. Nevertheless, it is better than other currently available combinations and anesthesia can be deepened with low concentrations of volatile agents or local anesthesia as discussed above.

Anesthetic Management
Monitoring
Anesthetic monitoring procedures in small rodents are essentially similar to those employed in larger species but the small physical size of these animals limits the techniques available. Assessing depth of anesthesia relies primarily on determining somatic reflex responses–tail pinch, toe pinch and ear pinch responses can be assessed and a barely perceptible or absent response indicates onset of a surgical level of anesthesia. Tail pinch response is often lost earlier than toe pinch and ear pinch responses. Ocular reflexes are of little value in these species since the loss of palpebral and corneal blink responses is quite variable both between individual animals and between different anesthetic agents. The globe does not rotate downwards as it does in dogs and cats during anesthesia with volatile anesthetics and some injectable agents. Eyes often remain central and open so it is important to protect them from damage by application of ophthalmic ointment and by being careful with positioning and handling. The globes are generally less protected by the bony orbit in these small rodents than in dogs and cats.

Clinical monitoring of cardiovascular and respiratory function relies on observation of respiratory rate and pattern and monitoring of heart rate. Changes that occur during induction of anesthesia with different agents are highly variable and it is important to gain familiarity with effects of specific agents. In general, respiration slows during anesthesia and magnitude of this change is exaggerated by the pre-anesthetic tachypnea shown by most animals. Gasping or labored respiration, very shallow respiration or a fall in rate by more than 50% of the estimated normal respiratory rate often indicate impending respiratory failure. Heart rate can usually only be assessed by palpating the thorax as the peripheral pulses are too weak to detect. A Doppler flow detector can be used on the chest to monitor heart sounds.

The small size of these animals limits use of capillary refill time as an assessment of circulatory function but the color of mucous membranes gives at least some indication of the adequacy of oxygenation. In white or pale coat animals, color of ears, eyes, nose and paws also provides an indication of oxygenation and degree of peripheral vasoconstriction or vasodilation.

Monitoring devices such as respiratory monitors, pulse oximeters and capnographs can be used but those designed for use with larger species may not function effectively in these very small animals. Respiratory rate monitors that rely on changes in sensor temperature may not be triggered by animals smaller than 400g and sensor positioning may be critical for successful functioning. Sensors may also produce excessive dead space in the circuit. Pulse oximeters may not detect the low signal strength in small species and this problem can be made worse by the use of ketamine/medetomidine because of the marked peripheral vasoconstriction and cardiovascular depression caused by this anesthetic combination. Even if a signal is detected, high heart rate may exceed the upper limits of the device. A number of manufacturers now produce pulse oximeters that function more effectively in very small animals and can register heart rates of up to 450 BPM. Even with these devices, it is necessary to experiment with probe placement. In most species the hind paw is a reasonably reliable site as is the tail in rats.

The small size of these animals results in low tidal volumes so that the gas sample rate of side-stream capnographs may prevent their use. Mainstream capnographs often cannot be used in small rodents because of the unacceptable increase in dead space that would result.

If signs of respiratory failure are noted, then possible causes should be identified and corrective action taken. Since underlying respiratory disease is relatively common and since all anesthetics depress respiration, oxygen should be administered to all animals as a routine. If the animal is intubated, it is easy to provide assisted ventilation but endotracheal intubation is difficult in small mammals. As a result, this is rarely undertaken. Nevertheless, ventilation can be improved by extending the head and neck, ensuring the oropharynx is free from obstruction and pulling the tongue forward. The chest can then be compressed between the anesthetist's finger and thumb, at a rate of 30 to 60 times per minute. As an alternative, a soft piece of rubber tubing or a syringe barrel can be placed over the nose and respiration assisted by gently blowing into the tube. Respiratory stimulants such as doxapram can also be used (5-10mg/kg IV, IM, SC, IP or sublingual).

If circulatory failure occurs, management is similar to that for larger animals but since venous access is more difficult, IV fluid therapy and IV administration of drugs to support the circulation may not be possible. With practice, an "over-the-needle" type catheter can be placed in the lateral tail vein in rats and the medial tarsal vein in guinea pigs. In these circumstances, it is also possible to transfuse whole blood from a donor animal to treat hypovolemia. Cross matching is not usually needed prior to an initial transfusion. More commonly, fluids will be given IP to provide a gradual correction of any deficit and early prevention of problems is thus particularly important. It is of great importance that blood loss during surgery is minimized. Blood volume of these species is approximately 70ml/kg body weight, so that a hamster would have a blood volume of only 7 to 8ml. Loss of only 1.6ml of blood (20% of circulating volume) could therefore be sufficient to cause circulatory disturbances. To monitor blood loss, swabs used should be weighed as a routine measure during all surgical procedures.

In addition to monitoring depth of anesthesia and cardiovascular and respiratory function, it is also important to monitor and maintain body temperature. Small mammals have a high surface area relative to their body mass and lose heat rapidly. Since most anesthetics depress thermoregulation and some cause vasodilation, heat loss can be rapid. When this is coupled with loss of insulation when fur is shaved to enable aseptic surgery and alcohol-based skin disinfectants are applied, it is not uncommon to see a 5 to10°C fall in temperature, unless efforts are made to prevent hypothermia. It is important to monitor rectal temperature and this is relatively easy in most small mammals using an electronic thermometer. All animals should be placed on a heat pad during anesthesia and warming measures must be continued in the recovery period. Any fluids given should be warmed to body temperature. The area of skin shaved and volume of skin disinfectant used should be kept to the minimum compatible with aseptic technique.

Recovery

Failure to provide high standards of post-operative care will delay recovery and may even result in death. As mentioned earlier, hypothermia must be prevented by continuing to provide supplemental heat. This is most easily achieved by placing the animal in an incubator, initially at approximately 35°C, with the temperature being lowered to 26-28°C as the animal recovers consciousness. All species should be provided with warm and comfortable bedding. Synthetic sheepskin products are ideal but shredded paper or tissues can also be used. Bedding should be absorbent. If the animal becomes soiled with urine, this will predispose to heat loss. Sawdust should be avoided as it can become crusted around the nose and mouth while the animal is recovering consciousness and its protective ocular and airway reflexes are depressed. A quiet area with subdued light is best to reduce stress during recovery.

Once the animal has recovered consciousness, food and water can be provided. Guinea pigs should be offered both good quality hay and fresh vegetables to encourage early resumption of feeding. Other rodents should be offered favored foodstuffs and their preferences should have been established when obtaining a case history. Rodents often readily eat softened diets and cereal mash which has the advantage of providing additional fluid as well as energy. Prior to recovery of consciousness, fluids should be administered to most animals by the SC or IP route (1 to 2ml/100g). Early resumption of eating and drinking is promoted by the provision of effective post-operative analgesia.

Pain Management

Postoperative pain relief should be provided as a routine either by use of pre-emptive analgesia or by administration of analgesics during anesthesia recovery. Assessment of pain in rodents is not easy but it is important to manage. If pain is not assessed accurately, it is not possible to determine whether analgesic therapy is proving effective. At present there are no controlled studies of pain assessment methods or analgesic therapies for small rodents, with the exception of the rat. In this species, it has been demonstrated that following abdominal surgery, a series of characteristic behaviors can be observed that are related to the degree of pain the animal is experiencing. The most easily recognized behaviors are back arching (Figure 6-8) and belly pressing–where the animal presses its abdomen towards the ground while walking. Rats also contract their abdomens, showing a characteristic "writhing" response (Roughan & Flecknell 2001). Preliminary studies suggest that mice show similar behaviors and that belly pressing and writhing are associated with abdominal pain. If these behaviors are observed, then additional analgesia should be administered.

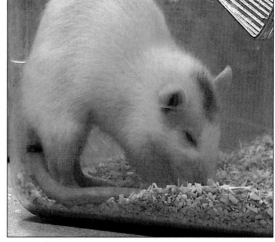

Figure 6-8 Rat showing back-arching behaviour, one of the signs of abdominal pain.

It is not certain how guinea pigs, hamsters and gerbils respond to post-surgical pain. They may become subdued and inactive and may also become aggressive when handled. Since pain is so difficult to assess, it must be assumed that pain will be present and an analgesic should be administered. Experience in the rat, where pain assessment can be carried out accurately, suggests that a single dose of buprenorphine or NSAID (Table 6-6) can provide sufficient analgesia after abdominal surgery. For more major procedures, administration of an opioid in combination with an NSAID (eg carprofen or meloxicam), repeated if needed at 12 to 24h intervals, is recommended.

All of the opioids and NSAIDs available for use in larger species can be given safely to small rodents. Many opioids appear to have a shorter duration of action in these species. It is therefore particularly advantageous to use buprenorphine which has an estimated duration of 6 to12hrs in these animals. Buprenorphine does have pronounced behavioral effects, causing increased activity in mice and sedation in rats. The drug has also been reported to cause rats to eat sawdust bedding. This side effect appears most common when large doses of analgesic are administered and is rare in most animals. If it is observed, then additional doses of the analgesic should not be given and alternative therapy selected.

All of the newer NSAIDs have undergone safety evaluation in rodents and these data enable one to estimate appropriate dose rates for post-operative use. No adverse reactions have been reported when NSAIDs have been administered perioperatively at the doses suggested in Table 6-6 but it seems appropriate to adopt similar precautions as in dogs and cats. Prolonged use should be avoided when possible and the drugs should be used with caution in animals with renal or hepatic impairment.

Table 6-6

Suggested Analgesic Dose Rates in Rodents

	Hamster	Gerbil	Guinea Pig	Mouse	Rat
Buprenorphine	0.1mg/kg SC	0.1mg/kg SC	0.05mg/kg SC	0.1mg/kg SC	0.05mg/kg SC
Butorphanol	?	?	2mg/kg SC	1-5mg/kg SC	2mg/kg SC
Carprofen	?	?	2.5mg/kg SC UID	5mg/kg BID SC or PO	5mg/kg BID SC or PO
Flunixin	?	?	?	2.5mg/kg SC BID	2.5mg/kg SC BID
Ketoprofen	?	?	?	?	5mg/kg IM
Meloxicam	?	?	?	4mg/kg SC daily	1.0mg/kg SC or PO daily
Morphine	?	?	2-5mg/kg SC or IM 4 hourly	2.5mg/kg SC or IM 4 hourly	2.5mg/kg SC or IM 4 hourly
Oxymorphone	?	?	?	0.2-0.5mg/kg SC or IM	0.2-0.5mg/kg SC or IM
Pethidine	?	?	10-20mg/kg SC or IM 2-3 hourly	10-20mg/kg SC or IM 2-3 hourly	10-20mg/kg SC or IM 2-3 hourly

Rabbits

Rabbits have increased in popularity as pets and are frequently kept as pairs or in small groups. To avoid aggression or unwanted offspring, these animals are often neutered. Female rabbits have a high incidence of uterine adenocarcinoma and neutering is often recommended as a preventive measure. As a consequence of this, the number of rabbits presented for anesthesia has increased dramatically. Providing safe and effective anesthesia has been regarded as challenging but rabbits should not be at increased anesthetic risk provided appropriate techniques are adopted.

Patient Preparation

A thorough clinical examination should be carried out with particular attention given to assessing respiratory function. Chronic bronchopneumonia which is often subclinical is relatively common and increases anesthetic risk. It is important to note that rabbits almost always have a marked, stress-induced tachypnea and tachycardia (> 250 breaths and beats per minute) when handled for examination. Gastrointestinal function should also be assessed and teeth should be examined. If this cannot be done pre-operatively, it can easily be completed after induction of anesthesia. Low grade dental disease is common in rabbits and inspection during routine surgery provides an opportunity to assess the teeth and correct problems. In addition, animals with dental disorders may have reduced food and water intake and supplemental fluids should be administered if abnormalities are detected. Many of the issues discussed earlier in relation to small mammals also apply to rabbits: if they are fed *ad libitum*, it may be difficult to assess food and water intake and if they are a child's pet, obtaining a good history may be problematic. Perhaps a more common problem than inappetance prior to elective surgery is obesity. This increases the risk associated with anesthesia and surgery and owners should be advised at an early stage of pet ownership to maintain their pet at an appropriate weight.

If the history or clinical examination is suggestive of fluid deficit, this should be corrected in the pre-anesthetic period. IV fluid access is relatively simple in the rabbit, either via the marginal ear veins (Figure 6-9) or the cephalic or jugular veins. The ear vein is easily accessible but the skin is sensitive causing the animal to jerk when a catheter is placed. Since the vein is very thin walled, resultant damage can make a subsequent attempt at catheterization difficult. This problem can be avoided by using a local anesthetic cream (e.g. EMLA, Astra-Zeneca). This is applied over the ear vein and covered with a plastic dressing and protective bandage. After 40 to 60 minutes, the dressing is removed. Full skin thickness anesthesia is produced for approximately 1 hour.

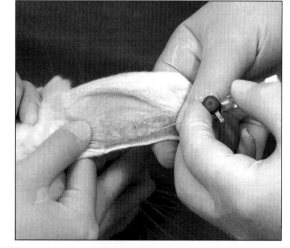

Figure 6-9 IV catheterization of rabbit ear vein.

Rabbits are easily stressed so their perioperative management must be tailored to reduce stress to a minimum. For elective surgeries, it should be possible to schedule the procedure to avoid the need to house the animal in close proximity to predators such as cats and dogs. If the rabbit is one of a pair but only one requires anesthesia, then consideration should be given to admitting both animals. This can reduce stress and improve post-anesthetic recovery but of course, it does result in unnecessary stress to the rabbit that does not require anesthesia.

There is no need to withhold food or water prior to anesthesia. This can be detrimental as it increases the risk of post-operative gastrointestinal disturbances. To further reduce stress associated with handling, restraint and the process of anesthetic induction, preanesthetic medication can be particularly useful in this species. A range of agents can be used to provide effective sedation (Table 6-7) and at higher dose rates, animals may become immobilized.

Preanesthetic Agents and Their Effects in Rabbits
(Analgesics are listed in Table 6-9)

Acepromazine	Provides heavy sedation in rabbits. Combining with butorphanol provides additional sedation and analgesia	1mg/kg SC or IM or 0.5mg/kg + 1.0mg/kg butorphanol IM or SC
Glycopyrrolate	Use in preference to atropine	0.01mg/kg IV or 0.1mg/kg SC or IM
Diazepam and midazolam	Sedation	1-2mg/kg IM
Medetomidine	Both agents produce sedation and analgesia. Higher dose rates	0.5-1mg/kg SC or IM
Xylazine	often immobiise the animal. Atipamezole can be used to reverse either agent (at 0.5-1.0mg/kg)	2.5mg/kg SC or IM

Restraint

Physical restraint for examination and undertaking minor procedures is relatively straightforward but must be carried out carefully to ensure the animal does not become frightened and make violent attempts to escape. This can result in injury to both the handler and the rabbit. It is particularly important to provide support to the rabbits back and hindquarters at all times as injuries to the lumbar vertebrae can have serious consequences.

Rabbits should be restrained by grasping the skin overlying the shoulders and as it is lifted clear of its transport box, the operator's other hand should be positioned under the animal's abdomen to support the hindquarters (Figure 6-10). Rabbits may kick out as they are placed onto the examination table so it is important not to release the animal until it is in firm contact with the table. Restraint by holding the scruff should be continued during examination and other procedures and it is best to have the hindquarters firmly against the examiner or supported by an assistant to prevent kicking. IM injections can be made into the quadriceps, posterior thigh and the lumbar muscles. SC injections are made into scruff of the neck.

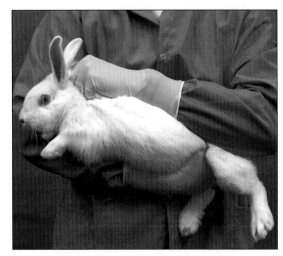

Figure 6-10 Proper positioning and restraint of the rabbit

Inhalation Anesthesia

All of the modern volatile anesthetics are safe for anesthetic maintenance in rabbits but induction with these agents can be hazardous. Rabbits respond to inhalation of halothane, isoflurane and sevoflurane with breath-holding that can be prolonged. This is accompanied by marked bradycardia and the animal may struggle violently before taking a breath. Administration of preanaesthetic sedatives does not prevent the breath-holding response but does minimize struggling. Since this enables the anesthetic to be given without need for firm physical restraint, the rabbit can be observed during induction and the mask removed if breath-holding occurs. Once the animal commences breathing again, the mask can be repositioned. This normally needs only be done on one or two occasions. Since breath holding is common, it is advisable to administer oxygen for 1 to 2 minutes before gradual introduction of the volatile agent. As an alternative to this technique, anesthesia can be induced by IV administration of an injectable agent such as propofol, intubation carried out and then anesthesia maintained with an inhalation anesthetic. Anesthetic potency of the different agents is similar to that in other species. MAC of nitrous oxide is high so that use of this agent is of little value in the rabbit.

Injectable Anesthesia

The relative ease of IV access enables more controlled use of injectable agents. However, two popular agents, propofol and alphaxalone/alphadolone, can only be used to produce light anesthesia in rabbits. Administration of higher doses to produce surgical anesthesia frequently results in apnea. Combining propofol with medetomidine produces surgical anesthesia and recovery time can be reduced by administration of atipamezole. Other options for anesthesia are listed in Table 6-8.

One of the most widely used anesthetic regimens is ketamine and medetomidine, administered as a combined injection. This combination produces surgical anesthesia in the majority of rabbits but also results in cardiovascular and respiratory depression. Provided oxygen is administered, this is not a significant problem in healthy rabbits. Initial suggestions of dose rates of this combination were too high and it was also recommended that the drugs should be given by IM injection. The volume of the lower doses listed in Table 6-8, administered by SC injection, are well tolerated. Use of the lower dose (15mg/kg ketamine, 0.25mg/kg medetomdine) results in less respiratory depression and usually provides sufficient relaxation to allow endotracheal intubation. Anesthesia can then be supplemented with low concentrations of volatile anesthetic to achieve a surgical plane of anesthesia. This is also the most preferable means of prolonging duration of surgical anesthesia when higher dose rates have been used, rather than by administering supplemental doses of ketamine and medetomidine.

Anesthetic Management
Monitoring

Depth of anesthesia can be assessed using the hind-limb pedal withdrawal response and ear pinch reflex. Both should be barely perceptible or absent at surgical planes of anesthesia. The fore-limb pedal withdrawal response is only lost at very deep planes of anesthesia. The eye remains fixed and central during anesthesia and loss of the palpebral and corneal reflexes is variable. At dangerously deep planes of anesthesia and following cardiac arrest, the globe rotates downwards. Since the eye remains open during anesthesia, it is important to protect it from accidental injury by either application of ophthalmic ointment or taping the eyelids closed with micropore tape.

Clinical monitoring of respiratory and cardiovascular function is similar to that for other species but it is difficult to palpate a peripheral pulse even in large rabbits. Capillary refill can be assessed on the gingiva and color of the mucous membranes provides some indication of circulatory and respiratory function.

Table 6-8

Anesthetic Dose Rates and Predicted Effects in Rabbits

Drug	Effects	Dose rate
Alphaxalone/Alphadalone	Light anesthesia, 5-10 min, apnea common at higher dose rates, sleep time 10-20 min	6-9mg/kg IV
Ketamine + Acepromazine	Surgical anesthesia, 20-30 min, good relaxation, sleep time 60-120 min	50mg/kg IM + 1mg/kg IM
Ketamine + Diazepam (or midazolam)	25mg/kg IM + 5mg/kg IM	Surgical anesthesia, 20-30 min, good relaxation, sleep time 60-120 min
Ketamine/Medetomidine	Surgical anesthesia, 30-40 min, good relaxation, sleep time 90-240 min, some of effects reversible with atipamezole	15mg/kg SC + 0.25mg/kg SC
Ketamine + medetomidine + butorphanol	Surgical anesthesia, 30-40 min, good relaxation, sleep time 90-240 min, some of effects reversible with atipamezole	15mg/kg SC + 0.25mg/kg SC + 0.4mg/kg SC
Ketamine + Xylazine	Surgical anesthesia, 20-30 min, good relaxation, sleep time 60-120 min, some of effects reversible atipamezole	35mg/kg IM + 5mg/kg IM
Ketamine + xylazine + acepromazine	Surgical anesthesia, 45-75 min, good relaxation, sleep time 100-150 min	35mg/kg IM + 5mg/kg IM + 1mg/kg IM
Ketamine + xylazine + butorphanol	Surgical anesthesia, 60-90 min, good relaxation, sleep time 120-180 min. some of effects reversible atipamezole	50mg/kg IM + 5mg/kg IM + 0.1mg/kg IM
Propofol	Light anesthesia, 5-10 min, apnoea common at higher dose rates, recovery smooth and rapid, 10-15 min sleep time	10mg/kg IV

Simple respiratory monitors generally function well in rabbits and monitors that function adequately when used on cats will also be suitable for use in rabbits. The high heart rate (> 250 bpm) can cause difficulties when using pulse oximeters not programmed for small animals but if xylazine or medetomidine are administered as part of the anesthetic regimen, the heart rate will usually be below 200 bpm. Placement of pulse oximeter probes can be difficult and some experimentation may be needed to find reliable sites for a particular instrument. Shaving the tail and placing the probe across the tail base can be effective if placement on the toe, tongue or ear proves unsuitable. Use of an angled probe across the surface of the tongue (Figure 6-11) seems particularly reliable in this species.

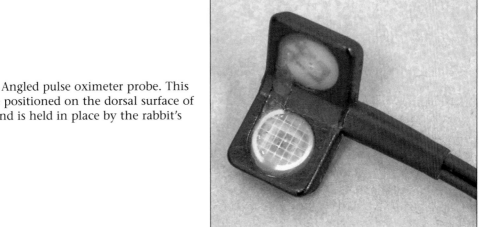

Figure 6-11 Angled pulse oximeter probe. This probe can be positioned on the dorsal surface of the tongue and is held in place by the rabbit's upper jaw.

Capnography is practicable in all but the smallest of rabbits. Automated NIBP measurement can be attempted and with proper cuff placement can be effective. Direct measurement of blood pressure is simple to undertake by cannulation of the central ear artery.

Management of cardiovascular or respiratory emergencies is by use of similar techniques to those applied in the dog and cat. The most commonly encountered problem is gradual or sudden respiratory failure and management of this is greatly facilitated if an endotracheal tube is in place. Attempting to assist ventilation using a face mask and compressing the reservoir bag on an anesthetic circuit is rarely effective.

Endotracheal intubation is simple to achieve. It can be accomplished either under direct vision or using a "blind" technique. Prior to attempting either method, the animal should receive oxygen by face mask for 1 to 2 minutes. To visualize the larynx, the rabbit is positioned on its back and the tongue pulled forward and to one side, to avoid damage to the tongue by the incisor teeth. Although a Wisconsin laryngoscope blade (0 or 1) can be used, it is simpler to view the larynx with an otoscope using a canine-sized speculum. The speculum should be inserted in the gap between the incisor and cheek teeth and advanced until the larynx is seen. The larynx should then be sprayed with local anesthetic and an introducer threaded down the speculum, through the larynx and into the trachea. The otoscope is then removed, and the endotracheal tube (size 3, 3.5 or 4mm ID in a 3-4kg rabbit) threaded over the introducer which is used to guide it into the trachea. The introducer is then removed. This is a very effective method of accomplishing difficult intubation in any small animal.

If "blind" intubation is to be attempted, the rabbit should be positioned on its chest and held around the base of the skull so that the head and neck are extended upwards (Figure 6-12). The endotracheal tube is introduced between the incisor and cheek teeth and advanced towards the larynx. When the tube reaches the larynx, some increased resistance can be felt. As the tube passes into the larynx, the animal usually coughs indicating successful intubation. If the tube passes into the esophagus, it should be withdrawn and repositioned slightly by adjusting the angle of the rabbit's head and neck, and then advanced again. The position of the tube can be monitored by listening for breath sounds directly at the end of the tube or by attaching it to the earpieces of an esophageal stethoscope. Another way to feel expired breaths in very small rabbits is to have the end of the tube very close to the anesthetist's cornea, which is sensitive enough to detect tiny puffs of air.

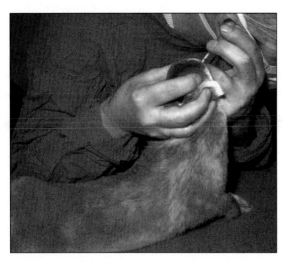

Figure 6-12 Positon of rabbit's head for "blind" endotracheal intubation. As the tube passes into the larynx, the animal usually coughs indicating successful intubation.

With both techniques, successful placement can be confirmed by checking for condensation of moisture in the tube with each breath or by placing a small piece of tissue paper across the end of the tube. The animal can then be connected to an appropriate semi-open anesthetic circuit, e.g., Bain's circuit or T-piece. Fresh gas flow rates are calculated as for other species.

Although the larger size of the majority of rabbits makes hypothermia less of a problem than in small rodents, it is important to monitor body temperature, to use a heat pad to maintain temperature and to continue these measures in the post-operative period.

Recovery

Rabbits should be maintained in a warm quiet environment and away from predators, during recovery from anesthesia. It is important to encourage animals to eat and drink as soon as possible after they have recovered consciousness. Metaclopramide (0.5mg/kg SC once daily) and cisapride (0.5mg/kg by mouth bid) may be given if there are any signs suggestive of gastrointestinal hypomotility or can simply be administered as a routine to help reduce the incidence of this problem. One of the factors that may contribute to inappetance and gut stasis is post-operative pain so provision of effective analgesia is of critical importance. Unfortunately, assessment of pain in rabbits is difficult with no pain scoring schemes being available at present. Rabbits appear to show little obvious pain-related behavior but after abdominal surgery some animals show occasional contractions of the abdominal muscles and pressing of the abdomen to the ground. Animals also show increased frequency of small postural adjustments. Other signs of pain are very non-specific with animals remaining hunched and immobile, a response that is also seen in rabbits that are simply apprehensive or frightened. Since a range of analgesics has been shown to be safe and effective in rabbits, it is preferable to assume that pain will be present and administer analgesics after all surgical procedures.

All analgesics available for use in dogs and cats can be used in the rabbit and suggested analgesic dose rates are given in Table 6-9. Buprenorphine appears to have a wide margin of safety in this species (Flecknell & Liles 1990) and also provides long-duration (6 to 12h) of analgesia. Although there have been few clinical trials of NSAIDs in the rabbit, meloxicam and carprofen have both been administered in controlled trials with no clinically apparent side-effects (Roughan, personal communication; Meredith, personal communication). Following routine neutering, use of NSAIDs may be sufficient, however, their use should be combined with an opioid when additional analgesia is required.

Table 6-9   Suggested Analgesic Dose Rates for Rabbits

Drug	Dose rate
Buprenorphine	0.01-0.05mg/kg SC
Butorphanol	0.1-0.5mg/kg SC
Carprofen	1.5mg/kg per OS UID, 4mg/kg SC UID
Flunixin	1.1mg/kg SC BID
Ketoprofen	3mg/kg IM
Meloxicam	0.2mg/kg SC daily
Morphine	2-5mg/kg SC or IM 4 hourly
Oxymorphone	0.05-0.2mg/kg SC or IM
Pethidine	10mg/kg SC or IM 2-3 hourly

UID = Once per day

Non-Domestic Carnivores
Exotic Cats, Foxes, Skunks, Ferrets, Raccoons, Others

The same general principals discussed elsewhere in this text for dogs and cats apply to wild and exotic carnivores. Biological variables such as anatomy and physiology as well as use of and response to drugs are generally very similar, as are the dosages used. Important differences relate to these non-domestic species being stressed by the proximity of humans trying to help them. This makes treatment and care challenging and potentially dangerous for animals and people involved. If the animal is a pet, it is not stressed as much as a wild animal. However, it is still more challenging to handle and treat than domestic dogs and cats which have been bred as companion animals for many generations. Predatory carnivorous species are usually more aggressive and do not seem as stressed by confinement and restraint as herbivorous prey species. They would normally either hide quietly or "defend" themselves by running away. Efforts to calm any animal prior to anesthetic administration will result in a smoother induction and recovery, whether sedation or anesthesia is needed. The intent of this text is to provide information needed to safely anesthetize a variety of animals.

There is an excellent text devoted exclusively to immobilization of wildlife (Kreeger et al. 2002) that goes into much greater depth and detail. There is also a comprehensive text on zoo and wildlife medicine that is an excellent reference for general care, restraint and handling of many non-domestic species (Fowler & Miller 2003). Some important differences from domestic species such as regulations and concerns for safety will be discussed before the actual anesthetic period is considered.

Preanesthetic Considerations

It is important to have a good working knowledge of the risks of disease for both the animal's well-being and those of the people involved. Patient preparation should include a good history and if the animal is a pet, vaccination status is important as most non-domestic carnivores are susceptible to many of the same viral diseases as dogs and cats.

A busy veterinary clinic is certainly a place where exposure potential is increased, along with overall excitement of all the other animals in the hospital. Handling non-domestic carnivores in a separate area of the building or before the regularly scheduled small animal day begins can help create a calmer environment for everyone. It might even be wise to treat exotic pets by making a house call. Wild, unvaccinated carnivores are at greater risk. The potential of zoonotic diseases, such as rabies in these patients makes it crucial that no one is bitten or scratched or more seriously injured. Veterinary staff working with potentially infected animals should be vaccinated for rabies to minimize risk and concern if exposure were to occur. Because there are no vaccine labels approved for most non-domestic carnivores, even a vaccinated pet, such as fox, raccoon or skunk is legally considered a non-vaccinate if there is human exposure. This would necessitate euthanasia of the animal to check the brain for the presence of rabies virus. Treatment of potentially exposed humans may be necessary with an initial dose of human anti-rabies immunoglobulin followed by a series of five rabies vaccinations over a one-month period. The post-exposure prophylaxis (PEP) treatment should start as soon as possible after exposure, and although quite expensive, prevents exposed humans from contracting rabies. Obviously, safe handling practices and pre-exposure vaccination of caretakers should negate the need to euthanize an animal for testing or PEP if the animal is not available for testing.

Owners of pet carnivores should be advised of the risks and liabilities of having an animal prone to bite or scratch for which there are no label approved rabies vaccines. This potential for health risk and expensive litigation are good justifications for not keeping these types of animals as pets. The fact that many of these carnivores are solitary and nocturnal makes them less suitable as an interactive pet and makes keeping them in captivity a practice some consider as inhumane.

Handling and Chemical Restraint

If there is a need to handle a potentially dangerous animal, safe protocols are tremendously important from start to finish. If the previously wild animal is being kept as a pet, it should have food withheld preanesthesia, similar to a dog or cat, to help minimize the risk of vomiting and aspiration. An accurate weight is important and easier to accomplish if the owner can weigh the animal or at least the cage it is transported in ahead of time. If the animal is a wild carnivore, there is less ability to control conditions prior to restraint and anesthesia induction. It is not uncommon for wild carnivores to be hit by a car while scavenging for road kill. Since these animals cannot be handled easily or safely without chemical restraint, it is often best to delay anesthesia unless immediate clinical treatment is necessary.

Chemical restraint may be needed to draw blood samples or identify the animal often follow live capture with a food bait. As a result, it is important to be prepared to deal with the potential for vomiting and aspiration just as in emergency situations with domestic small pets. If a wild carnivore is a game species that is hunted or trapped and potentially eaten by humans or other carnivores when returned to the wild after treatment, it is important to treat it as a "food animal." All drugs that are "labeled" for use on food animals have a withdrawal time established by the US FDA to assure the meat is safe for human consumption. Unfortunately, very few drugs are label-approved for use on exotic carnivores. Domestic carnivores are not considered food animals, so "withdrawal time" studies have not been done for the label-approved species. Because of these concerns of adverse reactions in humans due to residues in meat of game species after "extra-label" drug use and the lack of withdrawal studies in comparable species to use for guidance, it is recommended to be conservative.

There are some established guidelines and the Animal Medicinal Drug Use Clarification Act of 1994 (AMDUCA) which became law in 1996 in the U.SA, allows veterinarians to use FDA-approved drugs in species for which there is no label approval if certain requirements are met. If FDA approved drugs are used on non-food animals, their recorded use must be by or under the direct supervision of a licensed veterinarian involved in the treatment protocol (veterinarian/ client/ patient relationship). If these drugs are used in an extra-label fashion on food animals, the veterinarian must establish a safe withdrawal time and identify the animal treated to assure that it be held for that withdrawal time before release or tagged with instructions not to consume the meat before safe withdrawal time has passed. There is a database that helps provide guidance to veterinarians to prevent food animal drug residues. It is the Food Animal Residue Avoidance Database (FARAD), and it maintains a "hotline" in the US that veterinarians with questions on withdrawal times can call. All food animal species for which there are label-approved drugs and dosage recommendations are herbivores and FARAD recommends that certain drugs not be used in deer within 30 days of hunting season. This conservative withdrawal time of at least 30 days should be adequate for all drugs used for carnivore restraint and anesthesia. These conditions may not be practical and along with the previously mentioned disease risks and the stresses that clinical treatment and confinement put on the animal, euthanasia might be the most humane solution. This is especially true for common species or conditions with a poor prognosis requiring extensive handling and costly treatment.

If drugs are used for euthanasia, disposal of the carcass must address dangerous tissue residues to prevent risk to scavengers that might consume them. A well-placed bullet in brain is still considered a humane method of euthanasia (AVMA Panel Report 2001), but this method should be avoided if there has been any potential rabies exposure to people or pets requiring that the brain be checked for rabies. Many veterinarians can help local law enforcement officers, game wardens, wildlife biologists, and animal control officers with advice and even training on the use of drugs for restraint and euthanasia, thus fulfilling that veterinarian/ client/ patient relationship required for extra label drug use.

Nontraditional Concerns

There are situations when veterinarians must deal with the non-traditional patients in general terms. There is no way that specific disease risks, legal regulations or even specific drug dosages can be listed because they may vary by state, region or time of year. There are often varying regulations for treatment and care of wild animals that are enforced at the state and federal level. Veterinarians appropriately licensed to practice in a state are allowed to make critical decisions on treatment or euthanasia of protected wildlife. Even migratory birds and especially carnivorous raptors that are federally protected can be euthanized in an emergency situation for humane welfare reasons. A call to the local game warden or conservation officer should help clarify regulations for long-term housing and care or permission to euthanize threatened or endangered species with a poor prognosis for return to the wild. The environment and activities around a busy veterinary clinic generally make it a challenging place in which to house and care for a wild animal. A good working relationship with a local wildlife rehabilitator or nature center might allow the veterinarian to stop by and treat animals at the permitted facility or allow scheduled care for wildlife at the clinic at the end of the day when things have quieted down. This allows an interested veterinarian to provide much-needed professional service to wildlife without the veterinarian or clinic needing to go through the hassle of obtaining state and federal permits. Involvement with exotic pets and wildlife can be an exciting and challenging dimension of clinical practice. This can be personally rewarding and satisfying as well as enhance the image of the practice and profession in the local community.

Anesthetic Considerations
Inhalation Anesthesia

Once the decision to anesthetize a non-domestic carnivore has been made, the primary considerations are which drugs to use and to identify a safe dose. Many times, animals from the wild can best be induced in a chamber just as other small animals. This is the preferred method if equipment and facilities are available, as it is less risky to people administering the anesthetic than using an injectable agent. Some of the earliest accounts of anesthetizing wild carnivores describe sealing the live trap used to capture the animal with tarps and spraying ether into the chamber (Erickson 1957). This was successfully done with black bears in the field with diethyl ether, which was explosive and irritating to the respiratory tract. Field anesthesia with the newer, safer inhalation anesthetics can be accomplished with a portable vaporizer (Kreeger et al 1998). In addition, modern equipment can be used for induction and maintenance along with monitoring devices found in many veterinary clinics. As a result, safe inhalation anesthesia can be accomplished on most small carnivores.

Injectable Anesthesia

Injectable anesthetics are primary agents used for field anesthesia by wildlife professionals and there are many references available that list dosage ranges for many common species (Kreeger et al 2002; Norton 1998). Ketamine has been used extensively and safely for the longest time (Ramsden et al. 1976). Ketamine has a wide margin of safety and its undesirable side effects of salivation and nervous system stimulation can be controlled by combining ketamine with anticholinergics and sedatives. The combination of 100mg/ml ketamine and xylazine at a 5 to 1 ketamine/xylazine ratio has been suggested (Jessup 1982). It can be administered with a hand-held syringe if the animal is confined in a capture net or a pole syringe if it is in a cage or live trap. This mixture of ketamine and xylazine has been used successfully for chemical restraint at 0.5-1.0ml/10 lbs (0.02-0.05ml/kg) of body weight for immobilization of many species of non-domestic carnivores just as it has been used on dogs and cats. The high end of the dosage can be used on smaller species that have high metabolic rates or for longer procedures. This dose recommendation has a wide margin of safety and may need to be increased for very excited animals, but the combination of a dissociative agent with an alpha$_2$ agonist works well on all common carnivores encountered in a practice setting. The animal can be allowed to recover as the drug is metabolized or the xylazine can be antagonized with yohimbine at 0.125mg/kg. It should not be given unless the effects of ketamine have started to dissipate. If the tranquilizing effects of the alpha$_2$ agonist are reversed in less than 30 to 45 minutes, ketamine's CNS stimulating effects may cause seizure activity. Just as in dogs and cats, seizures can be controlled with diazepam, respiratory depression with doxypram and excessive salivation with atropine. Exotic animals do not require exotic anesthesia!

Another common injectable chemical immobilizing agent that is very useful in carnivores is Telazol®. It is given in the dose range of 5 to15mg/kg for all carnivores with a dose of 10mg/kg being appropriate for most small carnivores. Drug volumes for small carnivores easily fit in a syringe, but if they need to be injected with a dart, larger volumes required for larger species can be a problem. Freeze drying ketamine or starting with Telazol® powder and reconstituting it with 100mg/ml xylazine can decrease the volume so it fits into a dart for remote delivery. Most of the newer alpha$_2$'s come in concentrations that are useful for small animals but drug volumes become unwieldy as well as expensive for larger species. Kreeger et al. 2002 provided dosage suggestions for a wide variety of species from aardvarks to zebu and include many of the newer drugs and combinations. It suggested extrapolating from a related or similar species for which a dose is listed if the species is not included in the extensive published dosage guidelines. It also suggested ketamine and xylazine as the safest and most widely used combination for most species. The common injectable anesthetics and inhalation anesthesia machines plus the sophisticated monitoring equipment found in most veterinary practices, along with a rational, common sense approach to handling and anesthesia of small, non-domestic carnivores should allow practitioners to handle whatever challenge is presented. As new drugs become available to replace or to be used in combination with old standby drugs used on domestic species, the same drugs and techniques can be applied to all species.

Recovery

The biggest caution regarding recovery is to provide benign neglect. Animals must either recover in their own enclosure or in something that can be safely transported. Handling a non-domestic carnivore during later stages of recovery is not advisable and can be a significant danger to people involved. One must assure that animals are able to maintain an open airway and keeping them in a quiet area is paramount for a successful outcome.

Anesthesia of Freshwater and Saltwater Fishes

Immobilizing fish safely for capture, relocation or treatment present several challenges. The method selected must be effective, safe, easy to administer and should allow the animal to return to normal function within a relatively short time leaving no residual effects in its behavior or appearance. The purpose is to determine a safe and effective means for immobilizing or anesthetizing individual teleosts or elasmobranchs confined in large multispecies tanks to facilitate treatment and translocation. Teleosts and elasmobranchs can be conveniently immobilized using drugs when physical restraint is not possible or is inadvisable. Intramuscular anesthesia is also advantageous in reducing trauma or stress associated with capturing and transporting fast-moving fish and large specimens that are confined within large exhibit tanks.

Anesthesia comprises the triad of narcosis, analgesia and skeletal muscle relaxation. Anesthetics may be used alone or in combination with paralytics to immobilize animals. A wide range of drugs, some originally used to anesthetize humans and other mammalian species, facilitate handling, transport and surgery of fish—especially those in large exhibit tanks. The classic parameters of a well-balanced anesthetic regimen in fish are associated with minimal side-effects, render the patient unconscious, controls pain and stress and provide muscle relaxation. Regarding use of commercially available agents, less than 6ml, even for fish up to 15kg–is a requirement so that the drug can be administered by dart.

Preanesthesia
An advantage in anesthetizing fish compared to land mammals and birds is patient preparation. They don't have to be shaved, clipped, plucked, scrubbed or other preparation. The fish must either be captured by physical means or chemically immobilized. It is difficult to restrain fish without anesthesia; however when handling tuna for example, putting the fish in dorsal recumbency in a sling and covering the eyes will help make the fish lie still. The hardest challenge is hitting a moving fish in a column of water with a dart.

Types of Anesthetics
In teleosts and elasmobranchs, chemical immobilization is preferred over capture by electrical shock. Although shocking techniques have been used in streams to induce narcosis in trout, the effect lasts only a few minutes (Haskell 1940; Kynard & Lonsdale 1975). Higher currents are needed for the galvanonarcosis of marine fish because of higher conductivity of seawater. As a result, electric shock is usually used only in small freshwater holding tanks or in small streams (Tytler & Hawkins 1981).

Chemical anesthesia can be administered to various species of fish via several routes. The optimal route depends on size of fish, its behavioral and anatomical features and its physical location (e.g., whether it is in captivity or wild). Common routes of anesthetic administration include immersion, ingestion, or IM, IV and IP injection. The oral route is typically administered by gavage incorporating a capsule in food or by squirting anesthetic into a crevice. It cannot be employed in aquaria where contamination of water and other fish must be avoided.

Behavioral patterns of fish under anesthesia are classified into four major stages: (1) sedation; (2) loss of equilibrium; (3) loss of reflex reactivity; and (4) medullary collapse–a sequence similar to that described for higher vertebrates (McFarland & Klontz 1969). In fish, immersion anesthetics have been studied more extensively than those given IM (McFarland 1959; Stoskopf 1985).

Immersion Anesthesia
Immersion anesthesia is commonly used in small fish tanks. The anesthetic may be pumped or dripped over the gills or an appropriate dose may be added to a measured volume of water, whereupon the fish is immersed in the anesthetic solution. The four most common immersion anesthetics are benzocaine, tricaine methane sulphonate (MS 222, a derivative of benzocaine), metomidate (a derivative of etomidate) and quinaldine sulphate. CO_2 is also used, but is not recommended because of the Bohr Effect; in addition, the final concentration of CO_2 in the medium is difficult to control.

328 The Anesthetic Period: Other Small Animals

Tricaine Methane Sulphonate (MS 222)

Under the brand name of Finquel (Wyeth-Ayerst), this drug is licensed for fish by the US FDA and is the most widely used immersion anesthetic available. Induction and recovery are rapid at a dose of 70-100mg/L. This is commonly used when dealing with an individual fish as in a pet aquarium. It is available in powder form and reconstituted with water. A 10% solution is stable if stored in a brown bottle glass for up to 3 days. Solutions in sea water may become toxic if exposed to light. Dose depends on the level of anesthesia desired, species and size of fish, water temperature and water hardness. Solutions for gold fish are usually induced with 1:10,000 and then maintained with a more dilute solution of 1:45,000. It is important to check pH of the solution when first made up with distilled water. The pH will be about 3.7 and should to be titrated with NaOH to a pH of 7.0 to 8.0. When using saltwater, pH is usually closer to pH of 7.

A client will usually bring the fish for examination in a covered container or zip lock bag. It is recommended to have them bring a separate container of water from their home aquarium that can be used to recover the fish. Induction time at the above concentration will be about 5 minutes and recovery time will be about 4 minutes. MS 222 is carcinogenic so it is best to wear gloves for these procedures. A washout time of 21 days is required if harvesting fish for food with the drug.

Benzocaine

Benzocaine is popular as an immersion anesthetic and is less expensive than MS 222. Because it is not water soluble, it must be dissolved in ethanol; 100gm benzocaine per liter of ethanol. The Benzocaine-ethanol solution is then added drop-wise to the water in which the fish is immersed.

Metomidate

This drug has been used on trout and catfish at a concentration of 2.5 to 5.0mg/L. It has a long recovery time; increased muscle fasciculation's and causes an increase in pigmentation presumably due to increased production of melanocyte-stimulating hormone on the same primary protein as ACTH (Stoskopf 1985).

Quinaldine

Quinaldine, a quinoline compound, has become a useful agent for collecting fish from tidal pools, small lagoons and crevices. It is oily and like benzocaine, it is not water soluble. It must be dissolved in ethanol before being added to water. The dose is 15 to 70mg/L for warm-water species, 200mg/L for tropical marine species (Blasiola 1976) and 16mg/L for many other fish species. Quinaldine is irritating to gill tissue and causes increased bronchial mucus secretion. Corneal damage has been reported following its use with salmonids.

Isoeugenol

(2-methoxy-4-propenylphenol) is manufacufactured by Aqui-S New Zealand Ltd with brand name of Aqui-S. This drug is dispersed directly into seawater or fresh water. Dosage is 5 to 10ml/1000 liters for light sedation or 17 to 20ml/1000 liters for heavy anesthesia depending on the species and environmental conditions. Isoeugenol does not have FDA approval in the U.S.

Eugenol

Eugenol (4-allyl-2-methoxy-phenol) is the active compound (90 %) in clove oil. It has been used at concentrations of 25-100mg/L. The problem in using this in large tanks is disposing of the drug post anesthesia.

Injectable Drugs

Injecting drugs into fish is desirable in large bodies of water with multiple species where it is not feasible to add large amounts of anesthetic to the tank (Ross and Ross 1999). Small ornamental fish can be anesthetized by injecting the anesthetic IP on the ventral midline with the needle pointing in a rostrodorsal direction away from the spleen (Brown 1992). Large sharks can be given IV injections of anesthetics if they are placed in a sling in dorsal recumbency. IM injections of anesthetics can be made via dart into the dorsal musculature of fast-moving fish and large specimens in the wild or in large tanks.

Barbiturates
From an historical perspective, thiopental, methohexital and pentobarbital have been recommended for IP injection in fish (Walker 1972; Keys & Wells 1930). Lengthy anesthesia up to 24 hours is produced and associated with persistent ataxia, intense bradycardia and respiratory arrest. They have been used for anesthesia in tench *(Tinca tinca)* and roach *(Rutilus rutilus)* with IM injections of 20mg/kg (Shelton & Randall 1962). IP doses of 48 to 72mg/kg have been reported for trout (Oswald 1978). Because of undesirable side effects, they are not often used for anesthesia in fish.

Etorphine/acetylpromazine
Under the name of Immobilon, rapid immobility is provided with minimal effect on the primary sensory pathways and no evidence of neuromuscular blocking effects. Etorphine causes catatonia and loss of equilibrium but respiration and cardiovascular function remain nearly normal. Dose needed to anesthetize fish would be fatal to humans (Oswald 1978; Blane et al. 1957). Good anesthesia in rainbow trout is provided with 8 to 10mg/kg. After 1 hour, anesthesia was reversible within 5 minutes with diprenorhine (Revivon).

Magnesium Sulfate
IM injection of magnesium sulfate has been reported to anesthetize kelp bass but lethal dose and anesthetic dose are virtually the same. As a result, this drug does not have application in fish.

Propanidid
A dose of 325mg/kg IP are required for effective anesthesia in rainbow trout with duration of approximately 2.5 hours (Oswald 1978). Respiration does not appear to be greatly depressed.

Neuromuscular Blocking Agents
For muscle relaxation, d-tubocurarine (3-30mg/kg), gallamine triethiodide (Flaxedil) (0.5-1mg/kg) and succinylcholine (1-3mg/kg) have been reported for IM or IP injection in fish. These are paralytics without analgesic or anesthetic effects and should only be used if no other alternatives are available for safety of the animals and personnel. In sufficient dosage, these drugs stop movements of oxygenated water through the gill plates so forced ventilatory efforts may needed to prevent hypoxemia (Tytler & Hawkins 1981).

New Drugs and Combinations
Because of the lack of information regarding injectable anesthetics in fish, various drugs and combinations have been evaluated at the Monterey Bay Aquarium for potential use by IM injection and are listed in Table 6-10. The study had three major objectives: (1) identification of a dose response in fish to commercially available drugs and anesthetics used for IM injection in mammals.; (2) evaluation of safety and efficacy and (3) assessment of interspecies variation in response to specific drugs or combinations.

Fish were quarantined in an open system in which wastewater was discharged into a sewer and fish were observed for a period of 30 days prior to beginning the study. Subsequently, fish were kept in 12- and 20-foot-diameter tanks 4 feet deep; each tank had a Hartford loop. Water quality is listed in Table 6-11.

Individual fish were identified by insertion of a plastic colored floy tag next to the dorsal fin. Each experimental group was observed at 2, 5, 10, 15, 20 30, 40, 50, 60 minutes and thereafter every half hour until 8 hours post treatment; a final evaluation was made at 24 hours. Activity, appearance and equilibrium were recorded following introduction of a visual stimulus (placing a net in the water) and a vibration stimulus (tapping the side of the tank).

Two methods were used to deliver the darts non-traumatically to target fish. For slow-swimming fish, the dart was inserted into a special plastic holder[a] attached to the tip of a pole spear or a Hawaiian sling, while for faster fish a Mares[b] snub-nose pneumatic spear gun with a similar holder was used. Holders were designed to freely release the darts upon striking, allowing darts to remain embedded in muscle. Lightly barbed needles were used so that darts would remain attached to the subject long enough for the entire dose to be injected. To help cushion impact of the dart, shock absorbers made from rubber syringe plungers were installed on the needle shaft. A diver-using SCUBA allowed the target fish to swim past before shooting at an oblique (45-degree) angle to the sagital plane of the retreating fish. This procedure minimized damage from impact of the shaft. Fish injected from this angle were less aware of the impending impact and less likely to avoid the dart.

Table 6-10 Drugs Evaluated for Potential Use in Fish

Drugs Evaluated	Comments
Alphaxolone-alphadolone–Alphaxalone	Synthetic steroid anesthetic for long-term anesthesia.
Atipamezole hydrochloride	Alpha$_2$ adrenergic antagonist
Atracurium besylate	Nondepolarizing neuromuscular blocking agent
Azaperone	Butyrephenone tranquilizer
Carfentanyl–carfentanyl citrate	A synthetic opiate with a clinical potency 10,000 times that of morphine.
Diazepam	Benzodiazepine tranquilizer
Fentanyl	Potent mu opioid
Ketamine hydrochloride	Dissociative anesthetic
Medetomidine	Alpha$_2$ adrenergic antagonist
Metomidate	Imidazole-based nonbarbituate, hypnotic
Midazolam	Water soluble benzodiazepine
Neostigmine methylsulfate	Anticholinesterase
Succinylcholine chloride	Depolarizing neuromuscular blocking agent.
Tiletamine and zolazepam	Fixed combination of a dissociative anesthetic agent and a benzodiazepine tranquilizer
Vecuronium bromide	Non-depolarizing neuromuscular blocking agent.
Xylazine	Alpha$_2$ adrenergic agonist
Yohimbine hydrochloride	Alpha$_2$ adrenergic antagonist

Water Quality at Monterey Bay Aquarium

PH	8.0*
Water Temperature	48-58°F.
Salinity	32 PPT
Nitrogen	1-3 microbes of ammonia
Nitrite	0
Nitride	0
Dissolved Oxygen	> 95% **

*measured by ionic probe
**measured by oxygard probe
Note: The Monterey Bay Aquarium has an open seawater system. The water quality variables were analyzed for copper concentration by the porphyrin method (Hach Method 8143), nitrite concentration–colorimetric method (standard method 4500-N02B), nitrate concentration–UV method (standard method 4500-N03B) or cadmium reduction method (standard method 4500-N03E), ammonia concentration–oxidation method (manual of chemical and biological methods for seawater analysis).

IM injections of free-swimming fish utilized 3 to 5ml pneumatic darts manufactured by Telinject[C] Blue food dye (0.2ml) was added to ketamine to help ascertain that correct injection had occurred. If the dart did not inject properly, blue dye could be seen in the surrounding water indicating a miss.

Site for IM and IP injections are shown in Figure 6-13. Eighteen to 23 gauge, 2 to 4cm needles are recommended for larger fish and 25 to 28ga needles are preferred for smaller fish. Small drug volumes can be absorbed rapidly if introduced into the red lateral muscle, the quantity of which depends on the species of the fish. Because blood flow is approximately 10 times greater in red muscle, it is the preferred injection site for producing relatively rapid induction.

Drugs or drug combinations were administered IM to 15 species of temperate-water fishes (Table 6-10). Optimum dose was determined in a double dose process. Seven doses were evaluated: the recommended dose provided by the manufacturer for domestic animals and three double doses below and above that dose (e.g., 1/16, 1/4, 1/2, the domestic animal dose, 2×, 4×, 8×, 16×).

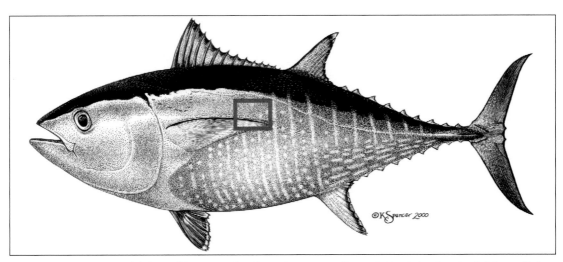

Figure 6-13 Picture of fish and location for dart placement. Entry is for injection in fish's medial epiaxial musculature.

a and c: Telinject,9316 Soledad Canyon Rd, Saugus, CA 91350 b: Sea Quest Inc, 2151-F Las Palmas Dr., Carlsbad, CA 92008

When an optimum dose was identified for a particular species, a group of fish was anesthetized (once a week at most). For example, striped bass (*Morone saxattilis*) were tested weekly with dosages ranging from 1 to 25mg/kg at various body sites using 100mg/ml and 200mg/ml concentrations of ketamine. Five rockfish (*Sebastes sp.*) and five Pacific mackerel (*Scomber japonica*) were given 1 to 5mg/kg of ketamine IM. White sturgeon (*Acipenser transmontanus*) and rainbow trout (*Salmo gairdnerii*) were given 20 and 18mg/kg, respectively. In this manner, a safe dose of ketamine could be established for each species. Once a safe dose was established, 40 striped bass, 1 giant sea bass (*Stereolepis gigas*), 1 sheephead (*Semicossyphus pulcher*), and 2 leopard sharks (*Triakis semifasciata*) were injected with ketamine at an average dose of 15mg/kg to facilitate their removal from the aquarium's 1,137,000 liter Monterey Bay Habitats exhibit. This was done safely with no fatalities.

Behavioral data were analyzed in relation to anesthetic doses and organized according to general categories of anesthesia (Table 6-12). Stages of anesthesia in fish are similar to those in mammals (McFarland 1959; Stoskopf 1985; Brown 1992). Level of anesthesia reached in each trial was classified according to the stages of anesthesia previously identified and are listed in Table 6-13 (McFarland 1959).

Time necessary for each fish to return to pre-anesthetic behavior and physical appearance was noted. Additionally, survivorship was determined for each dose (defined as percent of fish surviving). Deaths included those attributable directly to anesthesia as well as those possibly due to handling. Averages of the anesthetic categories were analyzed as X ± SEM and statistical analyses performed. Twenty-four drugs and drug combinations were evaluated using the IM route for a total of 411 trials (see Table 6-10).

Table 6-13 | Classification of Behavioral Changes in Fishes During Anesthesia

Stage 0	Normal behavior: reactive to external stimuli, equilibrium and muscle tone normal.
Stage I, Level 1	Light sedation: analgesia, slight loss of reactivity to external stimuli (visual and tactile), voluntary movement still possible, opercular rate normal.
Stage I, Level 2	Deep sedation: total loss of reactivity to external stimuli, slight decrease in opercular rate.
Stage II	Partial loss of equilibrium: partial loss of muscle tone, reactive only to very strong tactile and vibrational stimuli, rheotaxi present but swimming capability seriously disrupted, increase in opercular rate.
Stage III, Level 1	Total loss of equilibrium: total loss of muscle tone, reactive only to deep pressure stimuli, opercular rate below normal.
Stage III, (Level 2 -Surgery level).	Loss of reflex activity: – total loss of reactivity, opercular rate very slow, and slow heart rate.
Stage IV	Medullary collapse: respiratory movements cease, followed by cardiac arrest.

Drugs Recommended for IM Injection (Table 6-14)
Ketamine
Ketamine is commercially available in 100mg/ml concentration. It can also be concentrated from 100 to 200mg/ml by a compounding pharmacy so it can be delivered by dart syringe. A dose of

15mg/kg for a 15kg fish can be administered in 1.25ml of 200mg/ml concentration or 2.50ml of the 100mg/ml concentration. Induction time for ketamine will be about 8 minutes and fish should be fully recovered within 3 hours. It does not cause behavioral or pathological effects with good induction and recovery behaviors. The drug does not depress the respiratory system and is safe at doses up to 6 times the recommended dose.

Ketamine should not be used on ram-ventilator fish like tuna. When these fish are not moving through water, they require a flow of oxygenated water passing over their gills. Although a tube can provide oxygen via seawater, this additional procedure is considered undesirable. Medetomidine combined with ketamine and reversed with atipamezole is preferred in these species (Walker 1972).

Ketamine in dosages of 15 to 20mg/kg can be expected to be short-acting, easily administered and accessible immobilizing agent for IM injection in fish. It has wide margin of safety, short induction time and is available from Wildlife Pharmaceuticals in Fort Collins, CO at 200mg/ml. A disadvantage is that it is not rapidly reversible. In large fish, e.g., 50kg, two injections of the antagonist are required. A 15-minute delay should follow before administering a second injection if no effect was observed from the first injection. Fish anesthetized with the recommended dose exhibited no serious side effects. Deleterious effects occurred only at dosages above 50mg/kg. Sharks are more sensitive than teleosts and respond well to a dose of 15mg/kg. The tough epidermis and placoid scales of sharks require use of larger needles, which may result in a degree of leakage from the injection site. Eels can be anesthetized with ketamine at a lower dose but it appears that quinaldine sulphate is a better choice in this species.

Ketamine/medetomidine
The combination of medetomidine and ketamine, reversible with atipamezole, produced safe, effective anesthesia in bonito and mackerels (Williams et al. 2004). Significant interspecies variation can be expected between teleosts and elasmobranchs with IM ketamine. Ketamine produced safe anesthesia in teleosts at 15 to 20mg/kg but in elasmobranches, the dose was 10 to 15mg/kg. The combination of medetomidine and ketamine should be evaluated is specific species as variations can be expected.

Fish of the family Scombridae (bonitos, mackerels, and tunas) have unique physiology. These fish are also of great economic value in commercial fisheries and fish farming. The combination of ketamine and medetomidine produces anesthesia and hematological responses of bonito (*Sarda chilienesis*) and mackerel (*Scomber japonica*). Doses of 0.8mg/kg medetomidine and 2-4mg/kg ketamine appear to be equally safe and effective to achieve stage III anesthesia with 100% recovery after administration of 2.0mg/kg atipamezole. Ketamine at 4.0mg/kg in combination with medetomidine at a dose of 0.4mg/kg is the lowest effective dose that should be given IM and can be reversed with atipamizole at 2.0mg/kg. In mackerel, a dose of 1.1 to 2.3mg/kg of medetomidine and 57 to 222mg/kg ketamine is a safe and effective dose to achieve stage III anesthesia. The application of this injectable protocol can be used effectively in experiments to study the physiology of these fish or in husbandry of captive scombrids.

Studies on Morone saxattilis and Sebastes sp. using an IM dose of 50-100ug/kg combined with 1 to 2mg/kg ketamine showed an induction time of 30 minutes to reach stage III but this is unacceptably slow. Higher doses of medetomidine might produce more rapid induction and should be investigated.

Saffan
Saffan was ranked just below ketamine in efficacy and safety. In six species, induction time ranged from 4 to 17 minutes with duration of anesthesia from 4 to 16 hours.

Table 6-14

Trials of Drugs Administered by IM Injection in Fish

DRUG	DOSE RANGE mg/kg	SPECIES	IND TIME minutes	DURATION hours	FISH N	COMMENTS
Alphaxalone-alphadolone	0.02-0.59	A,B,C,D,I,K	4-17	4 to 16	41	Respiration close too normal; easily nettable at 0.1-0.2mg/kg; continues to get deeper into anesthesia.
Atracurium besylate	0.027-1.5	B,J	30	6-7	6	At does of 1.5mg/kg, one died after 17 hours; low safety factor.
Diazepam	0.227-1.51	A,B,C,D	25-50	48	18	2 died (at doses of 0.23 & 1.5mg/kg). Increased rate of respiration, protruding operculum, lack of coordination. No stage III. Fish became dark.
Ketamine hydrochloride	.45 to 45	All	3-21	2.7	104	Best nonreversible intramuscular anesthesia.
Ketamine & diazepam	9-18 ket & 0.23-.91 valium	A,B,J	70	22	18	No apparent synergistic effect.
Ketamine & midazolam (Versed)	14 ket & 2.27 versed	B	3-8	18-24	2	Anesthesia is too long.
Ketamine & xylazine	3.4-18 ket & 1.14-30 xyl	A,B,C,L,M	6-34	1-120	15	5 died
Medetomidine & atipamezole	0.02-0.18	A	22-34	0.8	10	Reversed within 24 min.
Medetomidine & ketamine & atipamezole	0.05 Med, 0.05 ket, 2.5 ati	A,L	17-47	3.45-4.0	18	Dose is too small should be Med 0.8 mg/kg and ket 4 mg/kg. Reversable
Metomidate	4.55-22.7	A,B,H,J	5-50	40 min. to 5 days	30	Black splotches worse; out for 24 to 48 hours; 10 died.
Neostigmine	0.11-0.20	A,B	90	>24	5	Hematoma at base of pectoral fin and operculum, slow respiration; 2 died. 0.1 mg/kg, no response; 0.2mg/kg, death.

Table 6-14 Continued

DRUG	DOSE RANGE mg/kg	SPECIES	IND TIME minutes	DURATION hours	FISH N	COMMENTS
Vecuronium bromide	0.02-1.36	A,B,D	3-140	>24	47	12 died. < 0.1mg/kg, no response; > 0.1 mg/kg, death. No safety factor.
Succinylcholine	.10,.15,.21	B,J	2-15	0.5	4	Dose of 0. mg/kg caused death in 35 min.
Tiletamine-zolazepam	0.45 to 9.1	A,H	6-24	24-120	8	Still affected at 48 hrs, shark died at 48hrs; twitching, flared operculum
Yohimbine	0.11-1.8	A,C,L	35-75	1.5	10	Black splotches where injected; swimming slow after 3hrs, 1 died
Atipamezole	4.54	A	No response		2	
Azaperone	0.91-15.9	A,D	No response		18	Dark splotches; < 12mg/kg, no response
Carfentanyl	4.54	B	No response		1	
Fentanyl	0.023-4.54	A,B	No response		9	No response; black mark at site of injection
Fentanyl & azaperone	0.011-0.068 fen & 0.054-0.27 az	B,C	No response		4	
Fentanyl & droperidol	0.036-0.58	B	No response		8	
Sterile saline	1-3ml	A	No response		6	Control
Tricainemethane sulfonate (MS 222)	4.54-45.45	A	No response		3	Dose of 45mg/kg caused death 4 days later
Midazolam Hcl	0.045-0.09	A	No response		4	Black splotches at injection site
Xylazine	0.45-.09	A,B	No response		20	One 2mg, 4mg & 5mg/kg fish died in 24 hours
					411	

A. STRIPED BASS *Morone saxatilis*, B. ROCKFISH *Sebastes sp.*, C. PACIFIC MACKEREL *Scomber japonicus*, D. WHITE STURGEON *Acipenser transmontanus*, E. RAINBOW TROUT *Oncorhynchus mykiss*, F. GIANT SEA BASS *Stereolepis gigas*, G. SHEEPHEAD *Semicossyphus pulcher*, H. LEOPARD SHARK *Triakis semifasciata*, I. SPINY DOGFISH *Squalus acanthias*, J. CHILIPEPPER *Sebastes goodei*, K. BLACK COD *Anoplopoma fimbria*, L. CABEZON *Scorpaenichthys marmoratus*, M. SALMON *Oncorhynchus tshawytscha*, N. KELP BASS *Paralabrax maculatofasciatus*, O. WOLF EEL *Anarrhichthys ocellatus*

Drugs NOT Recommended for IM Injection

Ketamine/midazolam

From these studies, several immobilizing or anesthetic drugs are inappropriate for IM administration in fish. Ketamine and midazolam has a short induction time but a long duration of effect, 18 to 24 hours. Addition of diazepam to ketamine increased induction time to 70 minutes and the duration of anesthesia to 22 hours.

Ketamine/xylazine

Ketamine and xylazine is associated with a long induction time and one-third of the fish died over periods ranging to 120 hours. As a result, this combination is not a good choice.

Medetomidine

This drug alone is not acceptable for immobilization or anesthesia (Jalanka 1991). Induction time will be about 30 minutes but response does not reach sufficient levels for capture. Medetomidine should be reversed with atipamezole at five times the injected dose (50ug/kg medetomidine and 250ug/kg atipamezole). Current formulation of medetomidine at a concentration of 1mg/ml is not acceptable for darting fish 15kg and larger because of the large volume required. The manufacturer now provides a higher concentration (20mg/cc) that will be used in future studies with yellow fin and blue fin tunas and striped bass. Recommended dose of this combination is 0.8mg/kg medetomidine with 4mg/kg ketamine depending on the species.

Metomidate

Metomidate has been used successfully as an immersion anesthetic but when administered IM, 33% of fish died. It also caused large black splotches at the injection site, which persisted more than 24 hours.

Neuromuscular Blocking Agents

Neostigmine, vecuronium, atracurium and succinylcholine had a poor safety factor including death. As a result, they should not be used alone.

Diazepam

Results with diazepam were not acceptable. This minor tranquilizer produced sedation for up to 48 hours, increased gill movement with protruded operculum and 11% of fish died. Length of sedation was its most deleterious effect.

Tiletamine/zolazapam

Telezol was used in two species of fish and effects were still noted 48 hours after administration. Thus this drug was not found to be acceptable.

Opioids (carfentanyl, fentanyl, fentanyl/droperidol)

Fish did not respond to any opioid given IM. Fish may lack opioid receptor sites commonly associated with anesthesia and pain in mammals nor do they have spinothalamic pathway as found in mammalian species. It is beyond the scope of this discussion whether fish feel pain or how they express their discomfort. It is known that fish react to physical and chemical stimuli, which make sedation and/or anesthesia a requirement for capture and surgery independent of pain perception.

Factors Affecting Anesthesia

Several factors affect rate of induction and depth of anesthesia in fish. These include individual and species variation, size, water temperature and water acidity. One variation of note in mackerel was that rate of induction and depth of anesthesia was different based on whether the injection was placed in red or white muscle.

With practice, both the pole spear and spear gun will allow consistent placement of the dart within the target fish's medial epiaxial musculature (Figure 6-13). The pole spear was found to be very effective at distances from 1 to 6 feet, depending on the amount of tension placed on the surgical tubing sling. The spear gun was effective at distances of 6 to 10 feet; at shorter distances, however, the spear gun was too powerful for the shaft to be effectively cushioned by the shock absorbers. Fortunately, it is not difficult to get sufficiently far away from the fish. Shots from the side or as a fish swims toward the diver create a higher risk of injuring the fish or failing to inject the entire dose of drug. Because darts cannot quickly release from the holder if fired head-on or perpendicular to the target, fish tend to thrash about in order to escape, causing the needle to slash from side to side or separate from the dart. With accurate injection, fish will likely rapidly swim straight ahead, pulling the dart from the holder. Other than the needle puncture, fish seldom show trauma at the site of injection.

Tranquilization or anesthesia should be constantly monitored throughout the procedure, and intervention should be prompt if problems are identified. Variables to observe include swimming activity, reaction to external stimuli, equilibrium, and respiratory rate. Respiratory rate in fish can be monitored by watching movements of the operculum. If the anesthetic appears too deep, oxygenated water can be pumped over the gills or the fish can be moved through the water head first. Anesthetic solutions and recovery tanks should be aerated constantly. When fish are under stress, they remove more oxygen from the water, a fact that must be taken into account during anesthetic procedures.

Anesthesia and Analgesia of Reptiles

Designing an effective and safe anesthetic protocol for the reptilian patient is often challenging due to their unique anatomy and physiology. The veterinary practitioner should have a good knowledge and understanding of reptilian anatomy, physiology and the pathophysiology of common diseases in order to select an appropriate anesthetic protocol. Reptiles are poikilothermic animals with species-specific preferred optimal temperature ranges and the patient's response to anesthetic and analgesic agents depends on environmental temperature.

All anesthetic agents affect cardiopulmonary variables and knowledge of normal respiratory anatomy and function is essential to monitor cardiopulmonary function of the patient throughout the anesthetic event. Comprehensive reviews on reptile anesthesia have been published previously (Bennet 1991; Heard 1993; Page 1993; Bennet 1996; Schumacher 1996; Heard 2001).

Anatomy and Respiratory Physiology

Anatomy and function of the reptilian respiratory system are unique among vertebrate species (Perry 1998; Wang et al. 1998). Anatomical differences can also be seen between orders and species and all reptiles have in common that they lack a functional diaphragm.

The glottis of snakes is located rostrally. The trachea consists of incomplete cartilagenous rings and bifurcates into short bronchi at the level of the heart (Wallach 1998). In carnivorous lizards, the glottis is located more rostrally while in herbivorous species it is found at the base of the tongue. The trachea of lizards also has incomplete tracheal rings and bifurcates at the base of the heart. In chelonians, the glottis is situated at the base of the tongue and the trachea has complete tracheal rings. At the thoracic inlet, the short trachea bifurcates into a left and right intrapulmonary bronchus. In snakes, lungs are sac-like structures extending into a caudal airsac lined with non-respiratory epithelium. A left lung is vestigal in most species, except in boid snakes. Lungs of most lizard species are single-chambered and may extend caudally into an airsac. In chelonians, lungs are paired, multi-chambered and located below the carapace. In crocodilians, the glottis is located behind an epiglottal flap and lungs are complex and multi-chambered.

Reptile respiratory physiology differs between orders, species and especially terrestrial and aquatic species. The primary organ for gas exchange is the lung, but aquatic species are capable of cutaneous gas exchange. During prolonged periods of apnea, many species have the capacity to utilize anaerobic metabolism. Reptilian lungs have high compliance values and minute volume is increased by an increase in respiratory rate. Although reptiles have large lung volumes, surface area for gas exchange is approximately 20% of a mammal of comparative body mass (Perry 1998). Reptilian respiration is controlled by hypoxia and hypercapnia and ventilation is increased during periods of low O_2 and high CO_2. Hypercapnia will result in an increased tidal volume while hypoxic events will increase respiratory rate. The stimulus to breath in reptiles comes from low oxygen tensions. Placed in an environment with increased oxygen concentrations, most species will decrease rate of breathing and tidal volume. Reptiles are known to develop intrapulmonary shunts which will reduce efficiency of gas exchange and result in a reduction of PaO_2 (Wang et al. 1998).

Patient Preparation

Standards and principles of small animal anesthesia also apply to reptiles. A thorough history, visual and physical examination, including accurate body weight and diagnostic tests should be performed. In many cases, reptiles are presented in poor body condition characterized by dehydration, anorexia and chronic secondary infections. Prior to anesthesia, the patient should be stabilized and supportive care measures including fluid therapy, nutritional support and effective antimicrobial therapy should be initiated. Rate and depth of respiration should be evaluated for evidence of respiratory disease (Schumacher 2003).

Collection of a venous blood sample for determination of hematologic and plasma biochemical variables is recommended prior to anesthesia, depending on the size and nature of the patient. Minimally, PCV, TP and glucose levels should be determined. Additional diagnostic tests may include fecal screens, collection of biopsy specimen and aspirates from masses for cytologic, microbiologic and histopathologic evaluation. Radiography and ultrasound can be performed in most species without anesthesia and may identify organ abnormalities.

Fluid therapy with a balanced electrolyte solution should only be initiated if there is indication of volume depletion, based on physical and laboratory findings. Fluid requirements and selection as well as treatment of disturbances of hydration status have been reported (Schumacher 2000).

Analgesia

Every effort should be made to evaluate the reptilian patient for evidence of pain or discomfort. Few studies have investigated effective pain management protocols in reptiles. However, conditions such as trauma, surgery and neoplasia will cause pain and discomfort in reptiles. Pain, stress and discomfort are closely related and effective pain management will reduce effects of pain on immune function, hematological, biochemical and metabolic disturbances (Muir 2002).

The clinician must be familiar with the normal behavior of the species in order to recognize signs of discomfort and pain such as restlessness, increased respiratory rate, anorexia and aggressiveness. In many cases, signs of pain are not obvious; however, abnormal body position, reluctance to lie down and abnormal gait and restlessness may indicate discomfort.

Few drugs are routinely used for treatment of pain and in many cases, drugs and dosages have to be adjusted from pharmacokinetic studies in domestic animals. Table 6-15 provides selected analgesics and anesthetics along with doses commonly used in reptiles. The most effective method of managing pain is preventing pain at the onset. Preemptive analgesic techniques are recommended in cases when the animal is undergoing elective surgery. Balanced analgesic techniques such as administration of systemic analgesic agents (opioid agonists) in combination with a long-acting local anesthetic, e.g., bupivacaine, are most effective in management of postoperative pain in reptiles. As part of a balanced anesthetic regimen, local anesthetic agents are given along with systemic analgesic agents. Lidocaine has a rapid onset of action while bupivacaine is more effective in controlling post-operative pain due to its long duration of action. Techniques for topical or regional anesthesia, local infiltration techniques and field blocks are applicable to most reptilian patients. Local anesthetics can directly be applied to surgical wounds, e.g., abscess debridement or injected into coeliotomy incisions. Toxic doses of lidocaine or bupivacaine have not been determined in reptiles. However, 4mg/kg bupivacaine and 10mg/kg lidocaine should not be exceeded in the reptilian patient in order to avoid potential side-effects such as arrhythmias and seizures.

Indications for management of acute pain include traumatic events such as shell fractures, fractures of the long bones in lizards, thermal burns and of course surgery. Acute pain in reptiles is most effectively treated with an opioid, e.g., butorphanol or buprenorphine. For elective procedures, analgesic agents should be incorporated into the anesthetic protocol to provide pre-, intra- and post-operative analgesia. Frequent clinical assessment of the patient for evidence of pain, especially in the post-operative period will often facilitate effective analgesic therapy.

Therapy of chronic pain in reptiles is in many cases neglected due to a poor understanding of the effects of NSAIDs. Chronic pain in reptiles is often associated with diseases such as metabolic bone disease, gout, renal disease as well as a variety of neoplastic diseases. Non-steroidal anti-inflammatory agents, e.g. ketoprofen and carprofen, should also be administered for the management of chronic pain. However, more research is indicated to determine effective dosages, dosage intervals and potential side-effects.

Table 6-15

Selected Analgesic and Anesthetic Agents Commonly Used in Reptiles

Agent	Lizards	Snakes	Chelonians
Bupivacaine (mg/kg)	1-2	1-2	1-2
Buprenorphine (mg/kg)	0.02-0.2 SC,IM,IV	0.02-0.2 SC,IM,IV	0.02-0.2 SC,IM,IV
Diazepam (mg/kg)	0.2-2.0 IM,IV	0.2-2.0 IM,IV	0.2-1.0 IM,IV
Isoflurane (%)	Induction: 4-5 Maintenance: 1.5-3	Induction: 5 Maintenance: 2-3	Induction: 4-5 Maintenance: 2-3
Ketamine (mg/kg)	5-20 SC, IM, IV	10-60 SC, IM	5-50 IM, IV
Medetomidine (µg/kg)	0.05-0.1 IM	0.1-0.15 IM	0.03-0.15 IM
Midazolam (mg/kg)	1-2 IM,IV	1-2 IM,IV	1-2 IM,IV
Propofol (mg/kg)	3-5 IV,IO	3-5 IV	2-5 IV,IO
Sevoflurane (%)	Induction: 7-8 Maintenance: 3.5-4.5	Induction: 7-8 Maintenance: 3.5-4.5	Induction: 7-8 Maintenance: 3.5-4.5
Tiletamine/zolazepam (mg/kg)	2-6 IM,IV	2-6 IM	2-4 IM

Restraint

Most snakes, except venomous species and large constrictors, are easy to handle and restrain. The head should be secured between the fingers of one hand while the other hand supports the body. Only experienced handlers should manipulate venomous snakes. Tongs, hooks, and plexi-glass tubes are valuable tools to facilitate handling and manipulation of venomous and large snakes. Venomous snakes should be induced with inhalant agents in an induction chamber or while being restrained in a clear plexi-glass tube. Large constrictors are dangerous, capable of inflicting a serious bite to the inexperienced handler and the head should be secured at all times. Small lizards are easy to restrain and the head should be secured with one hand while the other supports the body. Large lizards, including iguanas are capable of inflicting serious bite and scratch injuries without proper restraint. The head and body should be supported to avoid injury to the handler and patient. Use of leather gloves and towels will prevent serious bite and scratch wounds. Green iguanas may inflict serious injury with their tail. However, due to tail autonomy, they should never be held by the tail alone. Pet lizards accustom to frequent handling can easily be examined with minimal or no restraint. Chelonians may be challenging to examine, especially individuals that will retract into their shell. In order to avoid injury to the animal and/or the veterinarian, injectable agents may be necessary to perform a physical examination or for induction of anesthesia. Aquatic turtles especially, will deliver a painful bite and every effort should be made to secure the head. Large tortoises are capable of inflicting crushing injuries if not properly restrained. However, animals that are handled and manipulated fequently may allow a complete physical examination and administration of the immobilizing agent by an IV route, e.g., jugular vein or brachial plexus.

Preanesthetic Medication

Administration of anticholinergics, e.g.,atropine or glycopyrrolate, preanesthesia is not a common practice in reptiles. Agents routinely used for premedication in other animals often only have mild sedative effects in reptiles. If given in higher doses to produce sedation, cardiopulmonary depression is an undesirable consequence. However, potentially dangerous or large reptiles such as large lizards and crocodilians, boid snakes as well as chelonians, may require an injectable agent to faciliate safe handling prior to induction of anesthesia.

Reptile patients presented with evidence of pain or scheduled to undergo a surgical procedure should be administered pre-operative analgesic agents for a balanced anesthetic regimen to provide intra- and post-operative analgesia. Administration of butorphanol or buprenorphine may reduce maintenance requirements of the inhalation anesthetic. However, a study in green iguanas showed that administration of butorphanol (1mg/kg IM) prior to isoflurane anesthesia did not have isoflurane-sparing effects (Mosley et al. 2003). Although opioid's have minimal sedative effects in most reptile species, when administered prior to mask induction, less struggling and breath-holding may be seen especially in green iguanas.

Benzodiazepines including diazepam and midazolam have minimal sedative effects in most reptile species, however species differences are apparent. In red-eared slider turtles (*Trachemys scripta elegans*) midazolam (1.5mg/kg IM) resulted in a sedative plane suitable for minor manipulations (Oppenheim & Moon 1995). For most anesthetic protocols, benzodiazepines are combined with dissociative agents such as ketamine and/or opioids (butorphanol or buprenorphine).

Injectable Anesthesia

In reptiles, injectable anesthetics have been investigated for induction and maintenance of anesthesia but species differences are common. Most agents, especially when given IM are associated with pronounced cardiopulmonary depressant effects, prolonged induction and recovery times as well as poor muscle relaxation. In most reptiles, IM administration of anesthetic agents is most effective and practical. A renal portal system is present in reptiles, however, pharmacokinetics of injectable agents are minimally altered if injected into the caudal half of the body (Benson & Forest 1999; Holz et al. 1997).

In snakes, IM injections are given into the paravertebral muscles. IV injections are often difficult, especially in small specimens but can be given into the tail vein or the right jugular vein following a cut-down procedure. In lizards and chelonians, musculature of the front limbs is most accessible for IM injections. In turtles and tortoises, the jugular vein or the coccygeal vein can be used for IV injections. In lizards, the ventral coccygeal vein or ventral abdominal vein is used for IV administration. The ventral abdominal vein is a relatively large vessel which can be catheterized for IV injection of anesthetic agents and/or fluid therapy during anesthesia. Alternately, or if multiple sites are required for drug administration, an IO catheter can be inserted into the tibia.

Ketamine

Ketamine has a wide range of safety in most reptiles and can be administered IV or IM. Ketamine alone and at high dosages will produce immobilization; however poor muscle relaxation and prolonged recovery times are often seen. In order to lower the required ketamine dose and to improve quality of anesthesia, ketamine is commonly combined with diazepam, midazolam, butorphanol, buprenorphine or medetomidine). With these combinations, inductions as well as recoveries are more rapid and smooth, and muscle relaxation is improved. A study in snakes has demonstrated that ketamine alone will produce respiratory depression, hypertension and tachycardia (Schumacher et al 1997).

Tiletamine/zolazepam

Tiletamine/zolazepam (Telazol) has been reported to be a useful agent for immobilization and induction of anesthesia in different reptile species. At higher doses (> 6mg/kg IM), Telazol is often associated with prolonged recovery times (> 48-72hrs), especially in chelonians. Telazol is effective at a low dose (2-4mg/kg IM), to facilitate handling of large chelonians, lizards and snakes.

Medetomidine

Medetomidine has been investigated in combination with ketamine and/or butorphanol. These combinations appear useful to effectively immobilize potentially dangerous reptiles and to perform short procedures, especially chelonians, e.g., shell repair, collection of diagnostic samples (Lock et al. 1998). Administration of atipamezole at 5 times the medetomidine dose appears to effectively reverse the effects of medetomidine at the end of the procedure. Medetomidine alone will produce sedation, however at the high doses needed (150µg/kg IM), pronounced cardiopulmonary depressant effects will be seen (Sleeman & Gaynor 2000).

Propofol

Propofol is the injectable agent of choice in reptiles. It has minimal cumulative effects even after repeated injections and has been investigated in a variety of reptile species (Anderson et al 1999; Bennett et al. 1998). Propofol has to be administered IV or as an alternate route IO and placement of a catheter is recommended especially for CRI techniques. For induction of anesthesia, propofol should be titrated to effect since rapid bolus injections are often associated with apnea (Bennet et al. 1998). Cardiopulmonary depressant effects such as hypotension and respiratory depression are similar to other induction agents, however, they are of shorter duration. Propofol can be administered to induce anesthesia (2-5mg/kg IV or IO) and maintenance of anesthesia via CRI (0.3-0.5mg/kg/min) or with intermittent boluses (0.5-1mg/kg).

Administration of local anesthetic agents has similar indications as in domestic animal anesthesia. Lidocaine or bupivacaine can be administered along with systemic analgesics, especially for orthopedic procedures. Although techniques for local and regional anesthetic techniques have not been described in reptiles, nerve blocks or interpleural administration of local anesthetics is indicated for a variety of surgical procedures in reptiles. Bupivacaine (1-2mg/kg) appears to be effective in reptiles for controlling post-operative pain and can be repeated every 4-12 hours depending on the patient's needs.

Inhalation Anesthesia

Anesthetic protocols of most reptiles are based on inhalational agents for induction and mainte-nance of anesthesia. Parenteral agents, ketamine, benzodiazepines, opioids and alpha$_2$ agonists may be administered to facilitate handling and to decrease the amount of inhalation anesthetic required for induction and maintenance. Inhalational agents are administered with a precision vaporizer and a non-rebreathing/semiopen system is indicated in reptiles weighing less than 10kg. Induction and maintenance requirements of the anesthetic are determined by health status of the animal and amount of each preanesthetic agent administered.

Isoflurane

The anesthetic of choice for reptiles is isoflurane due to rapid induction and recovery times, minimal depressant effects on cardiopulmonary function as well as limited hepatic and renal toxicity. Despite its common usage, only few studies have determined the cardiopulmonary effects in reptiles. MAC and cardiac index of isoflurane has been reported for green iguanas (Mosley et al. 2003 a,b). For most reptile species, isoflurane concentrations for induction of anesthesia are 4-5% and maintenance requirements range between 1.5 and 3%.

Sevoflurane

Sevoflurane has been investigated in several reptile species with various results. Sevoflurane has low blood solubility resulting in short induction and recovery times and rapid changes of anesthetic depth. Species differences in response to sevoflurane are apparent and some reptile species may fail to reach a surgical plane of anesthesia.

Desert tortoises (*Gopherus agassizii*) induced and maintained with sevoflurane alone showed minimal cardiopulmonary depressant effects (Rooney et al. 1999). In green iguanas (*Iguana iguana*) induction and recovery times are shorter with sevoflurane compared to isoflurane. However, cardiopulmonary effects are similar to that produced by isoflurane (Hernandez-Divers et al. 2003). Most reptile species require concentrations of 7 to 8% for induction and 3.5 to 4.5% for mainte-nance of a surgical plane of anesthesia.

Anesthetic Management

Techniques for induction and maintenance of anesthesia depend on species of reptile, procedure to be performed and health status of the patient. Chronically sick patients in poor body condition will require less anesthetic agent for induction and maintenance of anesthesia.

Lizards

Butorphanol (1-2mg/kg IM) administered 30 minutes prior to induction is useful as a preanesthetic and will provide pre- and intraoperative analgesia. Although butorphanol alone has minimal sedative effects, most lizards will exhibit less struggling and breath-holding during induction with an inhalation anesthetic. Propofol (3-5mg/kg IV) administered to effect will facilitate endotracheal intubation. Alternately, lizards can also be manually restrained and anesthesia can be induced with isoflurane or sevoflurane via face mask. Maintenance of anesthesia in most patients, especially for long procedures should be with either agent.

Snakes

Small, non-venomous snakes should be premedicated with butorphanol (1-4mg/kg IM) and/or a low dose of ketamine (5-20mg/kg IM) prior to induction with 5% isoflurane or 8% sevoflurane by mask. Large snakes such as boid snakes can be premedicated with Telazol (2 to 4mg/kg IM) to facilitate handling, endotracheal intubation and induction with an inhalant. For IV administration propofol, 3 to 5mg/kg should be administered into the ventral tail vein. Clear Plexi-glass tubes are ideal for handling venomous snakes. They allow safe restraint and visualization of the snake and tubes are often provided with small holes and slits to allow injections and sample collection. Once restrained in the tube, isoflurane or sevoflurane can be administered into the tube to faciliate induction of anesthesia and endotracheal intubation. Alternately, the snake can be intubated awake and the anesthetic administered via positive pressure ventilation.

Turtles and Tortoises

Induction of anesthesia can be challenging in some tortoise species, especially large chelonians and aquatic species. In both small and large tortoises, it is often difficult to gain access to the head and limbs once retracted into the shell. Administration of inhalation anesthetics alone via face mask or induction chamber may result in prolonged induction times, especially in aquatic species capable of prolonged breath-holding. In most species, administration of an injectable anesthetic will facilitate handling and reduce the amount of induction agent required for induction. If a peripheral vein is accessible, it is preferable to give propofol IV for induction following premedication with IM butorphanol (1-2mg/kg). Propofol (2-5mg/kg) can be administered slowly to effect into the jugular vein or the coccygeal vein in most chelonians. In patients where IV access is not available, IM administration of immobilizing agents is indicated. Ketamine, if given alone for immobilization, requires high dosages resulting in prolonged recovery times and poor analgesia and muscle relaxation. A combination of ketamine (4-10mg/kg), butorphanol (0.5-1mg/kg) and medetomidine (40-150µg/kg) administered IM will facilitate handling and often allow endotrachael intubation and maintenance of anesthesia with isoflurane or sevoflurane (Lock et al. 1998).

Crocodilians

Most anesthetic regimen for crocodilians is based on injectable agents to provide immobilization and safe handling and facilitate induction and maintenance of anesthesia with inhalation anesthetics. For small crocodilians which can be manually restrained, propofol (3-5mg/kg IV) is the induction agent of choice and should be given into the ventral coccygeal vein.

Following induction, the animal should be intubated and maintained with isoflurane or sevoflurane. Large crocodilians require administration of IM anesthetic agents to provide safe handling. Tiletamine-zolazepam (5-10mg/kg IM) often provides sufficient immobilization to facilitate handling and endotracheal intubation. However, recovery times following tiletamine-zolazepam administration may be prolonged. A combination of ketamine (5-20mg/kg IM) and medetomidine (80-360µg/kg IM) induced effective and reversible anesthesia in American alligators (*Alligator mississippiensis*) (Heaton-Jones et al. 2002).

Following induction of anesthesia, the trachea should be intubated to maintain a patent airway and facilitate positive pressure ventilation during maintenance of anesthesia. Good jaw relaxation and the aid of an adequately sized laryngoscope blade will help visualize the glottis. For most species and procedures, an uncuffed endotracheal tube is recommended. Cuffed endotracheal tubes can be used but in order to minimize potential damage to the tracheal mucosa, high compliant cuffs are preferable.

All anesthetic agents commonly used in reptile anesthesia are associated with cardiopulmonary depression in reptiles. Minimal variables to be recorded to assess cardiopulmonary performance include depth and rate of respiration and heart rate. All reptiles require assisted or IPPV during anesthesia. Ventilators suitable for small animals can be used even in small reptiles at a rate between 4-8 breaths/min.

Fluid therapy should be administered throughout the anesthetic episode. Major fluid deficits or imbalances are most effectively treated IV and IO. Syringe pumps are invaluable to deliver accurate volumes at a constant rate, especially in small patients. For most reptiles, maintenance requirements for a balanced electrolyte solution range from 5-10ml/kg/hr. In critical patients, a venous blood sample for determination of PCV, hemoglobin, total protein and electrolytes should be collected during anesthesia in order to monitor effectiveness of fluid therapy.

Throughout the anesthetic event including the pre- and post-operative period, these animals should be kept within the preferred optimal body temperature of the particular species. Heating blankets and heat lamps are effective heat sources and should be used into the recovery period. Intra-operatively, the patient should be evaluated for effective analgesia and evidence of pain such as movement and/or increased heart rate in response to a painful stimulus, which may require additional analgesic therapy.

Monitoring

Reptiles should be closely monitored throughout anesthesia with corrective and supportive measures initiated as needed. The extent of monitoring depends on size of the patient, length of the procedure and available equipment. Monitoring systems suitable for even small patients include ECG, pulse oximetry and NIBP including the Doppler system and automated oscillometric devices.

In order to accurately assess anesthetic depth, presence or absence of several reflexes should be recorded. The righting reflex is the first reflex to be lost following induction and the last to return at the end of anesthesia. In a surgical plane of anesthesia, righting, palpebral and head-withdrawal reflexes will be absent, while corneal (except some lizard species and all snakes) and tongue withdrawal reflexes should be present.

A Doppler flow device is the most suitable monitor for reptiles and facilitates recording of flow rate and rhythm. The probe should be positioned at the level of the heart (snakes and lizards) or over the carotid artery (chelonians and lizards). In chelonians, a pencil probe placed at the level of the thoracic inlet will facilitate recording of an audible signal. ECG with leads attached in the same manner described in Chapter 4, is a useful monitoring device in all reptiles and will detect changes in heart rate as well as dysrhythmias. Direct arterial blood pressure measurements are difficult to obtain due to inaccessibility of peripheral arteries such as femoral or carotid artery. A cut-down procedure is necessary in most patients and catheterization may be difficult, especially in small patients. For the same reason, NIBP measurement in reptiles is difficult or impossible. All anesthetized reptiles will exhibit more or less pronounced respiratory depression, especially during a surgical plane of anesthesia. In mammals, pulse oximeters are useful devices to monitor trends in relative arterial SpO_2 and detect hypoxia ($SpO_2 < 90\%$). Calibration of pulse oximeters is based on the human oxygen hemoglobin dissociation curve, a potential source of error when using this device in reptiles. A study in green iguanas found no significant difference between pulse oximeter readings and arterial blood gas analysis (Diethelm 2001). Pulse oximetry is a useful device to monitor trends in arterial oxygen desaturation in reptiles. However, due to different respiratory physiology of reptiles, hypoxic events are difficult to define. Transmission and reflectance pulse oximeter probes are suitable for reptiles and in most species, an esophageal probe placed at the level of the carotid artery or a rectal probe will provide continuous readings.

Arterial blood gas analysis, to determine arterial blood oxygen tension and acid-base status of the patient is impractical in most reptiles. A cut-down procedure is often required to facilitate arterial access. Although blood gas analyzers directly measure PO_2, PCO_2 and pH, SaO_2 is calculated based on the human oxygen hemoglobin dissociation curve. The presence of intrapulmonary shunts in reptiles further complicates interpretation of arterial blood gas values. Venous blood gas analysis is of no value to assess pulmonary function in reptiles.

Capnography has become the standard monitoring technique to assess effectiveness of ventilation. Several error sources and complications limit the use of capnography in reptiles. Most analyzers have high sampling rates (> 100ml/min) and are inaccurate for small reptile species. However, analyzers with low sampling rates of 50ml/min and less are available. Furthermore, accuracy of capnography is limited by the fact that reptiles can develop cardiac shunts and readings may not accurately reflect $PaCO_2$. Cardiac shunts may affect arterial blood gas concentrations independent from pulmonary ventilation (Wang et al. 1998).

Recovery

The goal of post-anesthetic recovery is to return the patient quickly and pain-free to the pre-anesthetic state. Small animal incubators are commonly used to recover most small and medium-sized reptile patients from anesthesia. Temperature and humidity within the incubator should be within the natural range of the species. It is not recommended to increase temperature within the incubator above the preferred optimal temperature range for the species. An increase in temperature will increase metabolism resulting in increased oxygen demand by tissues, which may not be met due to respiratory depression of the patient.

Throughout the recovery period, heart rate, respiratory rate and pattern and return of reflexes (e.g. palpebral, corneal, foot and tail withdrawal reflex) should be recorded regularly. In most reptiles, respiration will be decreased and positive pressure ventilation (2-4 breaths/min) is indicated until the patient is breathing in a regular pattern. In reptiles, low oxygen concentrations are the stimulus to breath and high oxygen concentrations in the inspired air may prolong return to spontaneous respiration (Diethelm 2001). The animal should be extubated when oral and pharyngeal reflexes have returned. Reptiles with respiratory disease should receive respiratory support such as supplemental oxygen or IPPV. The air within the incubator may be enriched with oxygen or alternatively, a facemask may be used. In order to faciliate nasal insufflation, an adequately-sized catheter should be inserted into the nares and sutured or glued to the scales. Depending on patient size, supplemental oxygen at a rate of 0.5-5L/min should be delivered through a humidifier to prevent drying of the airway. Fluid therapy should be continued into the recovery period.

All reptiles recovering from anesthesia should be evaluated for signs of post-operative distress or pain and treated appropriately. Only fully recovered animals should be returned to their enclosure, especially aquatic species in order to prevent accidental drowning.

References

Abou-Madi N (2001). Avian Anesthesia. *Vet Clin North Amer: Exotic Animal Practice* 4:147-167.

Anderson NL, Wack RF, Calloway L, et al. (1999). Cardiopulmonary effects and efficacy of propofol as an anesthetic agent in brown tree snakes (Boiga irregularis). *Bulletin Assoc Reptile Amphib Veterin* 9:9-15.

Arnall L (1961). Anesthesia and Surgery in Caged Aviary Birds. *Vet. Rec* 73:139-145.

AVMA Panel on Euthanasia (2001). 2000 Report of the AVMA Panel on Euthanasia, *JAVMA*, 218:669-696, 2001.

Baert K, DeBacker P (2003). Comparative pharmacokinetics of three non-steroidal anti-inflammatory durgs in five bird species. *Comp Biochem Physiol Tox Pharm* 134:25-33.

Bennett RA (1991). A review of anesthesia and chemical restraint in reptiles. *J Zoo Wildl Med* 22:282-303.

Bennett RA (1996). Anesthesia. In: Mader DR (ed). *Reptile Medicine and Surgery*. W.B. Saunders Company, Philadelphia, p. 241-247.

Bennett RA, Schumacher J, Hedjazi-Haring K, et al (1998). Cardiopulmonary and anesthetic effects of propofol administered intraosseously to green iguanas. *JAVMA* 212:93-98.

Benson KG, Forrest L (1999). Characterization of the renal portal system of the common green iguana (Iguana iguana) by digital subtraction imaging. *J Zoo Wildl Med* 30:235-241.

Blane GP, Boura ALA, Fitzgerald AE, et al. (1957). Actions of etorphine hydrochloride (M99), a potent morphine-like agent. *J Pharmacol Chemother* 30:11-22.

Blasiola GC (1976). Quinaldine sulphate, a new anesthetic formulation for tropical marine fish. *J Fish Biol* 10(1):113-120.

Brown L (1992). Fish anesthesia and restraint. In: Stoskopf MK, ed. *Fish medicine*. Philadelphia: WB Saunders. pp 161-167.

Curro TG, Brunson DB, Paul-Murphy JR (1994). Determination of the ED50 of isoflurane and evaluation of the isoflurane-sparing effect of butorphanol in cockatoos (Cacauta spp.), *Vet Surg* 23:429-433.

Danbury TC, Weeks CA, Chambers JP, et al. (2000). Self-selection of analgesic drug carprofen by lame broiler chickens. *Vet Rec* 146:307-311.

Diethelm G (2001). The effect of oxygen content of inspiratory air (FIO_2) on recovery times in the green iguana (Iguana iguana). *Doctoral Thesis*, Universitaet Zuerich

Erickson AW (1957). Techniques for live-trapping and handling black bears. *Trans. N. Am. Wildl. Nat. Res. Conf.* 22:520-543.

Fedde MR (1980). Structure and gas-flow pattern in the avian respiratory system. *Poultry Sci* 59:2642.

Fitzgerald G, Cooper JE (1990). Preliminary studies on the use of propofol in the domestic pigeon (Columba livia), *Res Vet Sci* 49:334-338.

Flecknell PA and Liles JH (1990). Assessment of the analgesic action of opioid agonist-antagonists in the rabbit. *J Assoc Vet Anaesth* 17:24-29.

Fowler ME (1986). *Zoo and Wildanimal Medicine,* 2nd ed. WB Saunders Co., Philadelphia.

Fowler ME, Miller RE (2003). *Zoo and Wild Animal Medicine,* Fowler & Miller eds, 5th ed St. Louis, Missouri, USA, 2003, Elsevier Science.

Goelz MF, Hahn AW, Kelley ST (1990). Effects of halothane and isoflurane on mean arterial blood pressure, heart rate, and respiratory rate in adult Pekin ducks. *Am J Vet Res* 51:458-60.

Haskell DC (1940). Stunning fish by electricity. *Prog Fish-Cult* 49:33.

Heard DJ (1993). Principles and techniques of anesthesia and analgesia for exotic practice. *Vet Clin North Am Sm Anim Pract* 1301-1327.

Heard DJ (2001). Reptile anesthesia. *Vet Clin North Am Exotic Anim Pract* 83-117.

Heaton-Jones TG, Ko JCH, Heaton-Jones DL (2002). Evaluation of medetomidine-ketamine anesthesia with atipamezole reversal in American alligators (Alligator mississippiensis). *J Zoo Wildl Med* 33:36-44.

Hernandez-Divers S, Schumacher J, Read MR, et al (2003). Comparison of isoflurane and sevoflurane following premedication with butorphanol for induction and maintenance of anesthesia in the green iguana (Iguana iguana). *Proc Amer Assoc Zoo Vet,* Annual Conference, Minneapolis, Minnesota.

Holz P, Barker IK, Burger JP, et al (1997). The effect of the renal portal system on pharmacokinetic parameters in the red-eared slider (Trachemys scripta elegans). *J Zoo Wildl Med* 28:386-393.

Jalanka HH (1991). Medetomidine, medetomidine-ketamine combinations and atipamezole in nondomestic animals: A clinical, physiological, and comparative study. Academic diss. College of Veterinary Medicine, Helsinki, Finland.

Jessup DA (1982). Restraint and chemical immobilization of carnivores and furbearers. In Nielson L, Haigh JC, Fowler ME, editors: *Chemical immobilization of North American wildlife.* Milwaukee, Wisconsin, USA Wisconsin Humane Society, Inc.

Kobel R (1998). Comparative investigations on inhalation anesthesia with isoflurane (Forene) and sevoflurane (Sevorane) in racing pigeons (Columa livia) and presentation of a reference anesthesia protocol for birds. *Tierarztliche Praxis* 26:211-23.

Kreeger TJ, Arnemo JM, Raath JP (2002): *Handbook of Wildlife Chemical Immobilization*, International Edition, Fort Collins, Colorado, USA, Wildlife Pharmaceuticals.

Kreeger TJ, Vargas A, Plumb GE, et al (1998). Ketamine-medetomidine or isoflurane immobilization of black-footed ferrets. *J. Wildl. Manage.* 62:654-662.

Kynard B, Lonsdale E (1975). Experimental study of galvanonarcosis for rainbow trout (*Salmo gairdneri*) immobilization. *Can J Fish Res Board* 32:300-302.

Lock BA, Heard DJ, Dennis P (1998). Preliminary evaluation of medetomidine/ketamine combinations for immobilization and reversal with atipamezole in three tortoise species. *Bulletin Association Reptilian Amphibian Veterinarians* 8:6-9.

Ludders JW (1992). Minimal anesthetic concentration and cardiopulmonary dose-response of halothane in ducks. *Vet Surg* 21:319-324.

Ludders JW, Mitchell GS, Rode J (1990). Minimal anesthetic concentration and cardiopulmonary dose response of isoflurane in ducks. *Vet Surg* 19:304-307.

Ludders JW, Mitchell GS, Schaefer SL (1988). Minimum anesthetic dose and cardiopulmonary response for halothane in chickens. *Am J Vet Res* 49:929-934.

Ludders JW, Rode J, Mitchell GS (1989). Isoflurane anesthesia in sandhill cranes (Grus Canadensis): minimal anesthetic concentration and cardiopulmonary dose-response during spontaneous and controlled breathing. *Anesth Analg* (Cleve) 68:511-514.

Machin KL, Tellier LA, Lair S, et al (2001). Pharmacodynamics of flunizin and ketoprofen in mallard ducks (Anas platyrhynchos). *J Zoo Wildlife Med* 32:222-229.

Mansour A, Khachaturian H, Lewis M, et al. (1988). Anatomy of CNS opioid receptors. *Trends Nerurosci* 11:308-314.

McFarland WN (1959). A study of the effects of anesthetics on the behavior and physiology of fishes. *Inst Mar Sci* 6:23-55.

McFarland WN, Klontz GW (1969). Anesthesia in fishes. *Fed Proc* 28:1535-1540.

McGeown D, Danbury TC, Waerman-Pearson AE, et al. (1999). Effect of carprofen on lameness in broiler chickens. *Vet Rec* 144:668-671.

Mosley CAE, Dyson D, and Smith DA (2003a). Minimum alveolar concentration of isoflurane in green iguanas and the effect of butorphanol on minimum alveolar concentration. *JAVMA* 222:1559-1564.

Mosley CAE, Dyson D, and Smith DA (2003b). The cardiac anesthetic index of isoflurane in green iguanas. *JAVMA* 222:1565-1568.

Muir WW (2002). Pain and stress. In: Gaynor JS and Muir WW (eds). *Handbook of Veterinary Pain Management.* Mosby, St. Louis, p. 46-59.

Norton TM (1998): Carnivore anesthesia. *N. Am. Vet. Conf. Vet. Proc.* 12:885-886.

Oppenheim YC, Moon PF (1995). Sedative effects of midazolam in red-eared slider turtles (Trachemys scripta elegans). *J Zoo Wildl Med* 26:409-413.

Oswald RL (1978). Injection anesthesia for experimental studies in fishes. *Comp Biochem Physiol* 60c:19-26.

Paul-Murphy JR, Brunson DB, Miletic V (1999). Analgesic effects of butorphanol and buprenorphine in conscious African grey parrots (Psittacus erithacus erithacus and Psittacus erithacus timneh). *Am J Vet Res* 60:1218-1221.

Paul-Murphy JR, Ludders JW (2002): Avian Analgesia. *Vet Clin North Amer: Exotic Animal Practice* 4:35-43.

Page CD (1993). Current reptilian anesthesia procedures. In: Fowler ME (ed). *Zoo and Wild Animal Medicine Current Therapy 3.* W.B. Saunders Company, Philadelphia p. 140-143.

Perry SF (1998). Lungs: Comparative anatomy, functional morphology, and evolution. In: Gans C and Gaunt AS (eds): *Biology of the Reptilia Vol 19, Morphology G Visceral Organs,* St Louis, Society for the Study of Amphibians and Reptiles Pp. 1-92.

Ramsden RO, Coppin PF, Johnston DH (1976). Clinical observations on the use of ketamine hydrochloride in wild carnivores. *J Wildl Dis* 12:221-225.

Rooney MB, Levine G, Gaynor J, et al (1999). Sevoflurane anesthesia in desert tortoises (Gopherus agassizii). *J Zoo Wildl Med* 30:64-69.

Ross LG, Ross B (1999). *Anaesthetic and sedative techniques for aquatic animals.* 2d ed. Malden, MA: Blackwell Science. pp 1-159.

Roughan JV and Flecknell PA (2001). Behavioral effects of laparotomy and analgesic effects of ketoprofen and carprofen in rats. Pain 90:65-74.

Schumacher J (1996). Reptiles and amphibians. In: Thurmon JC, Tranquilli, Benson GJ (eds.): *Lumb and Jones' Veterinary Anesthesia 3rd ed,* Baltimore, Williams & Wilkins. p. 670-685.

Schumacher J, Lillywhite HB, Norman WM, et al (1997). Effects of ketamine HCl on cardiopulmonary function in snakes. *Copeia* 2:395.

Schumacher J (2000). Fluid therapy in reptiles. In: Bonagura JD (ed). *Kirk's Current Veterinary Therapy XIII Small Animal Practice.* W. B. Saunders Company, Philadelphia, p. 1170-1173.

Schumacher J (2003). Reptile respiratory medicine. *Vet Clin North Am Exotic Anim Pract* 6:213-231.

Sleeman JM, Gaynor J (2000). Sedative and cardiopulmonary effects of medetomidine and reversal with atipamezole in desert tortoises (*Gopherus agassizii*). *J Zoo Wildl Med*, 31:28-35.

Stoskopf MK (1985). *Manual for the aquatic animal workshop.* Washington, DC: AALAS National Capital Area Branch.

Tytler P, Hawkins AD (1981). Vivisection, anaesthetics, and minor surgery. In: Hawkins AD, ed. *Aquarium systems.* London: Academic Press. Pp 247-278.

Walker MD (1972). Physiologic and pharmacologic aspects of barbiturates in elasmobranch. *Comp Biochem Physiol A* 42:213-221.

Wallach V (1998). The lungs of snakes. In: Gans C, Gaunt AS (eds). *Biology of the Reptilia. Vol. 19: Morphology visceral organs.* St. Louis: Society for the Study of Amphibians and Reptiles, p. 93-295.

Wang T, Smits AW, Burggren WW (1998). Pulmonary function in reptiles. In: Gans C and Gaunt AS (eds): *Biology of the Reptilia. Vol 19, Morphology G Visceral Organs,* St Louis, Society for the Study of Amphibians and Reptiles, p. 297-374.

Williams TD, Rollins M, Block BA (2004). Intramuscular anesthesia of bonito and Pacific mackerel with ketamine and medetomidine and reversal of anesthesia with antipamezol. *JAVMA* 225:1-5.

Chapter 7
The "Nobody Wins" Period: Cardiac Arrest and Resuscitation

Veterinarians are in a distinctive position to treat cardiac arrest since such emergencies almost always occur in a clinical setting. Various support items are available including an oxygen source, equipment to provide IPPV, surgical instruments for internal resuscitation, emergency drugs and most important, technical support. Incidence of cardiac arrest associated with veterinary anesthesia is unknown because there are no central record systems available to provide such information. Nor are there details regarding success rate of cardiac and cerebral resuscitation in small animals but it likely is no better than the 5 to 20% rate for human patients. This would suggest that when an arrest occurs, the chance of complete return of neurological and other organ function is less than 1 in 10.

Although anesthesia in small animals is a relatively safe procedure with all the excellent drugs and monitoring systems available, it is not absolute. The state of anesthesia is a complex and often unstable physiological process that is considered to be an interval between life and death. By strict definition, any death associated with the procedure including preanaesthetic treatments, induction, maintenance or recovery is an anesthetic death. Some events may be explained by other causes such as uncontrolled hemorrhage but mortality during anesthesia is considered an anesthetic death if it occurs from surgery, pharmacological depression, physiological events or when not explainable, an unknown cause.

Cardiac emergencies fall into three major categories: adverse drug effects, those secondary to severe systemic disease and iatrogenic causes. Emergencies can result from mechanical failure of the anesthetic system or human error in either evaluation of the patient or conduct of the anesthetic procedure (De Young et al. 1979). Certainly the risk status of a patient in fair, poor or critical condition (P3, P4 or P5) is higher than for P1 and P2 patients with cardiac arrest the ultimate consequence. Prevention is the best means of avoiding a cardiac emergency and throughout this text, attempts have been made to provide information toward keeping anesthesia safe as possible.

Cardiac Emergency

A cardiac emergency implies a sudden cessation of heart function from a ventricular asystole, ventricular fibrillation or electro-mechanical dissociation (Sawyer et al. 1981). Asystole is reflected by a flat line on the electrocardiogram indicating no myocardial activity. Ventricular fibrillation is characterized by irregular electrical activity and no consistent pattern in the ECG (Figure 4-16); although there is muscle activity, it is uncoordinated and without effective contraction. Profound collapse or electrical-mechanical dissociation is distinguished by a discernible ECG pattern that may appear near normal but is associated with ineffective myocardial contraction, profound arterial hypotension and possible damage to vital organs if sustained. There are a number of other potentially dangerous dysrhythmias, as discussed in Chapter 4, which may lead to arrest.

Recognition

The most important part of the resuscitative process is prompt recognition of the emergency. Any delay may result in permanent damage to the brain and other vital organs even though successful return of myocardial function may occur (Lehman & Manning 2003a). Permanent brain damage is the consequence when brain hypoxia exceeds 5 minutes; thus immediate cerebral resuscitation is essential (Cole et al. 2002; Lehman & Manning 2003b). Even if cardiac resuscitation is successful, neurological recovery may be not be good. Cerebral postresuscitation syndrome may result, including failure of cellular energy and ion pumps, inadequate cerebral perfusion, production of free radicals, intracellular calcium loading and extracerebral organ injury (Evans 1999).

An important role of the technician anesthetist is to alert everyone that a cardiac emergency is imminent. Even if there is some doubt regarding signs of arrest, an alert should be sounded and resuscitation procedures started immediately; if it is a false alarm, assessment of the problem can be made and perhaps the procedure can be continued. Prompt recognition and alert may be life-saving.

Signs of an impending arrest include cyanotic or deep red blood in the surgical field, abnormal or absent breathing, irregular pulse, arterial hypotension and ECG changes including bradycardia, tachycardia and ectopic foci. Any abrupt change in heart rate or pulse rate may be the first sign. Often, an important sign is a washed-out or pale appearance of mucous membranes and unresponsiveness of pupils to light. Verification of cardiac arrest includes apnea, no detectable pulse, absence of measurable blood pressure, absence of heart sounds and cyanosis with dilated and fixed pupils. Presence of any or all of these signs should prompt the anesthetist to initiate resuscitation procedures.

Resuscitation

Resuscitation must be given in an organized manner and in definite sequence. Traditionally, the order has been the same as the beginning of the American alphabet; that is:

A: Airway
B: Breathing
C: Cardiac Resuscitation
D: Drugs

In recent years, it has become increasingly apparent that resuscitative ventilatory procedures, classically thought to be life saving, may have profound detrimental effects. Most assisted breathing techniques during resuscitation involve use of IPPV to inflate lungs for oxygentation and clearance of CO_2. A number of studies in humans have demonstrated that providing normal or overzealous ventilation with IPPV can significantly diminish both systemic and coronary circulation, most likely though interference of venous return (Sayre et al. 2003; Pepe et al. 2005; Fries and Tang 2005). Dramatic improvements in blood flow can be achieved, without loss of oxygenation, by delivering breaths infrequently, e.g., compression ratio of 15:2 during such low-flow states (Yannopoulos et al. 2005). Interrupting chest compressions, even to provide breaths, can be deleterious by abruptly or continually lowering aortic pressure to coronary arteries. Clinical studies in veterinary patients using infrequent PPV have not been published and some clinicians are even advocating use of drugs first to get the heart started. Realistically, one should begin resuscitative efforts first by making chest compressions, placing a tube flowing oxyen source in the mouth when time allows and then have some assessment of airway status with possibility of endotracheal intubation without or very brief interruption of chest compressions. Use of appropriate drugs should come sooner rather than later.

Airway and Breathing

A cardiac emergency may occur at any time and if the airway is not intubated, efforts to gain control of breathing must be considered. Adequate gas exchange will likely be provided by external cardiac compressions for the first 3 to 4 minutes. Oxygen by mask or from the delivery tube of the anesthesia machine placed in the patient's mouth will be helpful. Also, during these first few minutes, ET tube placement should be done if not present. Controlled breathing with oxygen will be beneficial thereafter with a tidal volume sufficient to raise the thorax one-third to half of vital capacity. Caution should be taken not to over ventilate the patient which can be detrimental to venous return and pulmonary blood flow and may cause profound hypocarbia.

External Cardiac Massage

The first attempt at cardiac resuscitation refers to external massage for the first 2 to 5 minutes. If a positive response cannot be achieved in the first 2 minutes, consideration must be given for internal massage. The earlier the switch to internal message, the better may be the outcome (Sanders et al. 1986). External CPR should be given minimally at a rate of 60 compressions per minute, e.g., one per second. This is less than the normal heart rate but 80-100 compressions per min are preferable. Compression and relaxation time should be evenly spaced. Simultaneous compression and ventilation may help improve blood flow in big dogs but this process has not been widely accepted as a way to improve outcome. Alternatively, a pause after 8 external compressions can be made to provide opportunity to ventilate or 15 compressions should be given and followed by 1 or 2 rapid breaths. Again, future studies may provide evidence to the contrary.

The animal should be placed in right lateral recumbency with the patient's back facing the resuscitator. The hand is placed between the 4th and 7th rib and an abrupt downward push is made keeping the elbow straight thus imparting force to the palm, followed by relaxation. Cats, puppies and toy breeds can be massaged effectively with the fingers of one hand whereas larger dogs require both hands. One must use judgement when applying force to the thorax during external massage. Complications such as rib fracture, hemopericardium, hemothorax, pneumothorax and laceration or rupture of the liver, spleen, stomach, esophagus or caudal vena cava may occur.

Whenever possible, intermittent abdominal compressions (IAC) should be provided by another person assisting with the resuscitation. IAC can be accomplished by alternating with every one to three chest compressions. The concept of IAC-CPR is to increase aortic flow and venous return from blood pooled in abdominal organs resulting in increased myocardial and cerebral blood flow. One must avoid trauma to abdominal organs from over vigorous compressions, especially liver and spleen (Kern et al. 1986).

An IV catheter must be in place for administration of isotonic fluids at a rate not to exceed 80ml/kg/hr. During these first few minutes of resuscitation, fluid drip should be rapid. Usually the vascular bed is dilated and added fluid volume is helpful, often essential for cardiac filling. This is one of the most important reasons for having an IV catheter in place even before the anesthetic procedure begins. Without an IV access, chances for resuscitation decrease by the minute. Alterative routes for administrating drugs are endotracheally, by femoral IO and by intracardiac injection (IC) (Evans 1999; Aeschbacher & Webb 1993).

Drugs

Drugs (D) given in the first few minutes are epinephrine, atropine, $NaHCO_3$ and lidocaine. There is new evidence that use of vasopressin may be more beneficial than epinephrine but this is not a drug commonly found in most small animal practices (Mayr et al. 2004; Schmittinger et al. 2005). It is important that components of the resuscitation process are initiated first and assessment of the situation is made; only then should drugs be given. As far as preference for an inotrope is concerned, epinephrine is the drug of choice to support ventricular function. Myocardial muscle tone will improve along with increased peripheral vascular resistance. High doses of dopamine produce alpha adrenergic effects but are not necessarily better than the mixed alpha and beta effects of epinephrine. Drugs not recommended are dobutamine and isoproterenol since their vasodilatory effects are detrimental to improving organ perfusion.

Asystole can be converted to either a normal conduction or ventricular fibrillation with epinephrine. Electrical-mechanical dissociation usually responds to external massage but if that is not effective in the first 2 minutes, response from administration of epinephrine should be positive if the myocardium is responsive.

Atropine has been used in resuscitative efforts for a long time. Although detailed studies have not been done to define the role of parasympathetic agents in cardiac arrest, clinical experience suggests that atropine should be part of the resuscitation protocol. In situations where severe bradycardia occurs and the ECG is not available, small doses of atropine (0.01mg/kg IV) might change the course of events.

Lidocaine is used in CPR protocols more commonly for treatment of postresuscitation tachycardia and ventricular dysrhythmias. To resolve persistent conduction abnormalities, CRI lidocaine at 25 to 80µg/kg/min may be required.

Sodium bicarbonate is used to treat metabolic acidosis but not necessarily in the first 10 minutes. When circulation starts to improve, 0.2-0.5mEq/kg should be given in anticipation of blood of low acidity returning to the heart. Refer to the section on blood gases and acid/base status in Chapter 4 for further information.

External Defibrillation

Interruption of ventricular fibrillation is most successful if the ECG pattern is coarse. Intracardiac injection of epinephrine may be used to change fine V-fibrillation to coarse. Defibrillation is accomplished with a direct-current countershock cardiac defibrillator. Passage of current through the heart causes the myocardium to depolarize and develop a refractory period. This allows the area of greatest pacemaker activity, preferably at the SA node, to provide a single source of myocardial stimulation. For small cats and dogs, 25 to 100 watt-seconds is used (1-5 watt-sec/kg). If unsuccessful, epinephrine (0.02mg/kg) can be given IV or a ¼ dose IC and the shock repeated. If this is still unsuccessful, lidocaine (2 to 4mg/kg) can is administered IV or IC to reduce myocardial irritability and then counter shock repeated.

Internal Massage and Defibrillation

If external massage is ineffective in the first 2-5 minutes, internal massage should be attempted (Benson et al. 2005). This is especially the situation in large barrel-chested dogs in which external CPR is more difficult to accomplish. If cardiac arrest occurs during surgery with an open abdomen, internal massage should be made immediately with an incision made through the diaphragm avoiding major vessels. If cardiac arrest occurs during thoracotomy, the pericardium should be incised and the ventricles compressed as described below.

When the decision has been made for internal CPR, the site over the left chest may be rapidly clipped and usually there is not time for much of a wet prep. A thoracotomy is made through the 5th left interspace, ribs are spread and pericardium opened. Care must be taken not to incise the lung, intercostal or internal mammary vessels when entering the chest or to damage the phrenic nerve when the pericardium is incised. This procedure must be done quickly and efficiently. Manual cardiac massage is begun by "milking" the heart from apex to base. If the right hand is used for massage, movement is made from the little finger to the thumb. To maximize blood flow to the heart and brain, the thoracic aorta may be intermittently compressed with the thumb of the left hand. Feeling blood passing through the aorta is a positive sign. Administration of epinephrine and $NaHCO_3$ should be continued and if ventricular fibrillation is evident, internal countershock should be attempted. Paddles are cupped on either side of the ventricle and 2 to 40 watt-sec are given based on body weight (0.1-0.5ws/kg). This procedure is then repeated at intermittent intervals with massage continued. If circulation is adequate, pupils will be reactive to light, signs of tissue perfusion will be evident and a peripheral pulse will be detectable.

Crash Cart or Box

For availability of drugs and supplies, a "crash cart" (Figure 7-1) or portable box, e.g., type used for keeping fishing tackle, may be used. For a large facility, the cart may be kept in the anesthesia prep area and either the arrested patient is brought to the room or cart taken to the arrest site. If a defibrillator is available, keeping it on the crash cart would be preferable. Alternatively, "crash boxes" should be located in each area of the hospital where arrests are most likely to occur, i.e., anesthesia, surgical preparation, surgery, intensive care, radiology, and special diagnostics.

The problem with more than one crash box in a hospital is keeping them properly stocked. It is essential that a specific person or section in the hospital be designated for that purpose. In addition, a paper tape should be wrapped around the box and dated. Once used and the tape broken, stock supplies should be replaced and a new paper tape applied. That way, there will be no surprises when time is of the essence.

Suggestion for contents is listed in Table 7-1. Everything in the cart or box should be clearly labeled and each place labeled as well so that anything missing can be identified. It is very handy to have a dosage sheet prepared with each drug listed by body weight to avoid having to make calculations on site. As an example, dosages for epinephrine, atropine, lidocaine, sodium bicarbonate and doxapram are provided in Table 7-2. This not only saves time but also helps avoid

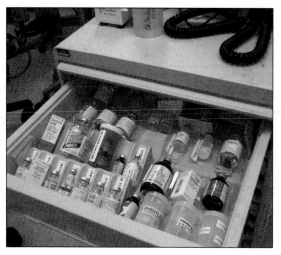

Figure 7-1 Drawer of a crash cart containing essential drugs. Note that drugs are clearly identified and the place for each drug is labeled. Syringes and other supplies identified in Table 7-1 are located in lower drawers. Veterinary Teaching Hospital, Michigan State University.

errors from having to calculate dosages under duress. Volumes instead of mg's by weight are very useful, e.g., at 5lb or 2.5kg increments. There are many stresses happening during such an event and giving the wrong drug is very easy if syringes are not properly identified. Any time a drug is drawn into a syringe especially during an emergency, it must be labeled. Syringes of atropine, epinephrine, and heparin flush all look the same so not putting labels on things is an accident just waiting to happen. Stick-on labels are commercially available or can be prepared in house.

There is one other precaution that will help everyone perform to the best of their ability. The veterinarian in charge should stay as calm as possible and it is best not to use a loud voice to provide directions to those involved in CPR. In addition, one person should be designated whose only job is to write down all events and all drugs administered. This allows for better tracking of elapsed time since the arrest and therefore may help with prognosis.

Assessment

If the resuscitative effort is successful, pupils will begin to show a response to direct light, mucous membranes will regain color and spontaneous respiratory efforts may be evident. Blood gas analysis will be helpful to determine the value of CO_2 and pH status. A positive response to a dose of doxapram to stimulate breathing may provide indirect assessment of cerebral responsiveness. Heart sounds should be strong and peripheral pulse should be easily detected with the pulse oximeter and NIBP monitor. As peripheral perfusion improves, blood pressure measurements should be possible. Cardiac dysrhythmias should be treated, oxygen continued and intensive care given for as along as deemed necessary. Continued intensive care and support of all major body systems may be required. Advanced monitoring procedures are required to resolve problems associated with renal, nervous and gastrointestinal function (Lehman & Manning 2003b). A success rate of 25%, that is, percentage of patients returned to a relatively normal condition, is considered outstanding. A 10% rate may be more realistic but it depends on the responsiveness of trained personnel, availability of drugs, whether or not an IV catheter has been in place before the arrest, and the patient's prearrest physical status. On occasion, the protocol for CPR should be rehearsed so that everyone in the hospital is prepared to deal with a cardiopulmonary emergency. Duration of resuscitation is quite variable and may last up to an hour with a successful outcome (Gilroy et al. 1980). However, experience would indicate that most successful resuscitations are accomplished within the first 5 minutes. Experience also shows that the longer it takes for resuscitative efforts, the lower the chances of survival. Even under ideal circumstances, survival rate may only be 10%. Prevention and preparation are without question the best way to achieve the best possible outcome.

Table 7-1

Drugs and Supplies Useful for Cardiac Emergencies

(These should be kept in a movable cart or box in areas where anesthetized animals would be in the hospital.)

Syringes	**Needles**
1ml	18 gauge
3ml	20 gauge
6ml	22 gauge
10ml	25 gauge
20ml	

Catheters	**Fluids**
18 gauge	Sterile water or saline
20 gauge	Lactated Ringers
22 gauge	5% Dextrose in water
23 gauge butterfly	Various sizes: 250ml, 500ml, 1 liter

Assorted Supplies	**Drugs**
Tube and rolled gauze	Solu-delta-cortef, 100 and 500
3-way stopcock	$NaHCO_3$ (1mEq/ml)
Scalpel handle & blade	Heparin
Tongue depressors	Lidocaine (20mg/ml)
Eye ointment	Atropine or Glycopyrrolate
ET tubes	Epinepherine (1mg/ml, 1:1000 amps)
	$CaCl_2$ or Ca Gluconate
	Doxapram (20mg/ml)
	Ephedrine (50mg/ml)
	Lasix (50mg/ml)
	Naloxone (0.4mg/m)
	Procainamide (100mg/ml)
	Diphehydramine (50mg/ml)

Note: Cart should have a laryngoscope with working batteries and bulbs and a supply of pens with a notebook for recording events. An AMBU bag should be available in those areas where oxygen may not be immediately available, e.g., in a recovery area when connection to oxygen may take a few minutes. Possibly also a supply of pre-made labels for quick application to syringes.

Table 7-2

Dosage Chart for Emergency Drugs Based on Body Weight (lbs)

Drug	Dose	5 lb	10 lb	15 lb	20 lb	25 lb	30 lb	35 lb	40 lb	50 lb	60 lb	70 lb	80 lb
Epinephrine 1mg/ml IC (1/4 dose)	1.0mg/20#	0.25ml	0.5ml	0.75ml	1.0ml	1.25ml	1.5ml	1.75ml	2.0ml	2.5ml	3.0ml	3.5ml	4.0ml
Atropine 0.4mg/ml	0.02mg/#	0.25ml	0.5ml	0.75ml	1.0ml	1.25ml	1.5ml	1.75ml	2.0ml	2.5ml	3.0ml	3.5ml	4.0ml
Lidocaine 20mg/ml	1-3mg/#	0.25ml	0.5ml	0.75ml	1.0ml	1.25ml	1.5ml	1.75ml	2.0ml	2.5ml	3.0ml	3.5ml	4.0ml
NaHCO3 1meq/ml	0.5mEq/#	2.5ml	5.0ml	7.5ml	10ml	12.5ml	15ml	17.5ml	20ml	25ml	30ml	35ml	40ml
Doxapram 20mg/ml	0.5-2mg/#	0.1ml	0.25ml	0.37ml	0.5ml	0.6ml	0.75ml	0.9ml	1.0ml	1.25ml	1.5ml	1.75ml	2.0ml

References

Aeschbacher G, Webb Al (1993). Intraosseous injection during cardiopulmonary resuscitation in dogs. *J Sm Ani Prac* 34:629-633.

Benson DM, O'Neil B, Kakish, et al. (2005). Open-chest CPR improves survival and neurologic outcome following cardiac arrest. *Resuscitation* 64:209-217.

Cole SG, Otto CM, Hughes D (2002). Cardiopulmonary cerebral resuscitation in small animals–a clinical practice review (part 1). *J Vet Emerg Crit Care.* 12:261-267.

De Young DJ, Evans AT, Sawyer DC (1979). Cardiopulmonary emergencies prevention and resuscitation. In Catcott EJ (ed). *Canine Medicine.* Santa Barbara, American Veterinary Publications, Inc.

Evans AT (1999). New thoughts on cardiopulmonary resuscitation. *Vet Clin North Amer, Sm Ani Prac* 29:819-829.

Fries M and Tang W (2005). How does interruption of cardiopulmonary resuscitation affect survival from cardiac arrest. *Curr opin Crit Care* 11:200-203.

Gilroy BA, Rockoff MA, Dunlop BJ, Shapiro HM (1980). Cardiopulmonary resuscitation in the nonhuman primate. *JAVMA.* 177:867-869.

Kern KB, Carter AB, Showen RL, et al. (1986). CPR-induced trauma: Comparison of three manual methods in an experimental model. *Ann Emerg Med* 15:674-678.

Lehman TL, Manning AM (2003a). Postarrest syndrome and the respiratory and cardiovascular systems in post arrest patients. Compendium on CE for Prac Vet 25:492-503.

Lehman TL, Manning AM (2003b). Renal, central nervous, and gastrointestinal systems in post arrest patients. *Compendium on CE for Prac Vet* 25:504-513.

Mayr VD, Wenzel V, Muller T, et al. (2004). Effects of vasopressin on left anterior descending coronary artery blood flow during extremely low cardiac output. *Resuscitation* 62:229-235.

Pepe PE, Roppolo LP, Fowler RL (2005). The detrimental effects of ventilation during low-blood-flow states. *Curr Opin Crit Care* 11:212-218.

Sanders AB, Kern KB, Ewy GA, et al. (1985). Importance of the duration of inadequate coronary perfusion pressure on resuscitation from cardiac arrest. *J Am Coll Cardiol* 6:113-117.

Sawyer DC, Evans AT, De Young DJ, Brunson DB (1981). Cardiopulmonary emergency. In *Anesthetic Principles and Techniques.* E. Lansing, Michigan State University Press.

Sayre MR, Swor R, Pepe PE, Overton J (2003). Current issues in cardiopulmonary resuscitation. *Prehosp Emerg Care* 7:24-30.

Schmittinger CA, Astner S, Astner L, et al. (2005). Cardiopulmonary resuscitation with vasopressin in a dog. *Vet Anaesth Analg* 32:112-114.

Yannopoulos D, Tang W, Roussos C, et al. (2005). Reducing ventilation frequency during cardiopulmonary resuscitation in a porcine model of cardiac arrest. *Respir Care* 50:628-635.

Chapter 8
The Recovery Period

Transition from anesthesia to recovery can be as unstable and unpredictable as the induction period. Total reversibility is the goal following any procedure even though anesthetics impose many physical and physiological changes. Throughout this text, there is information provided about recovery including specifics about individual drug groups, special breeds and unique needs of recovering animals other than dogs or cats.

The recovery period has three major components: recovery from anesthesia, recovery from surgery and management of perioperative pain. Surgical recovery is of variable length and proper management is very important for patient comfort and injury prevention.

When does anesthesia end and recovery begin? In most circumstances, it can be easily identified by a patient's subjective response to the endotracheal tube or pain and discomfort subsequent to the surgical procedure. Swallowing, head movement or chewing usually signals the onset of consciousness, which is an identifiable time following inhalation anesthesia. When pain has been managed properly, the patient may be slow to respond to the ET tube even though palpebral reflexes may be strong. The key judgment is to determine that the patient can protect its airway once the ET tube is removed. Until that happens, the patient must be cared for under direct observation. For the anesthetic record, time interval for anesthesia starts with induction and ends with extubation. If the patient wasn't intubated, judgment is made to an equivalent level of response during recovery such as head-lift.

Pain Management
Managing pain at the time of recovery really starts pre-anesthesia. If pain isn't treated before it begins, it is tough to catch later! As discussed in Chapter 1, preemptive analgesia is a process that cannot be emphasized enough. Pain is inevitable after surgery and can be managed in a number of ways. With the knowledge, drugs and experience available, there is no reason not to provide appropriate care and treatment for animals following anesthesia and surgery for as many days as necessary. Some animals may not appear to demonstrate pain or discomfort in a hospital setting while others show their pain in a variety of ways, especially after they are discharged to their owner. Morbidity from pain includes muscle splinting, inadequate ventilation, diminished cough predisposing to atelectasis, tachycardia, and hypertension. Therefore, preemption and treatment is an obligation, not an option.

Restlessness and Excitement
Agitation and excitement during emergence from general anesthesia may be quite severe and can result in damage to the surgical repair or other parts of the body. If proper assessment and appropriate premedication have been given, this is usually not a problem. Animals with psychomotor disturbances that are difficult to handle, those fearful of the hospital and staff and those that cannot tolerate even minor pain or discomfort are the most likely candidates. Agitation and restlessness may also result from hypoxemia, tracheal collapse or respiratory depression. Arterial hypotension may also contribute to restlessness. These conditions must always be suspected and appropriately corrected. As described for pain, the combination of a tranquilizer and an analgesic offer the best results. Hallucinations and convulsions may be associated with recovery from ketamine anesthesia and treatment with low doses of acepromazine, diazepam or midazolam may be indicated. When such reactions are anticipated, appropriate preanesthesia attitude adjustment will avert most of these problems (see Chapter 1).

Anesthesia Recovery
Dogs and cats recovering from anesthesia should be placed in an area specifically designated for that purpose. Padding of space on the floor of the prep room is sometimes used and is an excellent choice. Case in point is "The Beach" at the Animal Medical Center in New York City. Their first stage recovery area is in the prep room and then animals are moved to a ward area. Recovery cages may be located along one wall or part of a treatment area where staff can

monitor recovering animals (Figure 8-1). If it is a dedicated room or adjacent rooms allowing separation of dogs and cats, the recovery area should have visual and auditory components (Figures 8-2 and 8-3). That is, rooms should be warm, comfortable and interesting for animals and staff. Lighting should be muted since patients given an anticholinergic will have dilated pupils and bright lights are very irritating to recovering patients. It is also important that animals see people and hear voices. Obviously, that is not a problem if recovery is in a prep room but if in a separate room, one side might be open to the working area or with windows instead of enclosed walls. If it is possible to adjust temperature of the room, it should be a little warmer than other areas of the hospital. The room should be kept at around 22-24°C. When there is a chance to design a recovery area, incorporating heated cage bottoms is desirable.

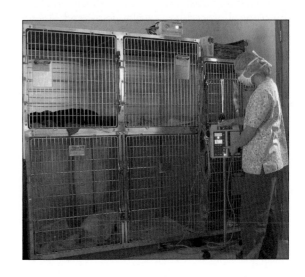

Figure 8-1 Recovery cages in prep/treatment room with technician checking monitor. Note electrical outlets below cages and ceiling lights are not directly over cages.
Courtesy of Dr. Doug Andrews, Falmouth Veterinary Clinic, Portland, ME

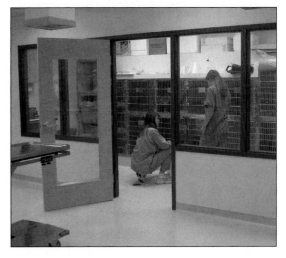

Figure 8-2 Recovery room for cats and dogs that opens to prep/treatment area. Lighting can be independently controlled and animals can see and hear activity in the adjacent area.
Courtesy of Dr. David Ramsey, The Animal Ophthalmology Center, Williamston, MI.

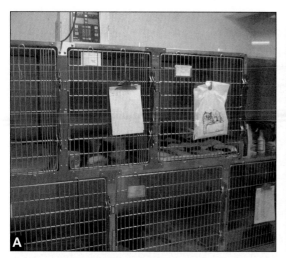
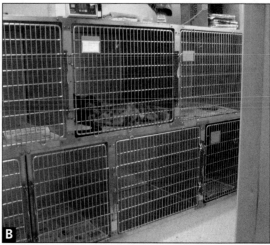

Figure 8-3A & B These two recovery rooms are side by side and connected separately to the prep room (doors not shown), one for cats (A) and one for dogs (B). A permanent wall, seen on the right side of 8-3A, separate the 2 rooms. Lighting is controlled by separate switches and windows (not shown) allow animals to see activity in prep room.
Courtesy of Dr. Kevin Harris, Haslett Animal Clinic, Haslett, MI.

For animals placed in a cage, a pad of absorbent material should be used since the recovering patient may defecate and urinate. Absorbent pads are available for this purpose and come in various sizes (Figure 8-4). To warm patients as they recover, animals should be placed on a heated circulating water blanket and covered with small blankets or towels that have been warmed in a microwave. Cats can damage water blankets during recovery so when they start moving around the cage, might be a good time for removal. In some situations, old towels or discarded mattress pads are very functional and may be washed for re-use.

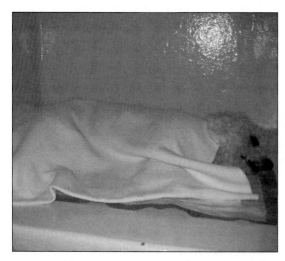

Figure 8-4 Recovering patient lying on warming pad and absorbent pad covered with an infant blanket.
Courtesy of Veterinary Teaching Hospital, Michigan State University.

Oxygen and suction outlets are advisable in recovery and sufficient electrical outlets at each cage site should be available for patient monitors, heated water blankets and other equipment (Fig 8-5). A selection of face masks and ET tubes should be readily available along with a laryngoscope that may be lifesaving in situations of airway obstruction. Emergency drugs, fluids and supplies should be on hand as listed in Table 7-1. If the recovery area is located next to the prep area, these supplies would be readily available.

As a general rule, when the patient is able to stand without ataxia, one may assume that anesthesia recovery is completed and that surgical recovery can continue. Pain medications often have a sedation component which means animals should be resting and not moving around very much. Also, there are animals that cannot become ambulatory, so one must determine when the patient is alert and responsive. As long as fluid needs have been met during anesthesia and the environment has been appropriate to prevent hypothermia during surgery and following operation, recovery should be without incident.

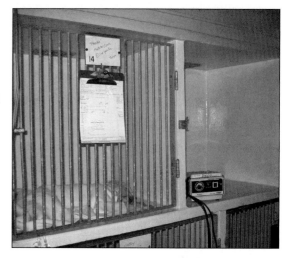

Figure 8-5 Warming system with pump and pad used for recovering patient (Gaymar Industries, Orchard Park, NY).
Courtesy of Veterinary Teaching Hospital, Michigan State University.

Recovery Procedures
Inhalation Anesthetics

When inhalation agents are used, the technician anesthetist has considerable influence and control over the length of time between end of anesthesia and onset of recovery. With agents of low solubility, e.g., isoflurane and sevoflurane, patients recover quickly. A specific timetable is difficult to establish because of the variability in length of procedures and use of various drugs but it is usually less than 10 minutes.

Caution should be taken not to turn off the inhalant too soon before the surgical procedure is completed. The time to begin the decrease depends on the length of the procedure, the size of the incision, speed of the surgeon, premedicants and whether the patient is breathing spontaneously or respiration is controlled. Because there is better alveolar ventilation with controlled breathing, maintenance (vaporizer) concentration is lower and therefore the decrease in concentration is begun later during closure. With the return of a slight palpebral reflex and an increase in jaw tension, the level should not be lowered further. Once judgment is made that only a few minutes remain, it is appropriate to turn the vaporizer off. In situations where N_2O has been a component of anesthetic management, it should be turned off 3 to 5 minutes before the patient is extubated. If extubation is premature, oxygen should be delivered by mask.

There are two options to follow as one approaches anesthesia recovery with an inhalation anesthetic. One is to maintain the same oxygen flow rate as that used for maintenance. Because of the volume in the circle anesthetic circuit, there will be anesthetic vapors retained as the washout proceeds. This will extend recovery a little longer than if oxygen flow is increased or flush valve is used to produce faster washout of anesthetic vapors. The option of increasing the oxygen flow will depend on how light the patient is and whether the procedure is completed. If either of these two procedures is not followed and the anesthetized patient is disconnected from the anesthetic system to be placed in recovery, there are a number of consequences that can occur including hypoxia (see Hypoxemia). Having the attendant sit on the floor with recovering patients increases exposure to waste anesthetic gases and should be avoided.

With a semi-open system (Bain circuit), the physical buffer or mechanical dead space of the circuit is essentially zero because fresh gases are delivered directly to the ET tube or mask. As a result, changes in vaporizer concentrations are more rapidly reflected in the alveoli and anesthetic levels need not be decreased as soon as is done with circle systems.

If thiopental or an injectable combination has been used for induction, recovery time will be slightly longer than if inhalation induction has been done by chamber or mask. For this reason, when inhalation anesthesia is used alone, the agent(s) should not be turned off until about 2 to 4 minutes remain for completion of the procedure. In some animals, recovery may be very abrupt and the anesthetist must be prepared by having monitoring equipment removed, cuff of the ET tube deflated, cuff of the blood pressure monitor removed (especially in cats not declawed), other monitors detached and the tie loosened that was used to secure the ET tube. When either isoflurane or sevoflurane has been used and a tranquilizer/analgesic combination has not been given, e.g., for non-surgical procedures, recovery from anesthesia will be much faster and reduction from maintenance concentrations should not be made until the procedure is finished. Caution must be taken to not place fingers in the mouth during this process. One must be careful not to allow the ET tube to be positioned between molar teeth since airway aspiration of a chewed off ET tube can happen. It is difficult to retrieve especially in cats and requires that the patient be reanesthetized. If for any reason it becomes necessary to place one's hand in the mouth of a recovering patient, it is best to position an object between the upper and lower jaw (small bite block, roll of tape or tube of gauze) to keep an inadvertent bite wound from happening.

Analgesics and Injectable Anesthetics
A small price to pay with use of analgesics is a slower recovery. With the exception of thiopental being used for the entire procedure, induction agents such as propofol or dissociative/benzodiazepine combinations are not usually associated with prolonged anesthesia recovery. Rate of metabolism, acid-base status, body temperature and degree of protein binding greatly influence recovery time. Recovery time will also be regulated by dosages of drugs given during the procedure and how soon before completion of the procedure drugs were given. In any case, time must be allowed for drug metabolism and return to consciousness. On occasion, the anesthetist may elect to reverse effects of the opioid or alpha$_2$ agonist only partially to the point that the patient is responsive to the ET tube and has adequate spontaneous breathing but is recovering quietly without struggle. This is not a common practice since the analgesic effects will be lost as well.

When recovering a narcotized dog, the patient should be responsive when aroused but would prefer to sleep. That is a good sign of effective pain management and a reason to not reverse the analgesic effects of the opioid. However, if this is not the case and there is a concern of respiratory depression as determined by pulse oximetry or blood gas analysis, naloxone should be given IV in 0.1mg increments depending on patient size. Usually not more than 0.8mg need be given to adequately reverse the opioid, depending on total dose administered. When sedatives or tranquilizers have been given with the opioid, only the effects of the analgesic can be reversed, not those of the tranquilizer.

Complications
Being prepared for the unexpected will pay big dividends especially for the recovering patient. An important protocol in this regard is to leave the IV catheter in place until the patient is removed from the recovery area. It is very difficult to obtain venous assess in the recovering veterinary patient that may be hypotensive and hypothermic.

Hypotension
The residual effects of premedication, anesthetics, unreplaced blood loss, motion and change of position from the operating table to the recovery area, cardiac arrhythmias, hypoxia, hypothermia, metabolic acidosis and electrolyte imbalance all contribute to the problem of hypotension in the

postoperative patient. The importance of continued monitoring of NIBP and adequate oxygenation in recovering animals especially for those at higher risk cannot be overemphasized. Arterial hypotension is evident when the peripheral pulse is weak or cannot be palpated and SAP is below 80mm Hg. Treatment is best given by first administering IV fluids and then proceeding to identify the specific cause and determine appropriate therapy.

Hypertension

Arterial hypertension in the recovering patient may be more common than is actually known. The most common causes of hypertension are pain, hypercarbia, hypoxia and over-replacement of fluid loss. A recommended protocol would be to measure blood pressure non-invasively during recovery and continue as needed. This is especially recommended for P3, P4 and P5 patients. Treatment such as analgesia, improved alveolar gas exchange and adequate oxygenation may be indicated.

Bradycardia

Low heart rate, e.g., slower than 70 BPM in the dog or 100 in the cat is usually not commonly observed in recovery, but if it is present, hypothermia and residual drug effects may be the cause. Treatment may not be needed as long as NIBP and tissue perfusion are within acceptable limits and the patient is recovering normally. An anticholinergic may be used along with identification and treatment of etiology. Dogs that are resting quietly with appropriate effects of analgesics in place should have a heart rate in the normal range of 60 to 90 BPM, cats a little higher.

Tachycardia

Tachycardia is much more common in recovery and may be the result of postoperative pain, hypercarbia, hypoxia or hypovolemia. Specific treatment for tachycardia is usually not necessary but it is important to identify the etiology. Attention should be given to controlling pain with appropriate analgesics, adequate oxygenation, fluid therapy and proper ventilation.

Hypoxemia

Airway obstruction, laryngospasm, accumulation of secretions and inadequate gas exchange may be evident. Residual neuromuscular block may also contribute to hypoxemia whenever muscle relaxants are used in the anesthetic regimen. Pneumothorax from any cause can definitely impair gas exchange. Hypoventilation is common postanesthesia because of reduced tidal volume, diminished forced expiratory volume and restricted cough due to pain. Secretions accumulate and atelectasis is usually present in recovering patients. Abnormal distribution of ventilation and perfusion and shunting during anesthesia may lead to hypoxemia immediately postanesthesia. For this reason, the anesthetized patient should breathe oxygen until it is responsive and swallowing prior to being moved to the recovery area. The practice of placing the anesthetized patient in a cage or on the floor, breathing room air when the ET tube has not been removed, is a practice that cannot be condoned. Providing high oxygen flow prior to extubation also allows time for post-extubation airway obstruction to be remedied before severe hypoxemia ensues.

Pneumothorax

Trapped intrapleural air may be present, especially following thoracic surgery. A chest tube should be placed prior to closure in all cases and the tube should not be removed until all evidence of pneumothorax is gone. Should pneumothorax from other circumstances such as alveolar rupture be present, prompt aspiration of the trapped air with a catheter or chest tube is essential. Decreased lung compliance and cyanosis may lead to the suspicion of pneumothorax. Use of a pulse oximeter during recovery in such cases has excellent utility.

Restrictive or Obstructive Dressings

Inadequate ventilation may result from excessively tight surgical dressings following different procedures including radical mastectomy or forelimb amputation. Obstruction to breathing may follow application of dressings around the head and neck. Dressings that encircle the throat should be applied with the neck flexed to ensure enough laxity when it is normally extended. Breathing of the recovery patient is assessed and the dressing is loosened as needed. Use of a pulse oximeter and NIBP will be useful in this assessment.

Aspiration

Vomiting during or following anesthesia may have serious consequences because of aspiration of stomach contents. The possibility of a partial or full stomach exists in any animal, especially if it has not been hospitalized the day before surgery. This is the prime reason for withholding intake of food for 10 to 12 hours preanesthesia and even longer for patients at risk. Problems with airway obstruction in recovery of brachycephalic breeds are discussed in Chapter 5 but aspiration pneumonia can also be a consequence during and following anesthesia (Lorison et al. 1997). Dogs with the most risk are English Bulldog, Pug, Boston Terrier and Cavalier King Charles Spaniel.

Aspiration is always a potential problem in emergency operations and special procedures indicated for these patients should be followed (see Chapter 2). The parturient and the trauma patient are particularly at highest risk because gastric emptying may be delayed by the processes of labor or by post-trauma shock.

When aspiration occurs or is suspected, tracheal intubation and suctioning are indicated. Tracheal lavage with saline, 3 to 5ml at a time, followed by suction is advocated to remove as much fluid and particulate matter as possible. One must be careful to provide oxygen to the spontaneously breathing patient in between suctioning to prevent hypoxemia. Antibiotics may be given for bacterial contamination and a brochodilator may be used to combat spasm.

Hypothermia and Shivering

Recovery from anesthesia may be associated with gross clonic movement that at times may mimic convulsions. Most often, shivering is seen in patients emerging from anesthesia with lowered body temperature. Shivering can be marked and may be associated with tachycardia, increased cardiac work and oxygen consumption, any of which can lead to hypoxemia. If cyanosis is detected, supplemental oxygen must be given while rewarming is aided by an incubator, heated water blanket, hot air blower or blankets. For small puppies, kittens and toy breeds, recovery in an incubator is strongly recommended. Fur or hair that is wet from saline-soaked gauze on cautery plates contributes to hypothermia and the animal should be dried as much as possible with towels immediately after surgery is completed, before being placed in recovery area.

Hypoglycemia

Withholding food prior to surgery contributes to hypoglycemia during the recovery period. Providing a small amount of food following recovery will help alleviate the problem. Low blood sugar is likely to be prevalent, especially in kittens and puppies, toy breeds and cats

Hemorrhage or Prolonged Oozing of Blood

In situations where there is a possibility of blood loss during recovery such as following thoracic or abdominal procedures and severe body wounds, vigilance of the recovering patient is very important. Use of automated NIBP is strongly recommended for these patients as decreasing SAP is very useful in detecting blood loss. For external wounds, a great deal of blood can be absorbed in bandage material so the patient must be examined closely to detect excessive oozing during recovery.

Summary

Successful management of the recovering patient begins in the preanaesthetic period. With proper patient evaluation and assessment, appropriate preemptive pain management along with the selected protocol for anesthesia will contribute to a successful outcome: anesthesia safe as possible.

References

Lorison D, Bright RM, White RAS (1997). Brachycephalic airway obstruction syndrome–A review of 118 cases. *Canine Pract* 22:18 -21.

Index

Page numbers followed by an *f* indicate figure; page numbers followed by a *t* indicate table.